Subsequent titles in the
Orthopaedics and Sports Medicine Series
Series Editor: David W. Stoller, MD, FACR

Stoller's Orthopaedics and Sports Medicine:
The Knee

Stoller's Orthopaedics and Sports Medicine:
The Hip

Stoller's Orthopaedics and Sports Medicine:
The Wrist and Hand

Stoller's Orthopaedics and Sports Medicine:
The Elbow

Stoller's Orthopaedics and Sports Medicine:
The Foot and Ankle

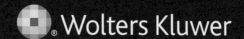

STOLLER'S
Orthopaedics and Sports Medicine

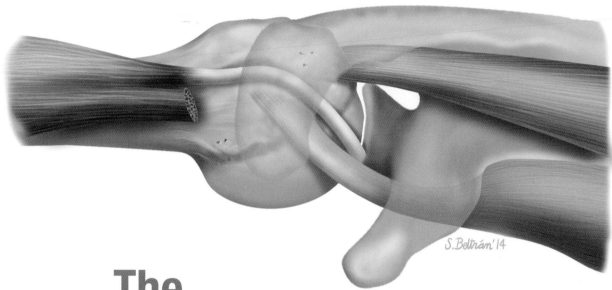

S. Beltrán '14

The
SHOULDER

David W. Stoller, MD, FACR

National Director
Orthopaedic and Musculoskeletal Imaging, RadNet
Medical Director
Orthopaedic and Musculoskeletal Imaging, Beverly Radiology, Northern California
San Francisco, California
Affiliate Member
American Shoulder and Elbow Surgeons

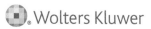 Wolters Kluwer

Philadelphia • Baltimore • New York • London
Buenos Aires • Hong Kong • Sydney • Tokyo

Acquisitions Editor: Ryan Shaw
Product Development Editor: Kate Marshall
Senior Production Project Manager: Alicia Jackson
Director of Creative Services: Doug Smock
Senior Manufacturing Coordinator: Beth Welsh
Marketing Manager: Dan Dressler
Prepress Vendor: Absolute Service, Inc.

9 8 7 6 5 4 3 2 1

Printed in the United States of America

Library of Congress Cataloging-in-Publication Data
Stoller, David W., author.
  Stoller's orthopaedics and sports medicine : the shoulder / David W. Stoller.
    p. ; cm.
  Orthopaedics and sports medicine
  Shoulder
  Includes bibliographical references and index.
  ISBN 978-1-4698-9298-6 (hardback)
  I. Title. II. Title: Orthopaedics and sports medicine. III. Title:
Shoulder.
  [DNLM: 1. Shoulder—injuries. 2. Magnetic Resonance Imaging. 3.
Shoulder—anatomy & histology. 4. Shoulder—pathology. 5. Shoulder
Joint—injuries. WE 810]
  RD557.5
  617.5'72044--dc23
                    2014040824

LWW.com

DEDICATION

To my family and friends for their support and understanding.

To my parents for their inspiration, love, and encouragement.

I have always been cognizant and thankful for the opportunity to contribute to the specialties of orthopaedics and radiology. The respect shown by my colleagues and students has and continues to be a humbling and motivating force in my life.

The veracity of truth is a trenchant ally against the consensus who follow convention as if dogma.

The model checklist:
- Honesty, humility in thought and action
- Excel for others through example
- Never compromise on the truth for without honesty we cannot build knowledge.
- Change of heart and mind through teaching others is the most powerful and natural healing force of the human spirit.

CONTRIBUTORS

Lesley J. Anderson, MD
Assistant Clinical Professor of Orthopaedic Surgery
University of California, San Francisco
Orthopaedic Surgeon
California Pacific Medical Center
San Francisco, California

Paul B. Roache, MD
Orthopaedic Surgery
California Pacific Medical Center
San Francisco, California

David W. Stoller, MD, FACR
National Director
Orthopaedic and Musculoskeletal Imaging, RadNet
Medical Director
Orthopaedic and Musculoskeletal Imaging, Beverly Radiology, Northern California
San Francisco, California
Affiliate Member
American Shoulder and Elbow Surgeons

Eugene M. Wolf, MD
Department of Orthopaedic Surgery
St. Mary's Medical Center
San Francisco, California

SCIENTIFIC/RESEARCH CONTRIBUTORS

Sophia D. Heber, MD
Johannes Gutenberg University of Mainz

Dave Hitt, MSc, RT (R) MR
MR Clinical Adoption Specialist
U.S. MR Marketing Department
Philips Healthcare

Adriana Kanwischer, BS
Medical Modality, UNISA
Advanced Applications Specialist, Global MR
GE Healthcare Technologies, Magnetic Resonance

Robert D. Peters, PhD
Manager
Global MR MSK
Applications & Physics/Core Technologies
GE Healthcare Technologies, Magnetic Resonance

PREFACE

Stoller's Orthopaedics and Sports Medicine: The Shoulder represents an ambitious and comprehensive undertaking for both myself and Wolters Kluwer. In order to organize this wealth of information and images in an accessible manner, a unique new format has been developed. A bulleted text that is concise provides for direct and rapid comprehension of orthopaedic advancements.

Special features include:

- Comprehensive collections of color illustrations and arthroscopic cases of orthopaedic pathoanatomy
- Key concepts section introductions to emphasize and reinforce critical information
- Detailed figure legends rich in content provide descriptive information and introduce novel concepts.
- 3T and high resolution MR images to demonstrate critical structures in functional shoulder anatomy and pathology.
- Evolved checklist approach as the keystone for accurate and reproducible image interpretation
- Updated concepts in the shoulder including:
    The rotator cable
    The superior glenohumeral ligament complex, IGLLC and BLC
    Proper cuff tensioning in rotator cuff repair
    PASTA lesions in the context of rotator cable anatomy
    Cadaver dissections highlighting anterior band and capsular variations

David W. Stoller, MD, FACR
National Director
    Orthopaedic and Musculoskeletal Imaging, RadNet
Medical Director
    Orthopaedic and Musculoskeletal Imaging, Beverly Radiology, Northern California
    San Francisco, California
Affiliate Member
    American Shoulder and Elbow Surgeons

ACKNOWLEDGMENTS

Undertaking the writing of this text has provided a unique opportunity to contribute to the emerging field of orthopaedic magnetic resonance imaging. Orthopaedic MRI has earned respect as a distinct subspecialty and is now a primary modality in the diagnosis of internal derangement of the joints. I would like to acknowledge the contributions of the following individuals:

> J.A. Gosling, MD, MB, ChB; P.F. Harris, MD, MB, ChB, MSc; J.R. Humpherson, MB, ChB; J. Whitmore, MD, MB, BS, LRCP, MRCS; and P.L.T. Willan, MB, ChB, FRCS, for providing quality gross anatomic color plates from their text, *Human Anatomy*, *Second edition*, Gower Medical Publishing.

The expert staff at Wolters Kluwer, for their efforts and appreciation of the necessary quality required to bring this text to fruition, including, Lisa McAllister, VP & Publisher, Medicine & Advanced Practice; Ryan Shaw, Acquisitions Editor; Kate Marshall, Product Development Editor; Doug Smock, Creative Services Director.

Crystal Perkins, West Coast Production liaison for Wolters Kluwer.

Sophia D. Heber MD, reference compilation and illustration research.

Dave Praz of Rapid, Restoration of DePalma cadaver dissections.

Robert Hoffman and Intelerad for their support in the storage of MR cases.

I would like to recognize the work of both **Stephen J. Snyder, MD and Stephen S. Burkhart, MD**. They deserve special recognition for their valuable contribution to the orthopaedic literature and collaboration in my understanding of shoulder surgical techniques.

Acknowledgement for the following masterful works:

Disorders of the Shoulder: Diagnosis and Management, Joseph P. Iannotti, MD, PhD; Gerald R. Williams Jr., MD; Anthony Miniaci; Joseph D. Zuckerman, MD

The Cowboy's Companion: A Trail Guide for the Arthroscopic Shoulder Surgeon, Stephen S. Burkhart, MD; Paul C Brady, MD; Ian KY Lo, MD, FRCS; Patrick J Denard, MD

The Master Techniques in Orthopaedic Surgery: The Shoulder, Edward V. Craig, MD

Surgery of the Shoulder, Anthony F. DePalma, MD

Controversies in Shoulder Instability, Joshua S. Dines, MD; Gerald R. Williams Jr., MD; Christopher Dodson; David Dines; Gilles Walch

Shoulder Arthroscopy 3rd Edition, Stephen J. Snyder, MD; Michael Bahk, MD; Joseph Burns, MD; Mark Getelman, MD; Ronald Karzel, MD

Atlas of Functional Shoulder Anatomy, Giovanni Di Giacomo, MD; Nicole Pouliart, MD, PhD; Alberto Costantini, MD; Andrea de Vita, MD

Technical Reference List

Bernstein MA, King KF, Zhou XJ. *Handbook of MRI Pulse Sequences*. Burlington, MA: Elsevier Academic Press; 2004.

Glover GH. Multipoint Dixon technique for water and fat proton and susceptibility imaging. *J Magn Reson Imaging* 1991;1(5):521–530.

Haacke EM, Brown RW, Thompson MR, Venkatesan R. *Magnetic Resonance Imaging: Physical Principles and Sequence Design*. New York, NY: Wiley-Liss; 1999.

Kuo MR, Panchal M, Tanenbaum L, Crues JV III. 3.0 Tesla imaging of the musculoskeletal system. *J Magn Reson Imaging* 2007;25(2):245–261.

Yoshioka H, Schlechtweg PM, Kose K. Magnetic resonance imaging. In: Weissman BN, ed. *Imaging of Arthritis and Metabolic Bone Disease*. Philadelphia, PA: Mosby; 2009.

CONTENTS

1
Practical Guide to Shoulder MR Imaging

Practical Guide to Shoulder MR Imaging

Key Factors to Clinical Diagnostics

■ **High Resolution**
Required for labrum, articular cartilage, and glenohumeral ligaments

■ **Flexible Contrast (T1, PD, T2)**
T1 (fat), PD/FSPD (articular cartilage + fluid) and T2 (cuff tear vs tendinosis)

■ **Uniform Fat Suppression**
Assessment of cuff tendon and muscle signal

Positioning

■ **RF Coils**
Shoulder coils are most commonly available as receive-only, phased array designs. Phased array coils are combined with multi-channel technology for increased SNR. A higher number of channels will improve SNR closer to the surface and enhance parallel imaging techniques. However, increasing the number of channels may compromise signal penetration since the coil elements will be smaller and penetration is directly proportional to the coil element size. Receive-only coils are paired with transmit coils that provide a uniform signal for the receive-coil to detect. Shoulder coils are typically paired with the whole-body transmit coil that is built into the system.

Shoulder coils can be exclusively for shoulder imaging or they can be flexible, designed for multiple anatomies. Dedicated coils will provide ease of use while flexible coils will better accommodate larger patients. Positioning will be crucial to avoid motion and proper anatomy signal coverage.

The region of interest must be positioned in the center of the coil. Identify the mark on the center of the coil provided by the manufacturer and landmark the patient accordingly.

■ **Immobilization**
Patient must be positioned supine, arm neutral. A wedge pad can be used under the opposite shoulder to the one to be imaged, keeping the side of interest relaxed on the coil and avoiding motion. Adjust straps firmly but never so tight to cause pain or discomfort.

■ **Off-Isocenter Scanning**
Patient anatomy placement must be as close as possible to the isocenter for best performance of B_0-dependent fat sat techniques. Special attention is required for the wide bore systems. Follow the operator manual recommendations and center the anatomy according to the system specifications.

Basic Pulse Sequences

■ FSE

The most used sequence for musculoskeletal imaging is the Fast Spin Echo. It provides spin-echo type contrast with faster scan times. Proton density, T1, or T2 image contrast is determined by the TR, TE, and ETL parameters. FSE protocols must focus on controlling echo spacing (time between echoes) to avoid blurring and flow artifacts. The minimum TE is an indicator of echo spacing and shorter values are desired to provide good image quality.

Parameter selections for decreasing Echo Spacing:			
⬆⬆ FOV	⬇⬇ Matrix	⬆⬆ Slice thickness	⬆⬆ Bandwidth

■ FRFSE

The Fast Recovery Fast Spin Echo sequence produces images with more T2 contribution. It is a modified FSE sequence using additional RF pulses after the acquisition window to drive preferential recovery of longitudinal magnetization from signal with long T2.

TR can be reduced at no expense to contrast to noise. SNR is improved and can be traded for spatial resolution.

FRFSE can be used to create highly T2-weighted images with decreased acquisition times.

Recommended TR, TE, and ETL values for FSE and FRFSE:			
Pulse Sequence	**TR**	**TE**	**ETL**
FRFSE PD	2000–3000ms	30–60ms	6–8
FRFSE T2	2000–3000ms	85ms	12–14
FSE T1	500–900	Min.	2–4

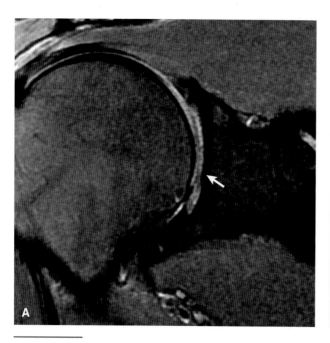 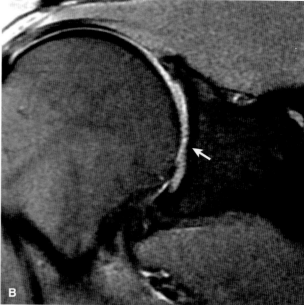

FIGURE 1.1   (A,B) Image on the left with an echo spacing = 8ms compared to an echo spacing = 16ms resulting in image blurring on the right.

■ **GRE**

The Gradient Echo sequence permits the use of pulse flip angles that control contrast. The flip angle is the angle by which nuclear spins are rotated from the direction of the static magnetic field. The contrast is strongly affected by the pulse sequence design. The most common uses for GRE sequences on musculoskeletal imaging are based on short repetition times and low flip angles to provide $T2^*$ contrast. The signal-to-noise ratio in musculoskeletal GRE sequences is proportional to the flip angle.

Sequence	Contrast	Flip Angle
2D GRE/SPGR	T1	40–60
	$T2^*$	20–30
3D GRE/SPGR	T1	25–45
	T2	5–8

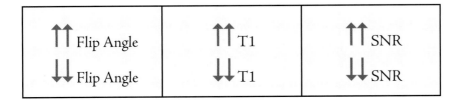

■ **IR**

Inversion Recovery is a sequence to adjust the T1 contrast between tissues by applying an inversion pulse before the normal pulse sequence. In musculoskeletal imaging, the contrast is usually adjusted to eliminate signal. The time between the inversion pulse and the image acquisition affects what tissue will be eliminated. This technique is most often used with FSE imaging and can provide uniform suppression of tissues (e.g., fat). Increased scan time is expected since there is an addition of the inversion pulse and inversion time. As tissue is suppressed, the signal-to-noise ratio will decrease.

Scan Parameters

■ **Spatial Resolution**

Determined by pixel size and voxel volume, resolution depends on the FOV, acquisition matrix, and slice thickness.

> **Calculating Pixel Size, Area, and Volume**
>
> $$\frac{FOV}{\#\ Phase\ matrix} = \text{Phase dimension}$$
>
> $$\frac{FOV}{\#\ Frequency\ matrix} = \text{Frequency dimension}$$
>
> Phase dimension $\times$ Frequency dimension = Pixel area
>
> Pixel area $\times$ Slice thickness = Voxel volume

High resolution may add valuable information for musculoskeletal imaging.

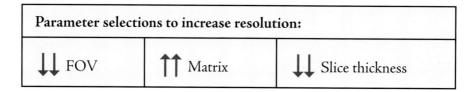

Parameter selections to increase resolution:		
⬇⬇ FOV	⬆⬆ Matrix	⬇⬇ Slice thickness

▪ Acquisition Time

Motion always represents a threat to good image quality. Faster acquisition times are desirable to reduce sensitivity to motion and are especially needed when scanning noncooperative patients. The parameters that affect image acquisition times are TR, Phase matrix, and NEX. When acquiring 3D images, the number of slices must also be considered.

Calculating acquisition time:
2D TR × Phase × NEX 3D TR × Phase × NEX × # slices

▪ SNR

Signal-to-noise ratio (SNR) is the ratio of amplitude of the MR signal to the amplitude of the noise. Noise is the undesirable signal that is generated from the patient, the environment, and the system electronics. Noise is difficult to control so it is more effective to try to increase the signal in order to increase the signal to noise ratio. Signal is proportional to field strength, voxel volume, and the time spent acquiring the signal. Of course, each method of generating an image has its own baseline for SNR.

There are resolution and acquisition time parameters that affect SNR.

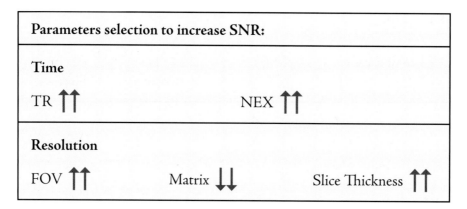

Parameters selection to increase SNR:		
Time		
TR ⬆⬆	NEX ⬆⬆	
Resolution		
FOV ⬆⬆	Matrix ⬇⬇	Slice Thickness ⬆⬆

▪ Trade-offs

In the clinical environment, the imaging protocol parameters will be determined according to many different goals. Understanding the parameter trade-offs is the only way to achieve good image quality, whether there is patient motion or anxiety, positioning limitations, anatomic variations, time restrictions, or any other challenges.

The table below is designed to provide guidance to adjust protocols without compromising the exam objectives.

Parameters	Resolution	Time	SNR
↑↑ TR	–	↑↑	↑↑
↑↑ TE	–	–	↓↓
↑↑ NEX	–	↑↑	↑↑
↑↑ Slice Thickness	↓↓	–	↑↑
↑↑ FOV	↓↓	–	↑↑
↑↑ Bandwidth	–	–	↓↓
↑↑ Frequency	↑↑	–	↓↓
↑↑ Phase	↑↑	↑↑	↓↓
↑↑ ETL	–	↓↓	–

Echo Train Length (ETL) and Bandwidth are parameters that affect protocols in a wider manner, deserving special mention.

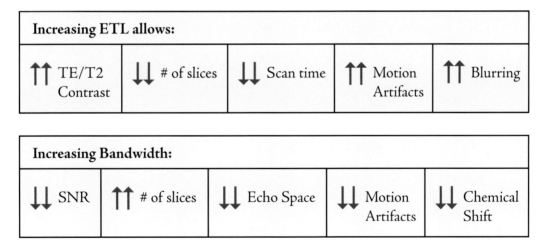

Increasing ETL allows:				
↑↑ TE/T2 Contrast	↓↓ # of slices	↓↓ Scan time	↑↑ Motion Artifacts	↑↑ Blurring

Increasing Bandwidth:				
↓↓ SNR	↑↑ # of slices	↓↓ Echo Space	↓↓ Motion Artifacts	↓↓ Chemical Shift

Advanced Applications

■ CUBE (GE Healthcare)

CUBE is a 3D FSE pulse sequence that applies modified refocusing pulses for better SNR and SAR efficiency. It can be used to generate PD and T2 contrast. It is always combined with acceleration techniques to avoid long scan times. CUBE allows isotropic volume acquisitions that can be reformatted in any plane with the same resolution as the original plane.

CUBE image quality is very dependent on protocol parameters. Settings enhanced for MSK provide for shorter gradients, reducing echo spacing and consequently decreased blurring. CUBE also allows a choice for the refocusing flip angle. Recommendations are 90 for 1.5T and 70 for 3-T, increasing SNR when relatively shorter ETL (~32 to 36) is used.

Whole volume excitation improves signal intensity uniformity across all slices. CUBE protocols allow NPW and multi-NEX. Fat saturation uses an adiabatic spectral inversion recovery technique (ASPIR) and the fat saturation efficiency can be modified by percentage, providing lighter to stronger fat suppression according to the user preference. Selecting fat saturation will minimize possible wrap artifacts in the slice direction that are visible in reformatted images. Banding or shading may be observed on off-center imaging so the anatomy must always be positioned as close as possible to the isocenter. Longer scan times when using NPW and multi NEX are expected.

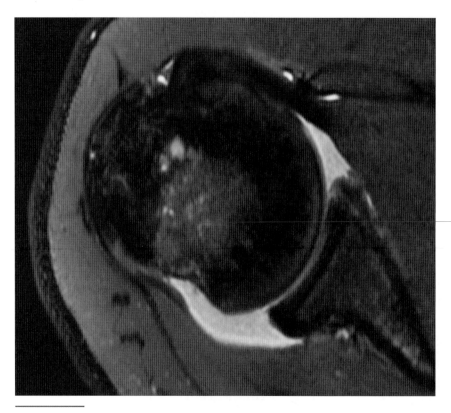

FIGURE 1.2   3D CUBE.

3-T										
PSD	TR (ms)	TE (ms)	BW (kHz)	ETL	NEX	FOV (cm)	MATRIX	Thick (mm)	Imaging Options	ARC (phase 3 slice)	Freq.
CUBE PD AXIAL	1500	25	50	40	2	16	224 × 224	0.8	Fat sat, EDR, Z512, Z2, FR	2 × 2	RL

IDEAL

IDEAL is a three-point Dixon technique that acquires three images at slightly different echo times to generate phase shifts between water and fat. The water/fat separation method is very efficient at providing homogeneous image quality.

One acquisition provides four contrasts: water, fat, in phase, and out of phase images. Available for 2D FSE, 2D FRFSE, 3D Fast GRE, and 3D Fast SPGR sequences, it can be combined with acceleration (ARC) for faster acquisition times. IDEAL is part of the imaging options list, and when selected, it will open a new tab on the protocol for a choice of which of the four contrasts should be reconstructed.

The typical IDEAL bandwidth is the pre-IDEAL sequence value multiplied by two. The FOV must include all the anatomy of interest since phase wrap artifacts may cause fat and water signal to be swapped.

To prevent blurring and maintain resolution, place the center of the effective TE between the Min and Max TE values by adjusting ETL to reduce the Max TE. The minimum and maximum TE values are annotated at the bottom of the protocol page. IDEAL reduces image artifacts caused by chemical shift and magnetic susceptibility.

3-T										
PSD	**TR (ms)**	**TE (ms)**	**BW (kHz)**	**ETL**	**NEX**	**FOV (cm)**	**MATRIX**	**Thick × Gap (mm)**	**Imaging Options**	**Freq.**
AXIAL PD FRFSE	2000	35	62.5	8	1	16	256 × 256	3.5 × 0.5	FC slice, TRF, ZIP512, IDEAL	RL

■ 3D MERGE

3D MERGE is a 3D Fast GRE pulse sequence that acquires multiple echoes at several different TEs and then average those echoes to form a single T2* weighted image. This technique can be used when susceptibility weighting is desired. It maintains visualization of ligaments while adding soft tissue contrast. Water excitation is available for robust fat suppression.

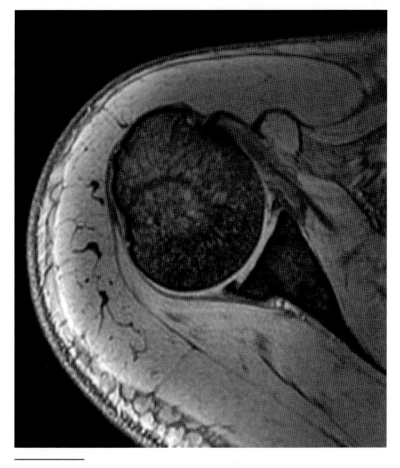

FIGURE 1.3　3D MERGE.

3-T										
PSD	TR	TE	Flip (deg)	BW (kHz)	ETL	FOV (cm)	MATRIX	Thick (mm)	Imaging Options	Freq.
AXIAL 3D MERGE	Minimum	Min Full	5	50	4	16	288 × 288	2.8	FC slice, Z2	LR

■ PROPELLER

PROPELLER is a pulse sequence designed for motion correction. The technique is based on periodically rotated overlapping parallel lines with enhanced reconstruction. It uses radial k-space filling with an arrangement of blades resulting in oversampling the center of k-space and providing images with high signal. The radial trajectory removes structured motion artifacts. Acceleration is used to increase blade width and reduce scan times. It can be used for any scan plane and it is an excellent choice of sequence when imaging through motion is needed due to breathing, flow, or uncooperative patients. It is compatible with Fat Saturation and it can produce PD and T2 contrast for MSK imaging.

PROPELLER image quality is very dependent of scan parameters. Blade width (ETL × Phase Acceleration), Over Sampling Factor, and Refocusing Flip Angle are concepts that deserve special attention for obtaining good image quality. The Over Sampling Factor (OSF) works as the analogue to NPW for PROPELLER.

Blade width must be adjusted properly to prevent streaking artifacts. Increase ETL, use acceleration, and decrease OSF to keep the minimum blade width equal to at least twelve for musculoskeletal imaging.

Contrast can be adjusted by modifying the refocusing flip angle value. Decreasing the refocusing flip angle will provide brighter cartilage signal. It will also allow higher TE and ETL values while still avoiding artifacts. Proper pre scan values must be obtained before scanning PROPELLER. Prescribe a shim volume on the area of interest for the series that will be scanned previously to PROPELLER.

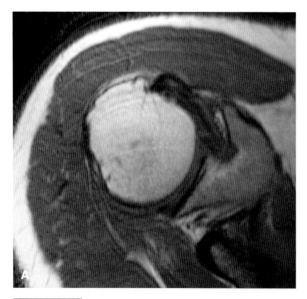 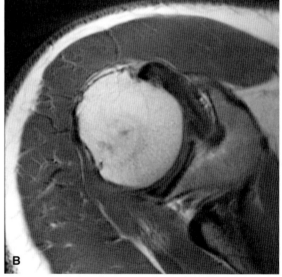

FIGURE 1.4   (A,B) Same study comparison of FSE image with motion and PROPELLER with motion correction in (B).

3-T										
PSD	BW (kHz)	ETL	NEX	FOV (cm)	MATRIX	Thick × Gap (mm)	Imaging Options	Refocus Flip (deg)	OVS	ARC
PROPELLER PD Fat Sat	83.3	14	2	14	288	3.5 × 1	Fat Sat classic, NP2.0	140	2	2

▪ **MAVRIC SL**

MAVRIC SL is a pulse sequence designed to reduce susceptibility artifacts. It is used for imaging soft tissue and bone near MR conditional metal implants. MAVRIC SL is a multi-spectral 3D imaging technique that acquires multiple 3D FSE images at discrete transmit and receive frequency offsets. All data acquired is then added together to form a final composite image.

The recommended protocol for MR conditional implant imaging includes MAVRIC SL PD, MAVRIC SL Fluid, and MARS (High bandwidth FSE) protocols.

The MAVRIC SL PD sequence is used for evaluating the tissue in the immediate vicinity of the implant. The MAVRIC SL Fluid (IR-based fat suppression) sequence is used as a low-resolution fluid detection mechanism replacing the conventional 2D FSE STIR sequence. A high-resolution MARS sequence is used for evaluating the soft tissue located away from the implant. The MARS technique is a 2DFSE protocol with a high bandwidth value.

Prescribing a wide enough FOV to cover the sensitivity region is recommended to avoid image wrap. Or, leave enough space away from the implant for fold over to occur without impinging on the metal-distorted region. Aggressive parallel imaging (ARC) is used to maintain low scan times and it is not limited by coil configurations like other applications. Residual metal artifacts may occur. They are different from conventional susceptibility distortions and could occasionally appear as "ringing" near the corners of the implants.

3-T											
PSD	TR (ms)	TE (ms)	BW (kHz)	ETL	NEX	FOV (cm)	MATRIX	Thick (mm)	Imaging Options	TI (ms)	Freq.
COR MAVRIC SL	3000	-	-	20	-	24	320 × 256	3.5	EDR, ARC	-	SI
COR MAVRIC SL FLUID	7000	-	-	20	-	24	256 × 160	3.5	EDR, IRp, ARC	175	SI
COR FSE MARS	4000	18	100	20	2	20	512 × 320	3.0	NPW, EDR, TRF	-	SI

3-T Imaging Considerations

▪ **Advantages**

High field MR imaging at 3-T allows for up to 100% SNR increase when compared to 1.5T systems. The extra SNR can be used to decrease scan times and increase resolution: increasing matrix, decreasing FOV, or decreasing slice thickness. Decreasing NEX will reduce scan acquisition time.

T1 relaxation times are longer at 3-T. Increasing the TR for acquiring the desired contrast must be considered.

Challenges

Chemical Shift:

Chemical shift is a mis-registration artifact in the frequency encoding direction caused by the frequency difference between fat and water signals. Precessional frequencies are proportional to the magnetic field and since they double from 1.5T to 3-T (220Hz /440Hz), chemical shift artifacts are twice as bad at 3-T.

Increasing the bandwidth reduces the number of pixels of the shift between fat and water, minimizing the appearance of the chemical shift artifact; therefore, 3-T protocols have higher bandwidth when compared to 1.5T protocols.

Magnetic Susceptibility:

The ability of the magnetic field to penetrate different substances is called susceptibility and it induces magnetic field perturbations resulting in distortion artifacts. The appearance of the artifacts is the result of the sum of surrounding tissues with different magnetic susceptibilities. Susceptibility artifacts cause signal loss and distortions and will be observed in interfaces like bone/tissue, air/tissue, and presence of metal. Since susceptibility is proportional to the magnetic field, the artifacts will be twice as severe at 3-T as at 1.5T.

Increasing bandwidth can help minimize susceptibility artifacts. Inversion recovery techniques are recommended since GRE sequences and fat suppression methods are more sensitive to susceptibility artifacts.

Specific Absorption Rate:

Specific Absorption Rate, SAR, is a measurement of the RF energy deposition.

SAR dependent is dependent on the square of the B_0 field strength; therefore, it is four times higher at 3.0T than at 1.5T.

SAR values may restrict minimum TR values and the number of slices per TR for FSE sequences. Increasing TR, decreasing refocusing flip angles, and the use of GRE sequences are efficient ways of decreasing SAR values.

Dielectric Effect:

Dielectric artifacts are represented by areas of inhomogeneity, shading, or lower SNR. They are caused by the interaction by the RF field and increased conductivity of the body tissue. Since the RF wavelength on the 3-T magnetic field strength is comparable to the patient diameter, the dielectric effect is more evident on 3.0T systems. The artifacts are seeing mostly on abdominal imaging and related to patient size, being more evident on smaller and thinner individuals. Presence of fluid can also exacerbate the shading, for example on patients with ascites. Multi-channel coils may also intensify dielectric effect due to the higher signal intensity, making nonuniformity areas more apparent. Dielectric pads may be used between the coil and the patient to minimize shading, but with limited success. They are made of a dilute Manganese Chloride solution. Also uniformity correction methods can be applied, reducing dielectric effect. Commonly used mitigation at 3T for reducing dielectric shading is "Dual Drive" or "RF shimming" which modifies the transmit RF field polarization.

Parallel Imaging

Parallel Imaging is a method that allows rapid MR data acquisition by using the spatial information in multi-channel coils combined with mathematical techniques such as ASSET and ARC. Acquisition times are shorter since only partial data is acquired. The rest of the information is completed using spatial information obtained by coil sensitivity. Parallel Imaging comes at the expense of SNR loss but it includes other benefits such as the reduction of image blurring, motion artifacts, and geometric distortion. Parallel Imaging performance is improved by optimized coil designs with more receiver channels and it is also dependent of the distance that separates elements in the phase encoding direction.

ASSET:
Array Spatial Sensitivity Encoding Technique is an externally calibrated parallel imaging method whose generic name is SENSE. The calibration acquisition provides the coil sensitivity maps and is acquired separately from the ASSET acquisition. Incomplete calibration coverage, calibration wrap, area of interest mismatch, and poor coil positioning are the most common causes of artifacts.

ARC:
ARC is an auto-calibrated Parallel Imaging technique that does not require a separated calibration series to acquire a coil sensitivity map. It simplifies workflow and it is extremely powerful against Parallel Imaging artifacts.

Parallel Imaging represents an important concept for MSK imaging. It allows acceptable acquisition times for several applications like CUBE, MAVRIC SL, PROPELLER, and other pulse sequences.

Fat Suppression Techniques

■ Spectral Selective Fat Saturation
Spectral Selective Fat Saturation is a method that applies a frequency selective saturation pulse at the frequency of fat before the imaging excitation pulse with the result being a signal measurement primarily from water. Since the fat and water frequency separation depends on the magnetic field strength (220Hz at 1.5T/440Hz at 3.0T), fat saturation techniques based on this method are more effective at higher field strengths because the saturation can more effectively distinguish fat from water. The disadvantage of this method is the dependency on the homogeneity of the B_0 field. Poor field homogeneity may cause the frequency-selective pulse to saturate water instead resulting in regions where water rather than fat will be saturated. Alternately, because of poor B_0 homogeneity (often caused by magnetic susceptibility artifacts), the frequency selective pulse may not saturate any signal at all.

■ STIR (Short TI Inversion Recovery)
STIR is an inversion recovery method that takes advantage the T1 difference between water and fat to allow selection of the signal to suppress. In order to eliminate the signal from tissues, the TI time must match exactly the null point of the tissue that needs to be suppressed. The TI time is approximately 69% of the T1 relaxation time of the tissue. Since this is an Inversion Recovery technique, the resulting image will be inherently T1 weighted, but at short TI time, T1 contrast will be inverted. It is also possible to acquire T2 contrast by using a long TE;

T2 contrast will not be inverted. STIR is very effective at suppressing fat signal since it can be made less dependent on field homogeneity by proper design of RF pulses and it is less dependent on the magnetic field homogeneity. The disadvantage of this sequence is longer acquisition time since Inversion Recovery techniques need longer TR times to give the spins enough time to recover.

■ SPIR (Spectral Pre-saturation with Inversion Recovery)

SPIR is a technique that uses both STIR and selective excitation of the fat signal. The TI value for the null point of a tissue follows the same rules as the STIR sequence. There will be no inherent T1 weighted contrast since only the fat signal is excited and water is not affected. The disadvantages include increase on scan acquisition times; it is sensitive to B_1 uniformity and it requires good separation of fat and water. SPIR can be improved by incorporation of an adiabatic pulse since adiabatic pulses are insensitive to B_1 nonuniformity. The result, SPAIR or ASPIR, is a fat suppression technique that is relatively insensitive to both B_0 and B_1 inhomogeneity.

■ SPAIR (Spectral Selective Adiabatic Inversion Recovery) or ASPIR (Adiabatic Spectral Selective Inversion Recovery)

SPAIR or ASPIR method is a solution for poor fat suppression due to B_1 inhomogeneity. It is based on the frequency and the relaxation fat behaviors.

Applies a spectrally selective adiabatic inversion pulse to excite the fat spins, imaging pulses are then applied after TI null time when longitudinal magnetization of fat crosses zero. The disadvantages include sensitivity to B_0 and longer scan times.

■ Dixon

The two-point Dixon technique is based on the difference between fat and water resonance frequencies, therefore they have different precession rates. With this method, two images are acquired, one with fat and water spins in phase and the other with them out of phase. When these images are added pixel by pixel, the result is a fat suppressed image and their subtraction a water suppressed image.

The three-point Dixon method is similar to the two-point technique, except that one extra image is acquired to correct phase effects like susceptibility or eddy currents. Dixon is a very robust fat suppression technique but scan times are longer since extra images are acquired. The final result is four images with four different contrasts: fat only, water only, in phase, and out of phase. The out of phase contrast is mostly used for abdominal imaging to evaluate the border between fatty and nonfatty tissues.

Uniformity Correction: Image Enhancement Filters

Signal intensity is most efficiently collected in the areas of the anatomy that are closest to the coil. This characteristic may cause nonuniformity of signal: the image will be brighter in the periphery close to the coil and relatively darker in the center away from the coil.

Intensity correction algorithms can be applied to the images to minimize the nonuniformity.

Phased array Uniformity Enhancement—PURE and Surface Coil Intensity Correction—SCIC (GE Healthcare) are two techniques designed to normalize the surface coil intensity variations. PURE or SCIC can be used with compatible surface coils.

PURE corrects field inhomogeneity using a low-resolution proton density weighted calibration scan while SCIC utilizes statistics from the actual image for inhomogeneity correction and does not require a calibration scan.

■ PURE: Phased Array Uniformity Enhancement

PURE corrects the field inhomogeneity by collecting a calibration scan from the (uniform) body coil and the (nonuniform) surface coil and calculating maps that relate the intensity correction values to the images. The correction is therefore stable across many image contrasts but is limited to the RF fields of the surface and body coil. It cannot correct for fat saturation uniformity.

Pure data can be automatically acquired during the exam acquisition or applied afterwards by post processing if a calibration series was acquired. PURE post processing will be available only for the series acquired after the calibration. Images are corrected by intensifying the signal. Areas of lower SNR will intensify the noise as well signal so the corrected images may appear "noisier" after correction on those areas. That is, both the detail and noise are amplified together in the process of making the average tissue intensity more uniform. To avoid the increased intensity of noise, prescribe your FOV in an area with proper coil coverage.

■ SCIC: Surface Coil Intensity Correction

SCIC is a method that uses statistics from the actual image for inhomogeneity correction. It uses an optimized set of parameters for tuning that are defined according to the different anatomies and coils. Since SCIC does not use an acquired reference image, the correction results will make the image contrast appear flatter when compared to images corrected by PURE. It compensates for smooth variations arising from any source and its performance can vary depending on the contrast of the image to be corrected. SCIC can also be applied automatically during acquisition or during post processing. The low SNR areas will appear slightly darker and noise enhancement is less noticeable than in images corrected with PURE.

SCIC and PURE methods are dependent on coil compatibility.

Sequences and Parameters Acronyms

The technical information provided in this chapter uses GE Healthcare sequence and parameters nomenclature as reference. The table below provides the list of acronyms from Siemens and Philips.

Pulse Sequences		
GE	**SIEMENS**	**PHILIPS**
FSE Fast Spin Echo	TSE Turbo Spin Echo	TSE Turbo Spin Echo
GRE	GRE	FFE
STIR	STIR	STIR
CUBE	SPACE	VISTA
PROPELLER	Blade	MultiVane
IDEAL	DIXON	DIXON
MAVRIC SL	syngoWARP	SEMAC
MERGE	MEDIC	MFFE

Parameters		
GE	**SIEMENS**	**PHILIPS**
Bandwidth BW ([kHz] ; $BW_{GE} = BW_{SIE}$ / 2 $\times$ Nb_points)	Bandwidth BW ([Hz/ pixel] ; $BW_{SIE} = 2 \times BW_{GE}$ / Nb_points)	WFS/BW Hz; Water Fat Shift (WFS) & (Hz/Pixel)
FR Fast Recovery	RST Restore	Drive (Driven Equilibrium)
ETL Echo Train Length	TF Turbo Factor	ES (Echo Spacing)
ARC/ASSET	GRAPPA/mSENSE	SENSE
SCIC/PURE	Normalize/Prescan Normalize	CLEAR (Constant Level Appearance)
NPW No phase wrap	Phase Oversampling	FO (FoldOver Suppression)
NEX	Average	NSA
FOV cm	FOV mm	FOV mm
ASPIR	SPAIR	SPAIR

Musculoskeletal MR Developments

The following items represent areas of active MSK development:
- Quantitative characterization of cartilage
- Advanced analysis and display: automated segmentation
- Faster Parallel Imaging: multiband excitation, compressed sensing
- Kinematic Imaging (advancements in kinematic and dynamic imaging)
- Automated scoring for RA
- Silent MSK
- Ultra Short TE
- Muscle and Fat quantification
- Surface Coil development
- Novel contrast mechanisms

Concept of Speed and Resolution (3T MRI)

Speed, High Resolution, and High Resolution with High SNR

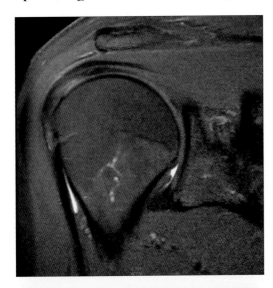

Speed
(Scan Time 2:44)

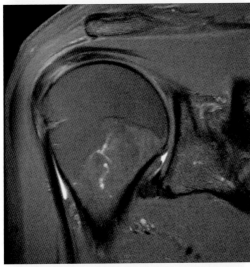

High Resolution
(Scan Time 5:43)

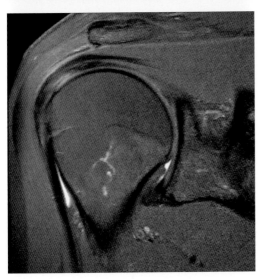

High Resolution
(Scan Time 11:51)

■ Speed protocols are achieved primarily through lowering the matrix and reducing the NEX.

2
Shoulder Anatomy

The Shoulder
MR Normal Anatomy

Coronal
pages 22 to 27

Axial
pages 28 to 33

Sagittal
pages 34 to 40

S.Beltrán '14

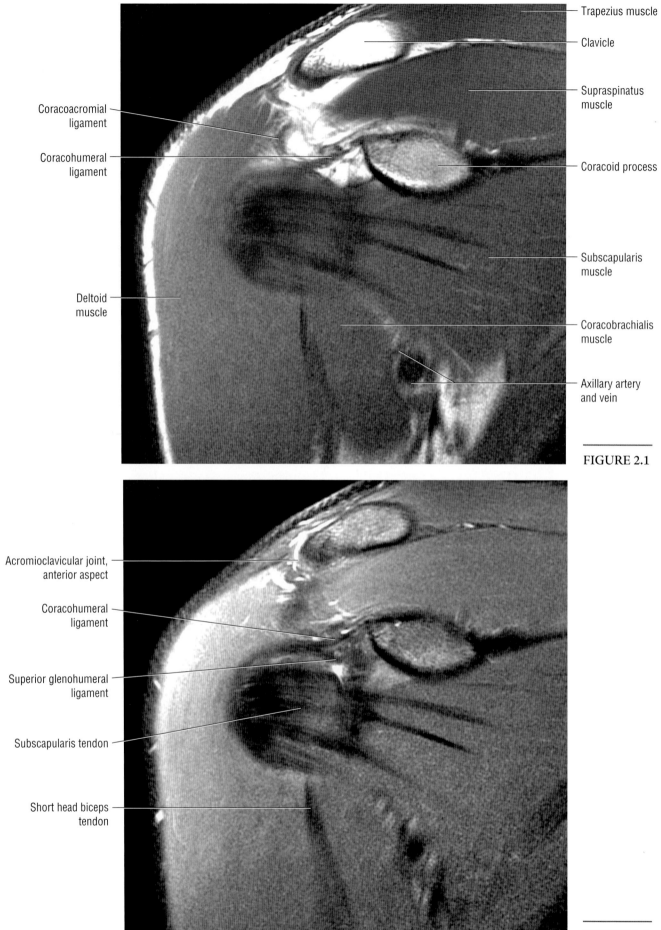

Trapezius muscle

Clavicle

Supraspinatus muscle

Coracoacromial ligament

Coracohumeral ligament

Coracoid process

Subscapularis muscle

Deltoid muscle

Coracobrachialis muscle

Axillary artery and vein

FIGURE 2.1

Acromioclavicular joint, anterior aspect

Coracohumeral ligament

Superior glenohumeral ligament

Subscapularis tendon

Short head biceps tendon

FIGURE 2.2

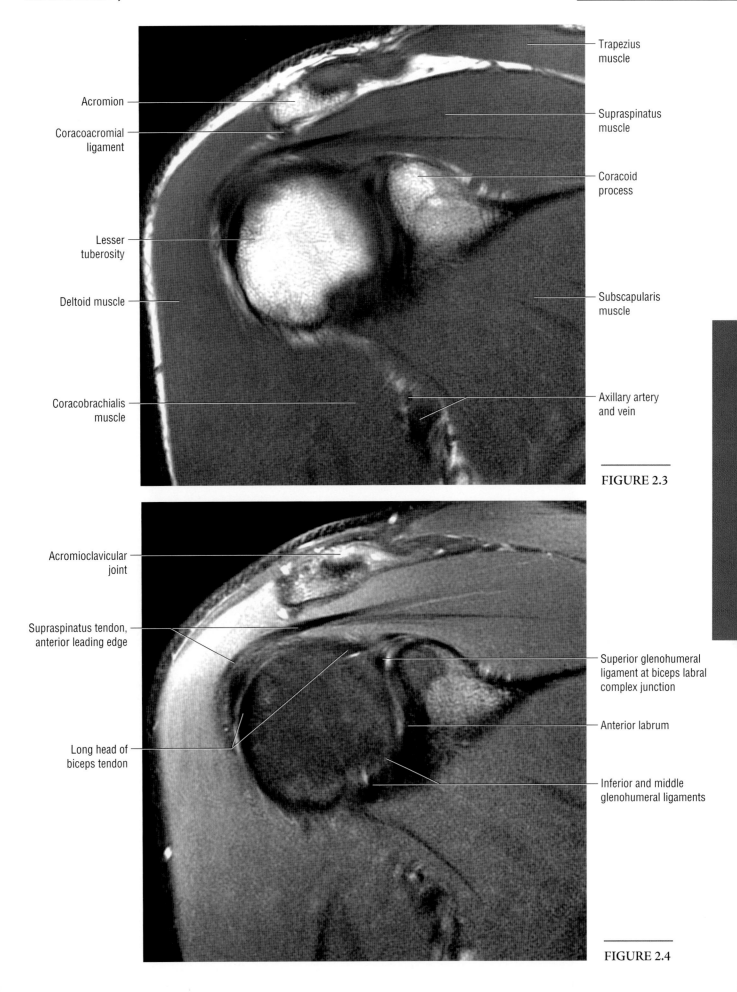

Trapezius
muscle

Acromion

Supraspinatus
muscle

Coracoacromial
ligament

Coracoid
process

Lesser
tuberosity

Deltoid muscle

Subscapularis
muscle

Coracobrachialis
muscle

Axillary artery
and vein

FIGURE 2.3

Acromioclavicular
joint

Supraspinatus tendon,
anterior leading edge

Superior glenohumeral
ligament at biceps labral
complex junction

Anterior labrum

Long head of
biceps tendon

Inferior and middle
glenohumeral ligaments

FIGURE 2.4

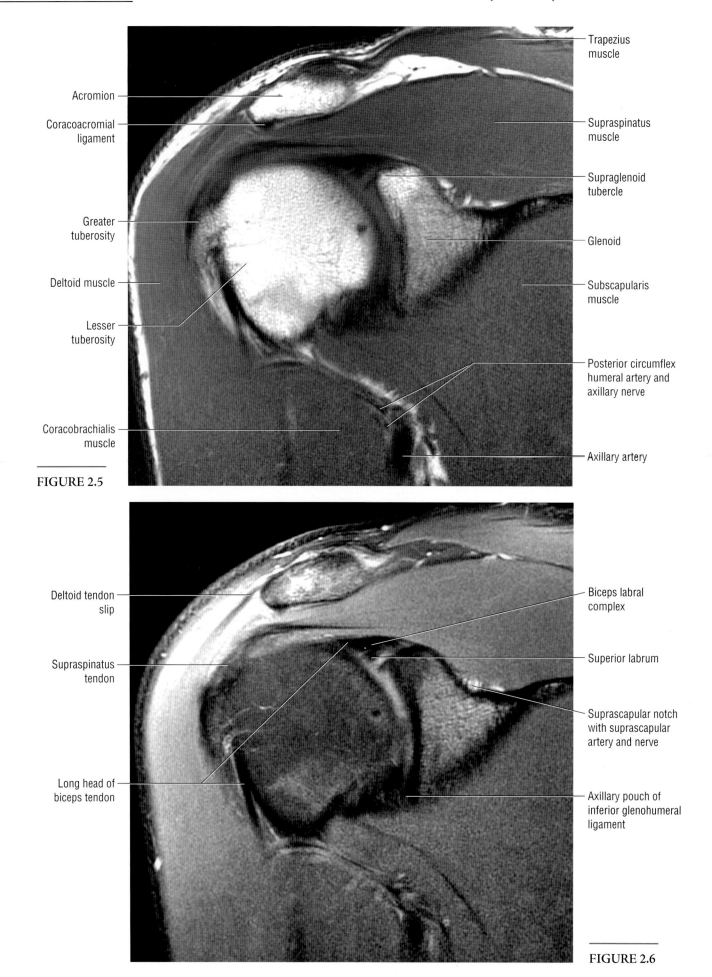

Acromion

Coracoacromial
ligament

Greater
tuberosity

Deltoid muscle

Lesser
tuberosity

Coracobrachialis
muscle

Trapezius
muscle

Supraspinatus
muscle

Supraglenoid
tubercle

Glenoid

Subscapularis
muscle

Posterior circumflex
humeral artery and
axillary nerve

Axillary artery

FIGURE 2.5

Deltoid tendon
slip

Supraspinatus
tendon

Long head of
biceps tendon

Biceps labral
complex

Superior labrum

Suprascapular notch
with suprascapular
artery and nerve

Axillary pouch of
inferior glenohumeral
ligament

FIGURE 2.6

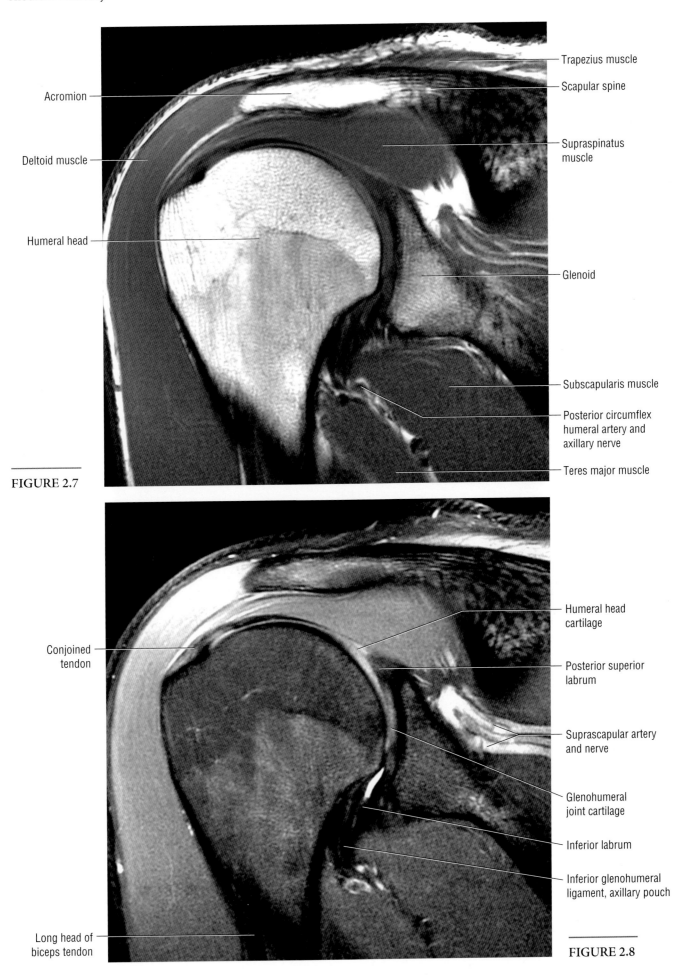

Trapezius muscle

Scapular spine

Acromion

Supraspinatus muscle

Deltoid muscle

Humeral head

Glenoid

Subscapularis muscle

Posterior circumflex humeral artery and axillary nerve

Teres major muscle

FIGURE 2.7

Conjoined tendon

Humeral head cartilage

Posterior superior labrum

Suprascapular artery and nerve

Glenohumeral joint cartilage

Inferior labrum

Inferior glenohumeral ligament, axillary pouch

Long head of biceps tendon

FIGURE 2.8

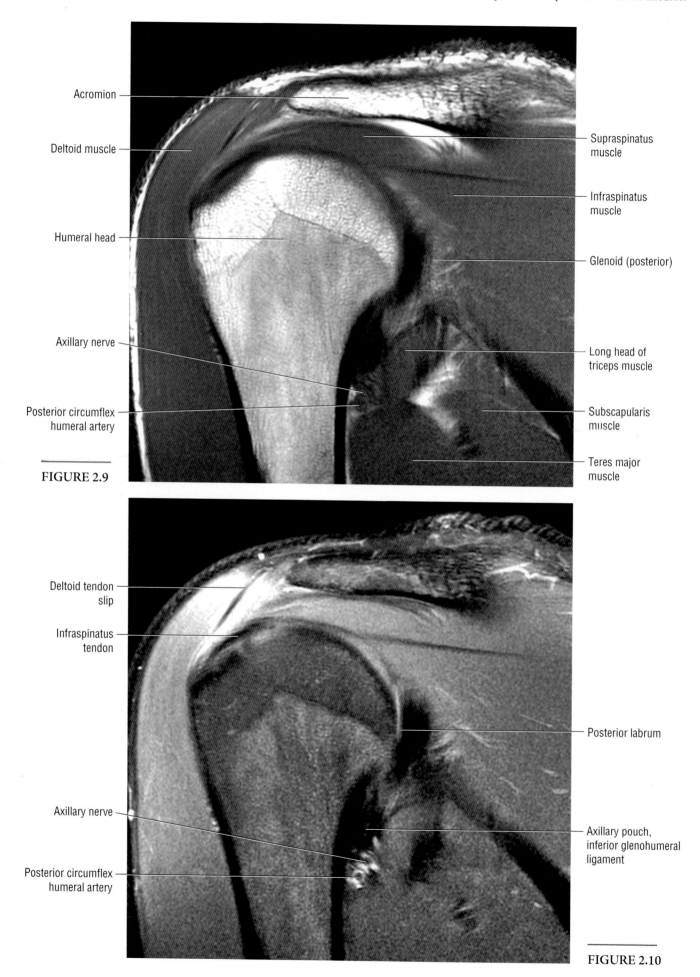

Acromion

Deltoid muscle

Supraspinatus
muscle

Infraspinatus
muscle

Humeral head

Glenoid (posterior)

Axillary nerve

Long head of
triceps muscle

Posterior circumflex
humeral artery

Subscapularis
muscle

Teres major
muscle

FIGURE 2.9

Deltoid tendon
slip

Infraspinatus
tendon

Posterior labrum

Axillary nerve

Axillary pouch,
inferior glenohumeral
ligament

Posterior circumflex
humeral artery

FIGURE 2.10

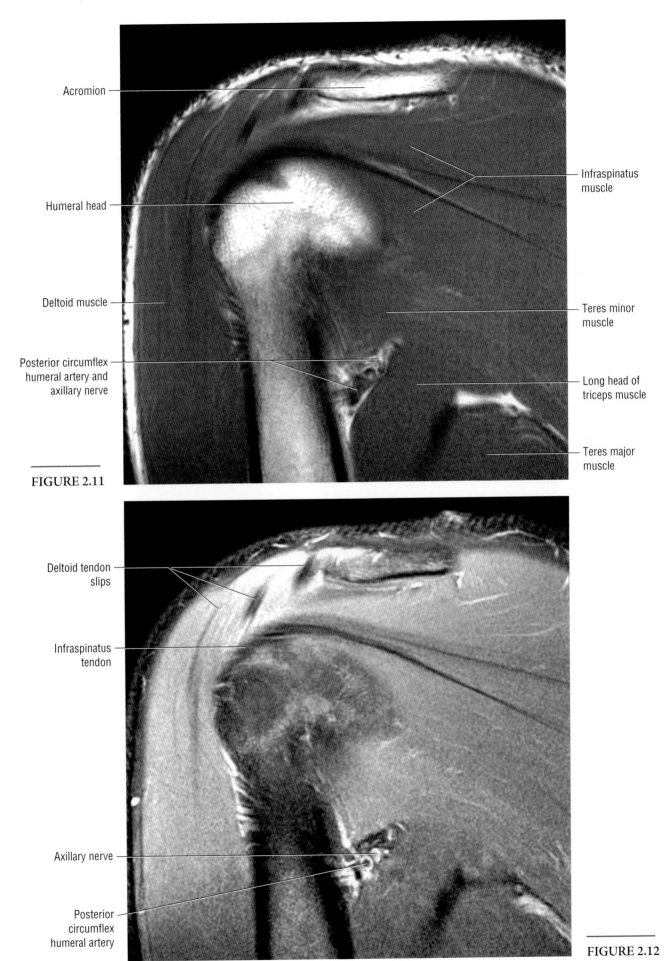

Acromion

Humeral head

Deltoid muscle

Posterior circumflex
humeral artery and
axillary nerve

Infraspinatus
muscle

Teres minor
muscle

Long head of
triceps muscle

Teres major
muscle

FIGURE 2.11

Deltoid tendon
slips

Infraspinatus
tendon

Axillary nerve

Posterior
circumflex
humeral artery

FIGURE 2.12

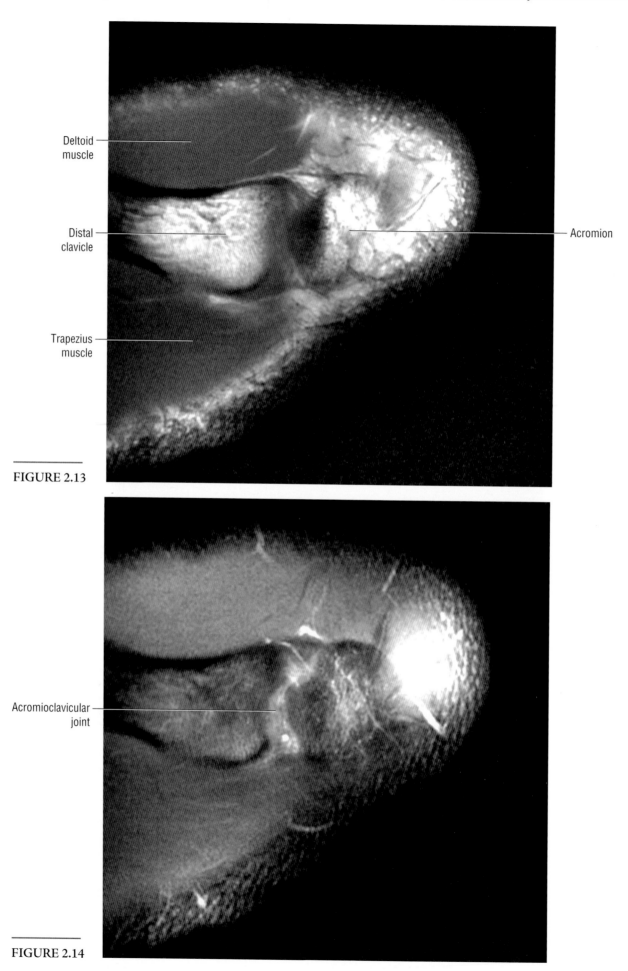

Deltoid muscle

Distal clavicle

Trapezius muscle

Acromion

FIGURE 2.13

Acromioclavicular joint

FIGURE 2.14

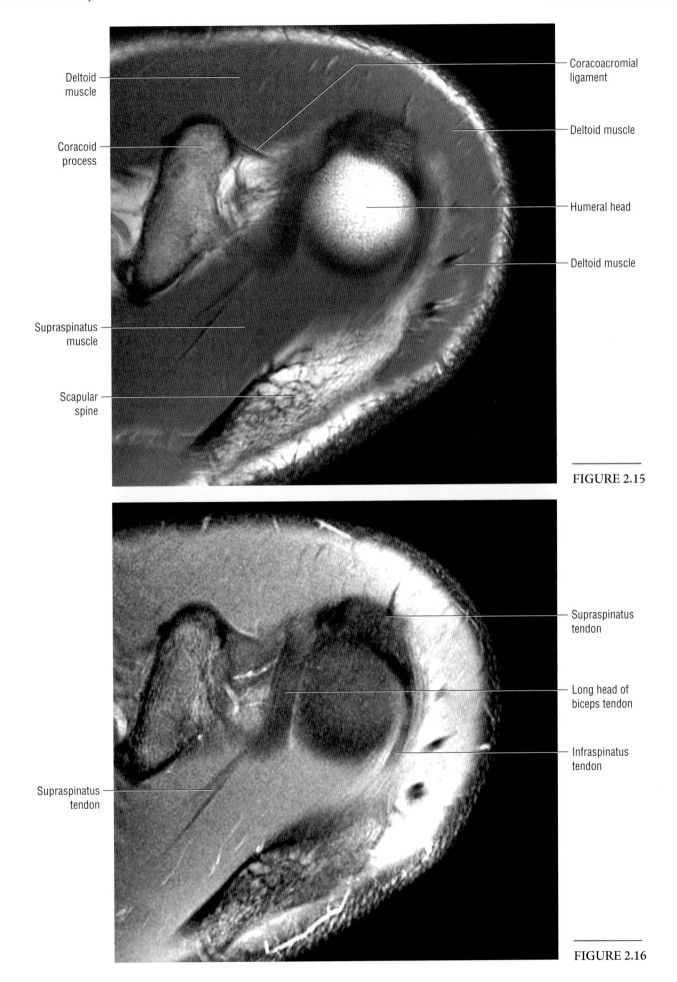

Deltoid muscle

Coracoid process

Supraspinatus muscle

Scapular spine

Coracoacromial ligament

Deltoid muscle

Humeral head

Deltoid muscle

FIGURE 2.15

Supraspinatus tendon

Long head of biceps tendon

Infraspinatus tendon

Supraspinatus tendon

FIGURE 2.16

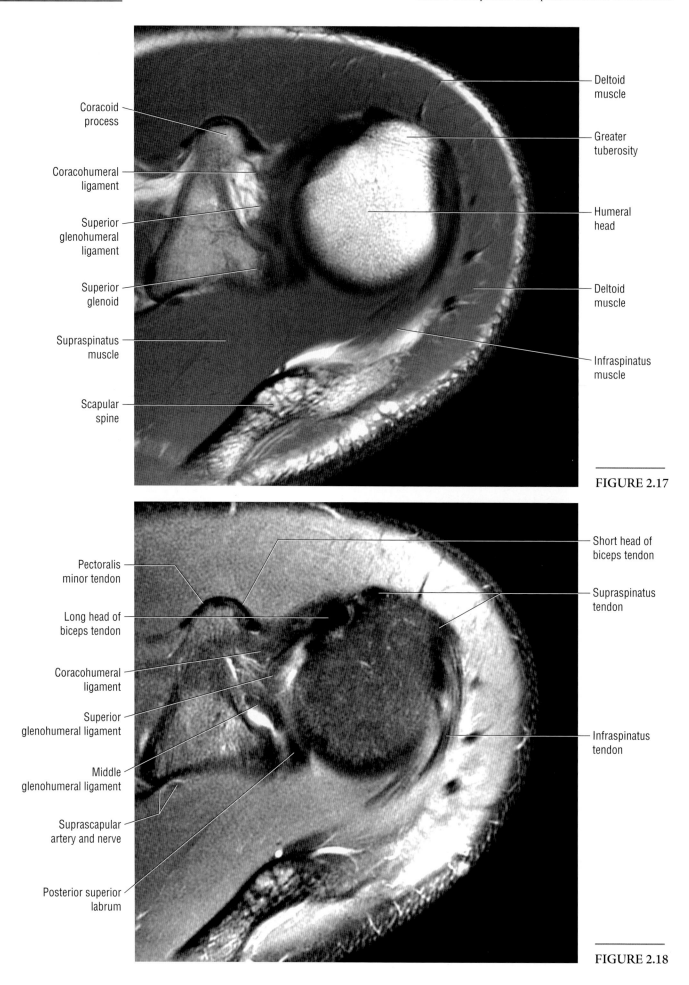

Deltoid
muscle

Coracoid
process

Greater
tuberosity

Coracohumeral
ligament

Superior
glenohumeral
ligament

Humeral
head

Superior
glenoid

Deltoid
muscle

Supraspinatus
muscle

Infraspinatus
muscle

Scapular
spine

FIGURE 2.17

Pectoralis
minor tendon

Short head of
biceps tendon

Supraspinatus
tendon

Long head of
biceps tendon

Coracohumeral
ligament

Superior
glenohumeral ligament

Infraspinatus
tendon

Middle
glenohumeral ligament

Suprascapular
artery and nerve

Posterior superior
labrum

FIGURE 2.18

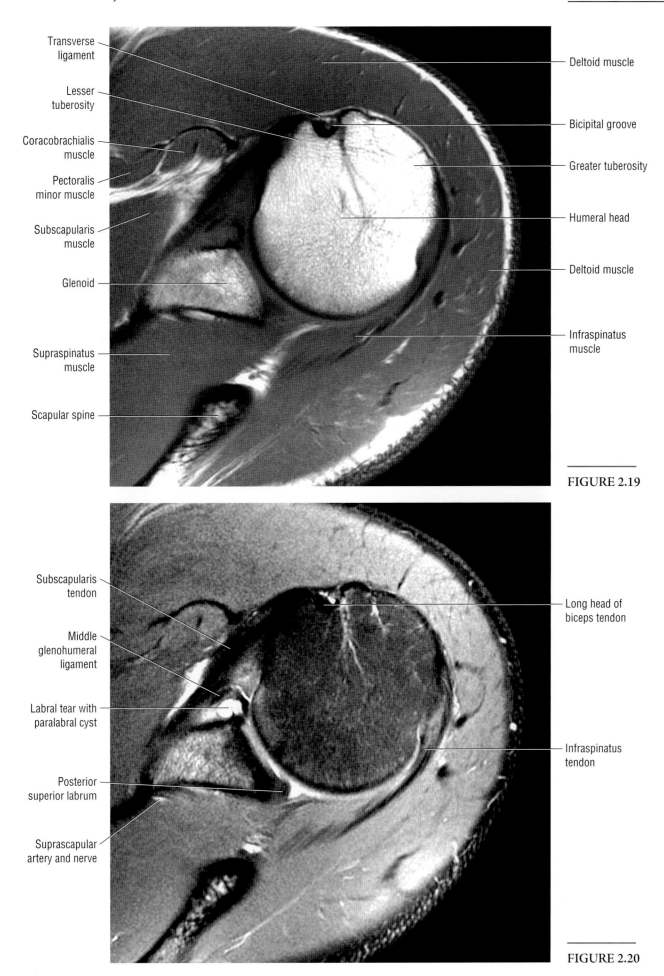

Transverse ligament

Lesser tuberosity

Coracobrachialis muscle

Pectoralis minor muscle

Subscapularis muscle

Glenoid

Supraspinatus muscle

Scapular spine

Deltoid muscle

Bicipital groove

Greater tuberosity

Humeral head

Deltoid muscle

Infraspinatus muscle

FIGURE 2.19

Subscapularis tendon

Middle glenohumeral ligament

Labral tear with paralabral cyst

Posterior superior labrum

Suprascapular artery and nerve

Long head of biceps tendon

Infraspinatus tendon

FIGURE 2.20

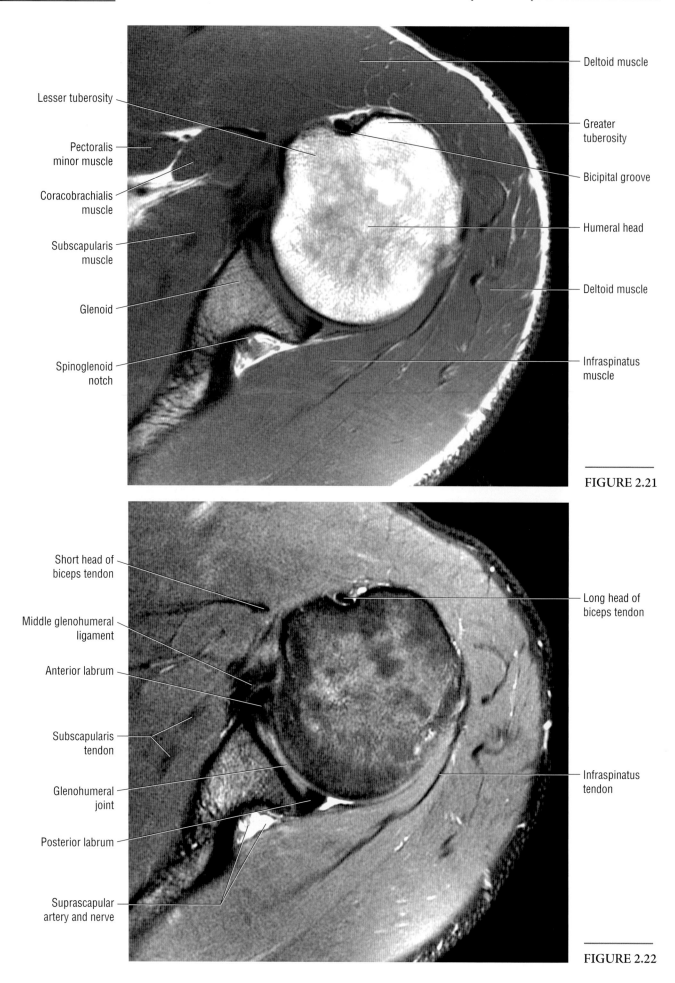

Lesser tuberosity

Pectoralis minor muscle

Coracobrachialis muscle

Subscapularis muscle

Glenoid

Spinoglenoid notch

Deltoid muscle

Greater tuberosity

Bicipital groove

Humeral head

Deltoid muscle

Infraspinatus muscle

FIGURE 2.21

Short head of biceps tendon

Middle glenohumeral ligament

Anterior labrum

Subscapularis tendon

Glenohumeral joint

Posterior labrum

Suprascapular artery and nerve

Long head of biceps tendon

Infraspinatus tendon

FIGURE 2.22

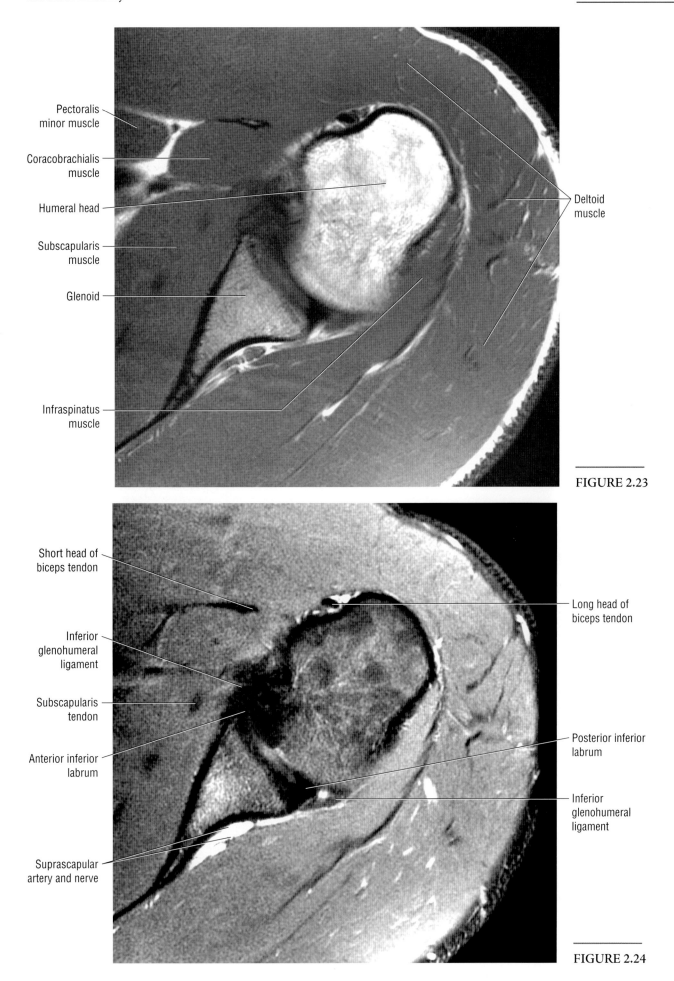

Pectoralis minor muscle

Coracobrachialis muscle

Humeral head

Subscapularis muscle

Glenoid

Infraspinatus muscle

Deltoid muscle

FIGURE 2.23

Short head of biceps tendon

Inferior glenohumeral ligament

Subscapularis tendon

Anterior inferior labrum

Suprascapular artery and nerve

Long head of biceps tendon

Posterior inferior labrum

Inferior glenohumeral ligament

FIGURE 2.24

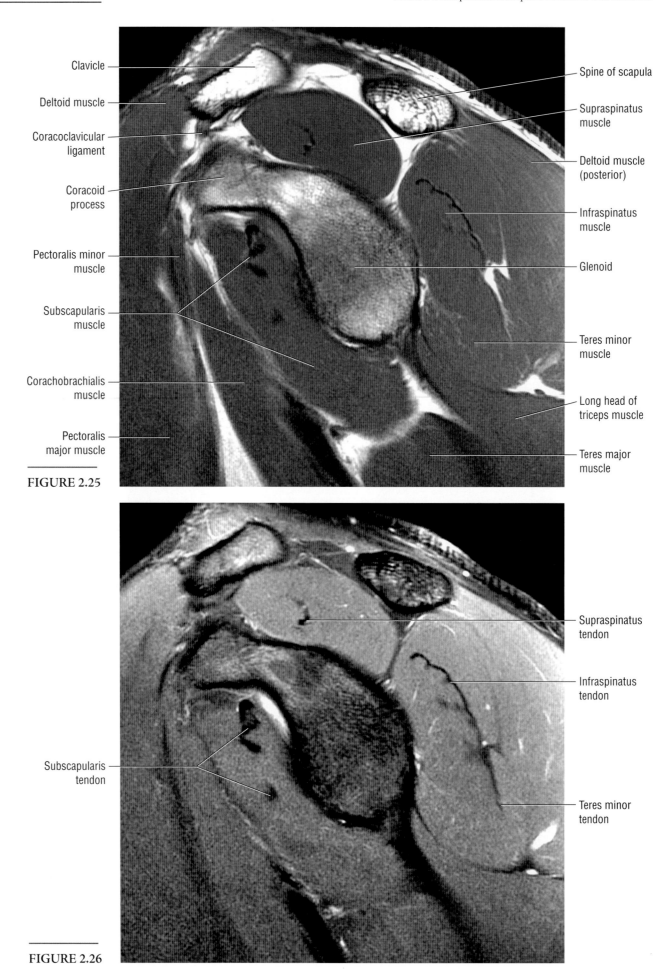

Clavicle

Deltoid muscle

Coracoclavicular
ligament

Coracoid
process

Pectoralis minor
muscle

Subscapularis
muscle

Corachobrachialis
muscle

Pectoralis
major muscle

Spine of scapula

Supraspinatus
muscle

Deltoid muscle
(posterior)

Infraspinatus
muscle

Glenoid

Teres minor
muscle

Long head of
triceps muscle

Teres major
muscle

FIGURE 2.25

Subscapularis
tendon

Supraspinatus
tendon

Infraspinatus
tendon

Teres minor
tendon

FIGURE 2.26

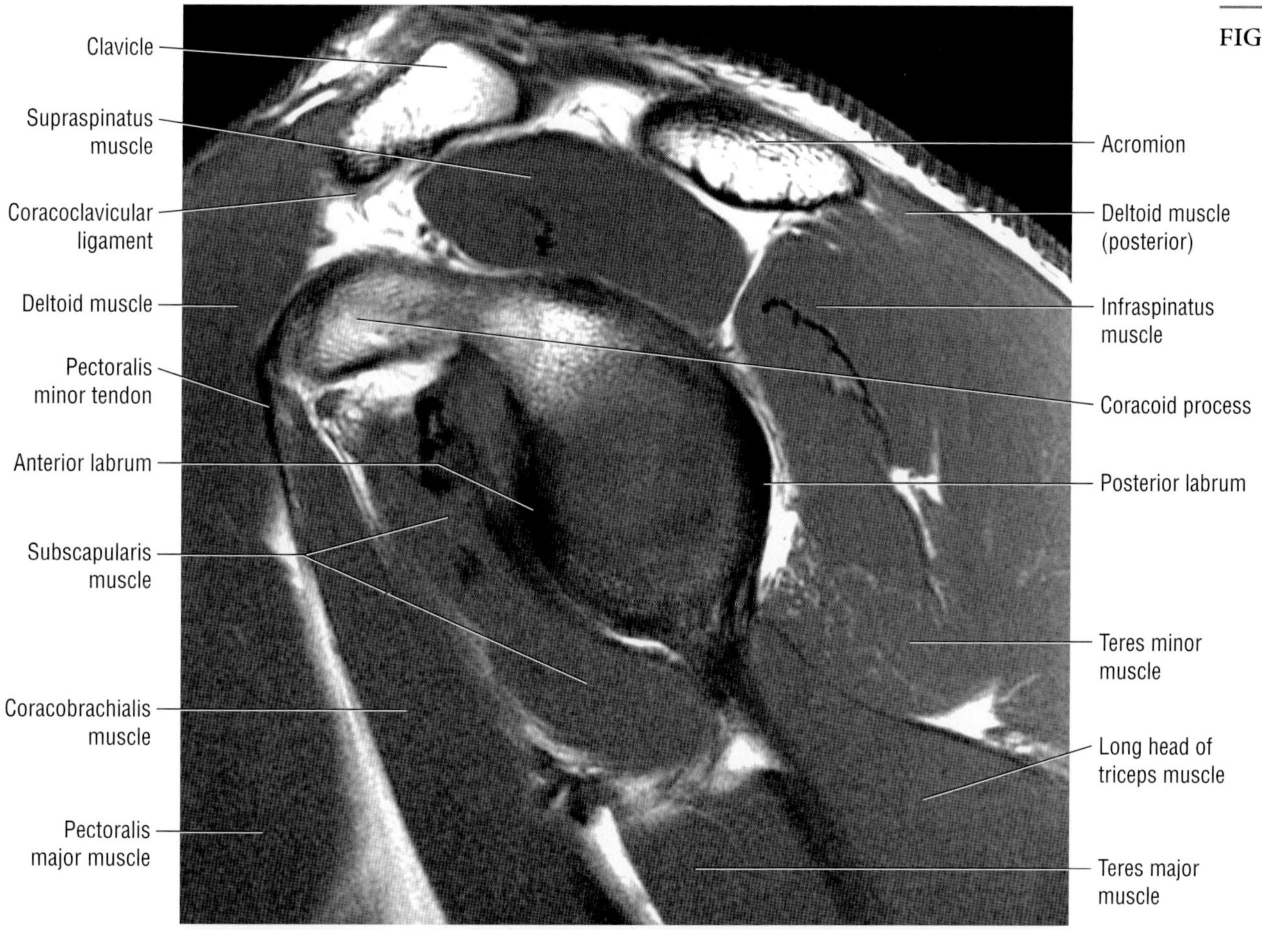

FIGURE 2.27

Clavicle

Supraspinatus muscle

Coracoclavicular ligament

Deltoid muscle

Pectoralis minor tendon

Anterior labrum

Subscapularis muscle

Coracobrachialis muscle

Pectoralis major muscle

Acromion

Deltoid muscle (posterior)

Infraspinatus muscle

Coracoid process

Posterior labrum

Teres minor muscle

Long head of triceps muscle

Teres major muscle

FIGURE 2.27

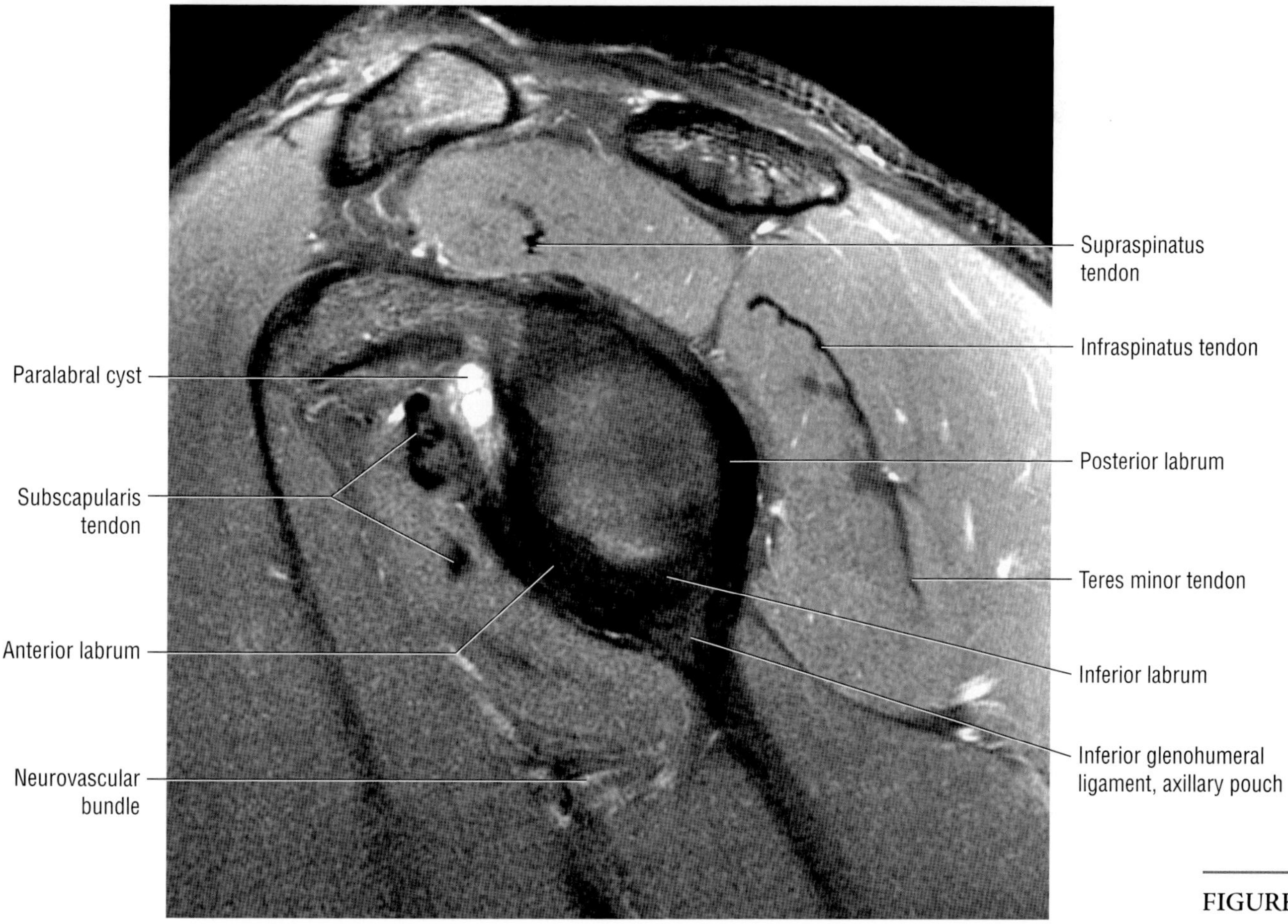

Paralabral cyst

Subscapularis tendon

Anterior labrum

Neurovascular bundle

Supraspinatus tendon

Infraspinatus tendon

Posterior labrum

Teres minor tendon

Inferior labrum

Inferior glenohumeral ligament, axillary pouch

FIGURE 2.28

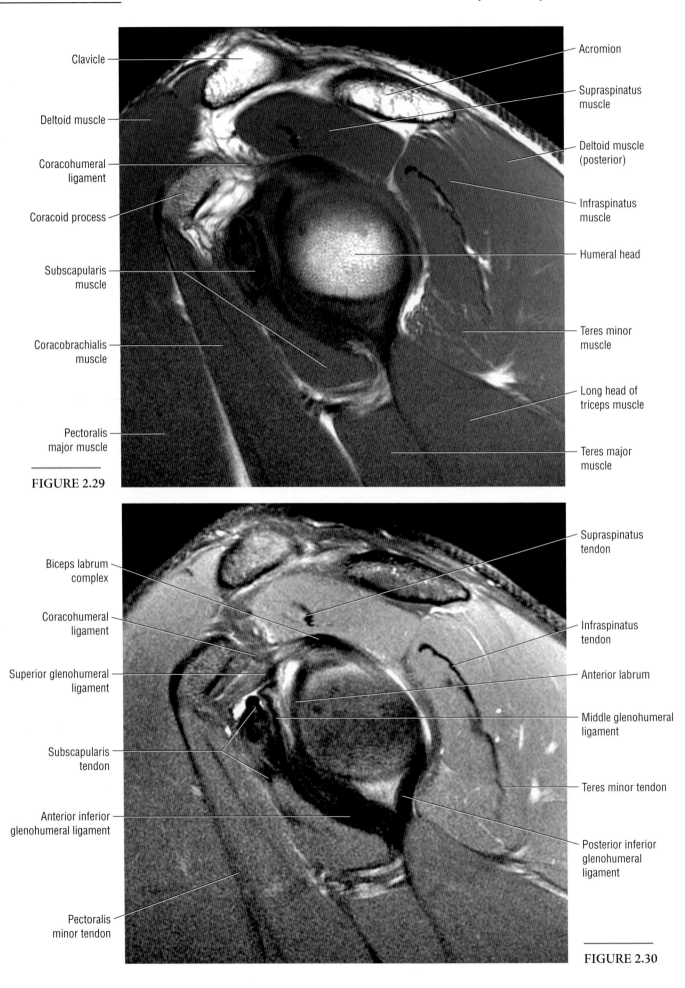

Clavicle

Deltoid muscle

Coracohumeral ligament

Coracoid process

Subscapularis muscle

Coracobrachialis muscle

Pectoralis major muscle

Acromion

Supraspinatus muscle

Deltoid muscle (posterior)

Infraspinatus muscle

Humeral head

Teres minor muscle

Long head of triceps muscle

Teres major muscle

FIGURE 2.29

Biceps labrum complex

Coracohumeral ligament

Superior glenohumeral ligament

Subscapularis tendon

Anterior inferior glenohumeral ligament

Pectoralis minor tendon

Supraspinatus tendon

Infraspinatus tendon

Anterior labrum

Middle glenohumeral ligament

Teres minor tendon

Posterior inferior glenohumeral ligament

FIGURE 2.30

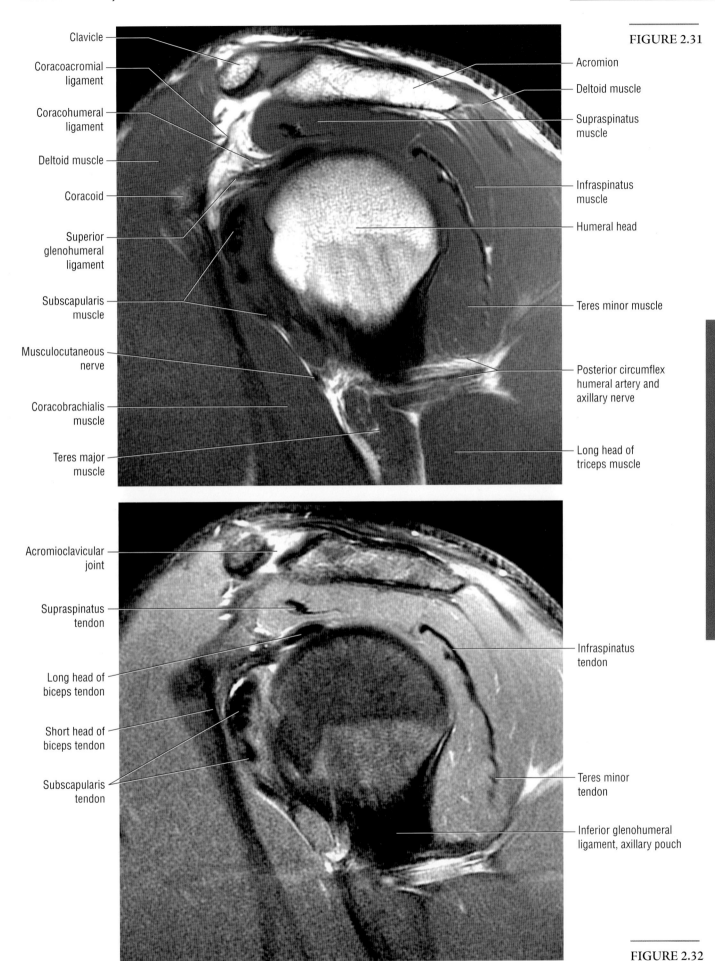

FIGURE 2.31

Clavicle

Coracoacromial ligament

Coracohumeral ligament

Deltoid muscle

Coracoid

Superior glenohumeral ligament

Subscapularis muscle

Musculocutaneous nerve

Coracobrachialis muscle

Teres major muscle

Acromion

Deltoid muscle

Supraspinatus muscle

Infraspinatus muscle

Humeral head

Teres minor muscle

Posterior circumflex humeral artery and axillary nerve

Long head of triceps muscle

Acromioclavicular joint

Supraspinatus tendon

Long head of biceps tendon

Short head of biceps tendon

Subscapularis tendon

Infraspinatus tendon

Teres minor tendon

Inferior glenohumeral ligament, axillary pouch

FIGURE 2.32

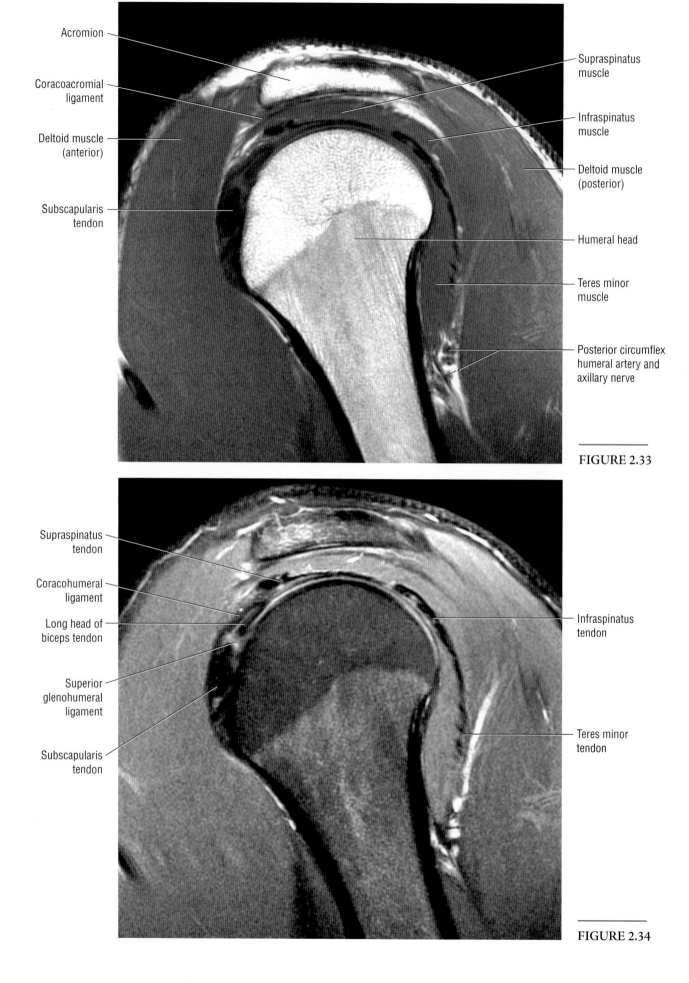

Acromion

Coracoacromial
ligament

Deltoid muscle
(anterior)

Subscapularis
tendon

Supraspinatus
muscle

Infraspinatus
muscle

Deltoid muscle
(posterior)

Humeral head

Teres minor
muscle

Posterior circumflex
humeral artery and
axillary nerve

FIGURE 2.33

Supraspinatus
tendon

Coracohumeral
ligament

Long head of
biceps tendon

Superior
glenohumeral
ligament

Subscapularis
tendon

Infraspinatus
tendon

Teres minor
tendon

FIGURE 2.34

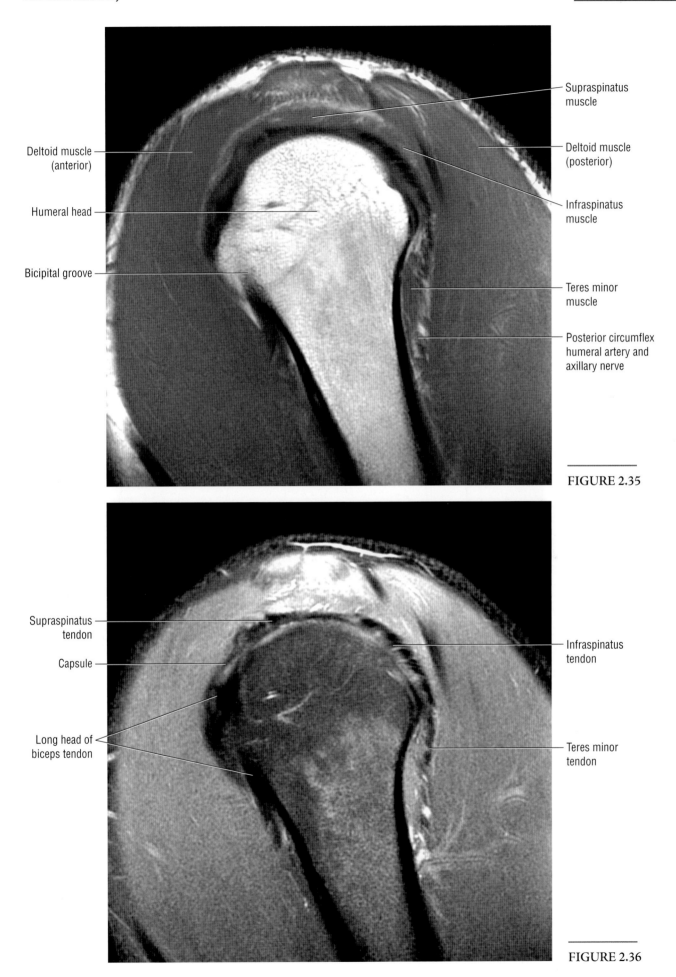

Supraspinatus muscle

Deltoid muscle (posterior)

Infraspinatus muscle

Teres minor muscle

Posterior circumflex humeral artery and axillary nerve

Deltoid muscle (anterior)

Humeral head

Bicipital groove

FIGURE 2.35

Supraspinatus tendon

Capsule

Long head of biceps tendon

Infraspinatus tendon

Teres minor tendon

FIGURE 2.36

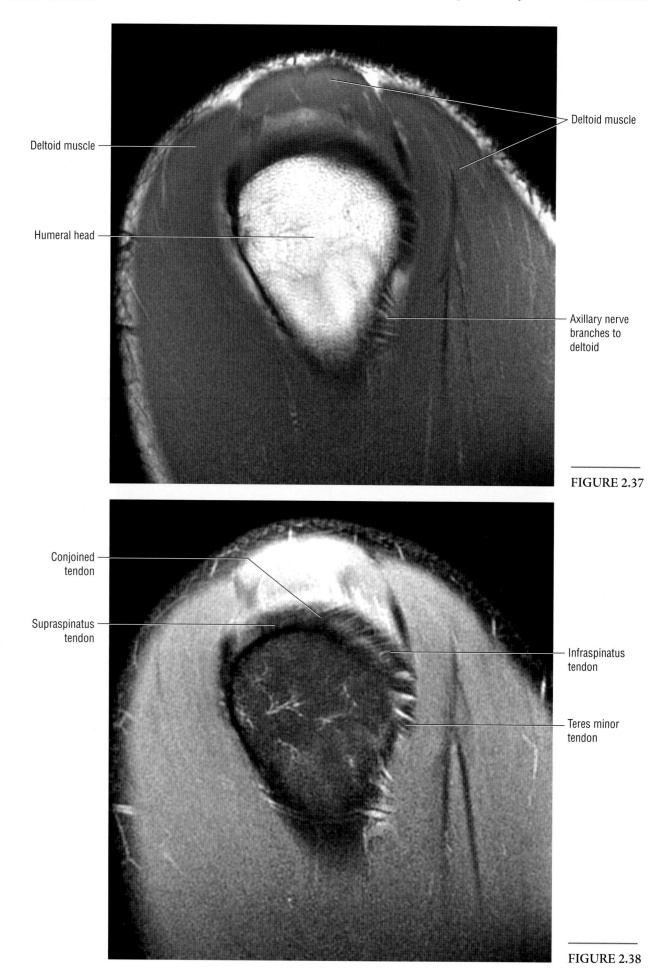

Deltoid muscle

Deltoid muscle

Deltoid muscle

Humeral head

Axillary nerve branches to deltoid

FIGURE 2.37

Conjoined tendon

Supraspinatus tendon

Infraspinatus tendon

Teres minor tendon

FIGURE 2.38

Shoulder and Related Muscles
Upper Arm Muscle Innervation

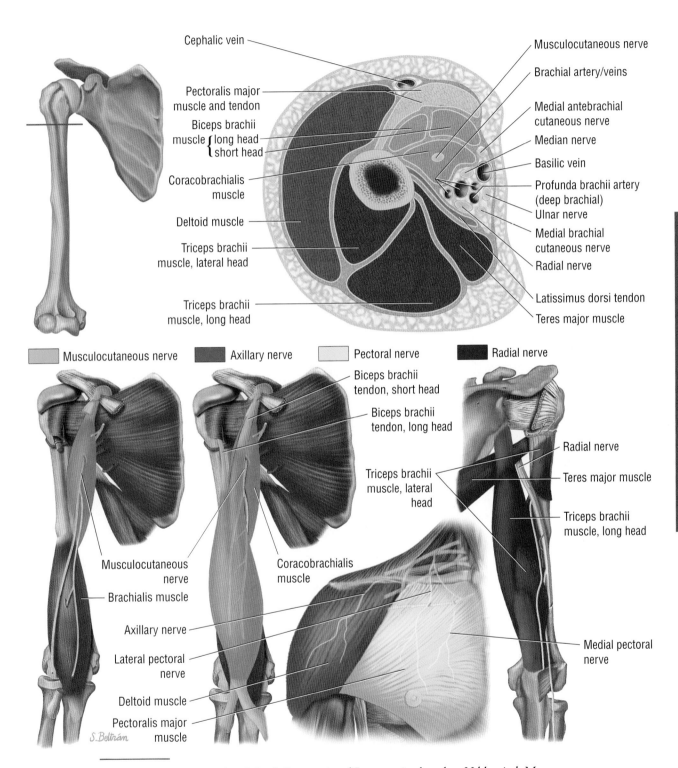

FIGURE 2.39 Upper Arm Muscle Innervation. (Cross-section based on Vahlensiech M, Genant HK, Reiter M. MRI of the Musculoskeletal System. New York/Stuttgart: Thieme, 2000.)

Mid Arm Muscle Innervation

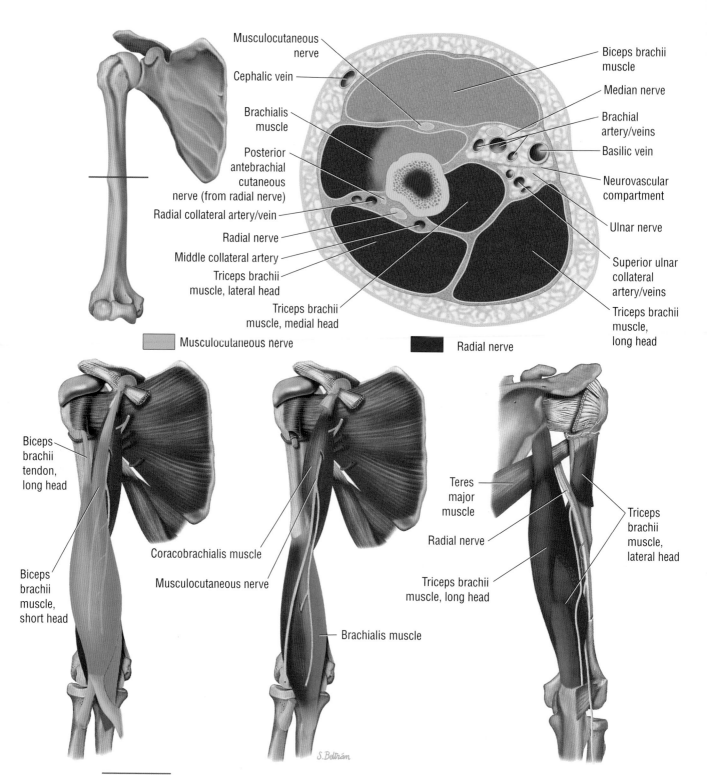

Musculocutaneous nerve

Cephalic vein

Brachialis muscle

Posterior antebrachial cutaneous nerve (from radial nerve)

Radial collateral artery/vein

Radial nerve

Middle collateral artery

Triceps brachii muscle, lateral head

Triceps brachii muscle, medial head

Biceps brachii muscle

Median nerve

Brachial artery/veins

Basilic vein

Neurovascular compartment

Ulnar nerve

Superior ulnar collateral artery/veins

Triceps brachii muscle, long head

Musculocutaneous nerve

Radial nerve

Biceps brachii tendon, long head

Biceps brachii muscle, short head

Coracobrachialis muscle

Musculocutaneous nerve

Brachialis muscle

Teres major muscle

Radial nerve

Triceps brachii muscle, long head

Triceps brachii muscle, lateral head

S.Beltrán

FIGURE 2.40 Mid-Arm Muscle Innervation. (Cross-section based on Vahlensiech M, Genant HK, Reiter M. MRI of the Musculoskeletal System. New York/Stuttgart: Thieme, 2000.)

Deltoid

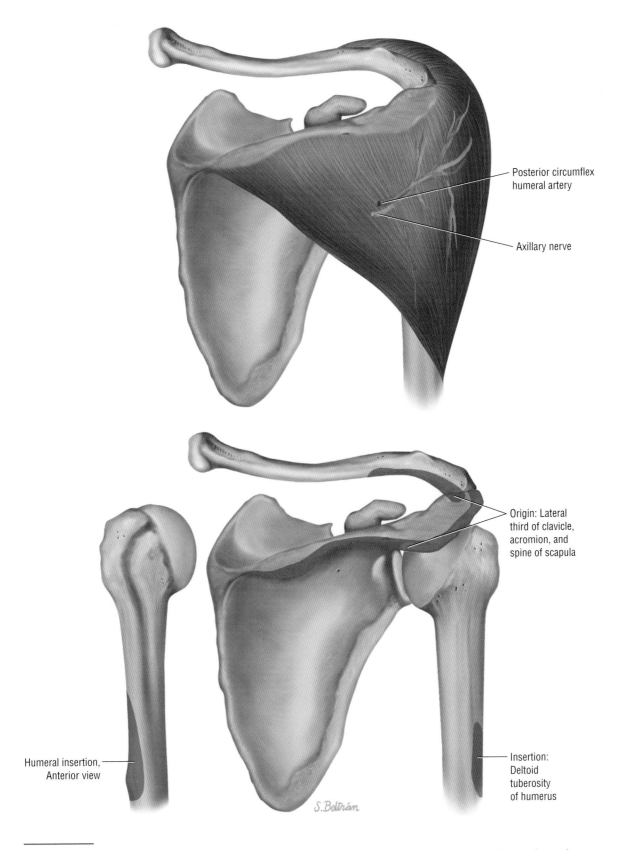

Posterior circumflex
humeral artery

Axillary nerve

Origin: Lateral
third of clavicle,
acromion, and
spine of scapula

Humeral insertion,
Anterior view

Insertion:
Deltoid
tuberosity
of humerus

S.Beltrán

FIGURE 2.41   DELTOID. The deltoid abducts the arm and represents the largest of the glenohumeral muscles.
The deltoid is multipennate, with an anterolateral raphe, and is important in any form of arm elevation. It is active
throughout the entire arc of glenohumeral abduction, even if the supraspinatus muscle is inactive.

Subscapularis

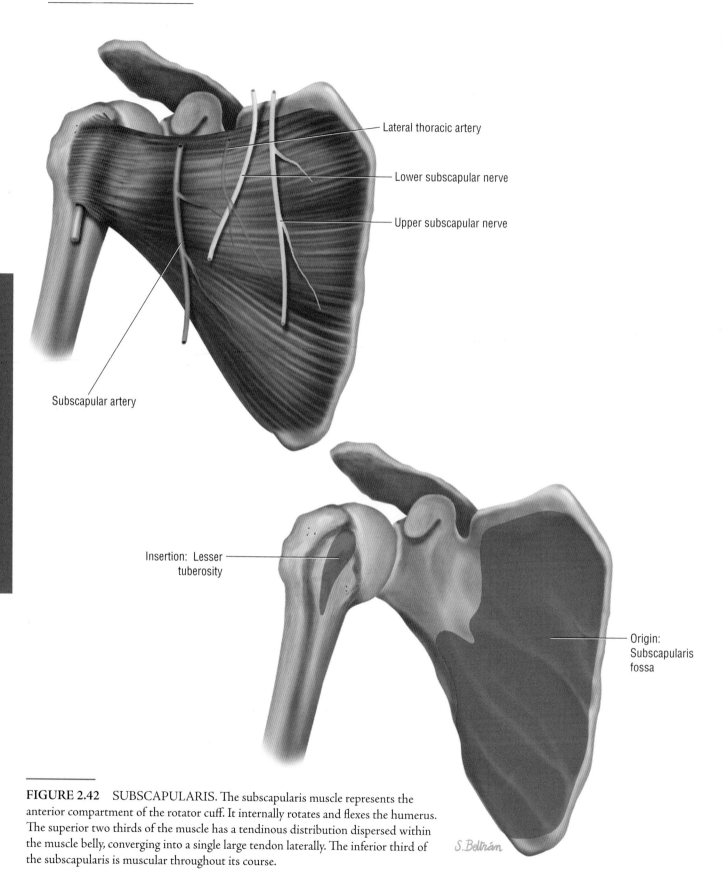

Lateral thoracic artery

Lower subscapular nerve

Upper subscapular nerve

Subscapular artery

Insertion: Lesser tuberosity

Origin: Subscapularis fossa

S.Beltrán

FIGURE 2.42 SUBSCAPULARIS. The subscapularis muscle represents the anterior compartment of the rotator cuff. It internally rotates and flexes the humerus. The superior two thirds of the muscle has a tendinous distribution dispersed within the muscle belly, converging into a single large tendon laterally. The inferior third of the subscapularis is muscular throughout its course.

Supraspinatus

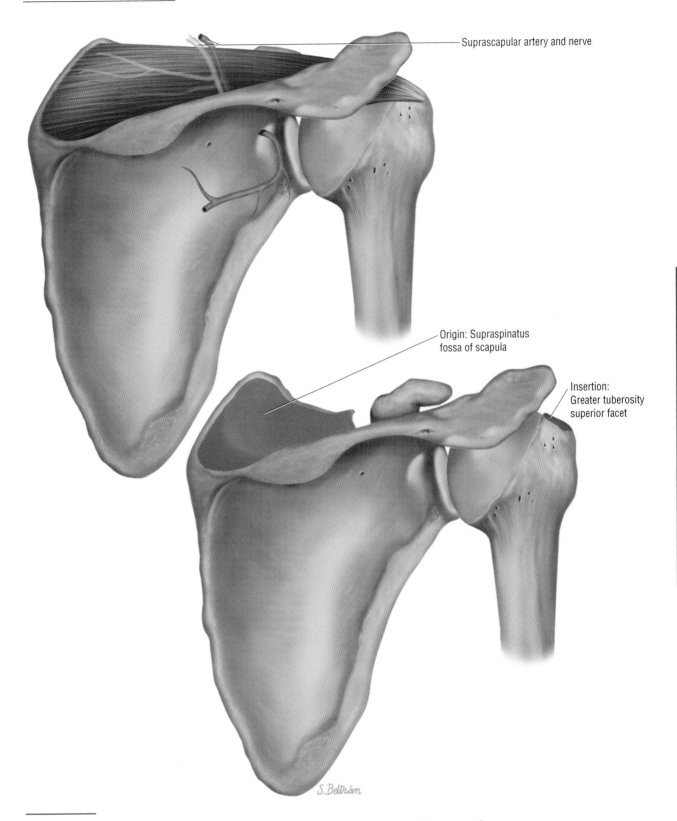

Suprascapular artery and nerve

Origin: Supraspinatus fossa of scapula

Insertion: Greater tuberosity superior facet

S. Beltrán

FIGURE 2.43 SUPRASPINATUS. The supraspinatus initiates abduction of the arm and is active during the entire arc of scapular plane abduction. The parallel independent collagen fascicles permit differential excursion of segments of the tendon. The supraspinatus exerts maximal effort at approximately 30° of abduction and functions with the rotator cuff as a humeral head depressor.

Infraspinatus

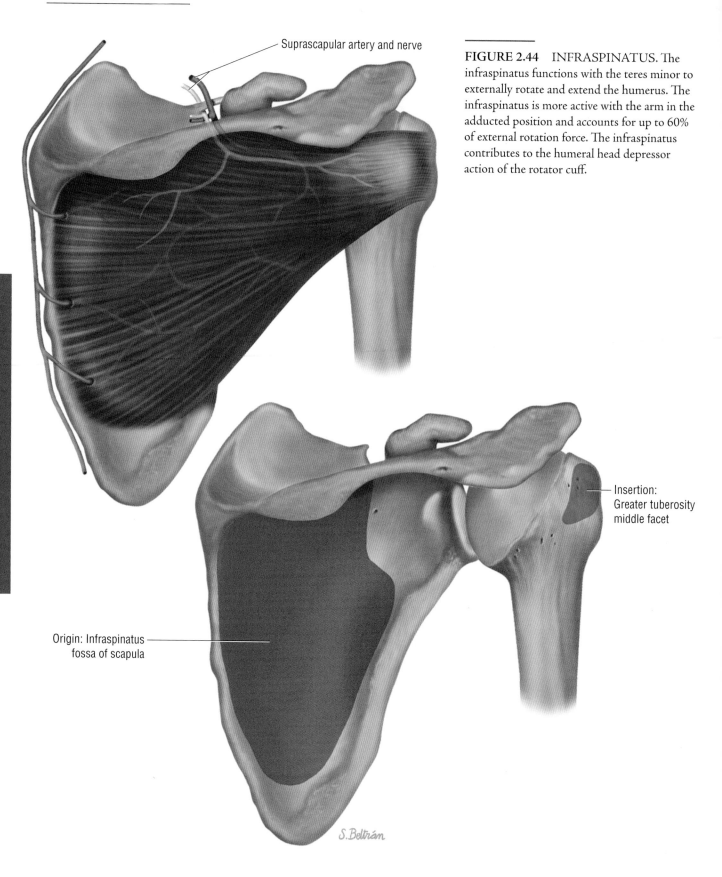

Suprascapular artery and nerve

FIGURE 2.44 INFRASPINATUS. The infraspinatus functions with the teres minor to externally rotate and extend the humerus. The infraspinatus is more active with the arm in the adducted position and accounts for up to 60% of external rotation force. The infraspinatus contributes to the humeral head depressor action of the rotator cuff.

Insertion:
Greater tuberosity
middle facet

Origin: Infraspinatus
fossa of scapula

S. Beltrán

Teres Minor

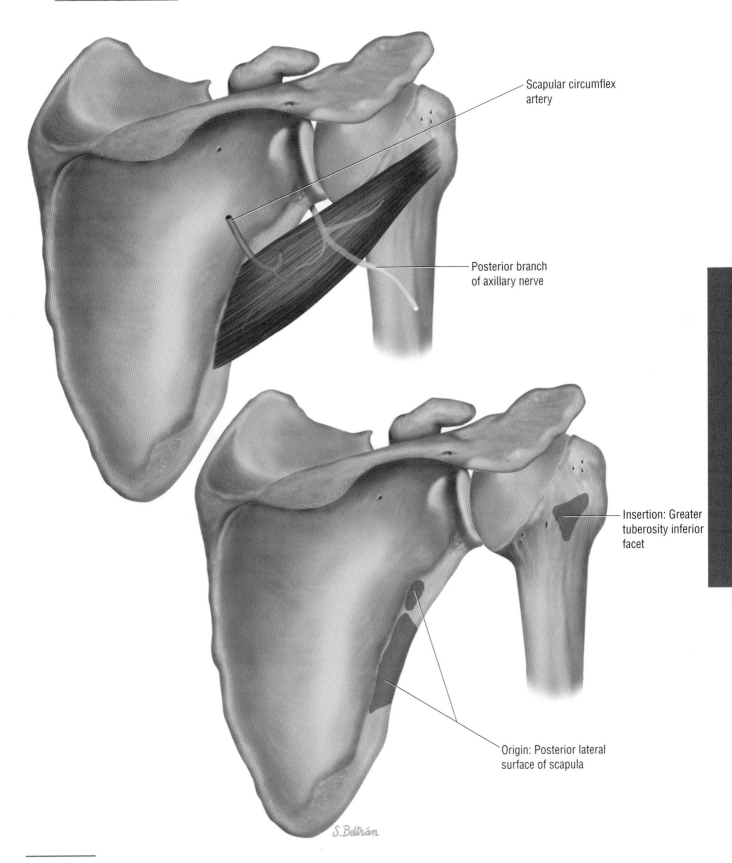

Scapular circumflex artery

Posterior branch of axillary nerve

Insertion: Greater tuberosity inferior facet

Origin: Posterior lateral surface of scapula

S.Beltrán

FIGURE 2.45 TERES MINOR. The teres minor functions with the infraspinatus to externally rotate and extend the humerus. The teres minor is active with the shoulder in 90° of elevation.

Teres Major

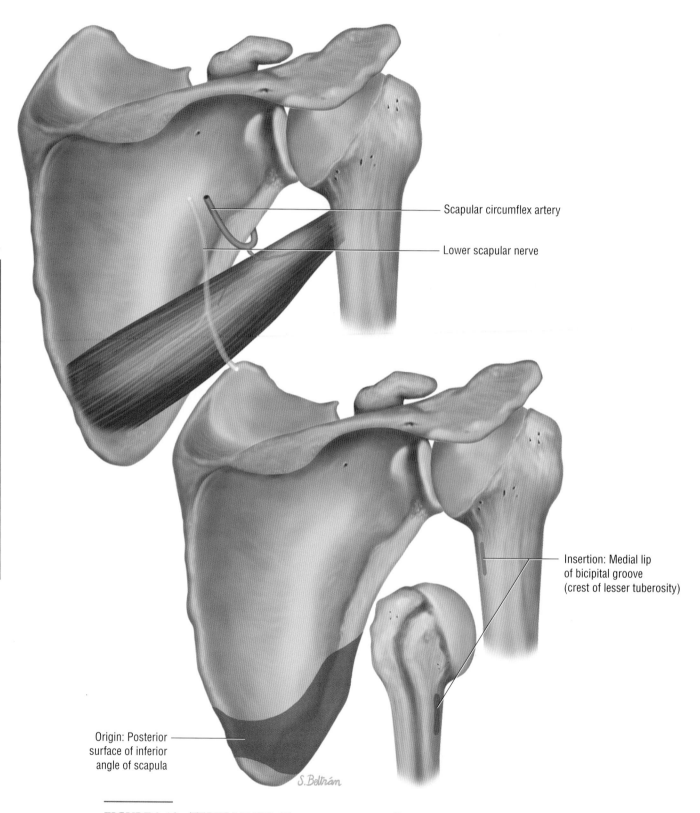

Scapular circumflex artery

Lower scapular nerve

Insertion: Medial lip
of bicipital groove
(crest of lesser tuberosity)

Origin: Posterior
surface of inferior
angle of scapula

S. Beltrán

FIGURE 2.46   TERES MAJOR. The teres major internally rotates and adducts the arm. The
axillary nerve and posterior humeral circumflex artery pass superior to the upper border of the teres
major through the quadrilateral space. The quadrilateral space is bordered also by the teres minor,
the triceps, and the humerus. The teres major functions with the latissimus dorsi muscle in humeral
extension, internal rotation, and adduction.

Coracobrachialis

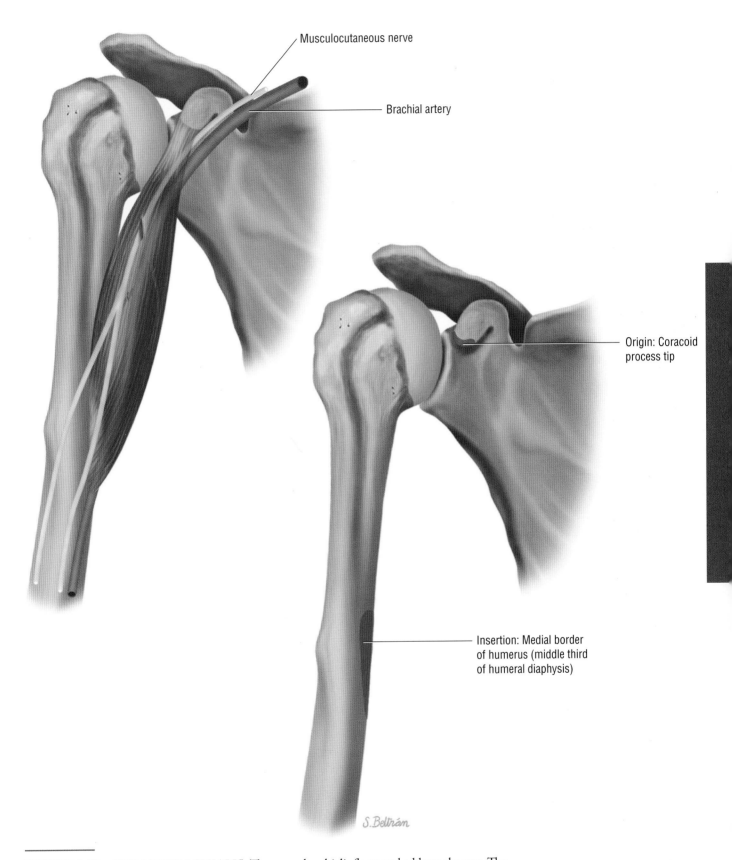

Musculocutaneous nerve

Brachial artery

Origin: Coracoid process tip

Insertion: Medial border of humerus (middle third of humeral diaphysis)

S. Beltrán

FIGURE 2.47 CORACOBRACHIALIS. The coracobrachialis flexes and adducts the arm. The coracobrachialis and the short head of the biceps have a conjoined tendon origin at the coracoid.

Biceps Brachii

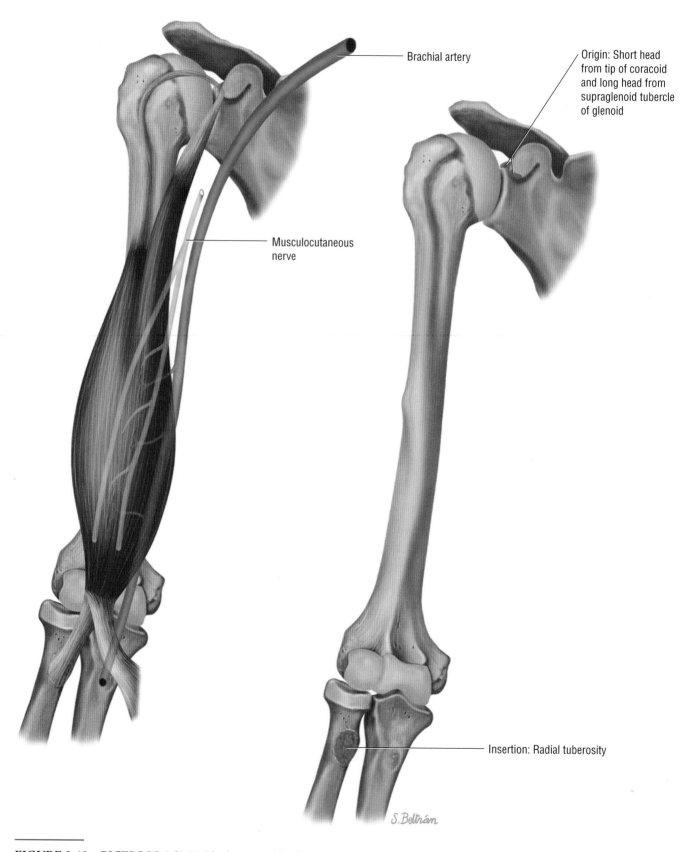

Brachial artery

Origin: Short head
from tip of coracoid
and long head from
supraglenoid tubercle
of glenoid

Musculocutaneous
nerve

Insertion: Radial tuberosity

S. Beltrán

FIGURE 2.48 BICEPS BRACHII. The biceps brachii functions to flex and supinate the forearm. The long head of the biceps tendon (LHBT) has origins at the superior pole of the glenoid and the posterosuperior labrum of the biceps labral complex. The LHBT extends within the synovial sheath of the glenohumeral joint. The long and short head muscle bellies join at the level of the deltoid insertion on the humerus.

Pectoralis Major

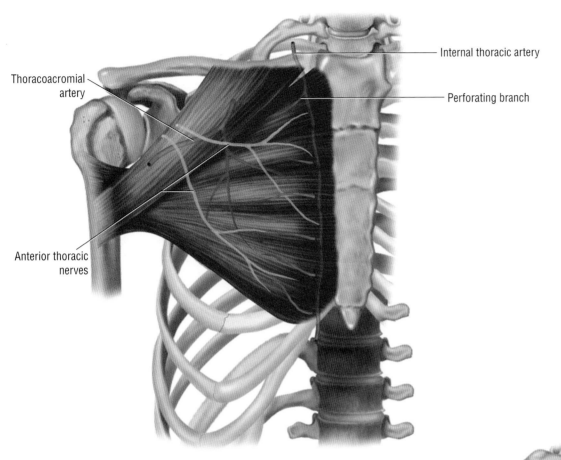

Thoracoacromial
artery

Internal thoracic artery

Perforating branch

Anterior thoracic
nerves

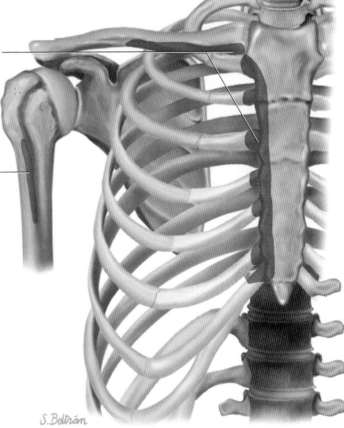

Origin: Sternal half
of clavicle and sternum
7th rib, costal cartilages
of true ribs and aponeurosis
of external oblique muscle

Insertion: Lateral lip
of bicipital groove

S. Beltrán

FIGURE 2.49   PECTORALIS MAJOR.
The pectoralis major muscle adducts the arm
and internally rotates the humerus. The pectoralis major has an upper clavicular and a lower
sternocostal head. The clavicular head contributes to the anterior lamina of the broad flat
tendon insertion to the humerus, whereas the
more distal and deep sternocostal head fibers
form the posterior lamina of the tendinous
insertion.

Pectoralis Minor

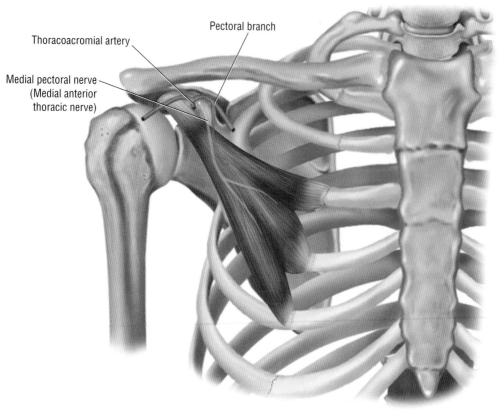

Thoracoacromial artery

Pectoral branch

Medial pectoral nerve
(Medial anterior
thoracic nerve)

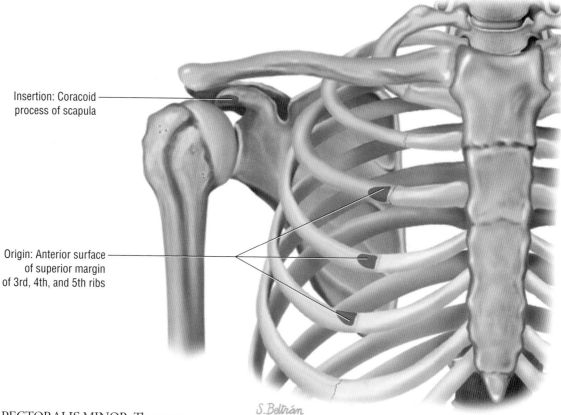

Insertion: Coracoid
process of scapula

Origin: Anterior surface
of superior margin
of 3rd, 4th, and 5th ribs

S.Beltrán

FIGURE 2.50 PECTORALIS MINOR. The pectoralis minor and major are internal rotators and flexors of the shoulder joint. The pectoralis minor helps stabilize the scapula.

Subclavius

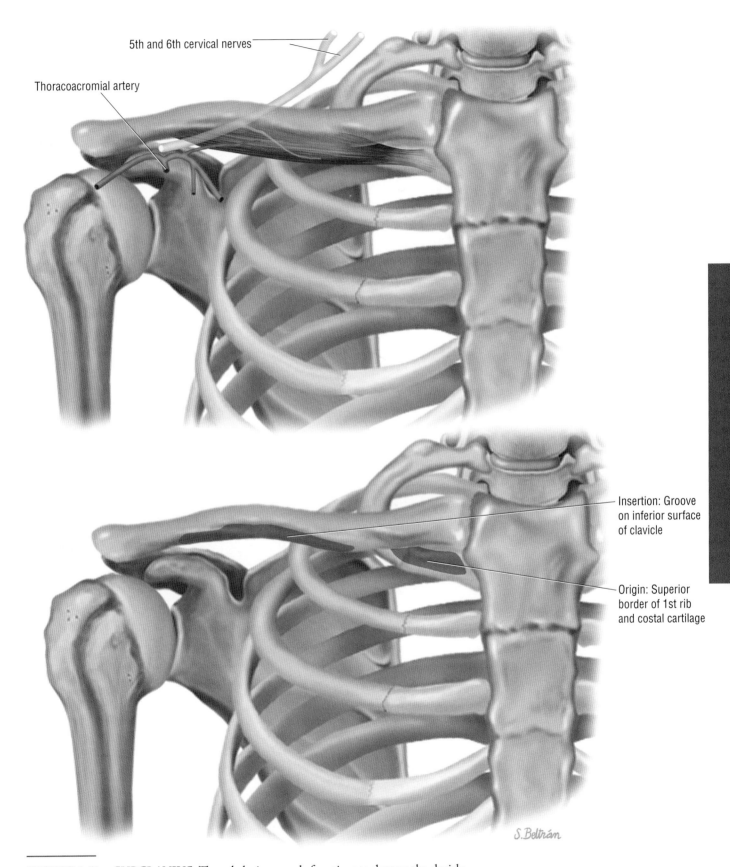

5th and 6th cervical nerves

Thoracoacromial artery

Insertion: Groove
on inferior surface
of clavicle

Origin: Superior
border of 1st rib
and costal cartilage

S. Beltrán

FIGURE 2.51   SUBCLAVIUS. The subclavius muscle functions to depress the clavicle.

Serratus Anterior

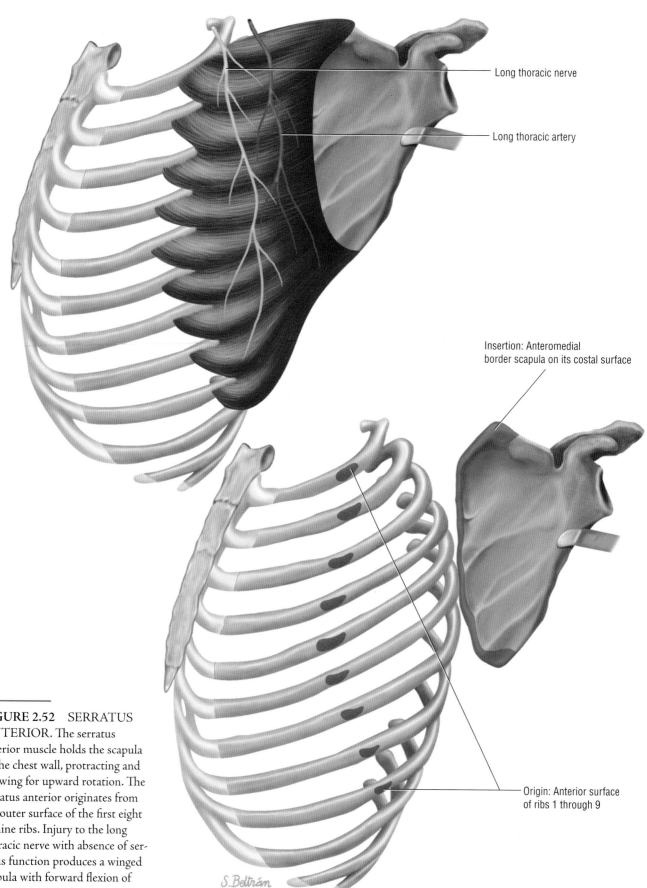

Long thoracic nerve

Long thoracic artery

Insertion: Anteromedial border scapula on its costal surface

Origin: Anterior surface of ribs 1 through 9

S. Beltrán

FIGURE 2.52 SERRATUS ANTERIOR. The serratus anterior muscle holds the scapula to the chest wall, protracting and allowing for upward rotation. The serratus anterior originates from the outer surface of the first eight or nine ribs. Injury to the long thoracic nerve with absence of serratus function produces a winged scapula with forward flexion of the arm.

Trapezius

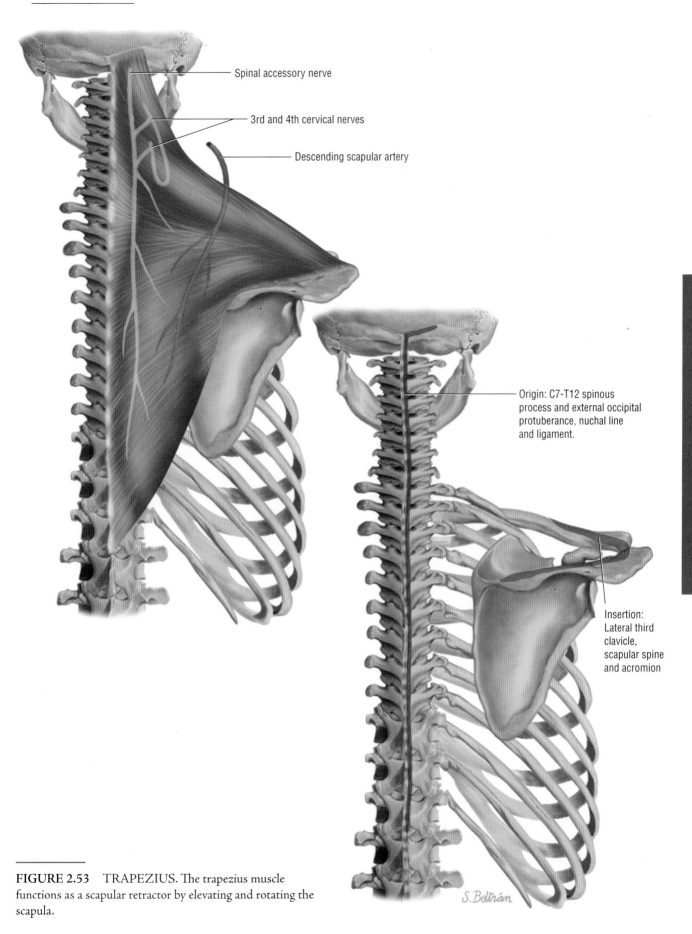

Spinal accessory nerve

3rd and 4th cervical nerves

Descending scapular artery

Origin: C7-T12 spinous process and external occipital protuberance, nuchal line and ligament.

Insertion: Lateral third clavicle, scapular spine and acromion

S. Beltrán

FIGURE 2.53 TRAPEZIUS. The trapezius muscle functions as a scapular retractor by elevating and rotating the scapula.

Latissimus Dorsi

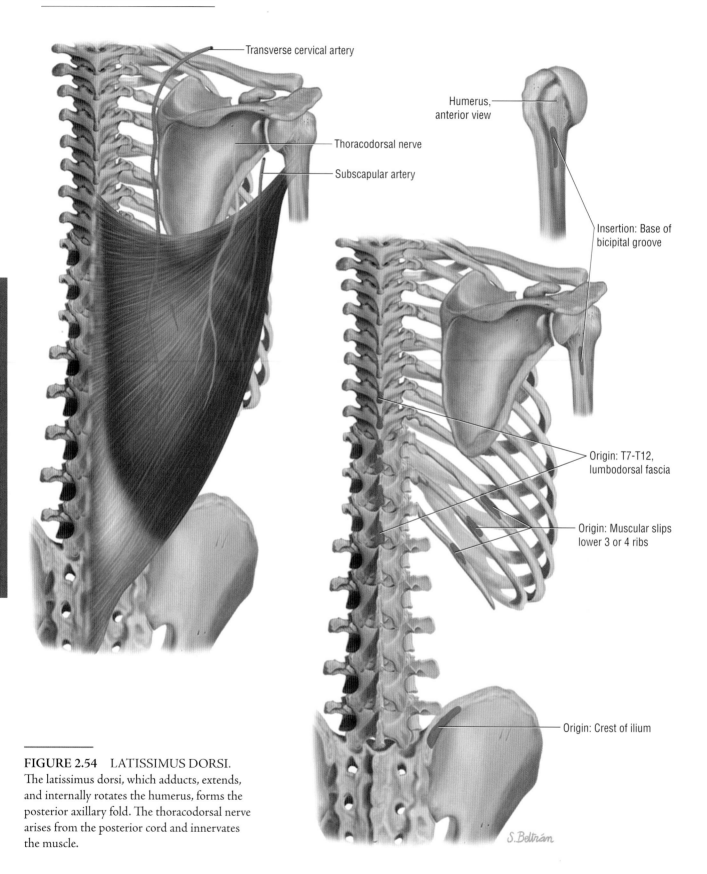

Transverse cervical artery

Humerus,
anterior view

Thoracodorsal nerve

Subscapular artery

Insertion: Base of
bicipital groove

Origin: T7-T12,
lumbodorsal fascia

Origin: Muscular slips
lower 3 or 4 ribs

Origin: Crest of ilium

S.Beltrán

FIGURE 2.54 LATISSIMUS DORSI.
The latissimus dorsi, which adducts, extends,
and internally rotates the humerus, forms the
posterior axillary fold. The thoracodorsal nerve
arises from the posterior cord and innervates
the muscle.

Rhomboid Major

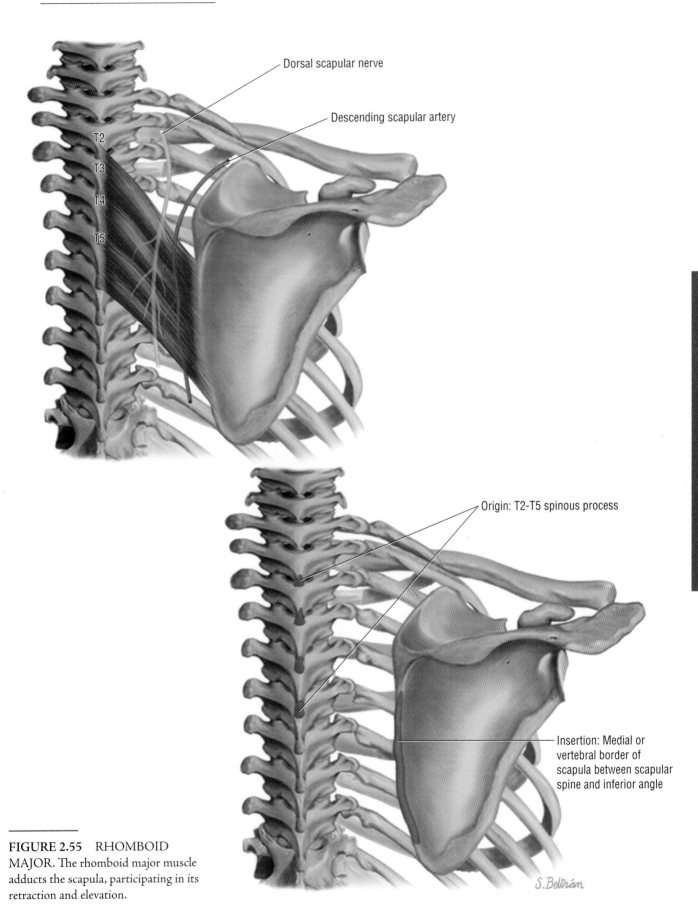

Dorsal scapular nerve

Descending scapular artery

T2
T3
T4
T5

Origin: T2-T5 spinous process

Insertion: Medial or vertebral border of scapula between scapular spine and inferior angle

S.Beltrán

FIGURE 2.55 RHOMBOID MAJOR. The rhomboid major muscle adducts the scapula, participating in its retraction and elevation.

Rhomboid Minor

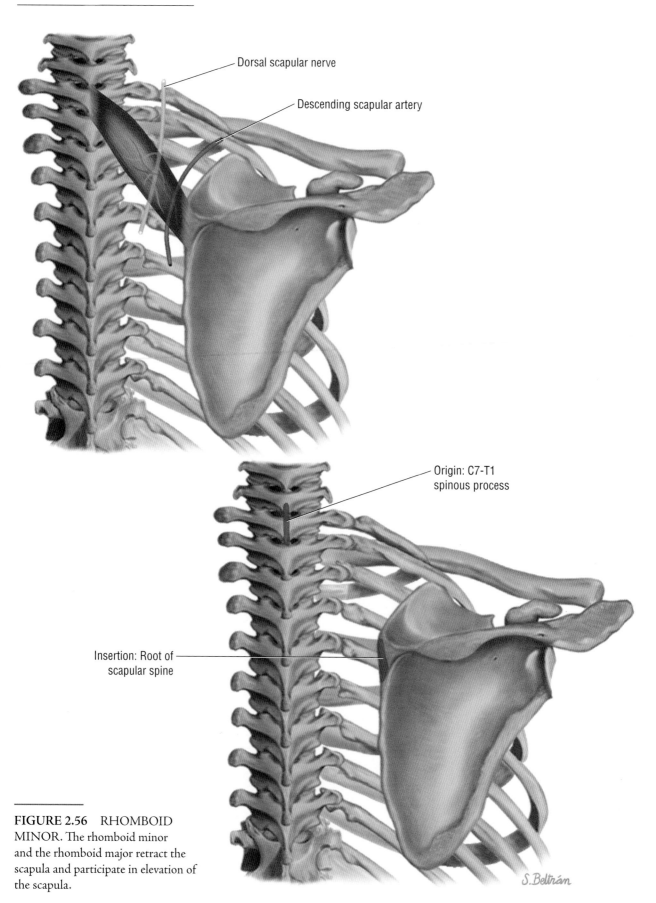

Dorsal scapular nerve

Descending scapular artery

Origin: C7-T1
spinous process

Insertion: Root of
scapular spine

S. Beltrán

FIGURE 2.56　RHOMBOID
MINOR. The rhomboid minor
and the rhomboid major retract the
scapula and participate in elevation of
the scapula.

Levator Scapulae

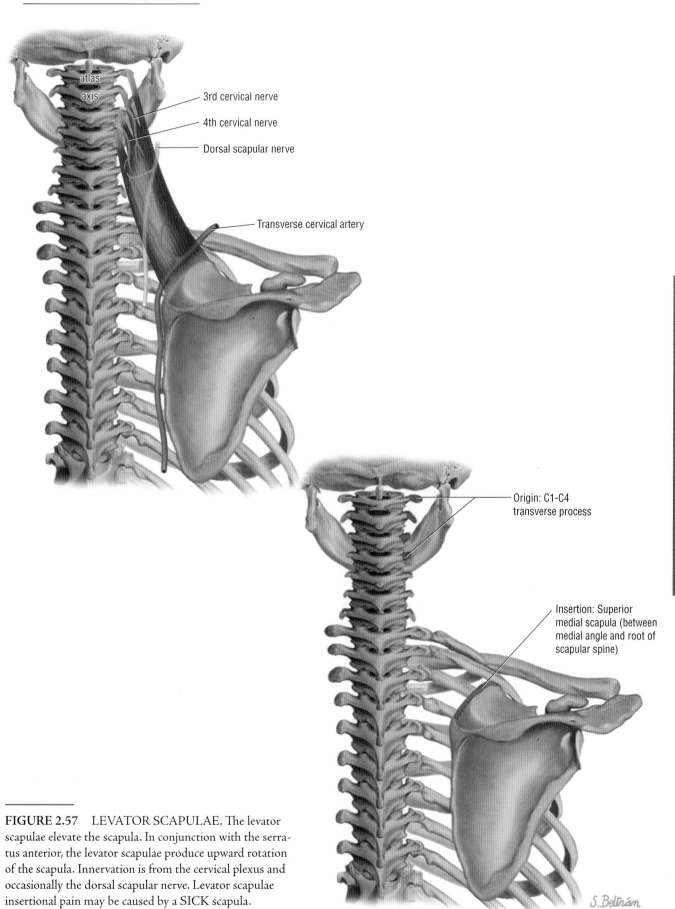

atlas
axis

3rd cervical nerve

4th cervical nerve

Dorsal scapular nerve

Transverse cervical artery

Origin: C1-C4
transverse process

Insertion: Superior
medial scapula (between
medial angle and root of
scapular spine)

FIGURE 2.57 LEVATOR SCAPULAE. The levator scapulae elevate the scapula. In conjunction with the serratus anterior, the levator scapulae produce upward rotation of the scapula. Innervation is from the cervical plexus and occasionally the dorsal scapular nerve. Levator scapulae insertional pain may be caused by a SICK scapula.

S. Beltrán

3
Stoller's Shoulder Checklist and Protocols

Stoller's Shoulder Checklist

Coronal

AC Joint (degenerative change)

Rotator Cuff (to include leading edge)

Biceps Labral Complex (SLAP diagnosis)

Humeral Head Articular Cartilage

IGLLC (inferior labrum and IGHL signal)

Axial

Anterior Labrum (below equator)

Anterior labrum and anterior band
    variations (above equator)

Posterior Labrum

Subscapularis/Biceps Tendon

Superior axial image to evaluate for
    os acromiale and AC joint

Humeral head position relative to
    glenoid fossa for centralization

Sagittal

Rotator Cuff

Acromion (slope, morphology and AC joint)

Glenoid Fossa (adaptive sclerosis vs OA)

Pulley Mechanism (mid-rotator cuff interval)

Secondary visualization of upper one-third
    of the subscapularis (bands + main tendon)

Assessment of mid-interval and
    subscapularis recess for synovitis

CORONAL

Acromioclavicular Joint and Humeral Head

AC Joint

+ Spectrum of AC joint arthrosis
  (mild, moderate, and severe)
     - Hypertrophy
     - Edema
     - Osteophytes
     - Loss of articular cartilage
+ AC joint capsule in AC joint dislocation

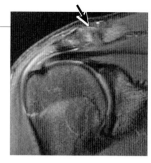

AC Joint

Os Acromiale

+ Synchondrosis
     - Edema
     - Fluid
     - Diastasis
+ May be mistaken for the AC joint
+ Always confirm on axial image

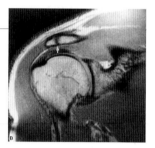

Asymptomatic os acromiale
(*arrow*) without associated
marrow changes on T1-weighted
coronal (oblique) image.

Mild, Moderate, and Severe AC Joint Arthrosis

+ Articular cartilage loss
+ AC hypetrophy
+ Cystic change across AC joint
+ Osteophytes with inferior spurring
+ Hypertrophy of AC joint

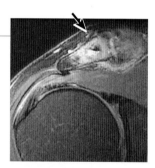

Severe AC Joint Arthrosis

Humeral Head

+ Articular cartilage loss
+ Subchondral sclerosis
     - Hypointense signal

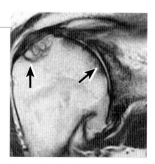

Severe Cartilage Loss,
Degenerative Arthrosis

CORONAL

Rotator Cuff

Anterior Coronal: Supraspinatus

+ Evaluate for the anterior leading edge of the
  supraspinatus tendon.

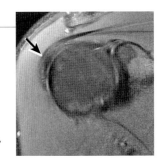

Anterior Leading Edge,
Supraspinatus Tendon

Mid Coronal: Supraspinatus

+ Assess the supraspinatus and conjoined cuff.
+ Evaluate tendon morphology and tendon signal intensity.

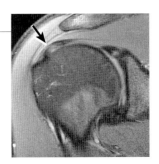

Mid Supraspinatus
Tendon

Posterior Coronal: Infraspinatus

+ The most posterior footprint of the infraspinatus is
  established to identify an isolated infraspinatus
  tendon tear.

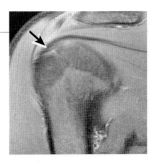

Infraspinatus Tendon

Tendinosis and Rotator Cuff Tear

+ Spectrum of cuff pathology

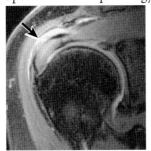
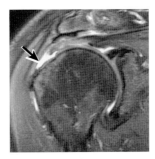
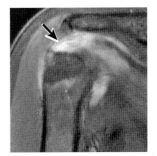

Supraspinatus Tendinosis   Full Thickness Tear, Supraspinatus   Full Thickness Tear, Infraspinatus

CORONAL

Biceps Labral Complex

12 o'clock

+ Superior labrum is isosceles in morphology in the 12 o'clock position.
+ A sulcus is present in a type 2 and 3 biceps labral complex.

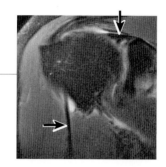

Biceps-Labral Complex and
Distal Bicipital Groove

Biceps Tendon in Bicipital Groove

+ Inferior to the rotator cuff footprint, the biceps is contained within the bicipital groove on corresponding axial images.
+ Medial dislocation in the axial plane

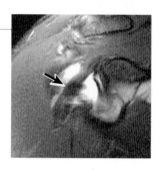

Medial Subluxation Biceps

Biceps Tendon Tear

+ Continuity of the biceps is evaluated on anterior coronal, axial, and sagittal images from the mid interval through its extraarticular course.

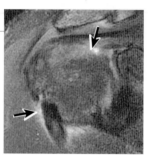

Torn Biceps with
Empty Rotator Interval

Normal Superior Labrum

+ Always evaluate the superior labrum in the 12 o'clock and peel-back locations.
+ Assessment of anterior superior labrum in the coronal plane should be made after the 12 o'clock position is evaluated to avoid false-positive interpretation.

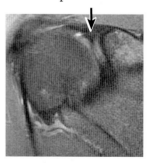

Normal Anterior Superior
Labrum

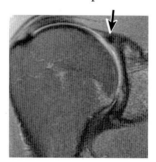

Normal Superior Labrum

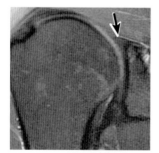

Normal Posterior Superior Labrum

Superior Labral Tear

+ Signal in labrum
+ Detachment of superior labrum from biceps
+ Inferior displacement of torn superior labrum
+ Fragmentation of superior labrum
+ Enlarged sulcus >5mm

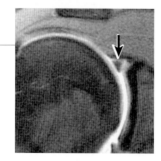

Superior Labral Tear

CORONAL

Inferior Glenohumeral Ligament (IGHL or IGL)

Anterior IGHL

+ Establish anatomic neck attachment (laterally) and inferior pole attachment (medially).

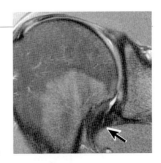

Anterior IGHL

Mid IGHL

+ Location of midcapsular tears

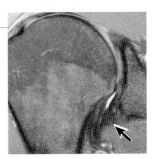

Mid IGHL

Posterior IGHL

+ RHAGL (Posterior neck and capsule)
+ Posterior labrum (medially)

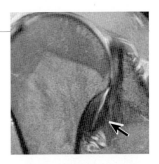

Posterior IGHL

Tear from Glenoid (GAGL) or Anatomic Neck of the Humerus (RHAGL)

+ Bankart lesion is more common than the GAGL.
+ IGL tears occur at the humerus, midcapsule, or inferior pole of the glenoid.

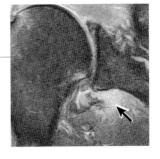

IGHL Tear from Glenoid (GAGL)

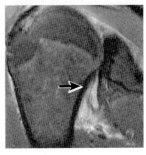

IGHL Tear from Humerus (HAGL)

Adhesive Capsulitis

+ Hyperintense ligament often associated with synovitis in the axillary pouch, mid interval, and subscapularis recess
+ Adhesive capsulitis findings need to be stated in impression and body of dictation.

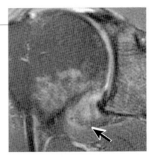

Adhesive Capsulitis

AXIAL

Acromioclavicular Joint and Labrum

Assess for asymmetric AC edema and presence of an os acromiale

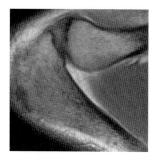

Normal AC Joint

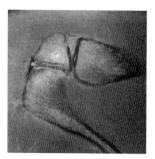

Os Acromiale

Labrum from BLC to anterior inferior and posterior labrum

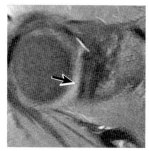

Superior Labrum

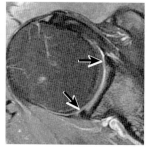

Mid Labrum

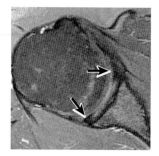

Mid Inferior Labrum

Instability Lesions

• Anterior inferior labrum (Bankart) and posterior labrum

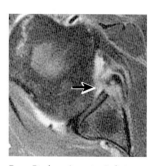

Bony Bankart Anterior Inferior
Glenoid Labrum

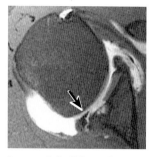

Posterior Labral Tear with
Posterior Chondral Defect

AXIAL

Biceps Tendon/Subscapularis

Superior Axial Identify Biceps Tendon and Subscapularis Tendon

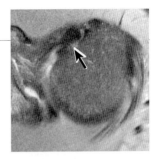

+ Partial tear superior distal subscapularis tendon

Superior Distal
Subscapularis Tendon,
Proximal Biceps

Mid Axial Biceps Tendon in Groove and Subscapularis Tendon Footprint

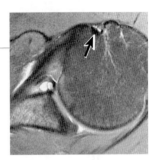

+ Document extraarticular biceps in groove.

Mid to Distal
Subscapularis, Biceps
in Bicipital Groove

Medial Subluxation Biceps and Subscapularis Tendon Tear

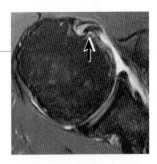

+ Biceps is perched or medial to the lesser tuberosity.
+ Biceps pulley is torn.
+ Biceps tendon changes morphology.
    Flattened

Medial Subluxation
Biceps, Complete
Subscapularis Tendon
Tear

Subscapularis Interstitial Tear

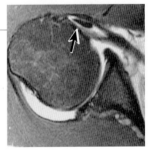

+ Associated with articular surface or deep
  margin articular sided tear and
  biceps pulley rupture

Medial Subluxation
Biceps into Interstitial
Tear Subscapularis

SAGITTAL

Rotator Cuff

Muscle Bellies

+ Supraspinatus, infraspinatus, and teres minor posteriorly, subscapularis anteriorly

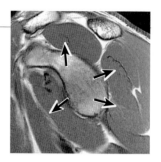

Rotator Cuff Muscle Bellies

Muscle Tendons

+ Convergence of rotator cuff tendons peripherally

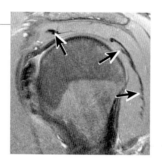

Myotendinous Junctions

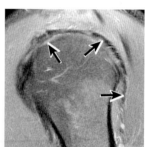

Rotator Cuff Tendons

Muscle Atrophy

+ Atrophy visualized on T1/PD weighted images while denervation is seen on fluid sensitive images

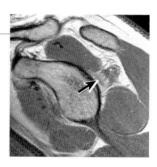

Severe Infraspinatus Atrophy

Supraspinatus Tear

+ Anterior to posterior measurements of tear in the sagittal plane and always follow torn tendon medially to its primary contributing muscle (supraspinatus vs infraspinatus)

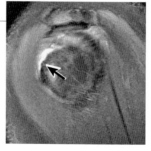

Supraspinatus Tear

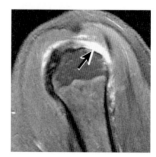

Infraspinatus Tear

SAGITTAL

Acromion

Medial Sagittal AC Joint

• Os acromiale vs AC joint

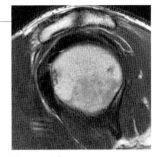

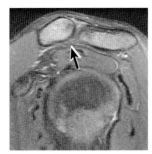

Os acromiale

Normal AC Joint (medial)

Mid Sagittal AC Joint

• Coracohumeral ligament attachment

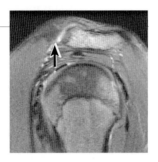

Normal AC Joint
(lateral)

Lateral to AC Joint

• Acromial morphology assessed
  lateral to AC joint

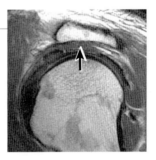

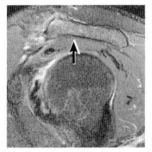

Type 2 Acromion

Type 3 Acromion

Arthrosis

• Spectrum of arthrosis and outlet narrowing
        Supraspinatus outlet

Severe AC Joint
Arthrosis with Inferior
Spurring

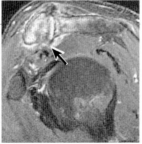

Enthesophyte/Type 3 acromion

• Which corresponds to the location of the
  anterior inferior keel osteophyte

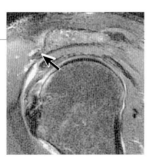

Anterior Acromial Spur

SAGITTAL

Glenoid Fossa

Normal Glenoid Fossa

+ Absence of spurring or sclerosis

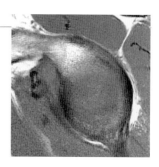

Normal Glenoid Fossa

Bony Bankart

+ Anterior inferior quadrant fracture or compression defect in osseous (bony) Bankart
+ Soft tissue Bankart assessment with intact anterior inferior glenoid rim

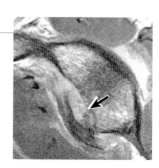

Bony Bankart

Posterior glenoid rim wear (sclerosis), remodeling or rim fracture + posterior labral tear

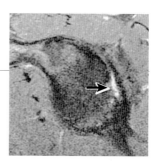

Posterior Labral Tear
and Rim Defect

Glenoid Deficiency

+ Osseous Bankart with >25% bone loss

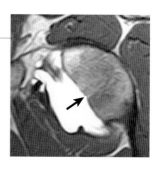

Inverted Pear
Morphology
Secondary to
Osseous Bankart

SAGITTAL

Biceps Pulley Mechanism

Normal Biceps Labral Complex

• Intraarticular biceps contributes significantly to the posterior labrum.

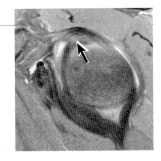

Biceps Labral Complex
at 12 o'clock

Biceps Tendinosis

• Evaluate biceps at and distal to mid-interval.

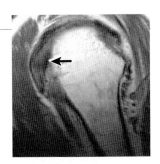

Severe Biceps Tendinosis
in Proximal Bicipital
Groove

Normal CHL and SGL

• Evaluate biceps pulley at mid-interval between supraspinatus and subscapularis.

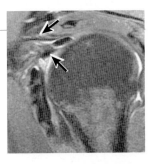

Normal CHL and SGL

Synovitis

• Typical location for synovitis at mid-interval with thickened CHL and SGL components of the biceps pulley

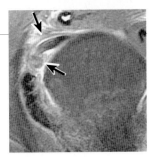

Adhesive Capsulitis
CHL and SGL

Tear of CHL and SGL

• Biceps instability with inferior displacement of the biceps in the sagittal plane (The corresponding axial images demonstrate medial dislocation of the bicep.)

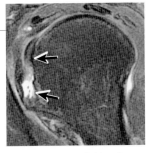

Biceps Tendinosis, Subluxed into
Subscapularis Tear

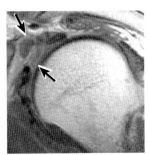

Tear CHL and SGL

Stoller's Shoulder Protocols

Protocols

- Position arm in partial external rotation.

- Coronal oblique images are performed parallel to the course of the supraspinatus tendon.

- FS PD FSE coronal oblique images are sensitive to rotator cuff degeneration and fluid signal, and T2 FSE coronal images are useful to distinguish between cuff tendinosis and tear.

- Axial FS PD FSE images are sensitive for the detection of small paralabral cysts as markers for labral tears.

- Rotator cuff tears should be measured in the coronal (medial to lateral) and sagittal (anterior to posterior) planes.

- The glenoid fossa is evaluated in the sagittal plane for patterns of glenoid rim osteophytes and glenoid fossa sclerosis associated with instability and osteoarthritis.

- ABER (abduction external rotation) positioning in conjunction with MR arthrography is helpful in evaluating the postoperative labrum and nondisplaced (e.g., Perthes) labral tears.

  - Improved visualization of articular surface and footprint of the supraspinatus and infraspinatus

- T2* weighted coronal oblique images are not used to evaluate the rotator cuff since areas of increased signal intensity may be seen in both cuff degeneration and tear, making the distinction between tendinopathy or tendinosis and rotator cuff tear difficult.

Protocols (continued)

■ T2* weighted axial images are, however, used to evaluate the glenohumeral capsule and labrum. Intralabral signal and sharpness of labral boundaries are optimized on GRE images. Postoperative susceptibility, subscapularis tendinosis, and the identification of calcific tendinitis is improved. The trabecular bone pattern of the proximal humerus is optimized on GRE images for improved assessment of bone architecture in cases of infection, fracture, tumor, or marrow replacement.

■ 3T MR imaging affords an increase in signal-to-noise ratio (SNR) as long as the proper coil is utilized and protocols are modified to reduce chemical shift, blurring, and adjusted to compensate for 3T sensitivity to motion and breathing.

■ Flexible phased array coils must be properly positioned to provide for proper SNR of deep structures including the anterior and posterior labrum.

■ Parallel imaging techniques reduce the number of phase encoding steps to speed up image acquisition time. T2 images have more than adequate SNR as these speed up techniques will diminish SNR in 3T imaging.

■ Techniques like PROPELLER to speed up imaging may be associated with blurring of articular cartilage and require precise protocol modifications to minimize these effects.

■ High resolution in the shoulder is needed to diagnose SLAP lesions, assessing humeral head articular cartilage loss, and accurately evaluating the integrity of the anterior inferior glenoid labrum. The glenohumeral joint chondral surfaces require high-resolution techniques as routinely utilized in the coronal and axial plane.

■ Flexible contrast techniques in the shoulder require the use of PD, FS PD FSE, and T2 FSE pulse sequences. T1-weighted images may be useful when replacement of fat needs to be appreciated as in infection, metastatic disease, primary tumors, marrow replacement disorders, or subchondral signal changes as seen in adaptive or degenerative sclerosis. PD or intermediate weighted images are sensitive to tendon degeneration. T2 FSE images (without fat suppression) are used in the coronal and sagittal planes and in conjunction with an even more fluid sensitive sequence (FS PD FSE).

■ Uniform fat suppression is required for accurate detection of tendinosis, edema, fluid, paralabral cysts, and muscle denervation.

MR Arthrography

■ Joint distension is used to outline intraarticular structures such as the labrum and glenohumeral ligaments.

■ Since capsular distension is the goal of arthrography, saline may be used in place of an MR contrast agent.

■ Improved detection of rotator cuff tears, including partial articular sided tears

■ Demonstration of communication between the joint and extraarticular abnormalities (e.g., paralabral cysts, bursae, and other fluid-containing masses or potential spaces)

Techniques of MR Arthrography

■ MR arthrography with intraarticular contrast is performed using either a paramagnetic contrast agent saline to facilitate capsular distension and to improve the contrast between fluid and the rotator cuff and glenohumeral joint capsule.

■ Preinjection or postinjection PD, FS PD FSE, and T2-weighted FSE coronal oblique images plus FS PD FSE axial images are performed to identify pathology that may not be appreciated on post-contrast FS T1-weighted images, including:

   ■ A bursal surface tear or intrasubstance degenerative cuff changes

   ■ A paralabral cyst that does not directly communicate with the joint (on T2* axial images) and may not be appreciated on post-intraarticular paramagnetic contrast injection FS T1-weighted images

   ■ Preexisting fluid secondary to an effusion or hemorrhage

Pectoralis Major Muscle

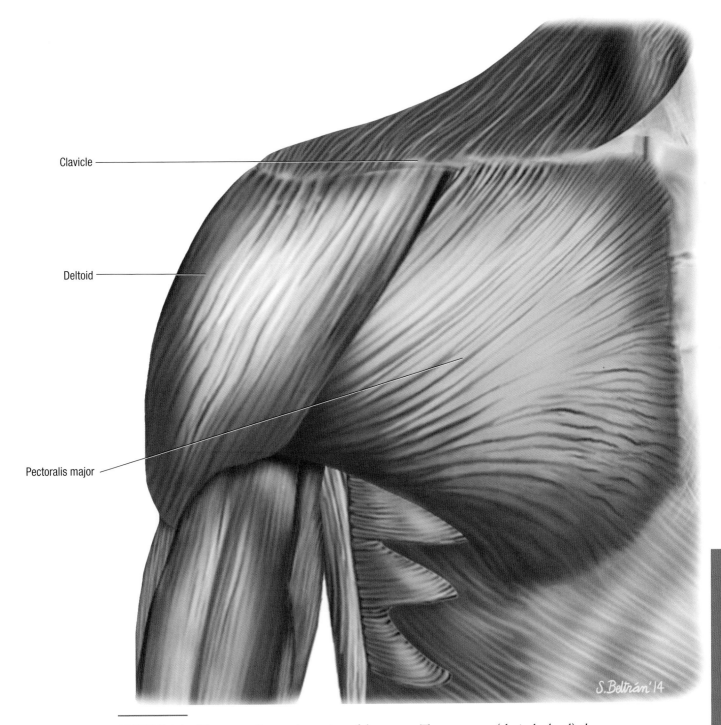

Clavicle

Deltoid

Pectoralis major

S.Beltrán'14

FIGURE 3.1   The pectoralis muscle consists of three parts. The upper part (clavicular head), the middle part (sternal), and the inferior part (distal sternal origin). The inferior fibers rotate 180° to insert higher on the humerus. Both the pectoralis major and the latissimus dorsi provide for glenohumeral stability.

Deltoid Muscle

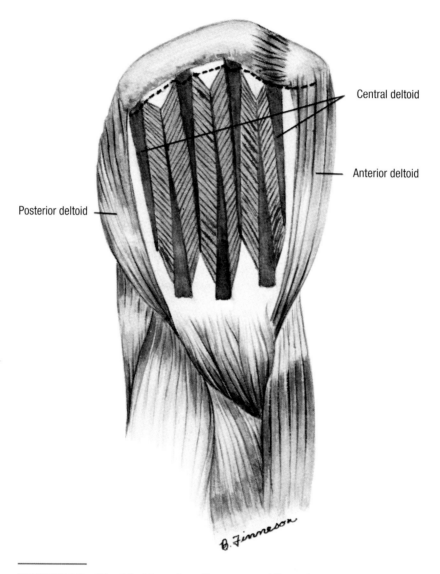

FIGURE 3.2   The deltoid consists of anterior, middle, and posterior deltoid muscle fibers. The deltoid is an anterior stabilizer of the shoulder with the arm positioned in abduction and external rotation. (Modified from DePalma AF. *Surgery of the Shoulder*. 3rd ed. Philadelphia, PA: JB Lippincott; 1983.)

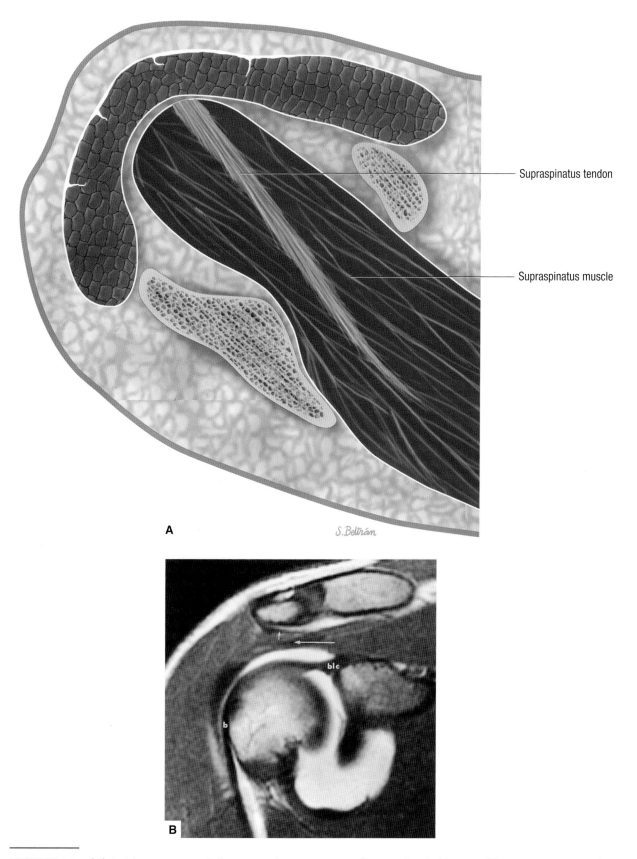

Supraspinatus tendon

Supraspinatus muscle

A

S. Beltrán

B

FIGURE 3.3 (**A**) Axial cross-sectional illustration showing a steeper (greater slope) obliquity of the supraspinatus tendon relative to the supraspinatus muscle. Coronal oblique MR images are correctly prescribed using image locations parallel to the supraspinatus tendon. Images improperly obtained parallel to the supraspinatus muscle and not the tendon will fore-shorten the supraspinatus tendon in the coronal plane and lead to a potential misdiagnosis of a rotator cuff tear. (**B**) A T1-weighted coronal oblique MR arthrogram shows the continuity between the supraspinatus muscle and tendon (*long white arrow*), biceps labral complex (BLC), biceps tendon (b), and coracoacromial ligament (*small white arrow*).

Rotator Cuff

■ MR arthrographic evaluation of the rotator cuff outlines the surfaces of the rotator cuff, with imbibition of contrast indicating surface fraying or tendinosis.

■ Contrast also insinuates into partial tears from the articular surface side. T2-weighted or FS PD-weighted images are needed for bursal surface evaluation since the bursal surface is not outlined by intraarticular contrast.

Labrum

■ MR arthrography outlines the anatomy of the glenoid labrum, identifies partial articular or full thickness tears of the rotator cuff, and demonstrates glenohumeral capsular ligaments not adequately appreciated in the nondistended joint capsule.

■ Capsular distension can "pull" on the labral attachment, revealing detachment.

■ Healing changes or fibrosis may prevent this pulling away and therefore prevent visualization of lesions, and for this application, the ABER technique may be helpful.

■ Intermediate signal intensity granulation tissue at chondrolabral interfaces or underlying bone reactive changes (hypointense sclerosis) or scarring of capsular ligament attachments can be associated with adjacent labral abnormalities.

■ Except for subtle cases of a humeral avulsion of glenohumeral ligament (HAGL), adherent Perthes lesion, or postoperative Bankart repair, MR arthrography is not routinely required if optimized MR studies with high signal-to-noise and adequate spatial resolution have been performed with the appropriate surface coil.

■ Partial chronic articular sided tears can be visualized with improved conspicuity without contrast provided image contrast is adjusted post acquisition to emphasize the boundary between a shallow partial surface tear and adjacent intermediate signal as seen in hypertrophic synovium or granulation tissue.

Biceps

- The long head biceps tendon (LHBT) is intraarticular but extrasynovial.

- The synovial sheath of the LHBT as visualized in its proximal extraarticular course communicates directly with the glenohumeral joint and ends in a blind pouch at the distal bicipital groove.

- Contrast outlines the biceps and the biceps labral complex, aiding in the detection and characterization of superior-labral anterior-to-posterior (SLAP) lesions.

- The biceps labral complex or BLC is visible without intraarticular contrast provided contrast and spatial resolution are optimized.

- Arthrography is also useful in visualization of the superior glenohumeral ligament (SGHL) and the coracohumeral ligament (CHL) components of the pulley, aiding in the detection and characterization of microinstability lesions.

- Maximum thickness of the LHBT is 3.3 to 4.7mm.[182]

- Supraglenoid tubercle is anatomic origin in 30% of shoulders.

- Origin of biceps is a Y-form from the anterior and posterior labrum in 45%.

- Origin from both the supraglenoid tubercle and labrum occurs in 25% of cases.

- Cross-sectional area of the LHBT tapers from its intraarticular course to its proximal extraarticular course.

- Labral attachment of the intraarticular biceps is posterior.

- Biceps degeneration and rupture can also be the result of primary pathology without requiring subacromial impingement and antecedent subacromial abrasion.

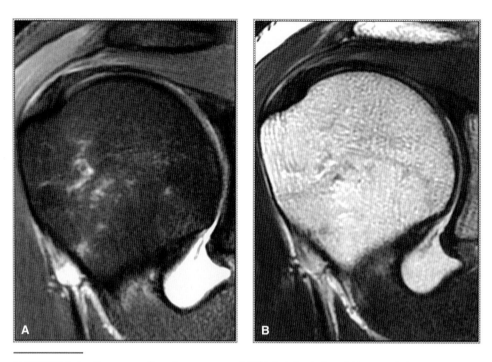

FIGURE 3.4   Rotator cuff tendon on coronal FS PD FSE (**A**) and T2 FSE (**B**) images using an eight-channel phased-array coil.

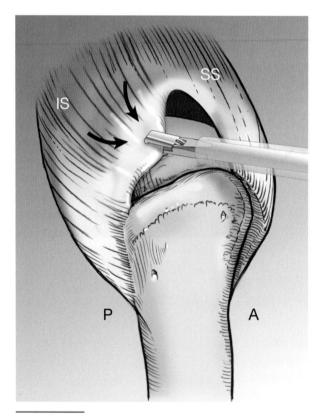

FIGURE 3.5   With an arthroscopic approach, rotator cuff tear pattern and mobility can be assessed from multiple angles of approach. In this schematic, a grasper introduced from an anterior portal is used to assess the anterior mobility of the posterior leaf. A, anterior; IS, infraspinatus; P, posterior; SS, supraspinatus. (Reprinted from Burkhart S, Lo IK, Brady PC, Denard PJ. *The Cowboy's Companion: A Trail Guide for the Arthroscopic Shoulder Surgeon.* Philadelphia, PA: Lippincott Williams & Wilkins; 2012, with permission.)

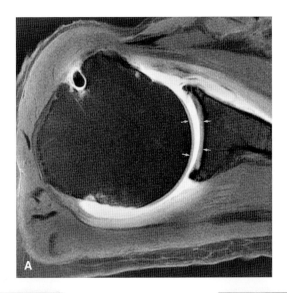

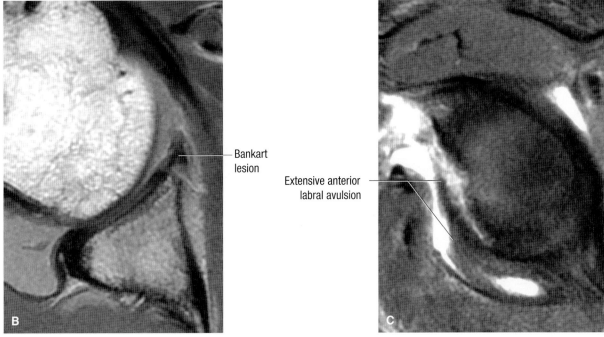

Bankart
lesion

Extensive anterior
labral avulsion

FIGURE 3.6 (A) Axial FS PD FSE image shows intact and congruous humeral head and glenoid articular cartilage surfaces (*arrows*), separate from the high-signal-intensity intraarticular contrast. (B) PD FSE contrast without FS is shown in an axial image of a Bankart lesion. Chondral surfaces are not as well demonstrated. (C) Excellent contrast is shown between the avulsed anterior labrum and the anterior glenoid rim on the corresponding sagittal FS PD FSE image.

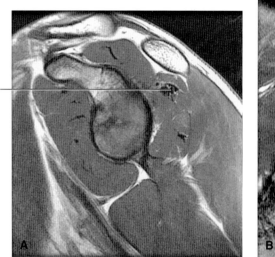
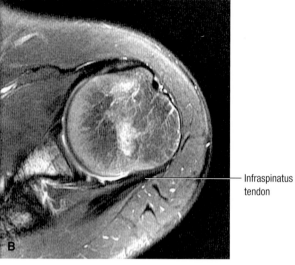

Infraspinatus
tendon

Infraspinatus
tendon

FIGURE 3.7   Pseudo-thickening of the infraspinatus tendon resulting from external glenohumeral joint rotation. This is not a cuff tear with retraction. (**A**) Sagittal PD image. (**B**) Axial FS PD FSE image.

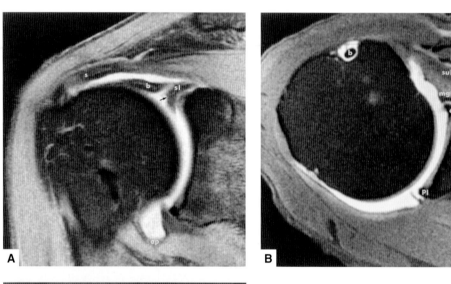
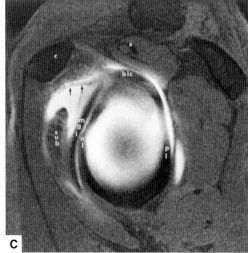

FIGURE 3.8   Routine MR arthrography with FS T1-weighted (**A**) coronal oblique, (**B**) axial, and (**C**) sagittal oblique (at the level of the glenohumeral joint) images. s, supraspinatus tendon; b, biceps tendon; SL, superior labrum; arrow, conjoined origin of the superior and middle glenohumeral ligaments; AP, axillary pouch; al, anterior labrum; PL, posterior labrum; MGL, middle glenohumeral ligament; sub, subscapularis tendon; c, coracoid; BLC, biceps labral complex; small arrows, superior glenohumeral ligament.

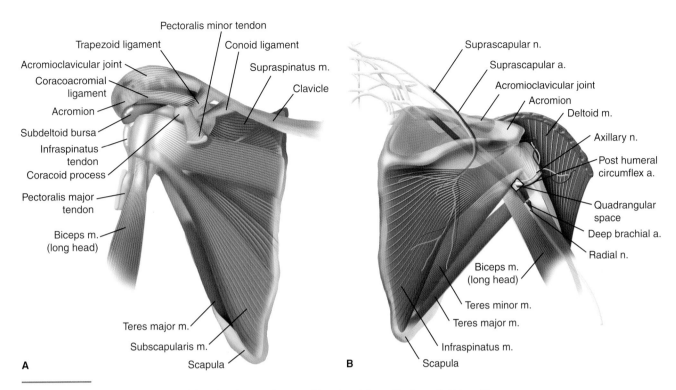

FIGURE 3.9 Gross anatomy of the glenohumeral joint. (Reprinted from Dodson C, Dines D, Dines JS, Walch G, Williams G. *Controversies in Shoulder Instability*. Philadelphia, PA: Lippincott Williams & Wilkins; 2014, with permission.)

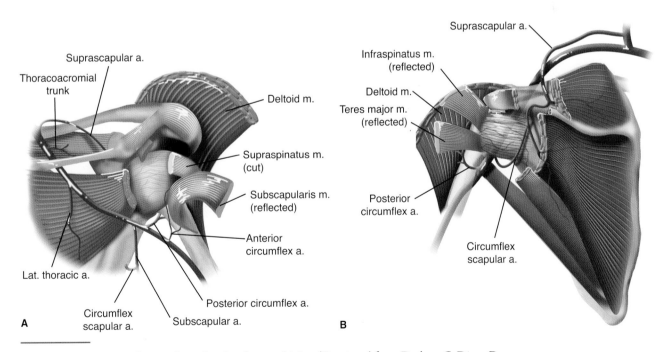

FIGURE 3.10 Vascular supply to the glenohumeral joint. (Reprinted from Dodson C, Dines D, Dines JS, Walch G, Williams G. *Controversies in Shoulder Instability*. Philadelphia, PA: Lippincott Williams & Wilkins; 2014, with permission.)

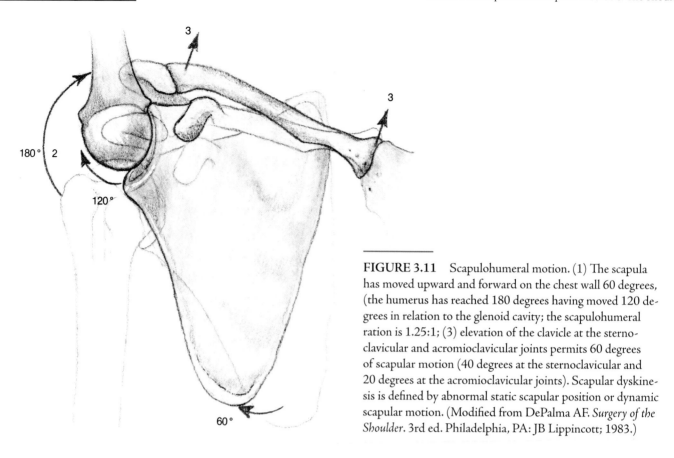

FIGURE 3.11 Scapulohumeral motion. (1) The scapula has moved upward and forward on the chest wall 60 degrees, (the humerus has reached 180 degrees having moved 120 degrees in relation to the glenoid cavity; the scapulohumeral ration is 1.25:1; (3) elevation of the clavicle at the sternoclavicular and acromioclavicular joints permits 60 degrees of scapular motion (40 degrees at the sternoclavicular and 20 degrees at the acromioclavicular joints). Scapular dyskinesis is defined by abnormal static scapular position or dynamic scapular motion. (Modified from DePalma AF. *Surgery of the Shoulder*. 3rd ed. Philadelphia, PA: JB Lippincott; 1983.)

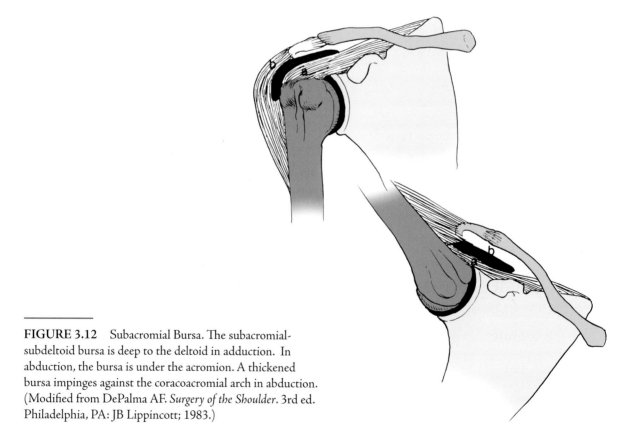

FIGURE 3.12 Subacromial Bursa. The subacromial-subdeltoid bursa is deep to the deltoid in adduction. In abduction, the bursa is under the acromion. A thickened bursa impinges against the coracoacromial arch in abduction. (Modified from DePalma AF. *Surgery of the Shoulder*. 3rd ed. Philadelphia, PA: JB Lippincott; 1983.)

ABER Technique

- ABER imaging was developed for evaluating glenohumeral anterior instability and multidirectional instability and to assess tears or laxity of the anterior band of the inferior glenohumeral ligament (IGHL).

- For ABER imaging, the arm is placed in abduction to tighten the inferior glenohumeral ligament labral complex (IGLLC) in the position of abduction and external rotation.

    - In the supine position the patient's hand is placed behind the head for the symptomatic shoulder to be studied on that side. This hand placement posterior to the head results in the desired abducted externally rotated position.

- Used historically for Perthes lesions and articular surface footprint tears

- Useful in assessment of Bankart soft tissue repairs

- Optional technique employed in conjunction with MR arthrography

    - Contrast should not extend between the anterior inferior labrum or IGL and the glenoid. Absence of the anterior inferior labrum adjacent to a taut IGL also indicates a labral tear.

- This technique places stress on the labral ligamentous complex to help reveal detachments that may not be seen on routine MR exams if the bulk of the subscapularis prevents displacement.

- It also relieves tension on the undersurface of the rotator cuff, thus revealing nondisplaced undersurface flap tears of the supraspinatus and helping to characterize the horizontal component of a partial articular side rotator cuff tear.

- The ABER technique may also be additionally supplemented with a flexed, adducted and internally rotated (FADIR) position to characterize posteroinferior labral tears.[37]

■ In SLAP lesions in throwing athletes, ABER positioning produces decentering of the humeral head, revealing biceps anchor detachment (the posterior peel-back subcategory type 2 SLAP lesions).

■ In subtle shoulder instability, ABER in aging may also reveal decentering of the humeral head from the normal central point of rotation.

    ■ The ABER position with the arm in abduction and external rotation may produce positive "apprehension" and "apprehension supression" signs in patients with MDI. Pain, apprehension or reflex guarding occurs as the arm is placed into external rotation.

■ ABER images were initially used to confirm IGHL tightening in the position of abduction and external rotation.

■ ABER imaging is usually performed in conjunction with MR arthrography.

■ In routine imaging, there is a greater reliance on coronal images to show the IGLLC without using ABER MR arthrography. Only in the position of function will the inferior glenohumeral ligament will be visualized taut and without laxity.

■ Non-arthrographic imaging in the ABER position, although less common, can still be used to evaluate the taut IGL and anterior band.

■ In the ABER position, the image showing the location of the taut IGLLC is the same image that demonstrates the anatomy of the posterior inferior labrum and infraspinatus footprint.

■ The supraspinatus footprint is located on the ABER image closest to the LHBT as it courses proximally to join the BLC superiorly.

    ■ Identify the percentage of the exposed cuff footprint in partial articular sided rotator cuff tears and evaluate the quality of the remaining tendon fibers.[559]

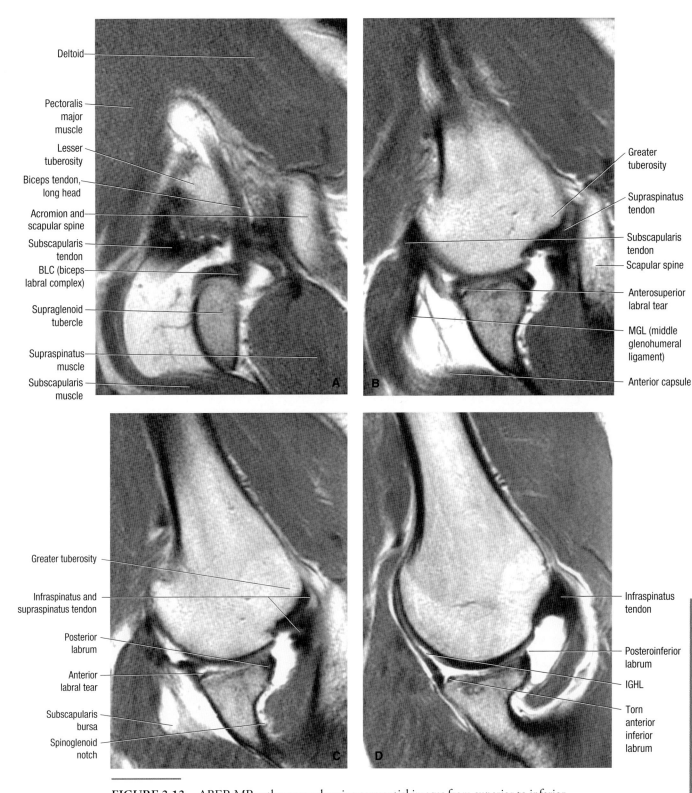

Deltoid

Pectoralis major muscle

Lesser tuberosity

Biceps tendon, long head

Acromion and scapular spine

Subscapularis tendon

BLC (biceps labral complex)

Supraglenoid tubercle

Supraspinatus muscle

Subscapularis muscle

Greater tuberosity

Supraspinatus tendon

Subscapularis tendon

Scapular spine

Anterosuperior labral tear

MGL (middle glenohumeral ligament)

Anterior capsule

Greater tuberosity

Infraspinatus and supraspinatus tendon

Posterior labrum

Anterior labral tear

Subscapularis bursa

Spinoglenoid notch

Infraspinatus tendon

Posteroinferior labrum

IGHL

Torn anterior inferior labrum

FIGURE 3.13 ABER MR arthrogram showing sequential images from superior to inferior. (**A**) Superior axial oblique image at the level of the biceps labral complex and the long head of the biceps tendon. (**B**) Anterosuperior axial oblique image at the level of the subscapularis tendon and supraspinatus footprint. (**C**) Mid-axial oblique image at the level of the conjoined insertion of the supraspinatus and infraspinatus tendons and the spinoglenoid notch. (**D**) Anteroinferior axial oblique image at the level of the IGHL and infraspinatus tendon.

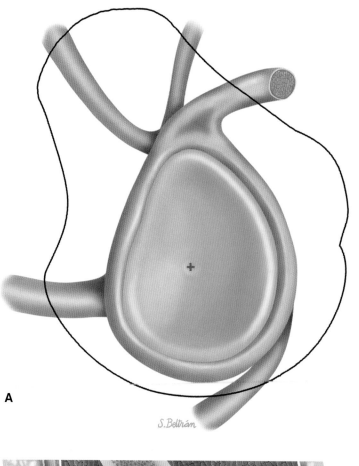

A

S. Beltrán

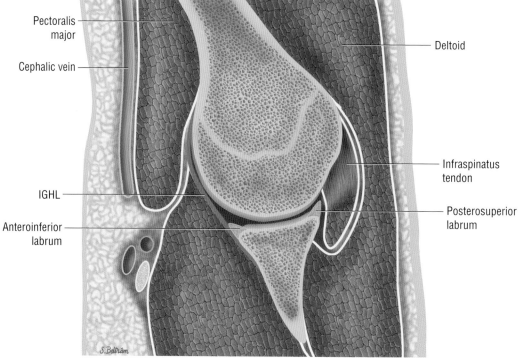

Pectoralis
major

Cephalic vein

IGHL

Anteroinferior
labrum

Deltoid

Infraspinatus
tendon

Posterosuperior
labrum

S. Beltrán

B

FIGURE 3.14   (**A**) Normal central point (*red cross*) of glenohumeral rotation with arm positioned in abduction and external rotation. (**B**) Axial oblique ABER (abduction and external rotation) anatomy illustrated at the level of the inferior glenohumeral ligament (IGHL) labral complex.

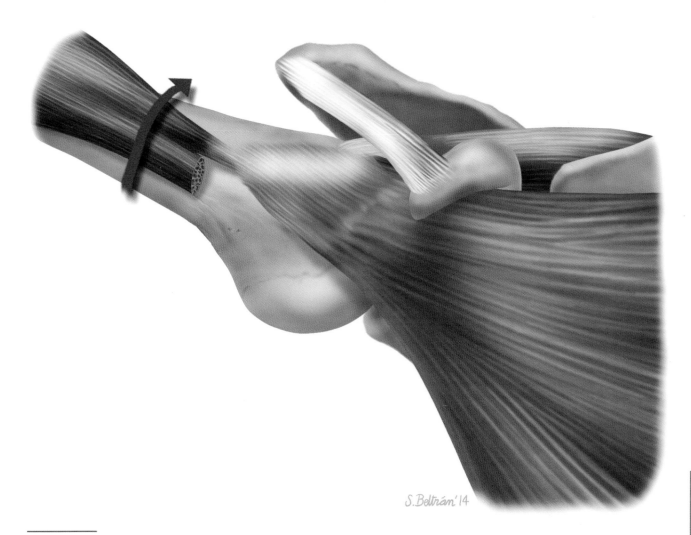

FIGURE 3.15 Three-dimensional view of ABER positioning from anterior prospective with subscapularis and supraspinatous visualized. Because the anterior band of the inferior glenohumeral ligament is taut or placed under tension in the ABER position the anteroinferior capsulolabral complex can be functionally evaluated. This technique is especially useful in postoperative Bankart repairs. The delamination or horizontal interstitial component of a partial articular sided tear of the supraspinatus may be more conspicuous in the ABER position.

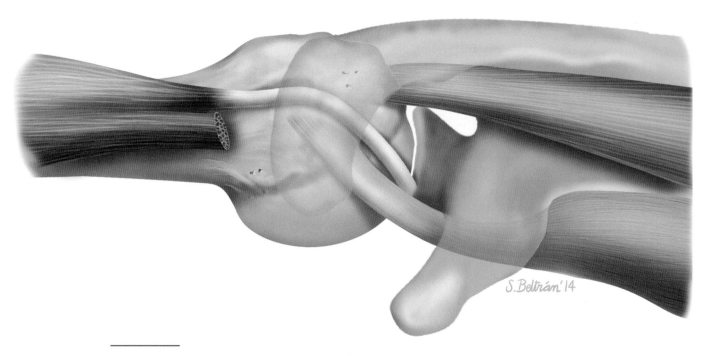

FIGURE 3.16   Superior view. ABER position from superior perspective viewing down on the supraspinatous tendon and the long head of the biceps at the level corresponding of the biceps labral complex.

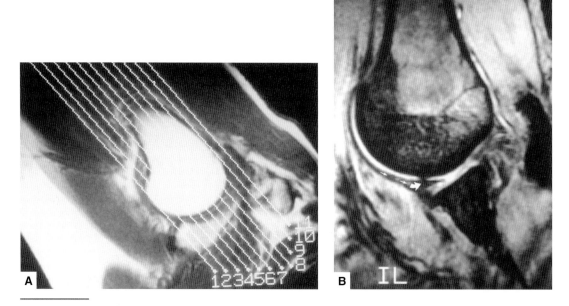

FIGURE 3.17   Functional anatomy of the inferior glenohumeral ligament (IGL). (**A**) A coronal localizer obtained with the arm placed in 90° of abduction (i.e., the position of function of the IGL) and external rotation. (**B**) The corresponding axial image through the glenohumeral joint shows a taut IGL (*small straight arrows*) and intact anterior labrum (*curved arrow*).

Marrow Imaging

■ Metaphyseal marrow inhomogeneity of the proximal humerus may represent a normal pattern of conversion from red to yellow marrow as a function of age-related changes in marrow distribution in the shoulder.

■ Red marrow may also extend medially and proximal to the physeal scar.

■ Red marrow has a characteristic intermediate signal intensity on T2 or progressive T2-weighted images and is not associated with aggressive characteristics such as cortical bone erosion or a soft tissue mass.

■ When there is both medial and lateral extension of red marrow proximal to the physis, further evaluation for a marrow disorder is warranted.

■ Myelodysplastic marrow produces uniform marrow replacement, hypointense on T1 and hyperintense on fluid sensitive images (FS PD FSE).

■ Gradient echo is used to assess trabecular architecture, taking advantage of increased susceptibility of underlying trabecular bone. CT with bone technique is an additional method used to document intact osseous architecture.

  ■ Since gradient echo is not a marrow sensitive technique, GRE contrast is best suited to evaluate the integrity of bony architecture in cases of excessive marrow edema as initially visualized on STIR or FS PD FSE images.

■ The marrow of the contralateral humerus can be imaged for comparison in cases of atypical marrow inhomogeneity.

■ Abnormal marrow identified on a fluid sensitive technique should always be compared to a corresponding T1-weighted image to appreciate the replacement of fat.

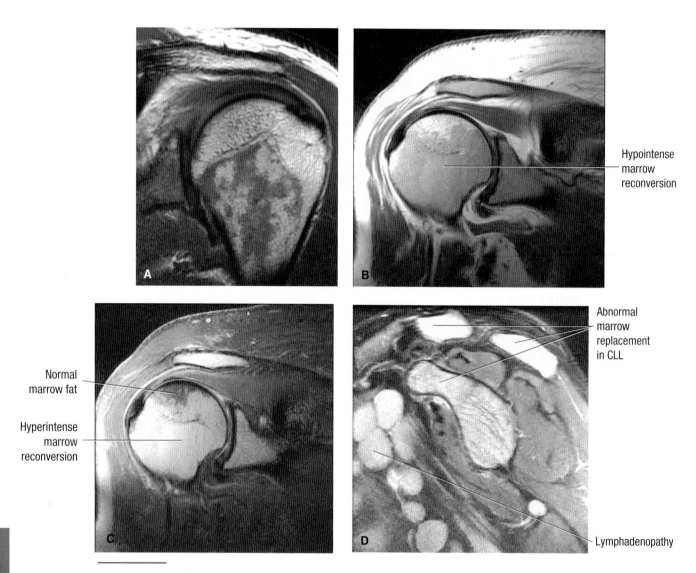

FIGURE 3.18 (**A**) Coronal PD FSE image showing normal hypointense red marrow signal distal to the proximal humeral physeal scar. Red marrow may partially exist in subchondral locations of the proximal humeral epiphysis, providing characteristic T1 and T2 signal intensities. (**B,C**) Marrow reconversion in polycythemia vera, a myeloproliferative disorder. Red marrow signal intensity is apparent proximal to the physeal scar. Red marrow demonstrates lower signal intensity than fat on coronal PD-weighted images (**B**) and is hyperintense relative to fat signal on coronal FS PD FSE images. (**C**) Red marrow associated with pathologic conditions tends to image with greater hyperintensity than normal areas of persistent red marrow. (**D**) Abnormal hyperintense marrow replacement in chronic lymphocytic leukemia (CLL) on a sagittal FS PD FSE image. CLL is not associated with high-dose radiation or benzene exposure.

Brachial Plexus

■ On axial images, the brachial plexus can be identified adjacent to the subclavian vessels, which are used as landmarks for off-axis coronal images.

■ Axial STIR (including fast STIR techniques) or T2-weighted images of both upper extremities are obtained to demonstrate any extrinsic effacement of the brachial plexus (from either soft tissue or osseous encroachment) or secondary increased signal intensity from an area of trauma.

■ Innervation of the Shoulder

　■ Suprascapular nerve is main sensory nerve for posterior joint capsule.

　■ The subscapular and axillary nerve send branches to the inferior part of the anterior capsule.

　■ The rotator cuff muscles have innervation from the subscapular nerve (C6 and C7) for the subscapularis muscle, suprascapular nerve (C4-C6) for the supraspinatus and infraspinatus muscles. The axillary nerve supplies the teres minor muscle.

　■ Deltoid-axillary nerve innervation[182]

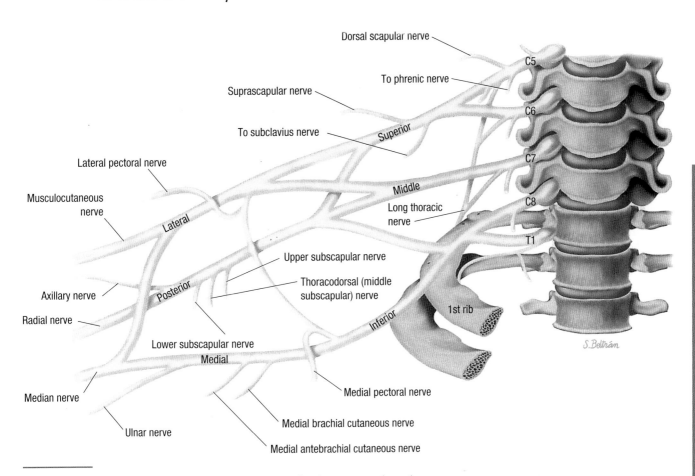

FIGURE 3.19　Brachial plexus with plexus roots, trunks, divisions, cords, and nerves.

- Latissimus dorsi-thoracodorsal nerve
- Biceps brachii-musculocutaneous nerve
- Triceps brachii-radial nerve
- Pectoralis major-pectoral nerves[182]

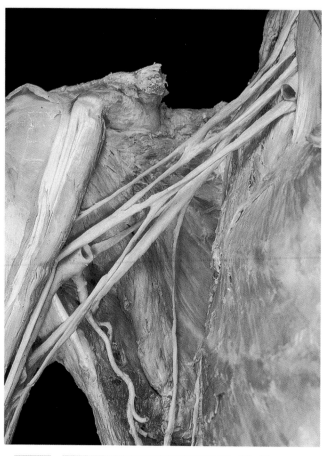

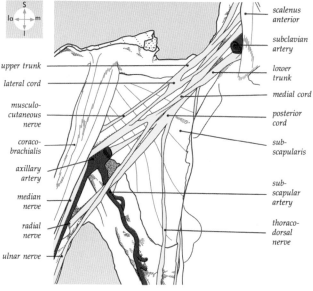

FIGURE 3.20   The components of the brachial plexus. The veins and most of the axillary artery have been removed.

4
Glenohumeral Joint and Capsular Gross Anatomy

Glenohumeral Joint and Capsule (pages 99-107)

Glenoid Labrum (pages 108-117)

Long Head of the Biceps Tendon and Biceps Labral Complex (pages 118-135)

Glenohumeral Ligaments Unifying Perspective (pages 136-159)

Rotator Cuff (pages 159-172)

Coracoacromial Arch (pages 173-183)

Glenohumeral Joint and Capsular Gross Anatomy

Glenohumeral Joint and Capsule

Key Concepts

■ The BLC is classified as type 1, 2, or 3.

■ Underneath the superior labrum, medial to the biceps labral complex the articular cartilage of the glenoid extends 2 to 3mm medial to the superior pole of the glenoid.

■ Type 1 BLC has the superior labrum firmly attached to the superior pole of the glenoid.

■ The superiorly located biceps labral sulcus in BLC types 2 and 3 should not be mistaken for the more anterior (anterosuperior quadrant) sublabral foramen (also known as the sublabral hole). Furthermore, the appearance of a sublabral foramen is in fact created by a high attachment of the anterior band of the IGHL.

■ The IGHL contributes to the anterior labrum through its anterior band. The anterior band may exist as a high attachment variant and will either overlay a small or absent (more common association) anterosuperior labrum as a normal finding.

■ The MGHL is cord-like, absent, thin, or redundant.

■ The superior glenohumeral and coracohumeral ligaments stabilize the long head of the biceps tendon by forming the biceps pulley or sling in the rotator cuff interval.[424]

■ Glenohumeral joint version or humeral retroversion projects the axis of the humeral head joint surface 25° to 40° from the coronal plane, whereas the glenoid surface is retroverted 4° to 12° with respect to the scapula.[407]

Posterior portal is the primary viewing portal for both the glenohumeral joint and subacromial space. The anterior portal is used for SLAP repair. Anterosuperolateral portal is used for SLAP and subscapularis repair, coracoid work and biceps tenotomy. This portal is used to view instability addressing the anteroinferior and posteroinferior labrum. The 5 o'clock portal is used in Bankart repair. The port of Wilmington is used to approach the posterosuperior glenoid (SLAP repairs). Posterolateral portal is used to address the posteroinferior labrum in posterior instability.

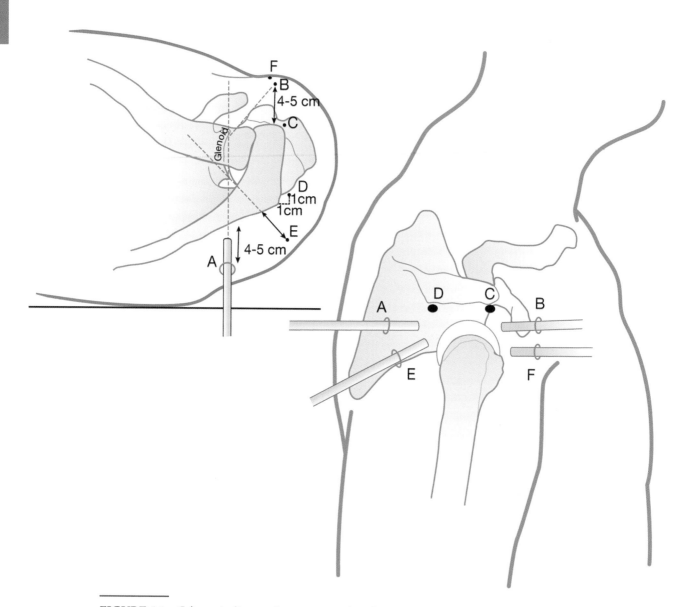

FIGURE 4.1   Schematic diagram demonstrating the relative positions of the most common glenohumeral portals. (A) posterior portal; (B) anterior portal; (C) anterosuperolateral portal; (D) Port of Wilmington portal; (E) low posterolateral portal; (F) 5 o'clock portal. (Reprinted from Burkhart S, Lo IK, Brady PC, Denard PJ. *The Cowboy's Companion: A Trail Guide for the Arthroscopic Shoulder Surgeon.* Philadelphia, PA: Lippincott Williams & Wilkins; 2012, with permission.)

The posterior portal provides access to the subacromial space. The lateral portal is used in rotator cuff repair. Modified Neviaser portal is utilized in SLAP repairs. The subclavian portal is used for retrograde passage through the anterior supraspinatus. With the use of antegrade suture passers the subclavian portal is not commonly used.

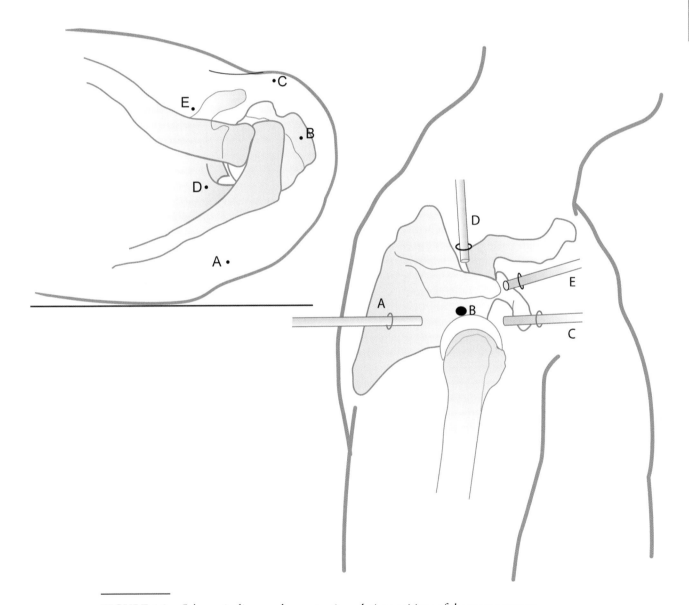

FIGURE 4.2   Schematic diagram demonstrating relative positions of the most common subacromial portals. (A) posterior portal; (B) lateral portal; (C) anterior portal; (D) modified Neviaser portal; (E) subclavian portal. (Reprinted from Burkhart S, Lo IK, Brady PC, Denard PJ. *The Cowboy's Companion: A Trail Guide for the Arthroscopic Shoulder Surgeon*. Philadelphia, PA: Lippincott Williams & Wilkins; 2012, with permission.)

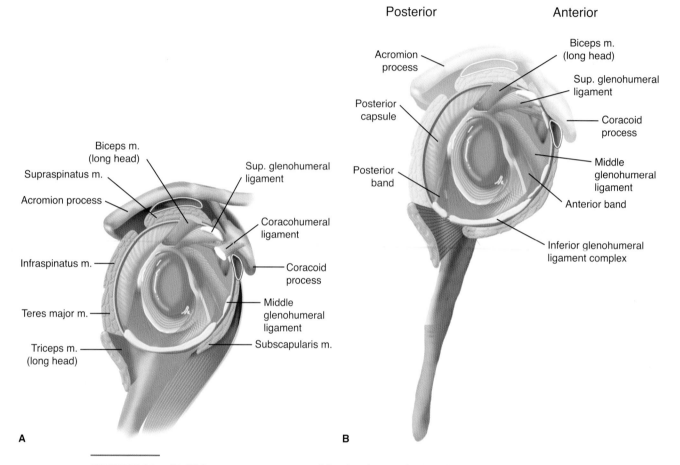

FIGURE 4.3 (**A,B**) Ligamentous anatomy of the glenohumeral joint. The middle glenohumeral ligament (component of the anterior glenohumeral capsuloligamentous complex) extends from the upper glenoid to the lesser tuberosity. The inferior glenohumeral ligament complex (IGLLC) consists of the anterior and posterior bands with an intervening axillary pouch. The IGLLC by forming a hammock cradles the humeral head and functions as the primary static restraint against anterior translation in abduction. The superior glenohumeral ligament and coracohumeral ligament are components within the superior (glenohumeral ligament) complex. (Reprinted from Dodson C, Dines D, Dines JS, Walch G, Williams G. *Controversies in Shoulder Instability*. Philadelphia, PA: Lippincott Williams & Wilkins; 2014, with permission.)

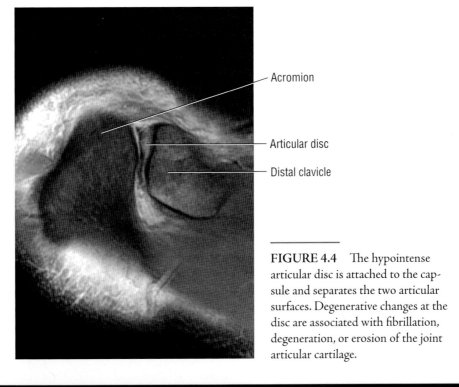

Acromion

Articular disc

Distal clavicle

FIGURE 4.4   The hypointense articular disc is attached to the capsule and separates the two articular surfaces. Degenerative changes at the disc are associated with fibrillation, degeneration, or erosion of the joint articular cartilage.

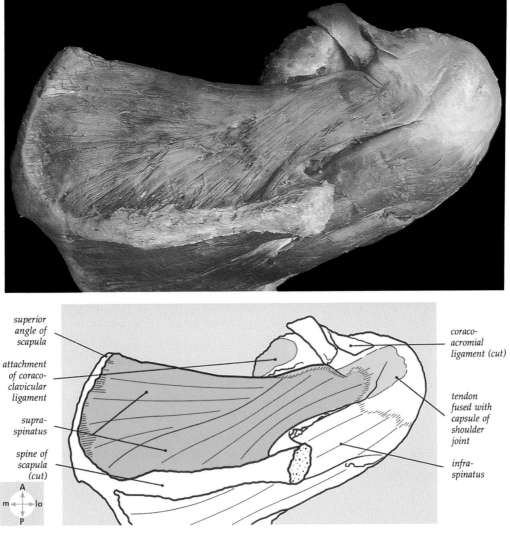

superior angle of scapula

attachment of coraco-clavicular ligament

supra-spinatus

spine of scapula (cut)

coraco-acromial ligament (cut)

tendon fused with capsule of shoulder joint

infra-spinatus

FIGURE 4.5   A superior view of the supraspinatus tendon after removal of the acromion of the scapula.

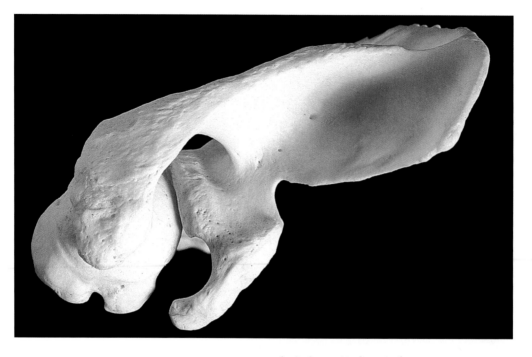

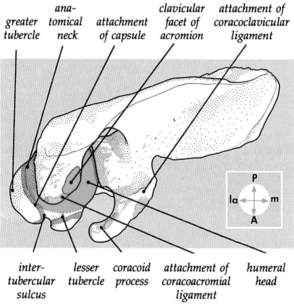

FIGURE 4.6   A superior view of the scapula and the upper end of the humerus. The acromion and the coracoacromial ligament prevent upward displacement of the humeral head.

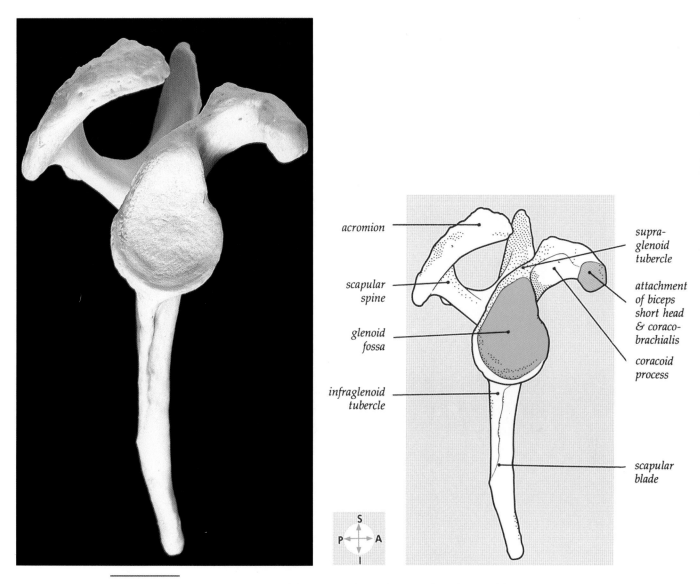

FIGURE 4.7 The lateral aspect of the scapula shows the pear-shaped glenoid fossa. The positions of the supraspinatus, infraspinatus, and subscapular fossae are shown.

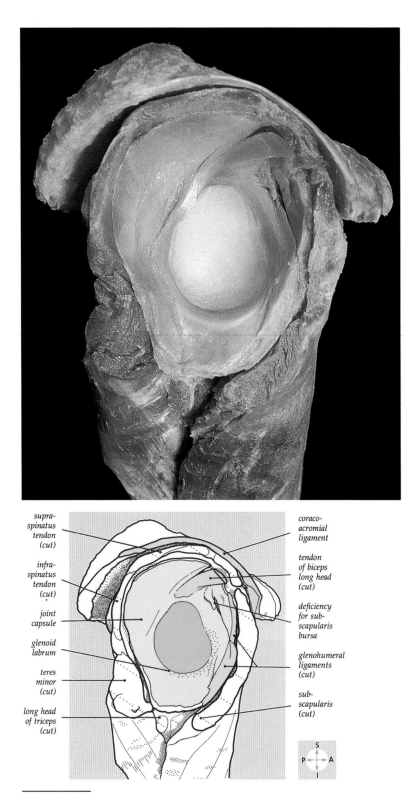

FIGURE 4.8   The scapular component of a disarticulated shoulder joint. The relations and internal features of the joint are seen.

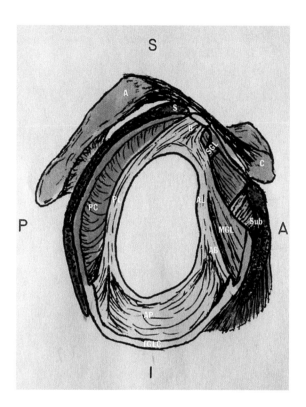

FIGURE 4.9 Glenohumeral capsular anatomy. A, acromion; AB, anterior band of IGHL; AL, anterior labrum; AP, axillary pouch of IGHL; B, biceps tendon; C, coracoid; IGLC, IGHL complex; MGL, middle glenohumeral ligament; PC, posterior capsule; PL, posterior labrum; S, supraspinatus tendon; SGL, superior glenohumeral ligament; Sub, subscapularis tendon.

Glenoid Labrum

- The Glenoid Labrum is:[231,424]

  - The fibrous attachment of the glenohumeral ligaments and capsule to the glenoid rim[138]

  - Typically 3mm high and 4mm wide but can vary considerably in size, shape, and configuration

    - The glenoid labrum is ovoid in shape and conforms to the kidney-shaped glenoid rim.

- The anterior glenoid labrum provides the major area of attachment for the anterior band of the inferior glenohumeral ligament (IGHL).[420]

- The middle glenohumeral ligament (MGHL) is a more variable capsular structure and may contribute fibers to the more superior aspects of the anterior glenoid labrum as it approaches the biceps tendon.

- The glenoid fossa and rim are divided into six quadrants (only descriptive locations should be used because sagittal images may be obtained from either the left or right shoulder).

- The superior pole is the 12 o'clock position and the inferior pole is the 6 o'clock position as these positions remain constant in reference for both right and left shoulders. [546,584]

Biomechanics and Vascularity of the Labrum

- The Glenoid Labrum

  - Makes up approximately 50% of the total depth of the glenoid fossa osseous socket

  - Increases the glenoid surface in the vertical and horizontal planes to better accommodate rotation of the humeral head[225,635]

  - The labrum is firmly attached inferior to the epiphyseal line and is continuous with the cartilaginous surface of the glenoid.

- The Posteroinferior Labrum absorbs the majority of the load in 90% of shoulder abduction with an applied compressive load.[260,635]

  - Thus, the posterior labrum is strong and usually more triangular in shape compared with the anterior labrum.

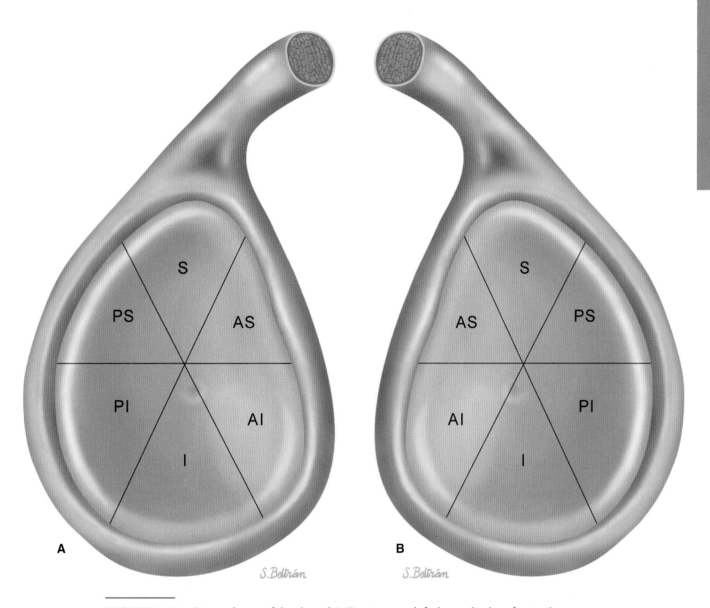

FIGURE 4.10 Six quadrants of the glenoid. MR units may default to a display of sagittal images of the shoulder from a left-shoulder perspective even if the right shoulder was imaged. It is accepted practice to describe a lesion by its quadrant. The description of the superior pole as 12 o'clock and the inferior pole as 6 o'clock is accurate for the right and left shoulders. To avoid mistaking right for left, however, use of the 3 o'clock or 9 o'clock positions should be avoided. (**A**) Illustration using a right-shoulder perspective. (**B**) Left-shoulder perspective. S, superior; AS, anteroposterior; AI, anteroinferior; I, inferior; PS, posterosuperior; PI, posteroinferior.

- Vascularity in the superior and anterosuperior labrum segments is decreased in comparison with the posterosuperior and inferior segments.

    - Decreased superior vascularity may be responsible for the development of superior labral degeneration with increasing age and may make the labrum more susceptible to SLAP lesions.[120]

Labral Types

- Classification[635]

    1. A labrum that is attached to the glenoid in its periphery through the fibrocartilaginous transitional zone

        - Above the physeal line or equator, the labrum may be mobile along its central border, with a meniscoid appearance (meniscoid superior labrum seen in type 3 BLC).

    2. A labrum that is firmly attached to the glenoid both peripherally and centrally

- Hypertrophy of the posterior glenoid labrum is associated with posterior glenoid (rim) hypoplasia.

    - Posterior humeral subluxation and an eccentric posterior glenoid fossa wear pattern may develop.[344]

- Posterior glenoid dysplasia may be graded as:

    - Mild

    - Moderate

    - Severe

- Retroversion of the osseous glenoid is greater than seen with measurements performed at the chondrolabral portion of the glenoid.

- Posterior subluxation is a function of the glenoid retroversion, which cannot be compensated for by an enlarged or hypertrophied labrum.

    - This excessive retroversion produces posterior instability.

- A hypoplastic posterior inferior labrum and a patulous capsule can be seen in multidirectional instability.

- The outer edge of the posterior labrum creates a chockblock-like border since the outer edge of the labrum is higher or proud relative to the edge of the glenoid articular cartilage.[559]

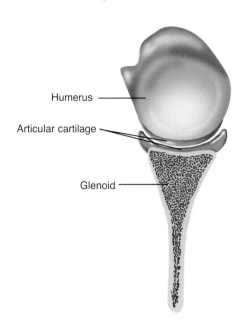

Humerus

Articular cartilage

Glenoid

FIGURE 4.11 Illustration demonstrating the conformity of the articular cartilage surfaces of the glenoid (G) with cartilage of the humeral head (H) despite the relative flat osseous glenoid. (Reprinted from Dodson C, Dines D, Dines JS, Walch G, Williams G. *Controversies in Shoulder Instability*. Philadelphia, PA: Lippincott Williams & Wilkins; 2014, with permission.)

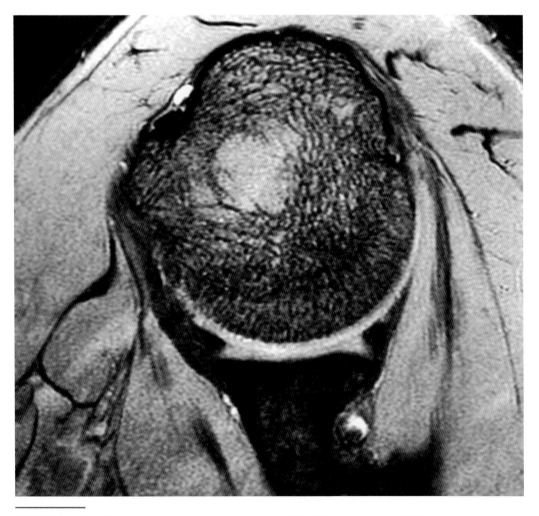

FIGURE 4.12 Glenohumeral joint contrast on axial T2* GRE image. Axial GRE images optimize visualization of intralabral signal and subscapularis tendinosis. FS FSE images are more sensitive to fluid collections, paralabral cysts, and articular cartilage. The humeral head is centralized.

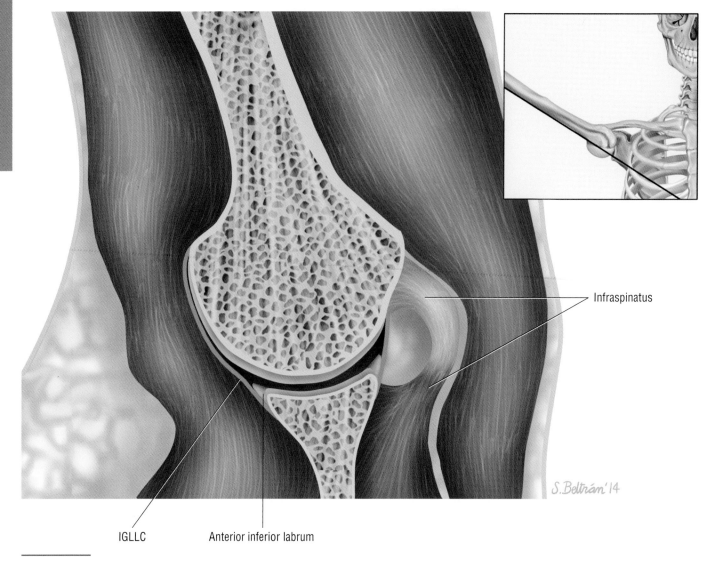

FIGURE 4.13   Two-dimensional view of the shoulder in ABER position demonstrating the taut relationship between the IGHL and the anterior inferior glenoid labrum. The posterior superior labrum is visualized on the same image that depicts the anterior inferior labrum. The IGLLC relationship and the infraspinatus footprint are displayed on the same ABER image. The anterior band of the IGLLC is placed under tension which improves visualization of anterior inferior labral tears. The articular surface of the supraspinatus and infraspinatus tendons is visible in the abducted externally rotated (ABER) position.

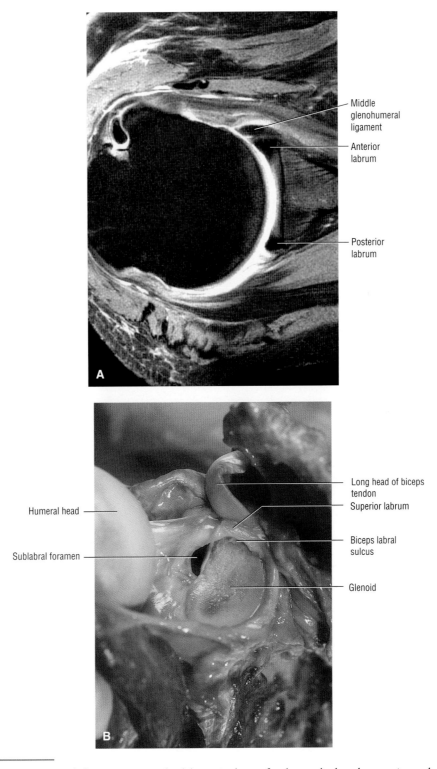

FIGURE 4.14 (**A**) A superior wedge labrum is shown firmly attached to the anterior and posterior glenoid rim. The anterior band of the IGL blends with the labrum to form one structure near the equator of the anterior glenoid rim. A sublabral foramen may exist in the anterosuperior quadrant in a superior wedge labrum. (**B**) A superior wedge labrum in which the free central edge of the superior labrum forms the biceps labral sulcus of the biceps labral complex type 2. A sublabral foramen (created by a high attachment of the anterior band) is an associated finding in the anterosuperior quadrant. Note the firm attachment of the anterior labrum (below the equator), posterior labrum, and inferior labrum.

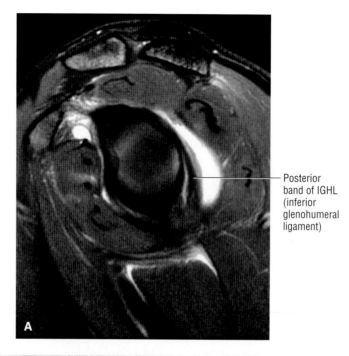

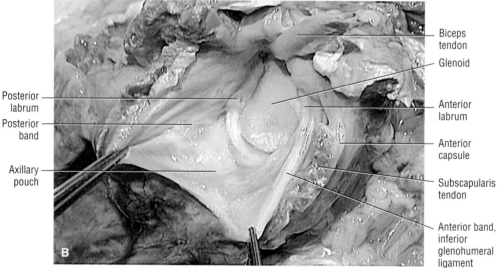

FIGURE 4.15 (**A**) A prominent or thick posterior band of the inferior glenohumeral ligament (IGL). Normally, the posterior band is not as well defined as the anterior band of the IGL. The posterior labrum may be relatively small underneath a prominent posterior band. Sagittal FS PD FSE image. (**B**) A posterior wedge labrum with central edge of posterior labrum overlapping the posterior glenoid rim. The anterior band (AB) is easily identified as a thickened band, attaching to the glenoid at 2–4 o'clock in this right shoulder specimen. The AB courses diagonally downwards to attach to the anatomic neck of the humerus. The posterior band originates at the 7–9 o'clock on the glenoid in this right shoulder specimen. Slight external rotation of the abducted humerus improves visualization of the PB. The axillary pouch is actually formed by the fasciculus obliquus medially and by the junction of the AB and PB on the humerus laterally.

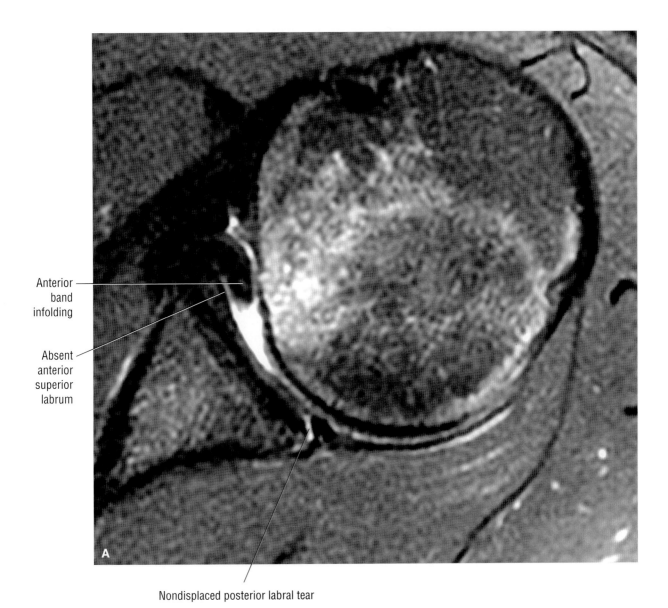

Anterior band infolding

Absent anterior superior labrum

Nondisplaced posterior labral tear

FIGURE 4.16 **(A)** Normal anterior infolding of the anterior band of the IGHL. There is the expected absence of the anterior superior labrum as a normal variation. The anterior labrum is either assent or attenuated in the presence of an AB with a high attachment. The slight posterior subluxation of the humeral head is related to the posterior glenoid labral tear. Axial FS PD FSE image.

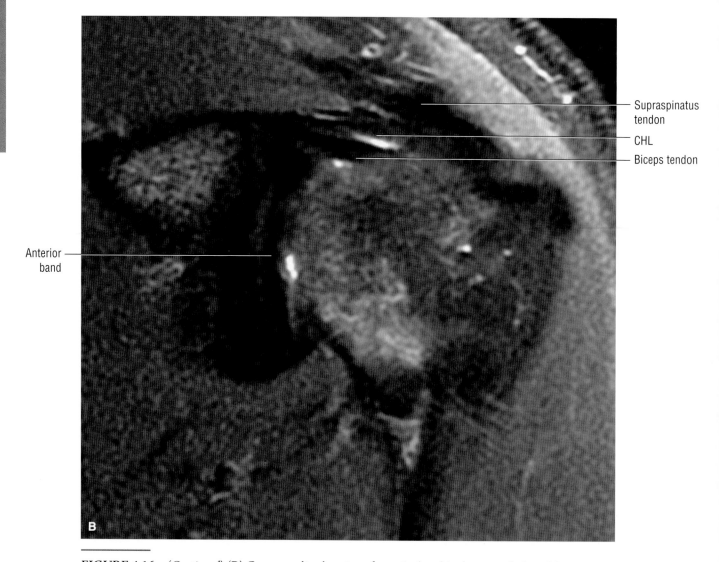

FIGURE 4.16   *(Continued)* (**B**) Corresponding location of anterior band in the coronal plane. Note the CHL is visible anterior to the supraspinatus tendon. The fasciculus obliquus (anterior to this image) does cross diagonally over and is anterior to the anterior band of the inferior glenohumeral ligament. The anterior band and the fasciculus obliquus merge with each other in the area where the two ligaments cross. Coronal FS PD FSE image.

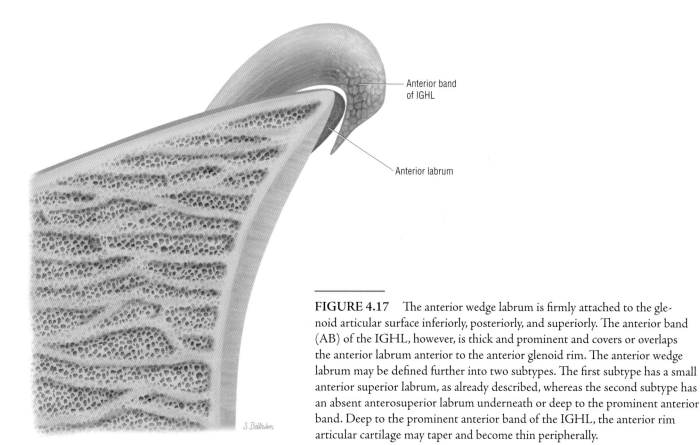

Anterior band
of IGHL

Anterior labrum

FIGURE 4.17   The anterior wedge labrum is firmly attached to the glenoid articular surface inferiorly, posteriorly, and superiorly. The anterior band (AB) of the IGHL, however, is thick and prominent and covers or overlaps the anterior labrum anterior to the anterior glenoid rim. The anterior wedge labrum may be defined further into two subtypes. The first subtype has a small anterior superior labrum, as already described, whereas the second subtype has an absent anterosuperior labrum underneath or deep to the prominent anterior band. Deep to the prominent anterior band of the IGHL, the anterior rim articular cartilage may taper and become thin peripherally.

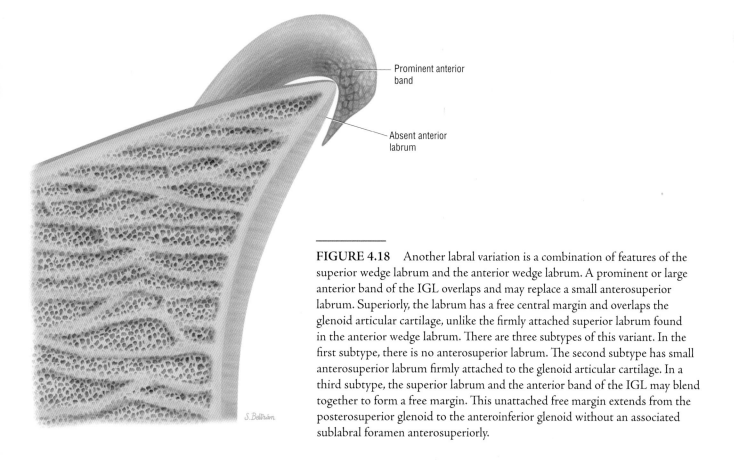

Prominent anterior
band

Absent anterior
labrum

FIGURE 4.18   Another labral variation is a combination of features of the superior wedge labrum and the anterior wedge labrum. A prominent or large anterior band of the IGL overlaps and may replace a small anterosuperior labrum. Superiorly, the labrum has a free central margin and overlaps the glenoid articular cartilage, unlike the firmly attached superior labrum found in the anterior wedge labrum. There are three subtypes of this variant. In the first subtype, there is no anterosuperior labrum. The second subtype has small anterosuperior labrum firmly attached to the glenoid articular cartilage. In a third subtype, the superior labrum and the anterior band of the IGL may blend together to form a free margin. This unattached free margin extends from the posterosuperior glenoid to the anteroinferior glenoid without an associated sublabral foramen anterosuperiorly.

Long Head of the Biceps Tendon and Biceps Labral Complex

Long Head of the Biceps Tendon

- The long head of the biceps tendon (LHBT)
  - Has four attachments:[546]
    - The supraglenoid tubercle (to the superior glenoid)
    - The posterior superior labrum
    - The anterior superior labrum
    - Extraarticular fibers that attach to the lateral edge of the base of the coracoid process
  - Exits the shoulder joint through a hiatus between the subscapularis and supraspinatus
  - Centralizes and stabilizes the joint in conjunction with the biceps labral complex (BLC), as does the rotator cuff
  - May be surrounded by multiple fine synovial bands (*vinculae biceps*) at the proximal entrance of the intertubercular groove, passing from the biceps to surrounding synovium and capsule

- The biceps tendon variations[142,654]
  - Presents with a large synovial mesentery attached to the articular side of the supraspinatus
  - As a "bifid biceps," in which one portion of the biceps attaches to the supraglenoid tubercle (normal attachment) and the second portion attaches to the rotator cuff cable/ridge

- The rotator cuff cable is a capsular tissue thickening of articular sided cuff tissue oriented perpendicular to the biceps tendon. This thickening represents the deep or articular sided extension of the coracohumeral ligament.

- The attachment of the glenoid labrum is variable above the epiphyseal line (i.e., the junction of the upper and middle thirds of the glenoid fossa).
  - The superior and anterosuperior portions of the labrum can be variably attached to the glenoid[63]

- Inferior to the epiphyseal line, the labrum is continuous with the glenoid articular cartilage and serves as the insertion site for the IGHL.

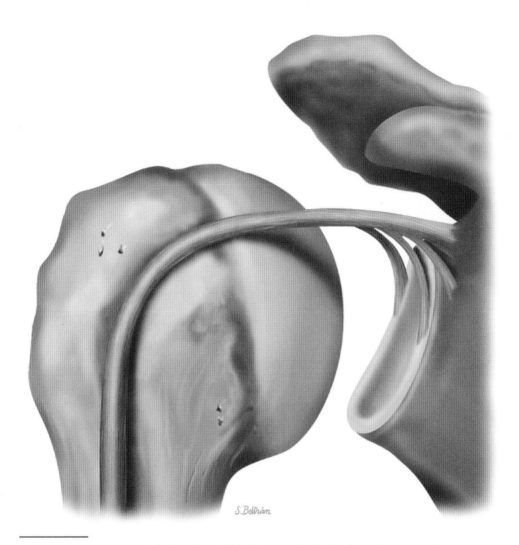

FIGURE 4.19 Origin of the long head of the biceps with idealized attachments to the posterior labrum, supraglenoid tubercle, anterior glenoid labrum, and base of the coracoid. The long head of the biceps (LHB) is intraarticular but extrasynovial. Fluid when present in the synovial sheath communicates directly with the glenohumeral joint. Fluid identified as tenosynovitis exists in the synovial sheath, which terminates in a blind pouch at the distal bicipital groove. (Based on Detrisac DJ, Johnson LL. Biceps and subscapularis tendons. In: Detrisac DJ, Johnson LL, eds. *Arthroscopic Shoulder Anatomy: Pathologic and Surgical Implications*. Thorofare, NJ: Slack; 1986:21–34.)

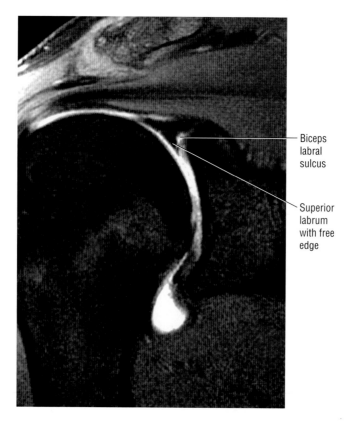

FIGURE 4.20   Unattached free margin of superior labrum in a type 2 biceps labral complex.

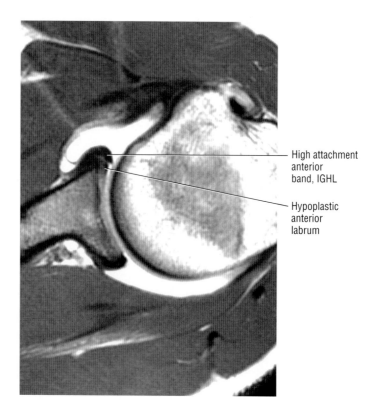

FIGURE 4.21   The anterior band of the IGHL overlapping a small anterior labrum. The anterior superior labrum is small because the anterior band attaches high. Axial T1-weighted MR arthrogram.

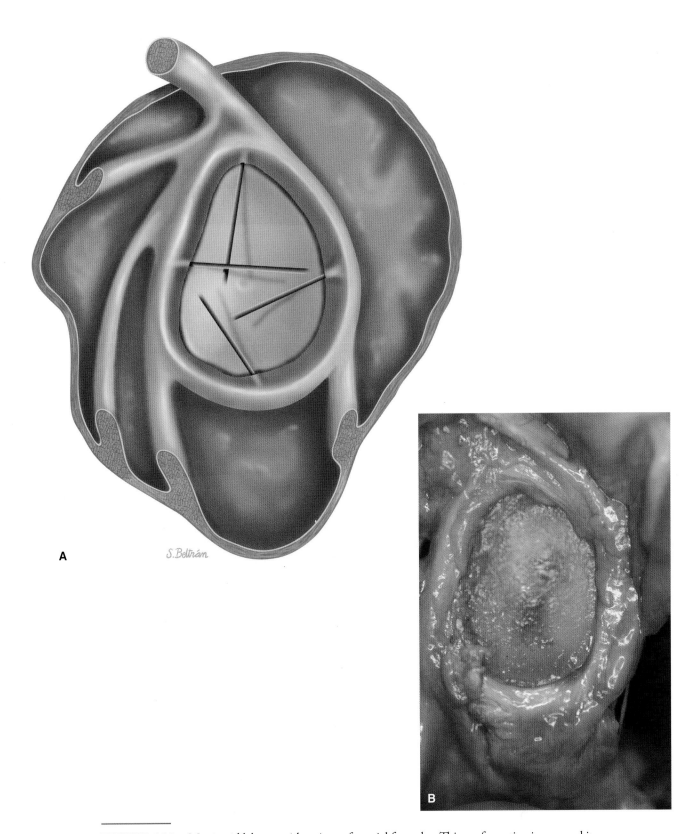

S.Beltrán

A

B

FIGURE 4.22 Meniscoid labrum with a circumferential free edge. This configuration is rare, and it is unusual to visualize an unattached free margin involving the inferior labrum on MR studies. Fluid between the inferior labrum and glenoid articular cartilage on coronal MR images thus represents labral tearing. (**A**) Lateral color illustration with probing of the free labral margin. (**B**) Corresponding gross specimen of meniscoid labrum.

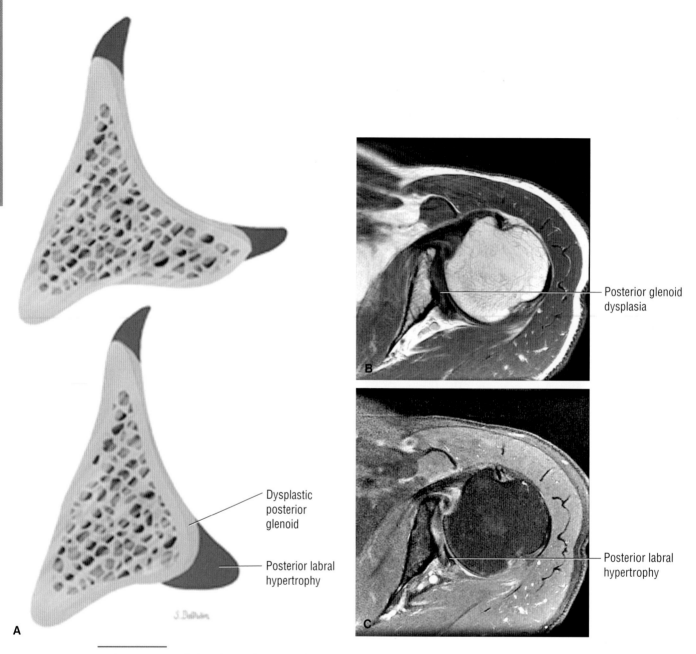

FIGURE 4.23 (**A**) Color axial section of normal posterior glenoid rim (top) compared to severe dysplastic posterior glenoid rim (bottom) with compensatory posterior labral hypertrophy. Axial T1 FSE (**B**) and axial FS PD FSE (**C**) images with severe posterior glenoid hypoplasia with thickened glenoid articular cartilage and posterior glenoid labral hypertrophy.

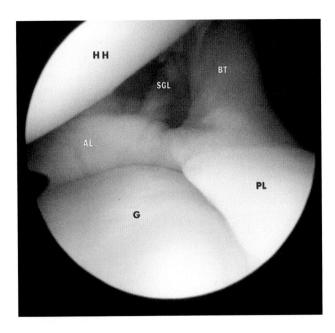

FIGURE 4.24 The biceps tendon (BT) contributes to the superior anterior labrum (AL) and the superior posterior labrum (PL) in the BLC. One component of the LHBT attaches to the supraglenoid tubercle. Extraarticular fibers attach to the lateral edge of the base of the coracoid process. The intraarticular portion of the LHBT is oriented at an approximate right angle to the surface of the glenoid (G). HH, humeral head; SGL, superior glenohumeral ligament.

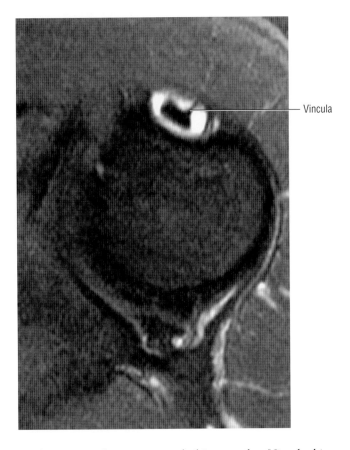

FIGURE 4.25 Vinculae biceps extending anterior to the biceps tendon. Vinculae biceps are small strands of mesentary-like synovium that extend from the biceps tendon to the adjacent synovium and capsule. Axial FS PD FSE image.

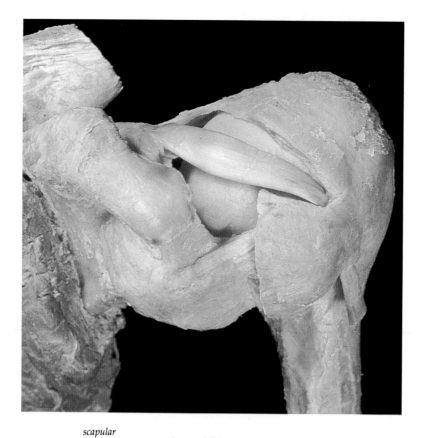

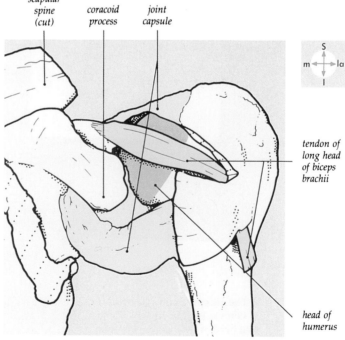

FIGURE 4.26   Removal of part of the shoulder joint capsule reveals the intracapsular but extrasynovial tendon of the long head of the biceps brachii.

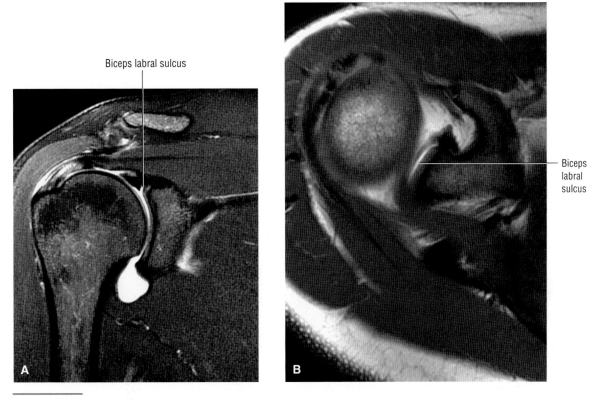

Biceps labral sulcus

Biceps labral sulcus

FIGURE 4.36 Type 2 BLC with normal superior sulcus on coronal FS PD (**A**) and axial PD (**B**) images with intraarticular contrast. This sulcus should not be mistaken for detachment of the superior labrum. Because the normal fluid-filled sulcus is seen in cross-section on axial images the diagnosis of SLAP tear should be restricted to review of coronal images only. The sulcus allows the superior labrum to function as an unconstrained extension of the upper glenoid fossa.

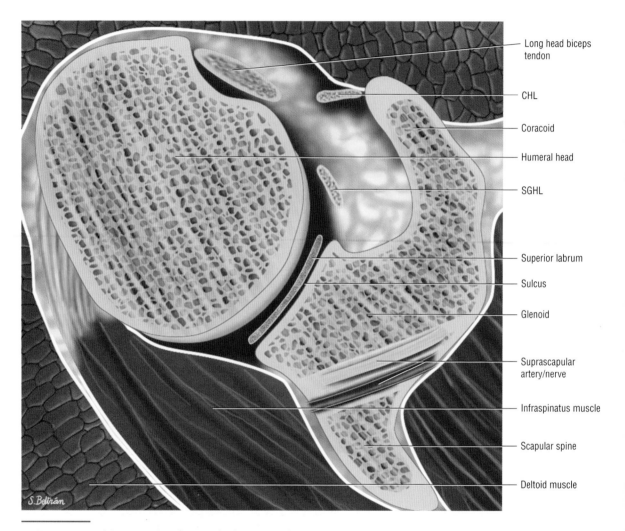

Long head biceps tendon

CHL

Coracoid

Humeral head

SGHL

Superior labrum

Sulcus

Glenoid

Suprascapular artery/nerve

Infraspinatus muscle

Scapular spine

Deltoid muscle

FIGURE 4.37   Type 2 BLC with normal sulcus on axial color cross-section. This sulcus should not be mistaken for detachment of the superior labrum. Although an extensive SLAP 2 lesion may be visualized in the axial plane it is more common for the axial image to section through the normal/biceps labral sulcus.

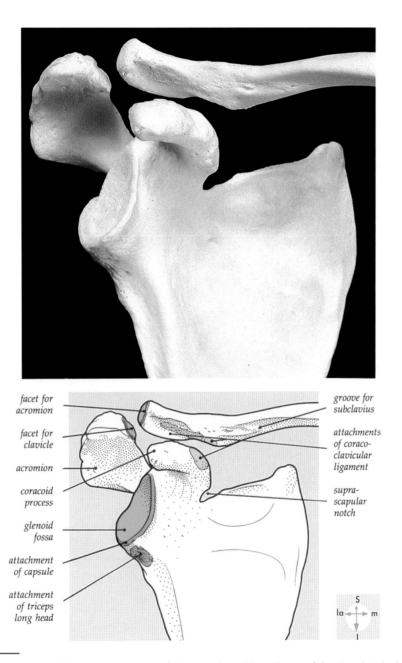

facet for
acromion

facet for
clavicle

acromion

coracoid
process

glenoid
fossa

attachment
of capsule

attachment
of triceps
long head

groove for
subclavius

attachments
of coraco-
clavicular
ligament

supra-
scapular
notch

S
la ← → m
I

FIGURE 4.38　An oblique anterior view of the scapula and lateral part of the clavicle. The bones have been separated to show the articular surfaces of the AC joint and the sites of attachment of the coracoclavicular ligament. The small area of the AC joint results in high AC joint stresses and potential compressive failure of the distal clavicle when subjected to increased compressive loads as transmittal by the humerus. Weightlifters may develop osteolysis of the distal clavicle for this reason.

Glenohumeral Ligaments Unifying Perspective

■ While the IGLLC has received much of the focus in understanding the relationship between the anterior band and the anterior labrum, a more global overview of the glenohumeral capsule requires appreciating the role and link that exists between the superior and inferior capsuloligamentous structures.[182]

Superior Capsuloligamentous Complex

■ Superior glenohumeral ligament

■ Coracohumeral ligament

■ Posterosuperior glenohumeral ligament

■ Coracoglenoid ligament

■ Transverse band (previous terminology) or rotator cable as an extension of the coracohumeral ligament

Inferior Glenohumeral Ligament Complex

■ Anterior band

■ Posterior band

■ Axillary pouch

■ Fasciculus obliquus

Link Between Superior and Inferior Complexes

■ Circular system

    ■ The glenoid labrum on the medial side

■ Semicircular system on the humeral side

    ■ Rotator cuff tendons

    ■ Fasciculus obliquus

    ■ Transverse band or rotator cable

■ Two diagonal cross-links

    ■ Fasciculus obliquus

    ■ Middle glenohumeral ligament

Function of Glenohumeral Capsular Labral Structures

- Superior complex
    - Acts as primary restraint in adduction
- Inferior complex
    - Primary restraint in abduction
- Stabilization of the long head of the biceps tendon through ligamentous reinforcements that form the biceps pulley as contributed by the superior capsuloligamentous complex
- Glenohumeral ligaments
    - Static stabilizers of the glenohumeral joint
    - Restraining effect at the extremes of motion
- Capsuloligamentous restraint to translation
    - Coracohumeral and superior glenohumeral ligaments
        - Against inferior translation in lower ranges of abduction as primary restraint
        - Secondary restraint against anterior translation and external rotation
- Middle glenohumeral ligament
    - Against anterior translation in the midrange of abduction
    - Secondary against inferior translation and external rotation
    - To limit external rotation rotation in the lower range of motion in abduction
- Inferior glenohumeral ligament
    - Anterior band restrains internal rotation.
    - Posterior band restrains internal rotation and forward flexion.
    - Secondary restraint against inferior translation in midrange of abduction
    - Limits abduction and external rotation
- Posterior capsule
    - Functions to limit posterior translation
    - Limits internal rotation during abduction
- Glenoid labrum as an indirect stabilizer against dislocation
    - Augmentation of glenoid fossa articular arc length from anterior to posterior

- Contributing to glenoid fossa-humeral head concavity-compression
- Maintaining negative intraarticular pressure
- The labrum serves as the anchor or point of direct attachment of the capsuloligmentous complex.[182]

The Superior, Middle, and Inferior Glenohumeral Ligaments

- The glenohumeral ligaments (superior, middle, and inferior)
  - Are thickened bands of the anterior joint capsule with attachments to both glenoid margins and the proximal humerus[138]
  - The normally lax ligaments are check reins on extremes of motion for the glenohumeral joint.[407]

Inferior Glenohumeral Ligament (IGHL or IGL)

- The Inferior Glenohumeral Ligament Complex (IGLC)
  - Largest and most important of the glenohumeral ligaments
  - Originates from either the glenoid labrum or glenoid neck and inserts onto the humeral neck at the periphery of the articular margin
  - Inserts onto the anatomic neck of the humerus in one of two configurations[420,623]:
    - Collar-like or V-shaped attachment
- The IGHL
  - Consists of anterior and posterior bands and an intervening axillary pouch, which have a role in anterior-posterior and superior-inferior instability. The fasciculus obliquus also contributes to the medial side of this complex.
    - The anterior band
      - Origin is located near the 3 o'clock position (2 to 4 o'clock) in the glenoid of the right shoulder[420,623]
      - Forms the anterior labrum at the medial attachment of the IGHL to the glenoid
        - Attaches to the labrum variably at or above the mid-glenoid notch
      - Fans out and supports the humeral head anteriorly, while the posterior band stabilizes the joint posteriorly

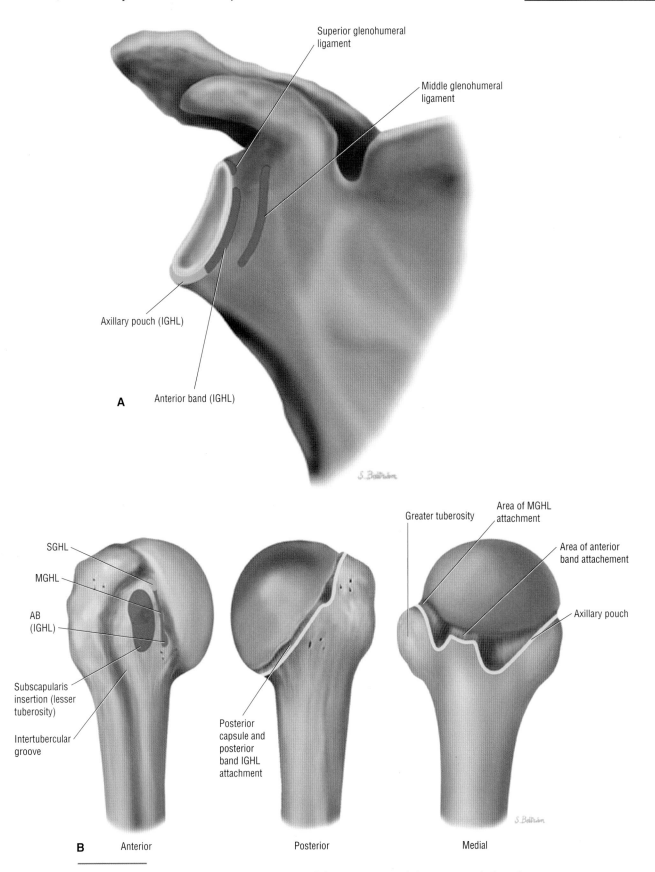

FIGURE 4.39 (**A**) The glenoid attachments of the anterior capsule ligaments including the superior glenohumeral ligament (SGHL or SGL), the middle glenohumeral ligament (MGHL or MGL), the anterior band of inferior glenohumeral ligament (IGHL or IGL), and the axillary pouch of IGHL. (**B**) Glenohumeral capsular and ligament attachments in anterior, posterior, and medial humeral projections. (**A** and **B** based on Detrisac DJ, Johnson LL. Biceps and subscapularis tendons. In: Detrisac DJ, Johnson LL, eds. *Arthroscopic Shoulder Anatomy: Pathologic and Surgical Implications.* Thorofare, NJ: Slack; 1986:21–34.)

▦ The posterior band

- Origin is located near the 9 o'clock (7 to 9 o'clock) position in the glenoid of the right shoulder

- Contributes to the formation of the posterior labrum

- Fans out and supports the humeral head posteriorly with the anterior band moving under the humeral head with internal rotation of the abducted arm

▦ The axillary pouch

- Located between the anterior and posterior bands; formed by medial part of the fasciculus obliquus on the glenoid side

- Extends inferior to the body of the glenohumeral joint as a redundancy of thickened capsular tissue

- Attaches to the inferior two thirds of the entire circumference of the glenoid by means of the labrum[420,573]

- Lax with the arm by the patient's side in the adducted position (as also shown with the anterior and posterior bands)

▦ Primary restraint for anterior and posterior dislocations at 90° of abduction[619]

▦ Lax in adduction and taut in abduction and external rotation

▦ Tightens with increasing abduction and the anterior and posterior bands move superiorly with respect to the humeral head

▦ Functions as a hammock, cradling the humeral head with increasing abduction[447]

- Different portions of the complex support the humeral head both anteriorly and posteriorly during 90° of abduction with internal and external rotation.[535]

▦ The fasciculus obliquus extends from the glenoid (5 to 7 o'clock) anteriorly and merges with the subscapularis tendon and the MGHL.

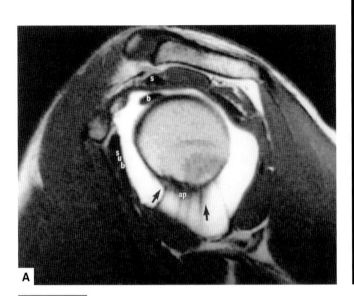

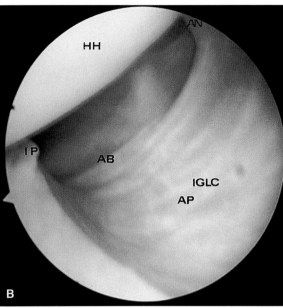

FIGURE 4.40 (**A**) The axillary pouch of the IGHL is seen on a T1-weighted sagittal MR arthrogram. Arrows and ap, axillary pouch of IGHL; b, biceps tendon; s, supraspinatus tendon; sub, subscapularis tendon. (**B**) The IGHL complex. An arthroscopic photograph shows the anterior band (AB) and axillary pouch (AP) components of the inferior glenohumeral ligament complex (IGLC). The inferior pole of the glenoid (IP) and the anatomic neck attachments of the IGLC (AN) are shown as viewed from the axillary pouch. HH, humeral head.

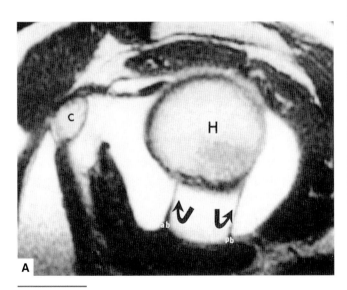

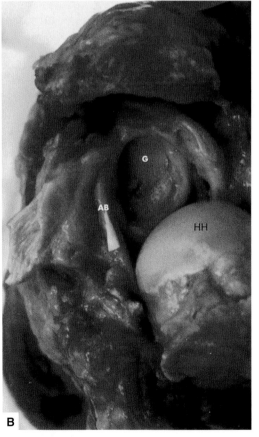

FIGURE 4.41 (**A**) The anterior band (ab) and posterior band (pb) of the IGHL (*curved arrows*) extend from the glenoid origin to the humeral attachment, as seen on an enhanced T1-weighted sagittal (oblique) image. C, coracoid; H, humeral head. (**B**) On a gross shoulder specimen, the superior course of the anterior band (AB) of the IGHL is identified (*triangular marker*). The glenoid (G) and humeral head (HH) are also identified.

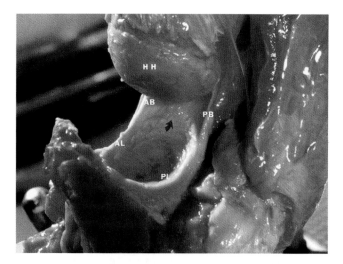

FIGURE 4.42   A gross shoulder specimen illustrates the structure of the inferior glenohumeral ligament (IGL) complex. With abduction of the humerus, the IGL structures are more prominent and taut in position. Coronal oblique MR images routinely show the lax axillary pouch of the IGL when the humerus is in the adducted position. Curved arrow, axillary pouch; AB, anterior band; AL, anterior labrum; HH, humeral head; PB, posterior band; PL, posterior labrum.

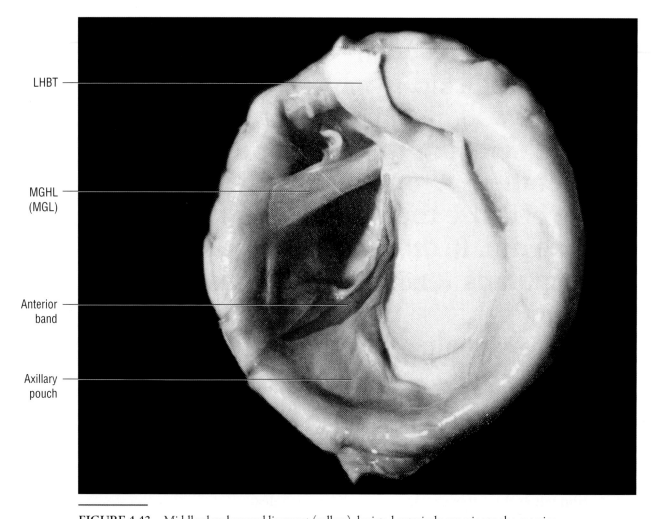

LHBT

MGHL
(MGL)

Anterior
band

Axillary
pouch

FIGURE 4.43   Middle glenohumeral ligament (yellow) depicted anteriorly superior to the anterior band (red) of the inferior glenohumeral ligament as it extends superiorly toward the biceps (blue) labral complex. Superior glenohumeral ligament in green anterior to LHBT. The anterior band attaches high replacing the anterior labrum above the equator. In contrast Figure 4.42 the anterior band is continuous with the anterior labrum at the equator. (Modified from DePalma AF. *Surgery of the Shoulder*. 3rd ed. Philadelphia, PA: JB Lippincott; 1983.)

Middle Glenohumeral Ligament (MGHL or MGL)

- The Middle Glenohumeral Ligament (MGHL or MGL)

    - Attaches to the anterior aspect of the anatomic neck of the humerus, medial to the lesser tuberosity[138]

    - Arises from the glenoid via the labrum and scapular neck

    - Passes across the subscapularis tendon and can be identified between the subscapularis tendon and the anterior labrum or anterior band of the IGHL

        - MGHL crosses the subscapularis tendon at an angle of 45 degrees.

    - The foramen of Weitbrecht

        - Located between the superior and middle glenohumeral ligaments

    - The foramen of Rouviere

        - Located between the middle and inferior glenohumeral ligaments

    - Demonstrates the greatest variation in size and thickness of the three glenohumeral ligaments[63]

        - DePalma originally described a poorly defined or absent MGHL in 30% of shoulders studied.[137]

    - Variation exists as thin ligamentous morphology or cord-like and as thick as the biceps tendon.

    - Role in the stability of the shoulder joint from 0° to 45° of abduction[63,535]

        - Contributes to anterior stability at 45° abduction, along with the subscapularis tendon and the superior part of the IGHL[604]

        - Limits external rotation in the lower to middle ranges of abduction

    - Secondary role in anterior stability of the shoulder in 90° of abduction when the anterior band of the IGHL is released[519]

    - Demonstrates a more vertical orientation with internal rotation

    - Assumes a more horizontal orientation with external rotation (elongation of the MGHL)

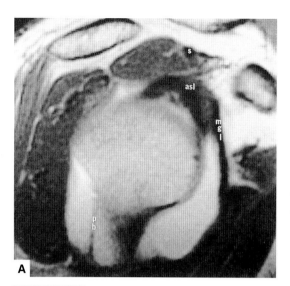

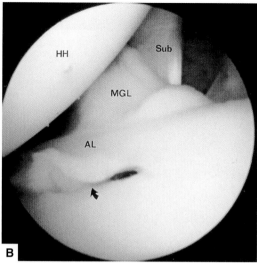

FIGURE 4.44 (**A**) A T1-weighted sagittal oblique arthrogram shows the attachment of the MGL (mgl) to the anterior superior glenoid labrum (asl). The MGL arises from the labrum below the superior glenohumeral ligament and from the neck of the scapula. The humeral attachment of the MGL is located medial to the lesser tuberosity. Normal variants of the MGL include the ligament arising only from the labrum or having no attachment to it. pb, posterior band of IGL; s, supraspinatus tendon. (**B**) Arthroscopic view of the middle glenohumeral ligament (MGL) anterior to the anterior labrum (AL) and posterior to the subscapularis tendon (Sub). An anterior superior quadrant sublabral foramen (*curved arrow*) exists as a normal variant although exists as a result of a high AB attachment. HH, humeral head.

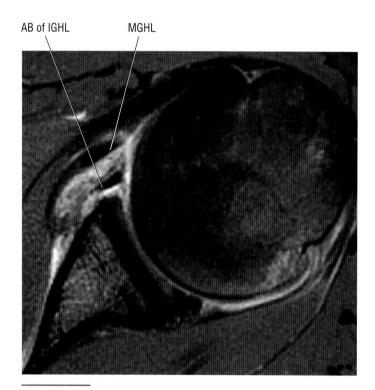

FIGURE 4.45 The anterior band (AB) is posterior to the subscapularis tendon and the MGHL. The AB is attenuated at the equator and absent in the anterosuperior quadrant. There is synovitis located between the MGHL and the AB. Axial FS PD FSE image.

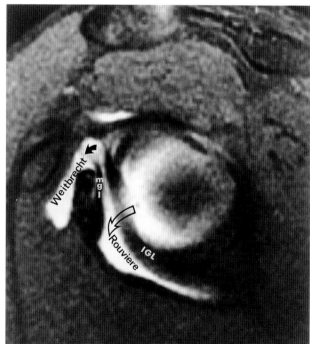

FIGURE 4.46 Normal foramen of Weitbrecht (*solid curved arrow*) is shown between the middle glenohumeral ligament (MGL) and the superior glenohumeral ligament. The foramen of Rouviere (*open curved arrow*) is located between the MGL and the inferior glenohumeral ligament (IGL).

Capsular Insertion Types (Relative to IGHL and MGHL)

- Three types of capsular insertions originally proposed:

    - Type 1 inserts near the anterior labrum.

    - Types 2 and 3 insert more broadly or medially on the scapular neck.[662]

        - These types of insertions, in fact, represent normal variations in the size and morphology of the subscapularis bursa and are dependent on the rotation of the shoulder.

            - With internal rotation, the recess is large and the capsule appears to insert more medially on the scapular neck.

            - Size variation of the subscapularis bursa is not the result of stripping of the capsule.

        - In a type 3 capsular insertion, the appearance of an anterior pouch does not predispose to anterior humeral subluxation or dislocation in this potential space.

        - However, medial to the subscapularis tendon and at the level of the IGHL, there may be stretching of the capsular complex in patients with a history of anterior dislocations.

            - It may be difficult to appreciate intraligamentous stretching of the IGHL in the absence of direct visualization of a tear or avulsion of the IGHL.

- Capsular elasticity and joint volume do not contribute to anterior shoulder instability.[543,565]

    - Recurrent dislocations do not produce irreversible capsular distention.

- Capsular tearing and or stripping that occurs with macroinstability does need to be addressed at the time of Bankart repair.

    - The inferior and medial displacement of the IGL associated with a Bankart lesion produces an inferior ALPSA-like morphology (in the coronal plane) of the labroligamentous complex.

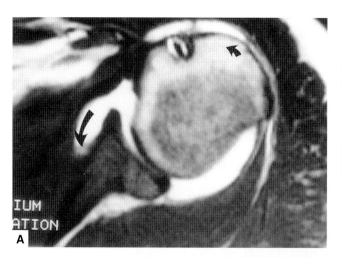

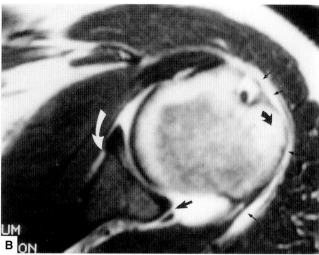

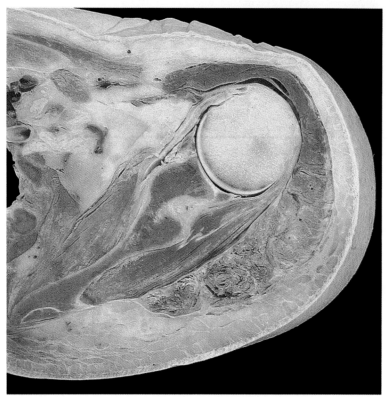

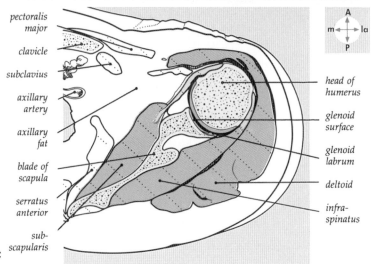

pectoralis major

clavicle

subclavius

axillary artery

axillary fat

blade of scapula

serratus anterior

sub-scapularis

head of humerus

glenoid surface

glenoid labrum

deltoid

infra-spinatus

C

FIGURE 4.47   Normal variation in morphology of the subscapularis bursa is seen with (**A**) internal rotation and (**B**) external rotation on gadolinium-enhanced T1-weighted axial images. The subscapularis bursa has the appearance of a type 3 capsular insertion (*long black curved arrow*) in internal rotation (*short black curved arrow*) and a type 1 capsular insertion (*long curved white arrow*) in external rotation (*short black curved arrow*). Gadolinium contrast between the posterior band of the IGHL and the posterior labrum (*large straight black arrow*) and gadolinium contrast lateral to the humeral head in the subacromial bursa (*small straight black arrows*) are indicated. (**C**) A transverse section at the level of the humeral head shows the relations of the glenohumeral joint.

Synovial Recesses

- Six anatomic types of the capsule based on the topographic arrangements of the synovial recesses with respect to the glenohumeral ligaments[137,420]

    - MGHL morphology determines the type of synovial recess.

- The six types of synovial recesses are best assessed on fluid sensitive sagittal oblique images where the MGHL and IGHL can be identified.

- Original work of DePalma (without the benefit of arthroscopy) did not identify the role of capsular variations as the result of a high attachment of the anterior band of the IGHL.

Superior Glenohumeral Ligament Complex (Superior Complex)

- Components of the superior complex (superior capsuloligamentous structure)

    - Superior glenohumeral ligament

    - Coracohumeral ligament

    - Coracoglenoid ligament

    - Posterosuperior glenohumeral ligament

    - Rotator cable or transverse band

- Superior capsule concept as a series of integrated structures

    - Anterior limb consisting of the coracohumeral, superior glenohumeral, and coracoglenoid ligaments

    - Posterior limb formed by the posterosuperior glenohumeral ligament

    - Anterior and posterior limbs fuse into the rotator cable or transverse band just proximal to their anterior and posterior attachment to the humerus.[182]

        - Superior ligaments merge with supraspinatus and infraspinatus tendons at the level of the rotator cable (transverse band).

- The functional unit of the coracoglenohumeral ligament represents the variable merging of three superior structures consisting of:
    - The coracohumeral ligament
    - The superior glenohumeral ligament
    - The coracoglenoid ligament
- The superior complex can be divided into the following categories:
    - Coracoglenohumeral ligament
        - Coracohumeral ligament
        - Superior glenohumeral ligament
        - Coracoglenoid ligament
    - Posterosuperior glenohumeral ligament
    - Rotator cable (transverse ligament)
- The rotator cuff interval and the biceps pulley are considered additional components of the superior complex.
    - The superior complex through its ligamentous reinforcements assist in stabilizing the long head of the biceps tendon.
        - Through the formation of the biceps pulley in the rotator cuff interval
- MR imaging in the axial plane can be used to identify multiple structures of the superior complex that exist between the plane of the supraspinatus muscle and the biceps tendon.
    - Because of the structures' course in more than one plane, not all the structures of the superior complex can be visualized on a single axial image.

Superior Glenohumeral Ligament (SGHL or SGL)

- Subdivided into direct fibers that course from the supraglenoid tubercle area to the lesser tuberosity and oblique fibers that cross superficial to the LHBT and contribute to reinforcing the rotator cable (transverse ligament) extension of the CH ligament
- Smallest of the glenohumeral capsular structures[138]
- Originates from the upper pole of the glenoid cavity and base of the coracoid process

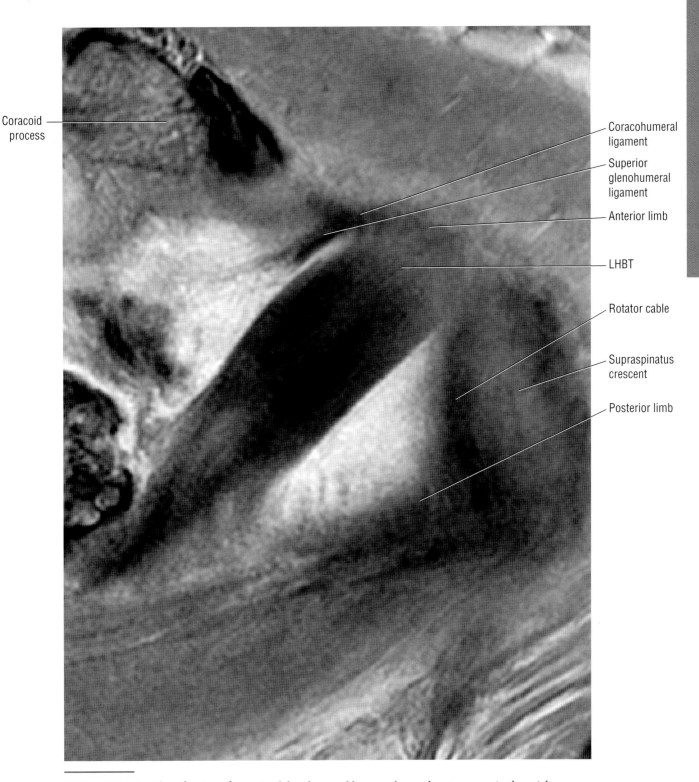

Coracoid process

Coracohumeral ligament

Superior glenohumeral ligament

Anterior limb

LHBT

Rotator cable

Supraspinatus crescent

Posterior limb

FIGURE 4.48 Identification of superior (glenohumeral ligament) complex structures in the axial plane on an FS PD FSE image at the superior surface of the LHBT. The rotator cable and its contribution from the posterior limb as formed by the posterosuperior glenohumeral ligament are shown. In addition, the coracoid process, coracohumeral ligament, superior glenohumeral ligament, and anterior limb component are also indicated as well as the region of the supraspinatus crescent laterally as it attaches to the greater tuberosity.

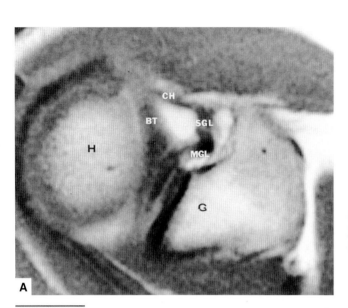
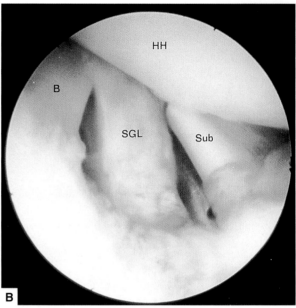

FIGURE 4.49   (A) The superior glenohumeral ligament (SGHL) is seen on an enhanced T1-weighted axial image above the level of the coracoid. The extraarticular coracohumeral ligament (CH) and intraarticular SGHL are closely related. The middle portion of the CH crosses the SGHL. The SGHL is oriented perpendicular to the middle glenohumeral ligament (MGL) as shown. BT, biceps tendon; G, glenoid; H, humeral head. (B) Arthroscopic photograph (posterior view) showing the lateral location of the biceps (B) relative to the superior glenohumeral ligament (SGHL). HH, humeral head; Sub, subscapularis tendon.

- ■ SGHL attaches to the MGHL, the biceps tendon, and the labrum.

- ■ Inserts just superior to the lesser tuberosity in the region of the bicipital groove[63]

- ■ Closely related to the extraarticular coracohumeral ligament, which originates in the lateral aspect of the coaracoid and inserts on the greater tuberosity

- ■ The SGHL and the coracohumeral ligament contribute to the stabilization of the glenohumeral joint and prevent posterior and inferior translation of the humeral head.

- ■ Represents the primary capsuloligamentous restraint to inferior translation of the unloaded, abducted shoulder

- ■ Disruption of the SGHL may be associated with a Hill-Sachs lesion that engages with the shoulder in a position of less than 45 degrees.

- ■ The SGHL (floor of the pulley) and CHL (roof of the pulley through the medial fibers of the CHL) have an important role in forming the biceps pulley of the rotator cuff interval.[63,626]

    - ■ Pulley floor consists of fibers from the posterior aspect of the subscapularis which blend with parts of the SGHL and CHL.

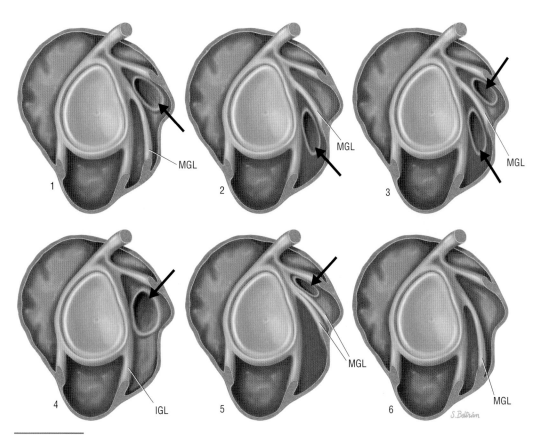

FIGURE 4.50 Six arrangements of synovial recesses (i.e., joint capsule variations, *arrows*) are described by DePalma. Type 1: One synovial recess exists above the middle glenohumeral ligament. Type 2: One synovial recess exists below the middle glenohumeral ligament. Type 3: Two synovial recesses exist, with a superior subscapular recess above the middle glenohumeral ligament and an inferior subscapular recess below the middle glenohumeral ligament. Type 4: No middle glenohumeral ligament. Type 5: The middle glenohumeral ligament exists as two small synovial folds. Type 6: Complete absence of synovial recesses.

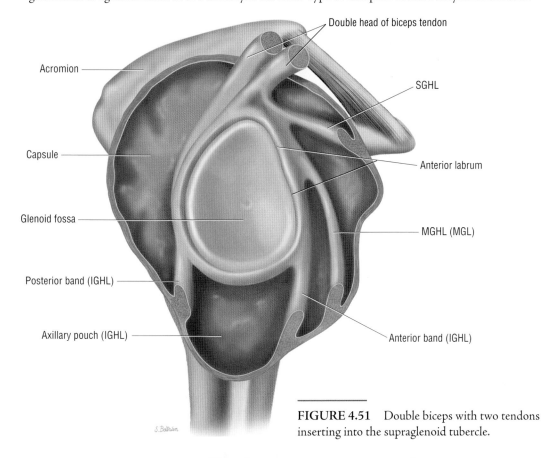

FIGURE 4.51 Double biceps with two tendons inserting into the supraglenoid tubercle.

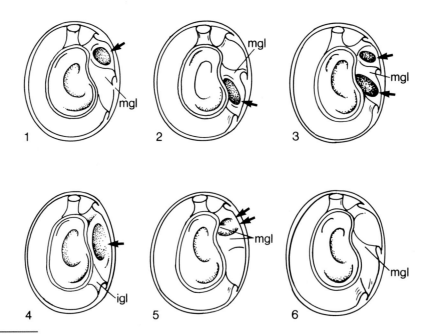

FIGURE 4.52   Six arrangements of synovial recesses (i.e., joint capsule variations, *arrows*) are described by DePalma. Type 1: One synovial recess exists above the middle glenohumeral ligament. Type 2: One synovial recess exists below the middle glenohumeral ligament. Type 3: Two synovial recesses exist, with a superior subscapular recess above the middle glenohumeral ligament and an inferior subscapular recess below the middle glenohumeral ligament. Type 4: No middle glenohumeral ligament is present, and one large synovial recess exists above the inferior glenohumeral ligament. Type 5: The middle glenohumeral ligament exists as two small synovial folds. Type 6: Complete absence of synovial recesses. (From DePalma AF. *Surgery of the Shoulder*. 3rd ed. Philadelphia, PA: JB Lippincott; 1983.)

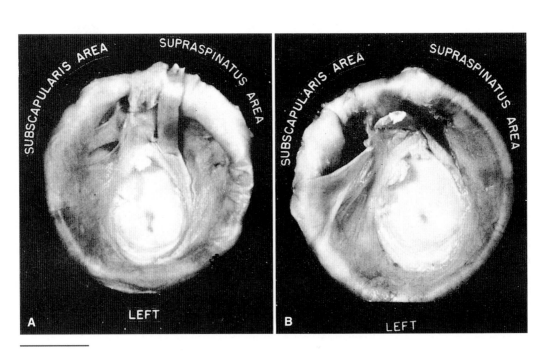

FIGURE 4.53   (**A**) Small synovial recesses above and below the middle glenohumeral ligament. (**B**) Large synovial recess above the middle ligament. This recess may be interpreted erroneously as a rent in the capsule. (From DePalma AF. *Surgery of the Shoulder*. 3rd ed. Philadelphia, PA: JB Lippincott; 1983, with permission.)

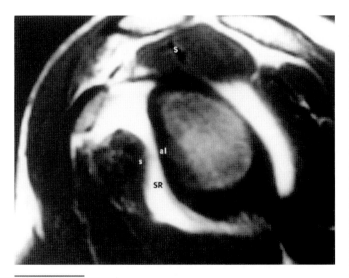

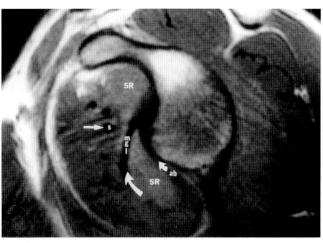

FIGURE 4.54 A single type 4 synovial recess. T1-weighted sagittal oblique arthrogram displays absence of the middle glenohumeral ligament, resulting in one large synovial recess above the inferior glenohumeral ligament. S, supraspinatus tendon; SR, synovial recess; s, subscapularis tendon.

FIGURE 4.55 Sagittal MR image with two synovial recesses. Synovial recesses are present above and below the middle glenohumeral ligament. SR, synovial recess; S, subscapularis; mgl, middle glenohumeral ligament; ab, anterior band; straight arrow, subscapularis tendon; small curved arrow, superior course of mgl; large curved arrow, superior course of anterior band.

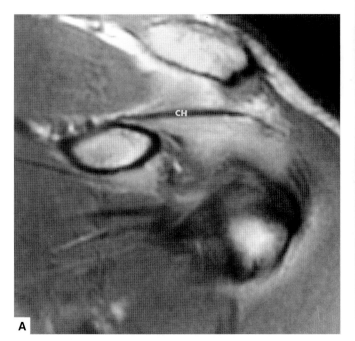

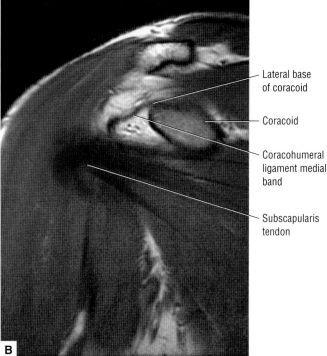

FIGURE 4.56 Coronal PD-weighted images showing (**A**) the lateral band of the coracohumeral ligament inserting on the greater tuberosity and anterior border of the supraspinatus and (**B**) the medial band of the coracohumeral ligament inserting on the lesser tuberosity, the superior fibers of the subscapularis, and the transverse ligament.

Coracohumeral Ligament (CHL)

- Originates in the lateral aspect of the base of the coracoid inferior to the origin of the coracohumeral ligament

- Inserts on the greater tuberosity on the lateral aspect of the bicipital groove[63]

- Overlies and is superficial to the SGHL at the anterior superior aspect of the shoulder

- Contributes to the restraint of inferior translation in external rotation in the abducted shoulder[119]

- Consists of both medial and lateral fibers
  - The medial fibers contribute to the biceps pulley and assist in the stabilization of the LHBT.[301]

- Sagittal images through the midportion of the rotator interval demonstrate the initial formation of the biceps pulley with a T-shaped junction between the CHL (forming the roof) and SGHL (forming the floor) of the pulley or biceps sling.
  - The anterior aspect of the biceps sling represents the confluence of the CHL and SGHL, which provides restraint to medial subluxation of the biceps tendon.

Coracoglenoid Ligament

- Origin superior or posterior surface of coracoid process between the limbs of the acromioclavicular ligament

- Inserts posterior to supraglenoid tubercle

- Corresponds to the superior medial border of the rotator cuff interval

- Receives fiber contribution from the pectoralis minor

Posterosuperior Glenohumeral Ligament

- Origin posterosuperior glenoid neck
  - Medial to the labrum
  - Medial and posterior to the origin of the LHBT

- Merges with circular system of linking fibers medial to the labrum and secondary insertion occurs with infraspinatus tendon to the greater tuberosity

Functional Role of the Superior Glenohumeral Ligament Complex Including the Cable

- The rotator cable provides stress shielding with rotator crescent.
    - To thinner capsular tissue
    - To rotator cuff tendons
    - Stress is transferred from the cuff to the cable.
    - Stress shielding effect is more evident and is important in older individuals to preserve cuff function.

- The coracoglenohumeral and posterosuperior glenohumeral ligaments
    - Create the medial anchorage for the cable

- The superior complex through its four-point attachment and its lateral extension in its anterior and posterior limbs
    - Allows for reciprocal tightening during rotation

- The superior complex functions as a suspension sling for the humeral head analogous to the hammock formed by the inferior glenohumeral ligament.

- The superior complex is effective as a primary restraint in adduction.
    - Secondary restraint in abduction which is the opposite of the function of the inferior glenohumeral complex

- There is synergy (reciprocal functional motion) between the superior capsuloligamentous complex and the inferior glenohumeral ligament complex.
    - Since the IGLC works in the opposite fashion
        - Primary restraint in abduction
        - Secondary restraint in adduction[182]

Posterior Capsule

- The posterior capsule
    - Includes the capsule posterior to the biceps tendon and superior to the posterior band of the IGHL
        - Represents the thinnest portion of the capsule[63,431]
    - Has a role in limiting both posterior and anterior translation of the glenohumeral joint
    - Torn in the reverse HAGL lesion[554]
    - Posterior dislocation does not occur with an intact anterior capsule, even with the division of the posterior capsule.[501]

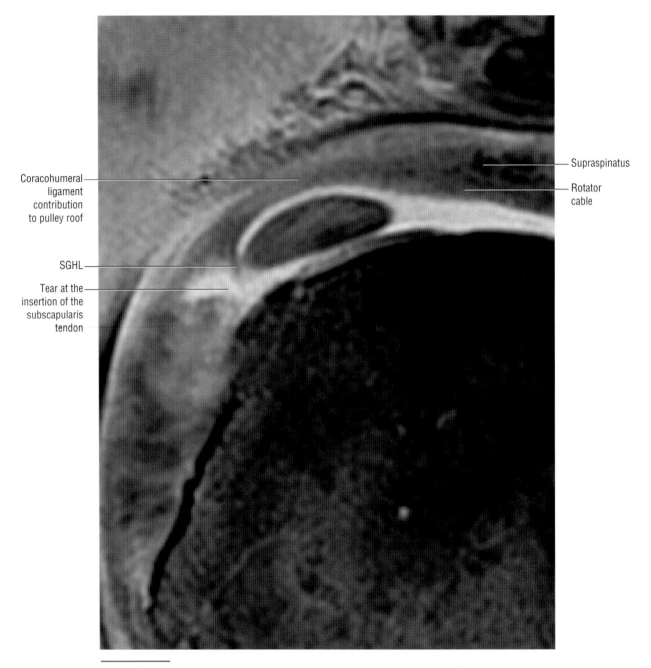

Coracohumeral
ligament
contribution
to pulley roof

SGHL

Tear at the
insertion of the
subscapularis
tendon

Supraspinatus

Rotator
cable

FIGURE 4.57   The SGHL forms a semicircular anterior support for the lateral aspect of the intraarticular long head of the biceps tendon (LHBT) in the rotator interval. The rotator interval represents the space between the anterior border of the supraspinatus tendon and the superior border of the subscapularis tendon. The subscapularis tendon inserts onto the lesser tuberosity anterior to the SGHL. There is a transition zone, however located laterally at the proximal bicipital groove where posterior fibers of the subscapularis tendon, anterior fibers of the SGHL and some fibers of the ventral CH ligament interdigitate at their insertion. Sagittal FS PD FSE image.

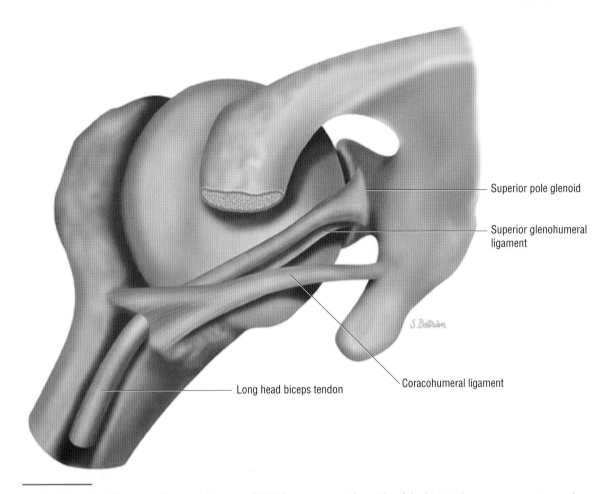

Superior pole glenoid

Superior glenohumeral ligament

Coracohumeral ligament

Long head biceps tendon

FIGURE 4.58 The coracohumeral ligament (CHL) inserts on either side of the bicipital groove rotator interval. The CHL and the superior glenohumeral ligament help stabilize the biceps tendon by forming a biceps pulley.

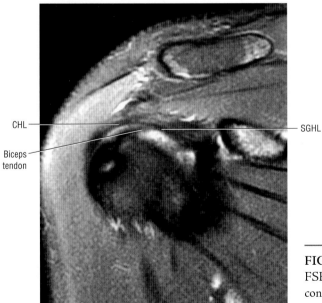

CHL

Biceps tendon

SGHL

FIGURE 4.59 An anterior coronal FS PD FSE image demonstrates the biceps tendon contained between the CHL and SGHL components of the biceps pulley.

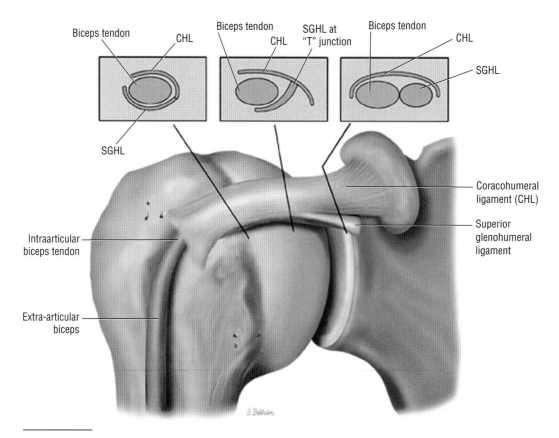

FIGURE 4.60   The biceps pulley complex is sectioned in the sagittal plane at the level of the proximal, middle, and distal rotator cuff interval. The confluence of the CHL and SGHL occurs at the middle and distal aspects of the rotator interval. A T-shaped junction is formed between the SGHL and CHL at the mid-interval, superior to the humeral head. An anterior U-shaped sling is shown at the distal interval at the entrance to the bicipital groove.

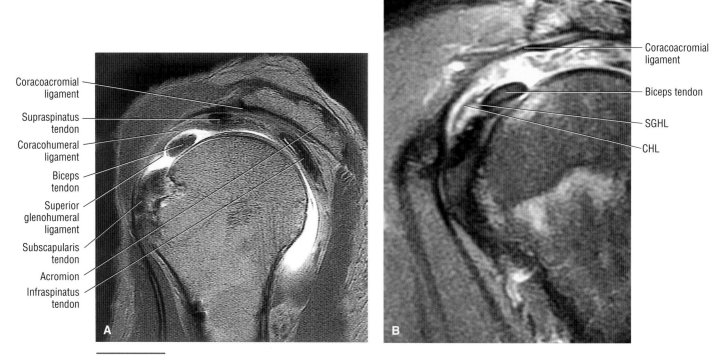

FIGURE 4.61   Sagittal MR arthrograms. (**A,B**) The T-shaped junction of the SGHL and CHL at the midportion of the rotator cuff interval.

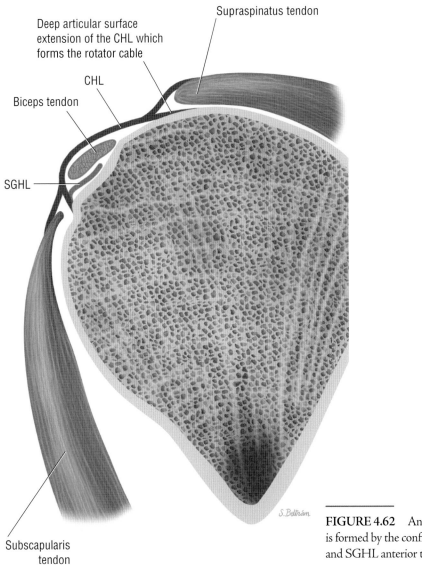

Deep articular surface
extension of the CHL which
forms the rotator cable

Supraspinatus tendon

CHL

Biceps tendon

SGHL

Subscapularis
tendon

S.Beltrán

FIGURE 4.62 Anterior biceps sling is formed by the confluence of the CHL and SGHL anterior to the LHBT.

Rotator Cuff

- The supraspinatus, infraspinatus, teres minor, and subscapularis muscles constitute the rotator cuff.

    - The rotator cuff's function is to centralize the humeral head, limiting superior translation during abduction.[546] Supraspinatus and infraspinatus are responsible for glenohumeral resting stability.

    - The supraspinatus, infraspinatus, and teres minor tendons insert on the greater tuberosity.

        - Tendons fuse into a single tendinous structure near their insertion to the tuberosity.

        - Supraspinatus and infraspinatus tendons join 15mm proximal to their insertion.

- The subscapularis tendon inserts on the lesser tuberosity.[229]
  - Greatest force-producing capacity
  - Role in glenohumeral stability in the position of apprehension
  - Teres minor and infraspinatus muscles merge proximal to the musculotendinous junction.

- The rotator cable is a condensation of articular-sided tissue.
  - The cable extends from anterior to posterior across the supraspinatus and infraspinatus insertions.[106]
  - The attachment points of the rotator cable:
    - Posterior cable attachment
      - Attachment of the lower infraspinatus
    - Anterior cable attachment
      - Bifurcates at superior bicipital groove[182]
      - Anterior attachment to supraspinatus and upper attachment to subscapularis

- The rotator crescent is the area at risk for most rotator cuff tears.
  - The crescent spans the conjoined tendon insertion lateral to the cable.[546]

- The supraspinatus muscle
  - Exists primarily in the supraspinatus fossa
  - Superior stabilizer of the humeral head against impingement on the undersurface (inferior surface) of the acromion
  - Insertion on both greater tuberosity and lesser tuberosity (through an accessory insertion)
  - Anterior edge forms superior border of rotator cuff interval.
  - Fusiform larger anterior muscle belly with intramuscular tendinous core
    - Proximal to the tendon insertion, the intratendinous supraspinatus tendon thickens and continues laterally toward the greater tuberosity as a tubular-shaped extramuscular tendon.

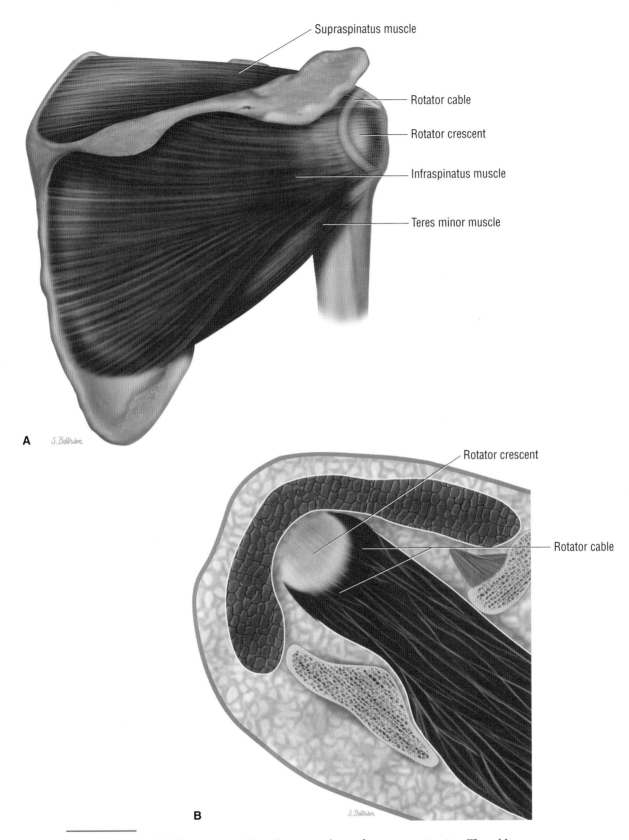

FIGURE 4.63 (A) The rotator cable and crescent shown from a posterior view. The cable represents thickened capsular tissue from the articular side of the cuff connecting the anterior and posterior tendon edges of the tendinous portion of the rotator cuff. An extension of the coracohumeral ligament contributes to the cable. The rotator crescent, especially the lateral portion of the supraspinatus peripheral to the cable, represents the concave portion of the cuff at risk for pathology. (B) A superior view of the rotator cuff ridge or cable.

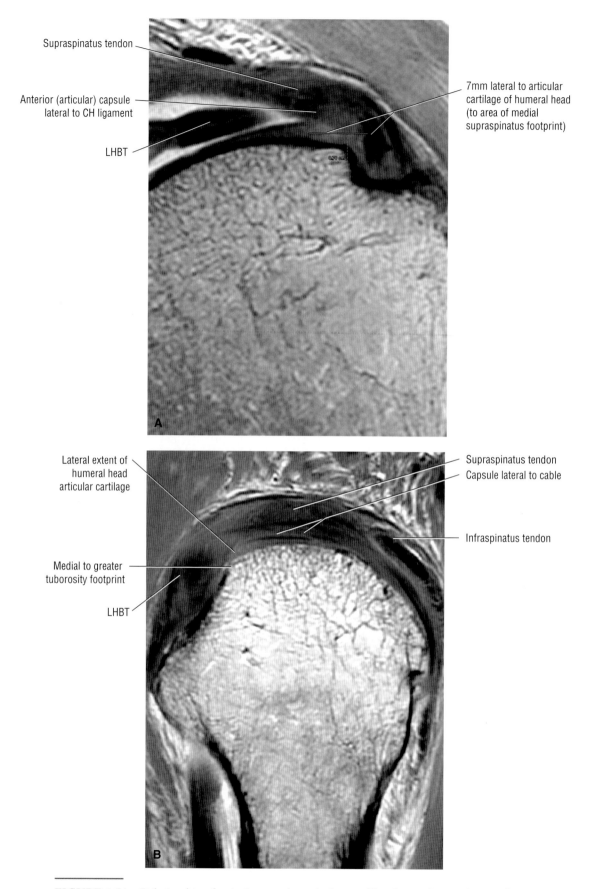

FIGURE 4.64 Relationship of articular capsule to the humeral head articular cartilage surface. The articular capsule is lateral to the rotator cuff cable. The capsule functions to reinforce the tendinous insertion and occupies a substantial portion of the cuff capsule/tendon insertion to the greater tuberosity. (**A**) Coronal, (**B**) Sagittal.

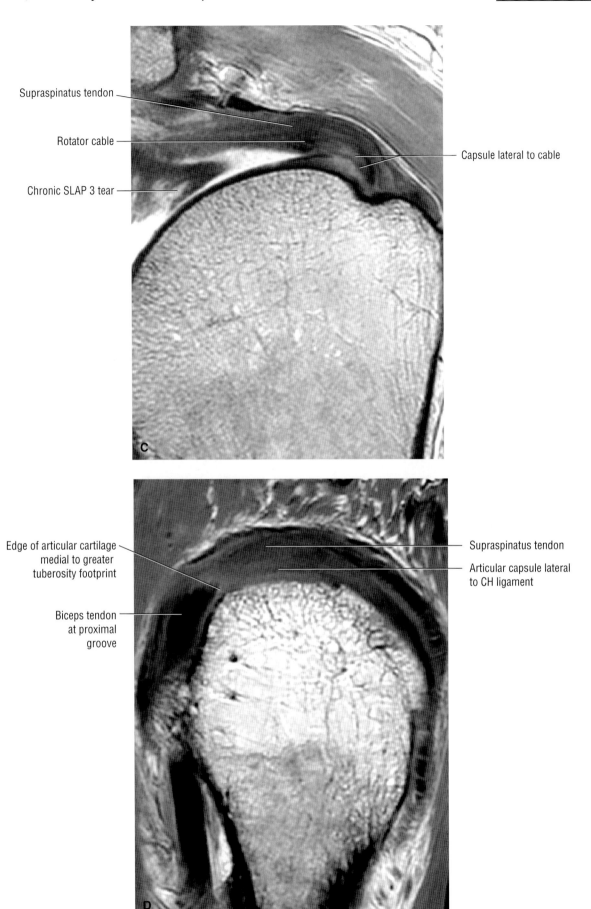

FIGURE 4.64   (*Continued*) (**C**) Coronal, (**D**) Sagittal.

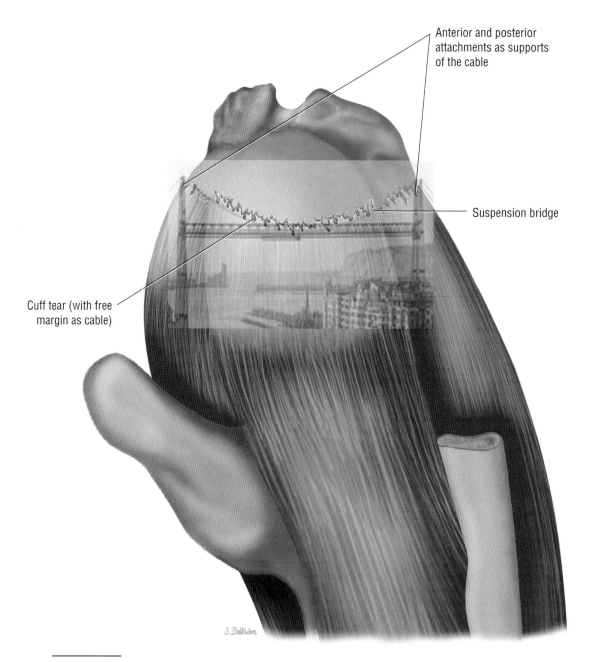

Anterior and posterior
attachments as supports
of the cable

Suspension bridge

Cuff tear (with free
margin as cable)

S.Beltrán

FIGURE 4.65   Rotator cuff tear with the free margin of the retracted cuff modeled after the cable
of a suspension bridge. A suspension bridge model can be used for the intact rotator cable-crescent
complex and rotator cuff tears. Even in the presence of rotator cuff tear, the supraspinatus muscle can
exert a compressive effect on the glenohumeral joint by means of its distributed load along the span
of the cable. Stress is transferred from the rotator cuff to the thick rotator cable. (Based on Burkhart
SS, Lo IKY, Brady PC. Burkhart's view of the shoulder. Burkhart SS, ed. In: *A Cowboy's Guide to
Advanced Shoulder Anthroscopy.* Philadelphia, PA: Lippincott Williams & Wilkins; 2006.)

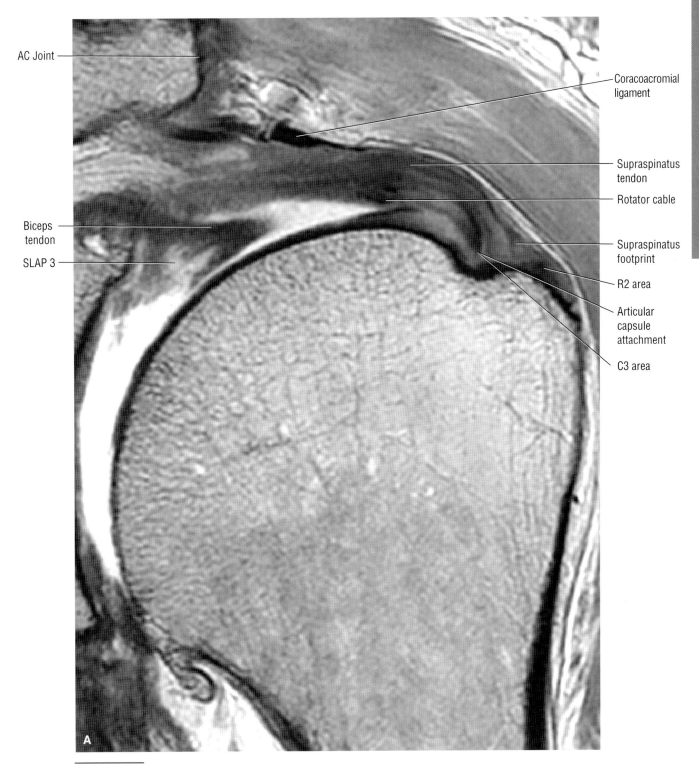

AC Joint

Coracoacromial ligament

Supraspinatus tendon

Rotator cable

Biceps tendon

SLAP 3

Supraspinatus footprint

R2 area

Articular capsule attachment

C3 area

FIGURE 4.66 **(A)** Articular capsule attachment (C3) at the margin of the greater tuberosity medial to the supraspinatus footprint (R2). C3 represents the area of the width of the capsule at the posterior margin of the supraspinatus tendon. The R2 portion of the supraspinatus footprint is indicated. The normal supraspinatus footprint spans from R1 (anterior) to R3 (posterior). Coronal T1 FSE.

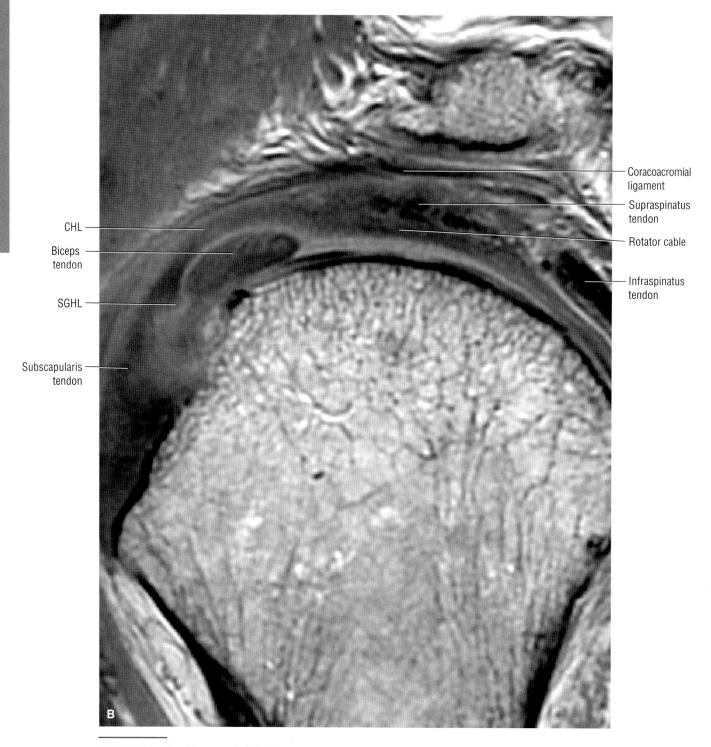

CHL

Biceps
tendon

SGHL

Subscapularis
tendon

Coracoacromial
ligament

Supraspinatus
tendon

Rotator cable

Infraspinatus
tendon

FIGURE 4.66   (*Continued*) (**B**) The CHL continues posteriorly as the rotator cable underneath the supraspinatus and infraspinatus tendons. The outer (anterior) surface of the subscapularis tendon is in close relationship with the coracohumeral ligament. The superior glenohumeral and coracohumeral ligaments and the subscapularis tendon all insert by the interdigitation of their fibers. The insertion of the subscapularis tendon inferior to the articular cartilage margin is medial to the insertion of the SGHL-CHL complex. T1 FSE sagittal MR arthrogram.

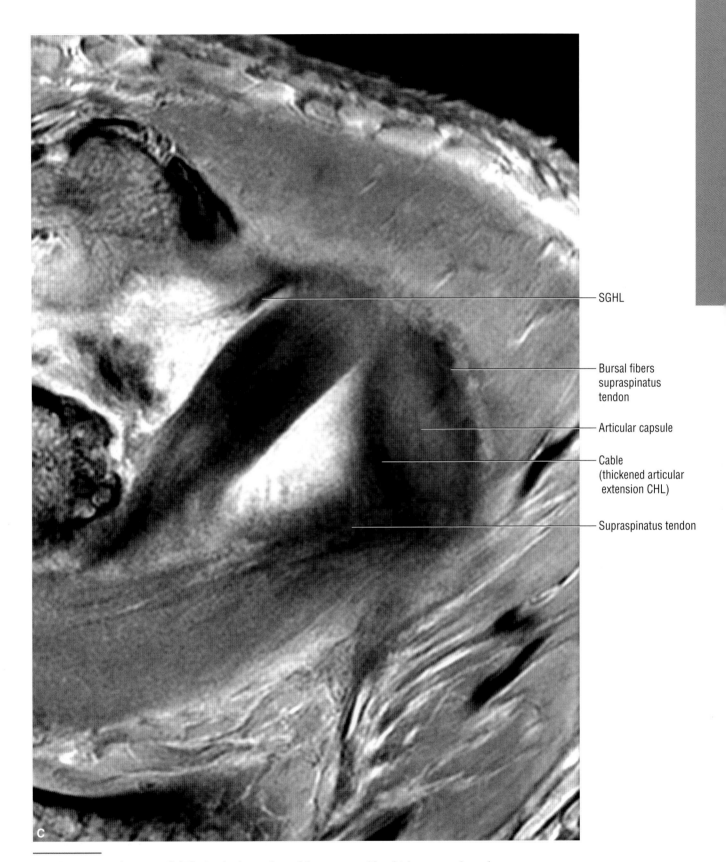

— SGHL

— Bursal fibers
  supraspinatus
  tendon

— Articular capsule

— Cable
  (thickened articular
   extension CHL)

— Supraspinatus tendon

FIGURE 4.66 (*Continued*) (**C**) Axial relationship of the rotator cable which courses along the articular side of the supraspinatus tendon and posterior to the biceps tendon. The rotator cable-crescent complex corresponds to the free margin of a cuff tear. The cable is thicker in older individuals where stress-shielding is more important in order to maintain proper cuff mechanics. Axial T1 FSE.

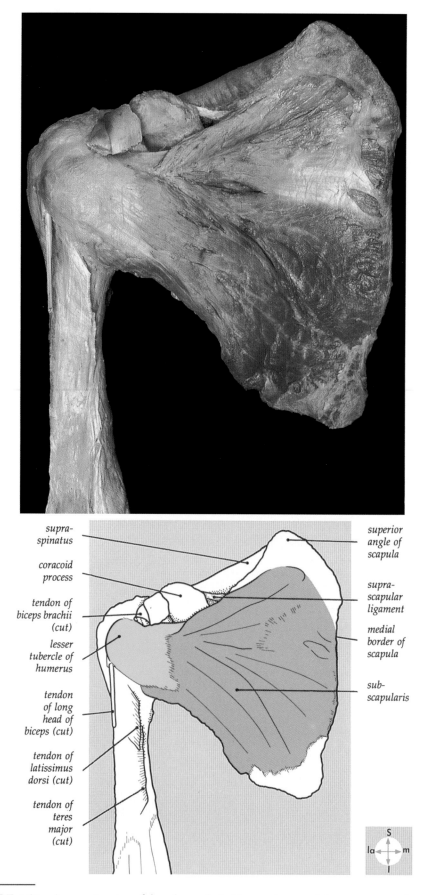

supra-
spinatus

coracoid
process

tendon of
biceps brachii
(cut)

lesser
tubercle of
humerus

tendon
of long
head of
biceps (cut)

tendon of
latissimus
dorsi (cut)

tendon of
teres
major
(cut)

superior
angle of
scapula

supra-
scapular
ligament

medial
border of
scapula

sub-
scapularis

FIGURE 4.67   An anterior view of the subscapularis. The attachment of the serratus anterior to the medial border of the scapula has been excised. In the position of internal rotation and adduction (along the articular side of the subscapularis) the fasciculus obliquus courses obliquely from its glenoid insertion with the long head of the triceps to its fusion with the MGHL and the subscapularis tendon.

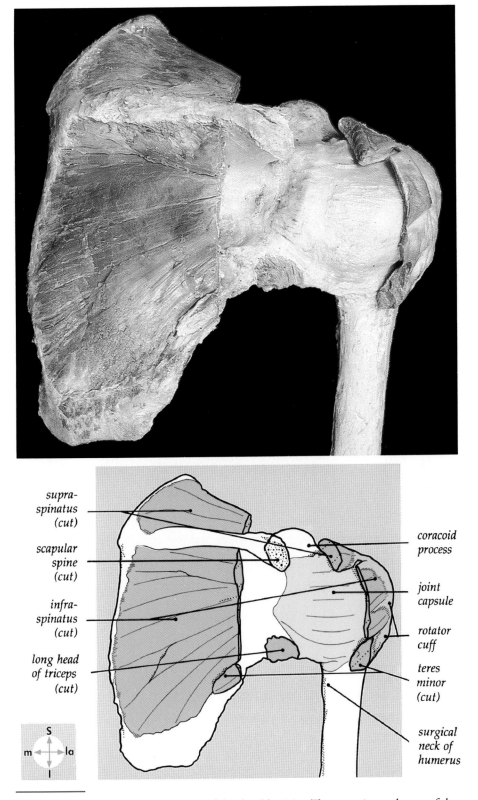

supra-spinatus (cut)

scapular spine (cut)

infra-spinatus (cut)

long head of triceps (cut)

coracoid process

joint capsule

rotator cuff

teres minor (cut)

surgical neck of humerus

FIGURE 4.68 The posterior aspect of the shoulder joint. The acromion and parts of the rotator cuff muscles have been excised to reveal the joint capsule. The axillary pouch of the inferior glenohumeral ligament (IGHL) is formed by the fasciculus obliquus medially and by junction of the anterior and posterior bands of the IGHL on the humerus laterally.

- The infraspinatus muscle which has been considered bipennate with a median raphe[339] actually has three pennate origins.
    - The infraspinatus is a thick triangular-shaped muscle.
    - A median raphe may be mistaken for the border between the infraspinatus and teres minor at surgery.
    - Tendinous fibers form ridges on the muscle surface.
    - Infraspinatus tendon inserts in the middle impression of the greater tuberosity.
- The subscapularis tendon lies on the anterior aspect of the anterior capsule of the glenohumeral joint.
    - The superior portion of the subscapularis tendon is intraarticular.
        - Tendinous bands converge laterally into a single large, flat tendon.
    - The lower third of the subscapularis is muscular while the upper third is tendinous.
- The subscapularis bursa lies between the subscapularis tendon and the scapula.
- The subscapularis muscle may be the cause of recurrent instability.[229]
    - Becomes attenuated from repeated dislocations
- The rotator cuff interval is located between the superior aspect of the subscapularis tendon and the inferior aspect of the supraspinatus tendon.[63] (Upper or superior fibers of the subscapularis tendon interdigitate with anterior fibers of the supraspinatus tendon to contribute to the rotator interval and transverse humeral ligament.)
    - Contains the coracohumeral ligament and the SGHL
    - A hidden lesion has been attributed to pathology of CHL–SGHL confluence, which forms the biceps sling/pulley.
    - Surgical closure of the interval appears to eliminate excessive inferior translation.
- The scapular circumflex vessels travel through triangular space formed by the teres major, the lower border of the teres minor, and the long head of the triceps.[229]
- The axillary nerve and posterior humeral circumflex artery travel through quadrilateral space (lateral to the triangular space) formed by the lower border of the teres minor, the upper border of the teres major, the lateral border of the LHBT, and the medial border of the humerus.

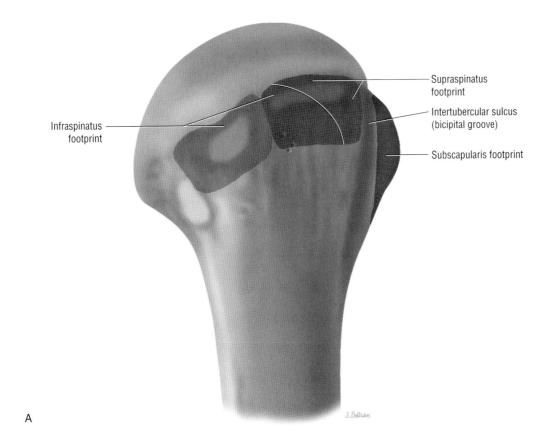

Supraspinatus
footprint

Intertubercular sulcus
(bicipital groove)

Subscapularis footprint

Infraspinatus
footprint

A

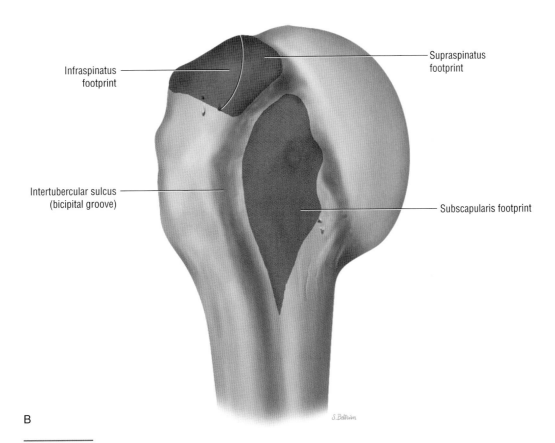

Infraspinatus
footprint

Supraspinatus
footprint

Intertubercular sulcus
(bicipital groove)

Subscapularis footprint

B

FIGURE 4.69 Footprints of the supraspinatus, infraspinatus, and subscapularis. (**A**) Lateral view. (**B**) Anterior view. The larger trapezoidal footprint of the infraspinatus tendon (lateral portion of the horizontal facet) actually extends and curves anterolateral to the posterior medial aspect of the triangular shaped footprint of the supraspinatus tendon on the greater tuberosity.

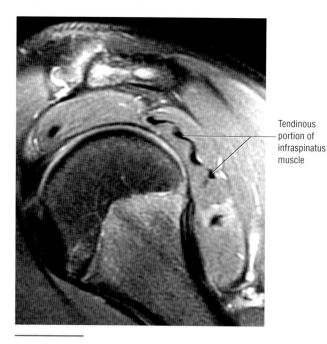

Tendinous
portion of
infraspinatus
muscle

FIGURE 4.70   The infraspinatus occupies the infraspinatus fossa and usually has three pennate origins. Superiorly, the footprint of the infraspinatus interdigitates and wraps around the posterior aspect of the supraspinatus tendon.[559]

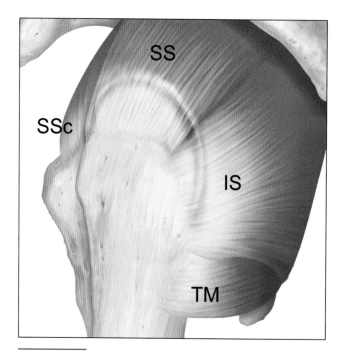

FIGURE 4.71   Schematic of the rotator cable in a left shoulder. The rotator cable has three attachment points that consist of the upper subscapularis and anterior supraspinatus anteriorly and the lower infraspinatus posteriorly. Thus, the infraspinatus also serves as an important attachment point for the cable posteriorly. IS, infraspinatus; SS, supraspinatus; SSc, Subscapularis; TM, teres minor. (Reprinted from Burkhart S, Lo IK, Brady PC, Denard PJ. *The Cowboy's Companion: A Trail Guide for the Arthroscopic Shoulder Surgeon.* Philadelphia, PA: Lippincott Williams & Wilkins; 2012, with permission.)

Coracoacromial Arch

Coracoacromial Ligament

- The coracoacromial ligament
    - Key structure of the coracoacromial arch
    - Triangular band of two fascicles
    - Originates from the lateral aspect of the coracoid and attaches to the anterior, lateral, and inferior surfaces of the acromion

- The coracoacromial arch stabilizes the humeral head and prevents superior ascent.

- The subacromial bursa
    - Located between the acromion, the coracoacromial ligament, and the rotator cuff[229]
    - Extends from the AC joint medially, under the anterior third of the acromion and coracoacromial ligament, to a line that extends approximately 4cm anterior to lateral to the anterolateral margins of the acromion

- Anterior acromial spurs may form within the acromial portion of the coracoacromial ligament associated with chronic irritation from the humeral head contact with the ligament.[407]
    - Anterior acromial spurs are frequently identified adjacent to the acromial attachment of the coracoacromial ligament.

- The normal low-signal-intensity acromial attachment of the coracoacromial ligament is frequently mistaken for an anterior acromial spur.
    - The additive thickness of the coracoacromial ligament and the inferior acromial cortex produces a hypointense pseudospur as interpreted in the coronal plane.

- The coracoacromial ligament and the anterior inferior margin of the acromion are resected in acromioplasty performed for chronic impingement.

- The LHBT
    - Attaches to the supraglenoid tubercle and exits the joint in the bicipital groove in the hiatus between the subscapularis and supraspinatus tendons[138]
    - Fibers contribute to the posterior and anterior superior labrum.
    - Has a synovial sheath as an extension of the synovial lining of the glenohumeral joint

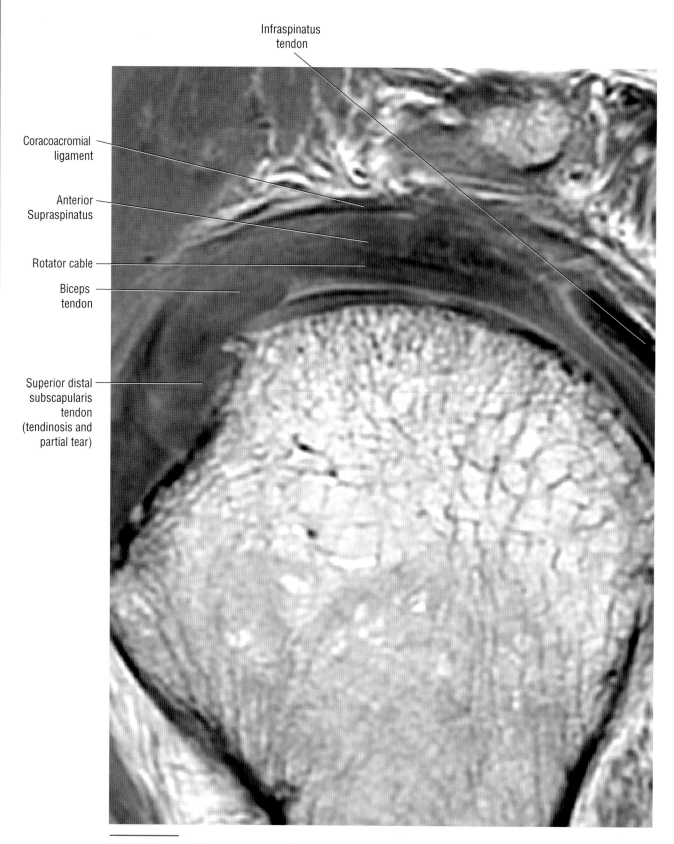

Infraspinatus
tendon

Coracoacromial
ligament

Anterior
Supraspinatus

Rotator cable

Biceps
tendon

Superior distal
subscapularis
tendon
(tendinosis and
partial tear)

FIGURE 4.72 The coracoacromial ligament is identified superior to the supraspinatous as it extends between the coracoid process and the acromion. This CA ligament is indirectly in contact with the supraspinatous tendon through an interposed bursa. The CA ligament may be quadrangular, Y-shaped, or broad in types. Sagittal T1 FSE image.

Coracoacromial
ligament

Lateral slip
of the deltoid

Supraspinatus
tendon

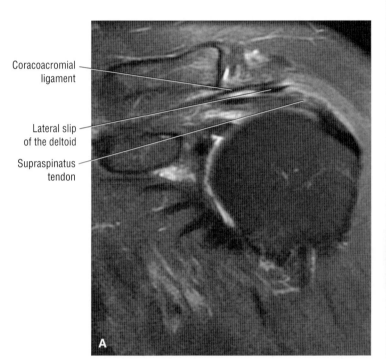

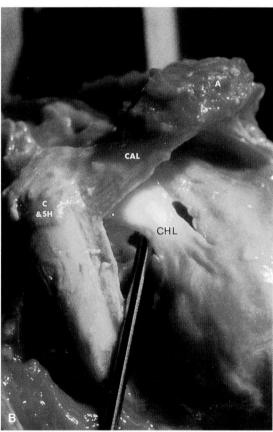

FIGURE 4.73   (**A**) Coronal FS PD FSE image demonstrates the course of the coracoacromial ligament to the undersurface of the acromion. The lateral slip of the deltoid extends between the coracoacromial ligament and the rotator cuff. (**B**) Gross specimen highlighting the anatomy of the coracohumeral ligament (CHL) and coracoacromial ligament (CAL). The coracobrachialis (C), the short head of the biceps (SH), and the acromion (A) are indicated. At arthroscopy the surface of the CAL should be smooth with a delicate synovial covering. In subacromial impingement there may be changes of CAL fraying or surrounding reactive bursitis.[559]

FIGURE 4.74 The anterior undersurface of the acromion and the coracoacromial ligament form the coracoacromial arch. The subacromial-subdeltoid bursa facilitates the passage of the rotator cuff and proximal humerus under the coracoacromial arch.

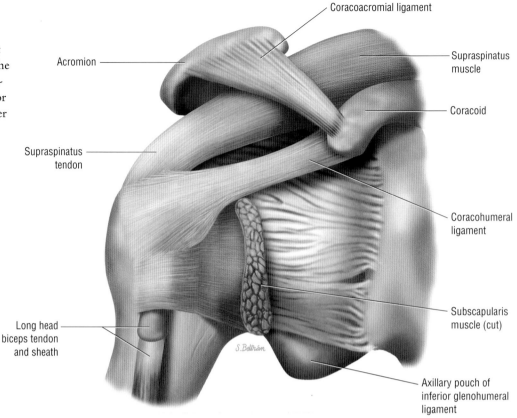

FIGURE 4.75 The coracoacromial ligament extends from the inferior surface of the acromion to the lateral aspect of the coracoid. The humeroscapular motion interface represents a relationship between the rotator cuff, the humeral head, the biceps, the coracoacromial arch, the deltoid and the coracoid muscles. Contact and load transfer occur between the rotator cuff and coracoacromial arch.

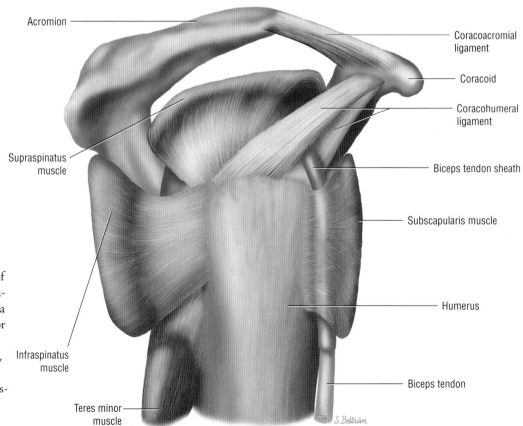

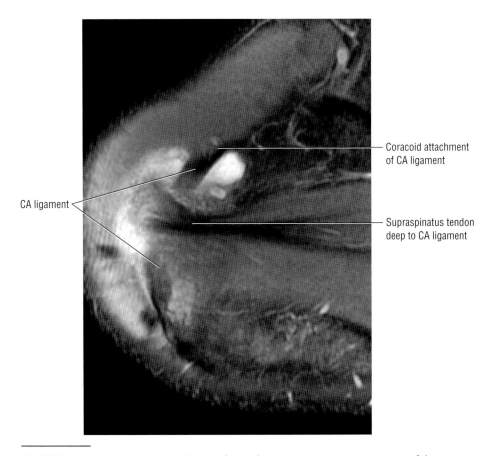

CA ligament

Coracoid attachment
of CA ligament

Supraspinatus tendon
deep to CA ligament

FIGURE 4.76   A superior axial image shows the anterior-to-posterior extent of the coracoacromial (CA) ligament perpendicular to the supraspinatus tendon. The fluid in the subacromial-subdeltoid bursa represents fluid between two serosal surfaces in contact with each other. One serosal surface is contributed by the undersurface of the coracoacromial arch and deltoid, and the other serosal surface is on the bursal side of the cuff.

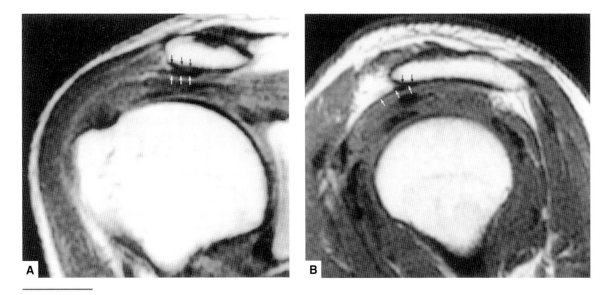

A   **B**

FIGURE 4.77   Pseudospur. The normal broad attachment of the coracoacromial ligament to the inferior surface of the acromion is shown on (**A**) T1-weighted coronal oblique and (**B**) sagittal oblique images. The low-signal-intensity acromial cortex (*black arrows*) and adjacent coracoacromial ligament and lateral slip of the deltoid attachment (*white arrows*) give the false impression of a small subacromial spur in the coronal plane. This pseudospur should not be misinterpreted as impingement; otherwise, unnecessary acromioplasties may be performed on patients with a normal coracoacromial ligament attachment and no associated acromial spurs.

Subacromial Bursa

- The subacromial bursa

    - Extends under the acromion and coracohumeral ligament

    - Lies over the superior surface of the supraspinatus and infraspinatus tendons laterally

    - Extends beyond the lateral and anterior aspects of the acromion under the deltoid

    - Represents sliding serosal surfaces lubricated by synovial fluid and serves as a gliding mechanism between the rotator cuff and coracoacromial arch[404]

        - Bursal tissue forms a layer under the acromion and over the superior surface of the cuff.

- Communication may exist (less common condition) between the subacromial and subcoracoid bursae.[223,394]

    - If MR contrast medium or saline is inadvertently injected into the subcoracoid bursa, visualization of the capsular structures will not occur because the subscapularis bursa is not distended.

- An obliterated peribursal fat plane has been used as an ancillary sign of shoulder disease.

- Fibrous bands may be seen within the subacromial bursa.[138]

- Arthroscopic Assessment[559]

    - The subacromial bursal cavity is identified inferior to the anterior half of the acromion and extends anterior and lateral.

    - A posterior bursal curtain (posterior border of bursa) separates the subacromial space into anterior and posterior compartments.

    - A lateral subacromial shelf divides the subacromial bursa:

        - Superior subacromial space

        - Lateral subdeltoid space

    - The subacromial and subclavicular space are demarcated by the medial wall of the bursa.

    - The anterior bursal portal is used to view the posterior cuff.

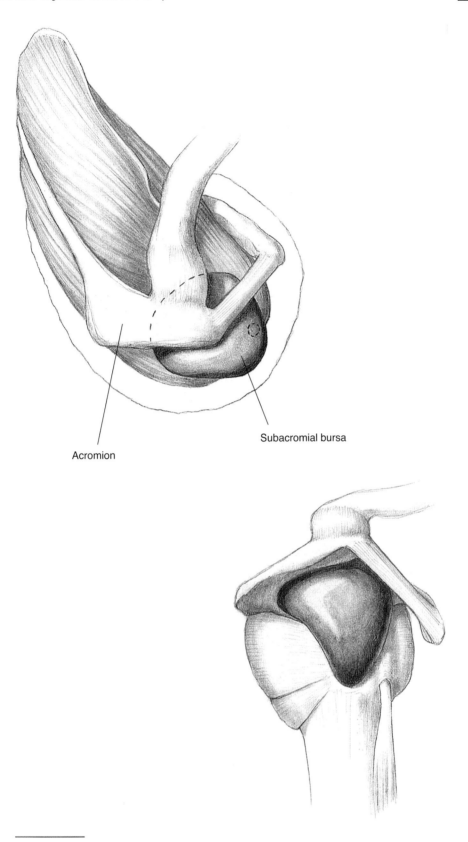

Acromion

Subacromial bursa

FIGURE 4.78   Subacromial bursa. The posterior aspect of this bursa acts as a veil of tissue that must be pierced by the arthroscope in order to visualize the anterior acromion. Note the anterolateral position of the bursa. (Reprinted from Craig, EV. *Master Techniques in Orthopaedic Surgery: Shoulder*. 3rd ed. Philadelphia, PA: Lippincott Williams & Wilkins; 2013, with permission.)

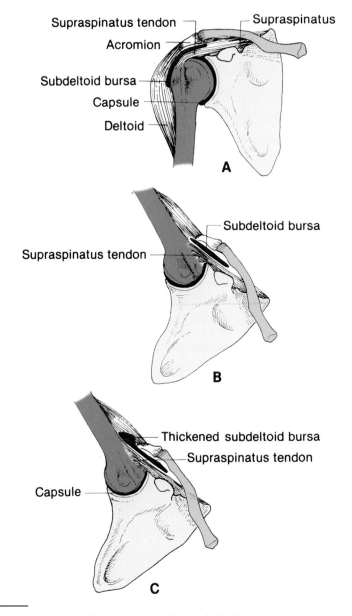

FIGURE 4.79   Subdeltoid or subacromial bursa. (**A**) With the arm at the side the greater part of the subdeltoid bursa lies under the deltoid. (**B**) With the arm abducted, the bursa migrates under the acromion; note the narrow interval between the acromion and greater tuberosity through which the supraspinatus must travel when the arm is widely abducted. (**C**) When the walls of the bursa are thickened as in acute or chronic bursitis, they impinge against the coracoacromial arch when the arm is abducted and thus restrict motion. (Modified from DePalma AF. *Surgery of the Shoulder*. 3rd ed. Philadelphia, PA: JB Lippincott; 1983.)

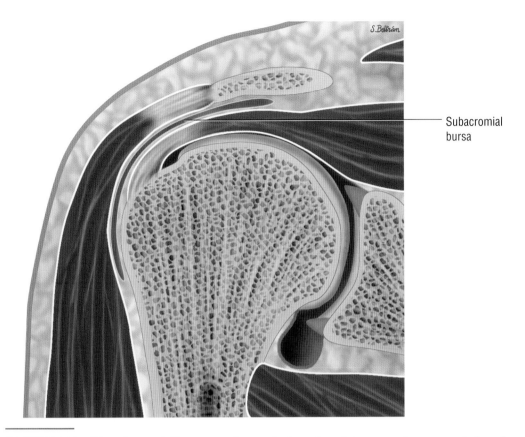

FIGURE 4.80 The subacromial bursa extends over the insertion of the supraspinatus superiorly and over the infraspinatus and teres minor posteriorly. The superior surface of the bursa is in contact with the undersurface of the acromion, the coracoacromial ligament, and the origin of the midportion of the deltoid muscle. The superior surface of the bursa extends medially adjacent to the deep surface of the acromioclavicular joint.

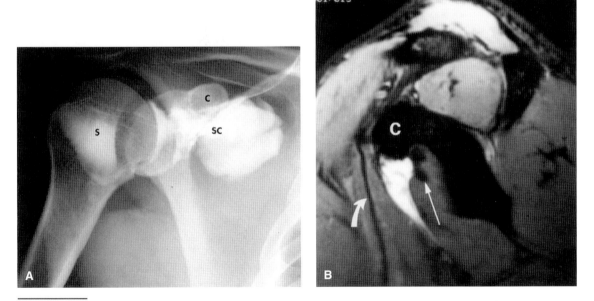

FIGURE 4.81 (**A**) After separate contrast injections into the subcoracoid (SC) and subscapularis (S) bursae, the subcoracoid and subacromial bursae are seen to communicate, whereas no communication occurs between the subacromial and subscapularis bursae. C, coracoid. (**B**) T2*-weighted sagittal oblique gadopentetate-saline subcoracoid bursagram demonstrates filling of the subcoracoid bursa anterior to the subscapularis tendon (*straight arrow*) and posterior to the conjoined tendon of the coracobrachialis and short head of the biceps (*curved arrow*). C, coracoid.

Acromioclavicular Joint

- The acromioclavicular joint (AC joint)

  - Is a synovial joint with articular surfaces covered by fibrocartilage similar to that in the sternoclavicular joint[348]

  - Superior and inferior ligaments reinforce the articular capsule.

    - The articular surfaces are separated by a wedge-shaped articular disc.

- The coracoclavicular ligament provides major stability to the AC joint with its conoid and trapezoid components.

  - The coracoclavicular ligament assists in controlling vertical stability and the AC joint restrains posterior translation of the clavicle.[229]

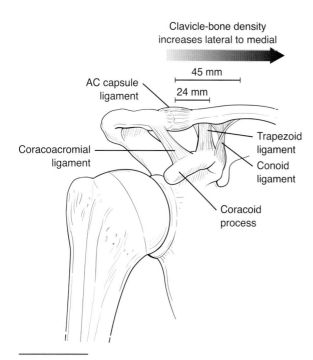

FIGURE 4.82 AC joint complex anatomy. Important static restraints that need to be considered during open surgical repair or reconstruction: AC joint capsule and coracoclavicular ligaments. (Reprinted from Miniaci A, Iannotti JP, Williams GR, Zuckerman, JD. *Disorders of the Shoulder: Sports Injuries.* 3rd ed. Philadelphia, PA: Lippincott Williams & Wilkins; 2014, with permission.)

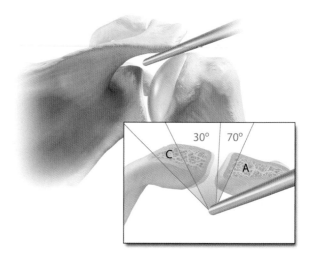

FIGURE 4.83 Schematic illustration of the view of the AC joint from a posterior portal. A 30° arthroscope provides a limited field of view (shaded in blue). The field of view with this arthroscope may not be sufficient to visualize the superior aspect of the joint, particularly when there is an oblique orientation of the joint. The 70° arthroscope provides a larger field of view (shaded in red), and with this arthroscope, the superior aspect of the joint can always be visualized. A, acromion; C, distal clavicle. (Reprinted from Burkhart S, Lo IK, Brady PC, Denard PJ. *The Cowboy's Companion: A Trail Guide for the Arthroscopic Shoulder Surgeon.* Philadelphia, PA: Lippincott Williams & Wilkins; 2012, with permission.)

- **AC joint functional anatomy**
  - AC joint has three types of motion at the normal AC joint:
    - Anterior and posterior gliding of scapula on clavicle
    - Abduction and adduction of the scapula on clavicle
    - Rotation of the scapula about the long axis of the clavicle[182]
  - AC joint motions limited to between 5 and 8 degrees in each direction.
  - Degenerative changes associated with
    - Rotational motion
    - Shear and compressive forces of the deltoid
    - Distance between acromion and clavicular articular surfaces is an important factor in normal AC joint biomechanics.
      - Normal 1 to 3mm
      - AC joint greater (wider) than 7mm in males and 6mm in females is pathologic.
      - Increased AC joint space associated with distal clavicle osteolysis or inflammatory AC joint changes
    - Evaluate for edema of the distal clavicle and adjacent acromion as well as subchondral cystic changes and erosions in both the coronal and axial imaging planes.
    - The axial imaging plane is more accurate in depicting asymmetry of involvement between the distal clavicle and the acromion that might not be evident on coronal images.
    - Pain localized to the AC joint[559]
      - Tenderness, crepitus, and pain with overhead and or pushing exercises
    - Concomitant pathology may exist.
      - Rotator cuff tears
      - Labral tears
    - AC joint injection test
      - Evaluate for relief of pain using 1mL lidocaine + 1mL corticosteroid.
    - Chronic symptomatic AC joint arthritis and osteolysis
      - Arthroscopic distal clavicle excision

5
Shoulder Impingement Syndrome

Shoulder Impingement

Shoulder Impingement

Key Concepts[27,579,601]

- Impingement syndrome is characterized by a range of MR findings from tendinosis to rotator cuff tears.

- Intrinsic impingement is associated with shoulder instability.

- Primary extrinsic impingement is associated with abrasion of the rotator cuff against the inferior surface of the acromion.

- Subacromial keel spurs are located on the anteroinferior lateral portion of the acromion.

- Acromial thickness is important in planning subacromial decompression procedures.

- The AC joint may hypertrophy, but symptoms of impingement may be absent.

- Hypertrophy of the coracoacromial ligament correlates with fraying or fragmentation of the ligament in association with impingement.

- A symptomatic os acromiale is associated with marrow edema on either side of the synchondrosis.

- Degenerative tendinopathy or intrinsic tendon degeneration associated with eccentric tensile overload may be the primary pathology in impingement.

- Rotator cuff tendinosis is conspicuous on FS PD FSE images.

  - Tendinosis is not hyperintense on T2 FSE images. (Justifying the use of this sequence to increase specificity for tendinosis versus partial tear diagnosis).

- Partial and full thickness tears are hyperintense on both FS PD FSE and T2 FSE sequences unless associated with chronic scarring or granulation tissue.

Shoulder Impingement Syndrome

- Consists of a continuum from mild tendinosis to massive rotator cuff tears
- Supraspinatus tendon predisposed to mechanical injury from overlying structures during movement of the shoulder joint into forward flexion and rotation

    - Acromion

    - Coracoacromial ligament

    - Acromioclavicular joint

- Condition of middle age, with the exception of throwing athletes

    - Age-related degeneration is an important risk factor in the progression and development of rotator cuff pathology.

- Causes an insidious onset of pain with overhead activities (usually without history of specific injury)

- May cause stiffness, catching, and local or referred pain to the deltoid insertion

    - Night pain and weakness are usually associated with rotator cuff tears, not impingement.

- Clinical assessment includes evaluation for atrophy and range of motion as well as direct palpation.[444]

    - In *Neer's impingement test,* pain is elicited by forcible evaluation of the arm and is caused by impingement of the critical area of the supraspinatus tendon.

    - Injection of lidocaine into the subacromial space relieves or decreases pain.

    - The Hawkins' test (impingement reinforcement) is performed by flexing the humerus 90° and then forcibly internally rotating the shoulder until pain is reproduced by cuff impingement.

    - Weakness is evaluated in the supraspinatus (weakness with abduction), subscapularis (weakness with internal rotation), and infraspinatus (weakness with external rotation).[201]

Related Anatomy

- The coracoacromial arch includes:
    - The coracoid
    - The coracohumeral ligament
    - The anterior inferior acromion[339]
- These structures can impinge on:
    - The subacromial bursa
    - The LHBT
    - The rotator cuff (especially the supraspinatus)
    - The proximal humerus
- Anterior inferior acromial spurs and acromioclavicular osteophytes (to a lesser extent) are related to impingement.

Pathogenesis

- The supraspinatus tendon
    - Anatomically confined under tension
    - Compressed between bony structures at its inferior and superior surfaces
    - At risk for acute injury and chronic wear
- Bursal inflammation and tendinosis, produced by compression, may cause pain, leading to disuse atrophy of the supraspinatus and infraspinatus in the subacromial space.
- A hooked type 3 acromion and muscle weakness lead to loss of centralizing forces and increased compression.
- Controversy exists as to whether chronic mechanical impingement precedes the development of complete rotator cuff lesions or whether primary degeneration of the cuff results in tears, leading to chronic impingement syndrome.[67,158,272,399,524]
- The most common location for impingement is between the anterior third of the acromion and the underlying tendons.
- A decrease in the subacromial space, secondary to anatomic or pathologic changes, is usually associated with a large tear that has compromised the centralizing ability of the cuff.[609]
    - Loss of the cuff centralizing function allows for proximal humeral migration (superior ascent).

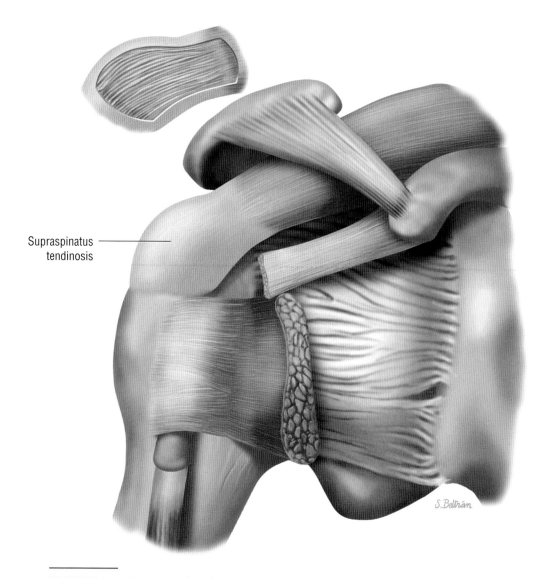

Supraspinatus
tendinosis

FIGURE 5.1   Rotator cuff tendinosis is seen as collagen degeneration without the influx of inflammatory cells. The thickened distal cuff tendon is viewed in an anterior coronal perspective.

Etiology

- Causes of painful shoulder syndrome include[46,479]:

  - Hypovascularity in the supraspinatus tendon

  - Mechanical wear

  - Acute trauma

  - Repetitive microtrauma from overuse (this is especially common in throwing athletes or those whose work activities emphasize overhead motions)

- Factors contributing to bony supraspinatus outlet compromise include[47,404,436]:

  - Anterior acromial spurs

  - Acromion shape (a curved or overhanging edge)

  - The slope of the acromion (a flat or decreased angle)

  - The morphology of the AC joint (hypertrophic bone, callus formation)

- Nonoutlet impingement includes:

  - Prominence of the greater tuberosity (fracture, malunion, nonunion)

  - Loss of humeral head depressors as seen in rotator cuff tears and biceps tendon rupture[531]

  - Loss of glenohumeral joint fulcrum function from articular surface destruction or ligamentous laxity

  - Impaired scapular rotation from trapezius paralysis or AC joint disruption

  - Lesions of the acromion, including an unfused anterior acromial epiphysis (apophysis)

  - Fracture malunion or nonunion

  - Subacromial bursa thickening (chronic bursitis or cuff thickening in calcific tendinitis)

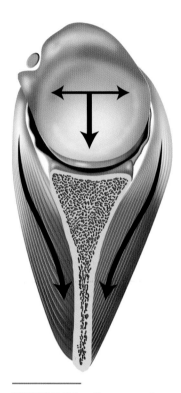

FIGURE 5.2 Co-contraction of the rotator cuff musculature results in compression of the humeral head onto the glenoid surface to improve dynamic stability of the glenohumeral joint. Rotator-cuff strenghtening exercises (using elastic cord or cable) is a key part of the conservative treatment of impingement syndrome. (Reprinted from Dodson C, Dines D, Dines JS, Walch G, Williams G. *Controversies in Shoulder Instability*. Philadelphia, PA: Lippincott Williams & Wilkins; 2014, with permission.)

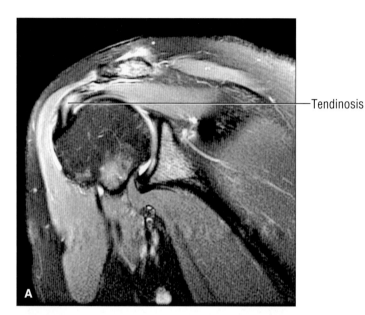

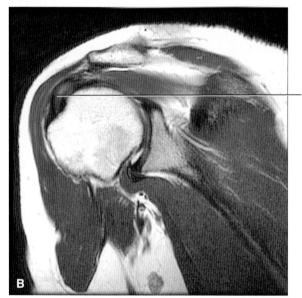

FIGURE 5.3 Rotator cuff tendinosis is seen as collagen degeneration without the influx of inflammatory cells. The thickened distal cuff tendon is viewed in an anterior coronal perspective. Moderate to severe rotator cuff tendinosis demonstrates hyperintensity on a coronal FS PD FSE image (**A**) and intermediate signal intensity on a coronal T2 FSE image (**B**).

Classification of Shoulder Impingement

- Rotator cuff impingement can be grouped into structural and dynamic factors:

  - Structural etiologies lead to mechanical obstruction and decreased space for rotator cuff clearance within the supraspinatus outlet.

    - Mechanical obstruction is associated with tendon degeneration and tears.

  - Dynamic etiologies are associated with superior migration of the humeral head during arm elevation, which leads to the abutment of the greater tuberosity against the coracoacromial arch, resulting in rotator cuff tendon injury.

    - Dynamic imbalance is attributed to rotator cuff dysfunction and fatigue.

  - Structural causes of subacromial pathology include:

    - Abnormal acromial morphology

    - Calcific tendinitis (thickening of the rotator cuff)

    - Severe AC joint arthrosis with hypertrophy and osteophytes

    - Coracoacromial ligament degeneration (hypertrophy)

    - Os acromiale

    - Inflammatory bursitis

    - Malunion of the greater tuberosity, distal clavicle or acromion

    - Partial or full thickness tears of the rotator cuff

  - Dynamic causes of subacromial pathology include:

    - Scapular dysfunction

    - Primary tendon overload

    - Glenohumeral instability

    - Repetitive microtrauma

    - Imbalance of shoulder musculature

Intrinsic and Extrinsic Impingement

- Impingement may also be classified as intrinsic or extrinsic to the glenohumeral joint.

  - Intrinsic impingement (also referred to as secondary extrinsic impingement) is associated with instability and represents secondary or nonoutlet impingement. Intrinsic impingement includes:

    - Posterior peel-back

    - Microinstabilities of the glenohumeral joint

    - Scapular dyskinesia

    - Greater tuberosity malunion

    - Loss of humeral head depressor function

  - Primary extrinsic impingement is the painful abrasion of the rotator cuff against the underside of the acromion with arm elevation.

    - Primary extrinsic impingement may be caused by:
      - Variations in anterior acromial shape
      - Slope of the acromion (lateral or anterior downsloping)
      - A low-lying acromial position
      - AC joint osteophytes
      - Anterior inferior acromial spurs
      - Coracoacromial ligament thickness
      - Os acromiale

  - Tendon dysfunction is the cause of both impingement and rotator cuff tears.

Pathogenesis of Extrinsic Impingement

- Extrinsic impingement can exist between:

  - The acromion and the rotator cuff

  - The AC joint and the rotator cuff

  - The anterior acromion and the biceps tendon

- There is no gap between the superior cuff and the coracoacromial arch as superior translation compresses the cuff tendon between the humeral head and the arch.[339]

  - Superior displacement is opposed by a downward force exerted by the coracoacromial arch through the cuff tendon to the humeral head.[656]

- In extrinsic impingement, the superior surface of the rotator cuff abrades the undersurface of the acromion during elevation and/or overhead motion.

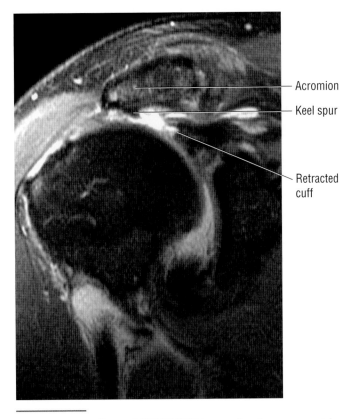

FIGURE 5.4   Coronal FS PD FSE image showing an acromial "keel" spur associated with a full thickness rotator cuff tear with retraction.

Acromial Morphology in Impingement

- **Shape of the Acromion[47]**

  - Type 1 acromion has a flat or straight undersurface.

  - Type 2 acromion has a smooth, curved inferior surface that approximately parallels the superior humeral head in the sagittal oblique plane.

  - Type 3 acromion has an anterior hook or beak.

    - The acromiohumeral distance is narrowed relative to the remainder of the acromion at the site of the hook.

    - Type 3 acromion is thought to be associated with greater predisposition to rotator cuff tears (i.e., tears involving the critical zone immediately proximal to the greater tuberosity insertion of the supraspinatus tendon).[385]

  - Type 4 acromion has a convex inferior contour.[616]

    - There may be partial narrowing of the subacromial space near the midposterior aspect of the distal acromion.

    - There is no correlation between a type 4 acromion and impingement.

  - Radiographic views to correlate with MR imaging[559]

    - Axillary view

      - Os acromiale

    - Modified scapular Y view (arch view) with the X-ray tube aligned with scapular spine and angled 30 degrees caudally

      - Acromial morphology types I–IV

    - AP view

      - Shoulder and glenohumeral joint

    - AC joint view with the X-ray angled in a cephalad direction

- Bursal-sided partial cuff tears correspond to anterior inferior acromial impingement.[173]

- Type 1 and 2 acromions are more common than type 3 in general population.

- Morphologic changes in type 2 and 3 acromions may be acquired rather than developmental.[649]

- Acromial hooks that lie within the coracoacromial ligament may be traction spurs.

- Dependence on the coracoacromial arch for superior stability and traction loads increase in the presence of cuff degeneration.

- The acromial hook lies within the coracoacromial ligament and points toward the coracoid and corresponds to the location of the anterior inferior acromial spur.[423]

- A subacromial keel, however, is an aggressive inferior acromial spur shaped like the keel of a sailboat.[556]

  - The subacromial keel spur may result in severe damage to the bursal surface of the cuff.

- The acromial keel spur can be found on the anterior edge between the lateral border of the acromion and the AC joint, continuing posteriorly to midway under the acromion.

- Thickness of Acromion

  - Measurement of the thickness of the osseous acromion helps prevent inadvertent acromial fracture caused by overly aggressive burring.[556]

  - Acromial thickness assessed at the posterior margin of the AC joint:

    - Type A acromion: thin, less than 8mm

    - Type B acromion: 8 to 12mm

    - Type C acromion: thick, more than 12mm

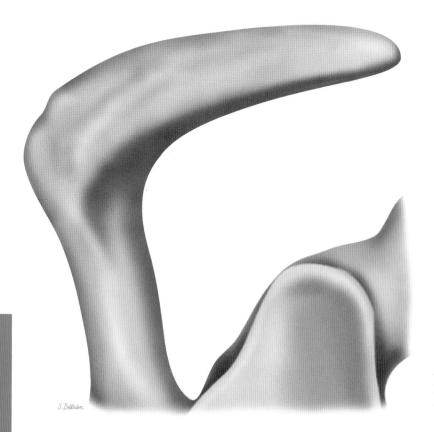

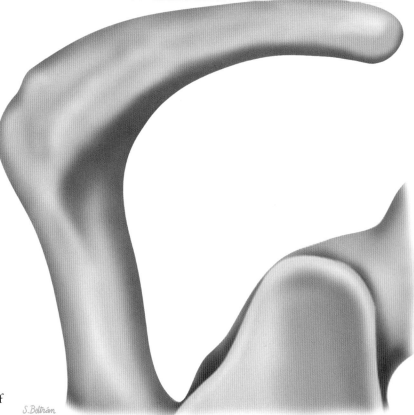

FIGURE 5.5   Type 1 acromion with flat acromial undersurface.

FIGURE 5.6   Type 2 acromion with a curved convex inferior surface that parallels the contour of the humeral head.

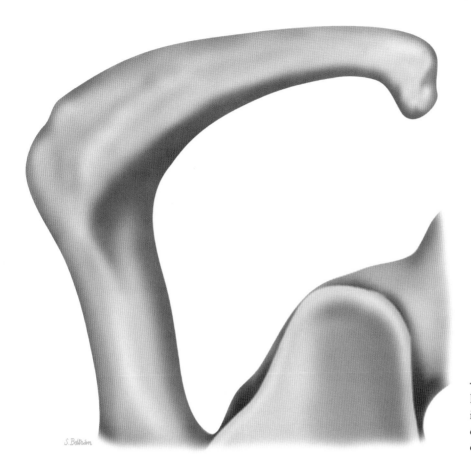

FIGURE 5.7   Type 3 acromion with an inferiorly directed beak or hook, which contributes to narrowing of the supraspinatus outlet for the supraspinatus tendon.

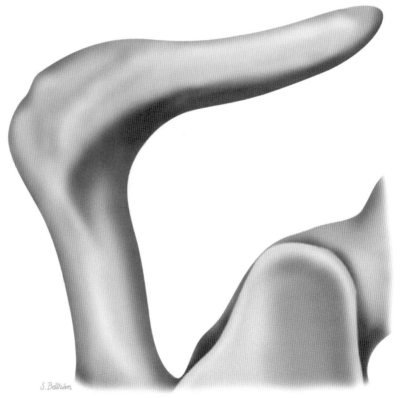

FIGURE 5.8   Type 4 acromion with upward or superior convexity of its inferior border. There is no association with cuff impingement.

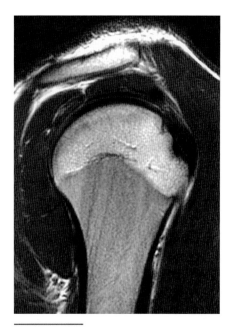

FIGURE 5.9 Type 1 acromion with straight inferior margin as seen on a sagittal T2 FSE image.

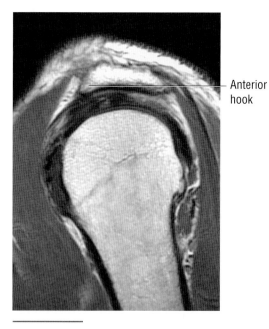

— Anterior hook

FIGURE 5.10 Sagittal PD FSE image of the type 3 or hooked acromion. The type 3 acromion is assessed on at least 1 to 2 images lateral to the AC joint. In fact, the anterior inferior acromial spur often corresponds to the hook of a type 3 acromion.

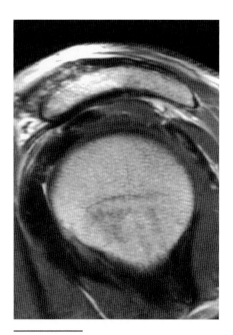

FIGURE 5.11 Type 2 curved acromion on a sagittal PD FSE image.

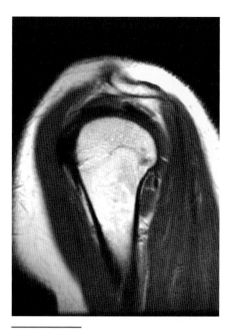

FIGURE 5.12 Sagittal PD FSE image of type 4 acromion with upper or superior convexity of its inferior border.

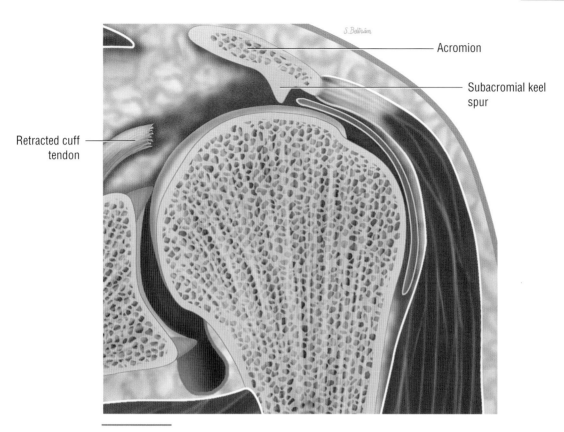

FIGURE 5.13   Acromial "keel" spur associated with a full thickness rotator cuff tear with retraction.

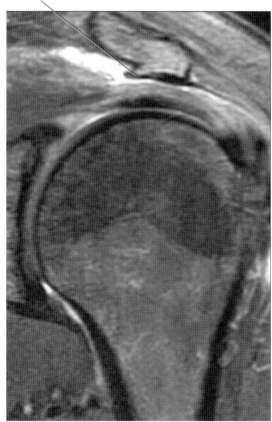

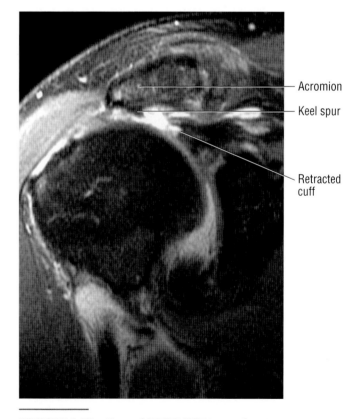

FIGURE 5.14   Keel osteophyte corresponds to the coracoacromial ligament attachment on the undersurface of the acromion. Cuff tendinosis with preferential involvement of the bursal surface. Coronal FS PD image.

FIGURE 5.15   Coronal FS PD FSE image showing an acromial "keel" spur associated with a full thickness rotator cuff tear with retraction.

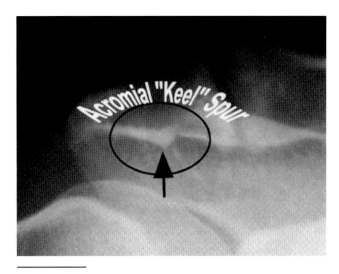

FIGURE 5.16   A subacromial keel is an aggressive spur that appears as a convexity under the acromion on the anterior-posterior radiograph. The location of the keel osteophyte corresponds to the inferior surface attachment of the coracoacromial ligament. (Reprinted from Snyder SJ, Bahk M, Burns J, Getelman M, Karzel R. *Shoulder Arthroscopy.* 3rd ed. Philadelphia, PA: Lippincott Williams & Wilkins; 2014, with permission.)

■ Acromial Slope

- ■ The normal acromial slope approximates the horizontal plane or slopes superiorly from posterior to anterior.

  - ▨ Anterior downsloping of the acromion is assessed in the sagittal plane.

  - ▨ Lateral downsloping of the anterior acromion as assessed in the coronal plane may narrow the supraspinatus outlet.

    - Does not correlate with impingement pain or rotator cuff tears

- ■ A low-lying acromion relative to the distal clavicle may predispose to impingement and degenerative changes of the acromion.[37]

Acromioclavicular Joint Disease in Impingement

- Extrinsic impingement may cause the humeral head to no longer be centered or contained on the glenoid fossa.[339]

- The unbalanced elevating force of the deltoid pulls the superior cuff into contact with the anterior acromial undersurface.

- True impingement secondary to the undersurface of the AC joint is not equivalent to the hypertrophic osseous spurs on the undersurface of the acromion.

- AC osteophytes are usually sufficiently medial that they do not compromise the rotator cuff.

- A symptomatic AC joint may require resection.[499]
    - Tests to identify the symptomatic AC joint include:
        - Cross-chest adduction (increasing symptoms)
        - Adduction, internal rotation, and extension (to isolate posterior AC facet pain)
        - Direct superior tenderness reproducing the pain
        - Tenderness on anteroposterior translation
        - Localized pain in the AC joint with impingement testing

- Distal Clavicle Osteolysis
    - Young patients
    - High stress on AC joint
    - Weightlifters, wrestlers, football players

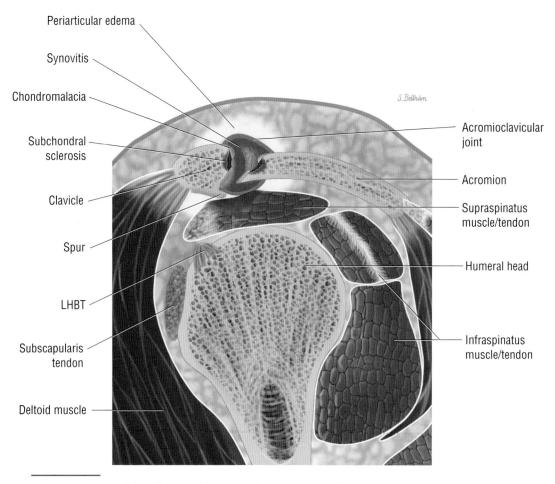

Periarticular edema

Synovitis

Chondromalacia

Subchondral sclerosis

Clavicle

Spur

LHBT

Subscapularis tendon

Deltoid muscle

Acromioclavicular joint

Acromion

Supraspinatus muscle/tendon

Humeral head

Infraspinatus muscle/tendon

S. Beltrán

FIGURE 5.17   Although AC arthrosis may be concurrent with impingement, it is the more lateral acromial spurs that are directly associated with symptomatic bursal-sided cuff damage.

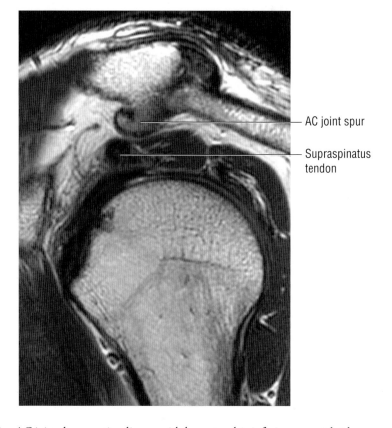

AC joint spur

Supraspinatus tendon

FIGURE 5.18   AC joint degenerative disease with hypertrophic inferior acromial side spur.

Coracohumeral Ligament and Arch in Impingement

■ In impingement, the coracohumeral ligament is usually frayed and fragmented with surrounding synovitis.

■ Increased contact and abrasion occur within upward displacement of the humeral head as the rotation of the cuff is squeezed against the acromion and the coracohumeral ligament.

    ■ Further upward displacement of the humeral head is associated with abrasion of the humeral head articular cartilage and rotator cuff arthropathy.[339]

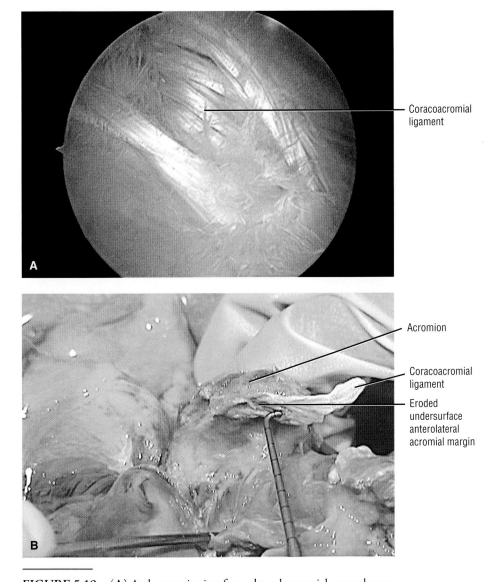

FIGURE 5.19 (A) Arthroscopic view from the subacromial space shows the fascicles of the coracoacromial ligament as they attach to the inferior aspect of the acromion. The coracoacromial ligament attaches to the anterior, lateral, and inferior surfaces of the acromion and originates as a triangular band of two fascicles from the lateral aspect of the coracoid. (B) The corresponding coracoacromial ligament has been cut, with the acromial attachment intact.

Os Acromiale in Impingement

- Os acromiale is a normal variation that may be present in patients with impingement syndrome.

    - A congenital os acromiale may be unstable inferiorly causing rotator cuff impingement.

- Os acromiale is failure of the acromial ossification centers to fuse (normally complete by 22 years of age).

    - The pre-, meso-, meta-, or basiacromion may fail to fuse.[309]

- Meso- and meta-acromion failure (failure of the fusion of the mesoacromion and the meta-acromion) is more common.

- The synchondrosis-like articulation may contain fibrous tissue, periosteum, or synovium.

- The os acromiale may be relatively mobile with shoulder abduction, causing impingement.[309]

- An unstable degenerative os acromiale is often associated with AC joint degeneration.

- The coracoacromial ligament inserts onto the os acromiale, and thus the os acromiale is susceptible to instability.

- Symptomatic os acromiale

    - Preacromion

    - Mesoacromion (most common)

    - Metaacromion

    - Os acromiale pain can be confused with AC joint symptoms.

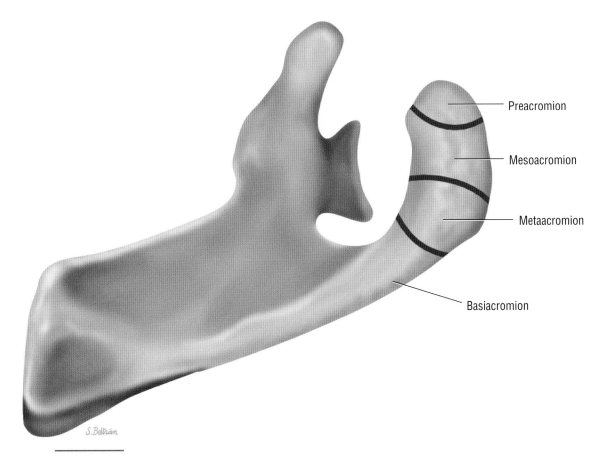

Preacromion

Mesoacromion

Metaacromion

Basiacromion

S.Beltrán

FIGURE 5.20 Superior view of os acromiale subtypes from distal to proximal. These unfused ossi-fication centers include pre-, meso-, meta-, and basiacromion based on the location of the articulation. The mesoacromion-metaacromion type is most common.

Clinical Classification of Impingement

- The stages in Neer's classification system are[399,400]:
    - Stage 1: Tendon edema and hemorrhage
    - Stage 2: Fibrosis and tendinitis (now referred to as tendinosis)
    - Stage 3: Partial or complete rupture or tear of the rotator cuff, often in association with anterior acromial spurring or greater tuberosity excrescence
        - When present, radiographic changes include greater tuberosity sclerosis and hypertrophic bone formation.
        - Bursal thickening, fibrosis, and partial tears of the superficial rotator cuff may be present.

- Rotator cuff tendons display areas appearing gray, dull, edematous, and friable at surgery.[366]

- Degenerative changes, including angiofibroblastic hyperplasia without inflammatory cells, are seen on correlative histologic examination.

- The progressive stages of impingement are more accurately described[609]:

  - Type 1: Rotator cuff degeneration or tendinosis without visible tears of either surface

  - Type 2: Rotator cuff degeneration or tendinosis with partial thickness tears of either articular or bursal surfaces

  - Type 3: Complete-thickness rotator cuff tears of varying size, complexity, and functional compromise

- Most rotator cuff tears do not begin at the bursal surface of the tendon, as tears secondary to impingement had originally been described.

- Partial tears of the rotator cuff involving the articular surface of the rotator cuff adjacent to the tendon insertion are more commonly seen.[606,609]

- Articular cuff lesions may be the result of tensile strength failure from overuse.

- Bursal lesions are more commonly associated with impingement.[423,606]

- Rotator cuff degeneration has been observed in the absence of anteroinferior acromial spurs.[423]

- Bursal-sided and full thickness rotator cuff tears can be correlated with degenerative changes of the coracoacromial ligament and anterior third of the inferior acromion.[436]

- Articular surface partial tears, however, can be associated with normal acromial morphology and histology.

- Most tears of the rotator cuff are attributed to degenerative lesions that were associated with increasing age, and the acromial changes present were secondary.[606]

- Relative rotator cuff hypovascularity in the critical zone of the supraspinatus (the distal 1cm) may be associated with tendon degeneration or may exacerbate changes associated with mechanical impingement.[45,366]

MR Appearance of Impingement

■ Rotator cuff disease is evaluated on the basis of tendon morphology and changes in the observed signal intensity within the specific cuff tendons.

■ Pathologic processes in the coracoacromial arch, including the acromion, the AC joint, and the subacromial-subdeltoid bursa, may be identified in the spectrum of findings in impingement lesions.[272,386,524,657,664]

■ MR Appearance of Subacromial-Subdeltoid Bursitis

　■ The normal subacromial-subdeltoid bursa is small with a flat and noninflamed synovial lining.[252]

　■ Identification of this structure and of signal intensity within the peribursal fat can be used to describe subacromial bursitis on MR images.[524,659]

　■ Although the changes of subacromial bursal inflammation are usually associated with tendinosis or cuff tears, small amounts of subacromial bursal fluid may be seen without abnormal cuff morphology or signal intensity alterations.

　　■ Impingement is associated with fraying and fragmentation of the CA ligament, synovitis, and bursal tissue thickening.

　■ The subacromial bursa may be distended with fluid in both partial and complete rotator cuff tears.

　■ FS PD FSE images have a high sensitivity for small amounts of fluid, making assessment of loss of peribursal fat no longer relevant.

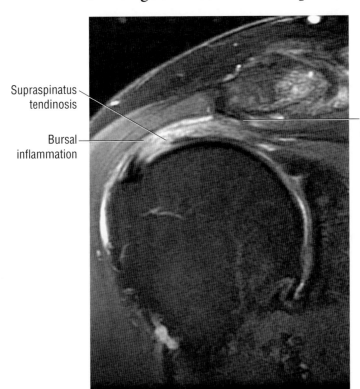

Supraspinatus tendinosis

Bursal inflammation

Acromial spur

FIGURE 5.21　Coronal FS PD FSE image showing severe tendinosis with greater bursal-side involvement and an anterior inferior acromial spur.

■ MR Appearance of Impingement Lesions of the Rotator Cuff

- ■ The normal rotator cuff tendons display low signal intensity.

- ■ Areas of intermediate signal intensity or signal inhomogeneity, especially in the distal extent of the supraspinatus tendon on T1- and PD-weighted images[287,408]

  - ▣ Attributed to a magic-angle phenomenon, partial volume averaging of the distinct components of the supraspinatus muscle and tendon, or histologic degeneration (eosinophilic, fibrillar, and mucoid)[484]

- ■ In the magic-angle phenomenon, tendon orientation at the magic angle of 55° to B_0 contributes to increased signal intensity in the supraspinatus tendon on short-TR/TE sequences.[589]

  - ▣ These signal effects may also be seen on GRE and FS images.

  - ▣ The routine use of T2-weighted images and observation of cuff morphology should minimize misinterpretation of these affected segments of the rotator cuff.

- ■ The pseudogap is a zone of increased signal intensity seen adjacent to the supraspinatus tendon attachment in asymptomatic subjects.

- ■ The pseudogap has been attributed to distinct portions of the supraspinatus muscle,[611] including the anterior fusiform portion, containing the dominant tendon of the supraspinatus, and a strap-like posterior portion.

  - ▣ The orientation of the tendon differs from the main muscle by 10°.

- ■ In cuff tendon degeneration, areas of intermediate signal intensity on T1- and PD-weighted images display intermediate to high signal intensity on T2*, FS PD-weighted FSE, and STIR sequences in both asymptomatic and symptomatic patients.

  - ▣ On T2 or T2-weighted (non-FS) FSE images, however, these regions of altered signal intensity are diminished or remain unchanged and are used to increase specificity in differentiating between tendon degeneration and partial tears.

- ■ Additional pitfalls in the interpretation of MR findings:

  - ▣ The subacromial peribursal fat plane may be effaced by bursal surface inflammation in the absence of a rotator cuff tear.[524]

  - ▣ Intrasubstance degeneration may also be associated with intrasubstance tears without bursal or articular surface extension.

▪ Rotator Cuff Degeneration in Impingement

▪ MR findings in degeneration and partial tears may overlap, and tendon pathology must be evaluated on the basis of bursal, intrasubstance, and articular surface morphology and on signal intensity changes.

▪ Evaluation is best accomplished with coronal oblique and sagittal oblique planar images.

▪ In rotator cuff degeneration, there is intermediate signal intensity on PD-weighted images, with no increase in signal intensity on T2- or T2-weighted FSE images.

▪ FS PD-weighted FSE sequences (TEs of 40 to 50ms) are sensitive to changes of degeneration and, in the absence of a partial or complete rotator cuff tear, display areas or regions of hyperintensity.

▪ Changes of cuff degeneration may be associated with intermediate to increased signal intensity on short-TE or T1 and PD weighted images without further increase in signal intensity on T2-weighted images.

▪ Fraying of the cuff may be seen as a surface contour irregularity of the articular or bursal surface.[471]

▪ Damage to the collagen fibers is associated with an increase in absorbed water.

  ▪ In severe degeneration and tears, there is a greater amount of free water within the affected tendon.

▪ Signal intensity in the supraspinatus tendon on PD-weighted images represents degeneration (eosinophilic, fibrillar, and mucoid) and scarring and not active inflammation.

▪ MR images often demonstrate increased subacromial fluid and bursal irregularity of the supraspinatus in patients with impingement.

- Tendinous enlargement associated with homogeneous or nonhomogeneous increased signal intensity is a more specific finding in symptomatic shoulders with tendinosis.

  - Tendinous enlargement, or the increased signal intensity of tendon degeneration, may also characterize the reparative process and healing of an interstitial tear.

- The term "tendinosis" is accepted (compared to tendinitis); it is acceptable to characterize an area of increased signal intensity on intermediate-weighted images and intermediate signal intensity on T2-weighted images as tendon degeneration.

- Impingement, however, is a clinical diagnosis, not an MR diagnosis.[533]

  - The tendon findings or osseous changes seen in impingement syndrome may be identified and described on MR images in conjunction with the patient's clinical presentation.

- In arthroscopic correlations of MR imaging and findings, degenerative tendon wear may be identified on the bursal or articular surface of the rotator cuff.

  - Not all cuff tears are initiated on the bursal surface as a result of impingement.

  - Most tears begin in the articular surface of the rotator cuff, adjacent to the tendon insertion on the greater tuberosity.

  - In early impingement (pretear tendinosis), there is relative preservation of articular and bursal tendon surface outlines.

  - A keel osteophyte of the inferior surface of the acromion can be visualized at arthroscopy in the subacromial bursa.[559]

  - "Room with a view" of the subacromial bursa obtained between the overlying acromion and the underlying rotator cuff tendon

  - Diagnosis of mechanical impingement confirmed with fraying on the undersurface of the coracoacromial ligament and irregularity of the bursal surface of the supraspinatus tendon

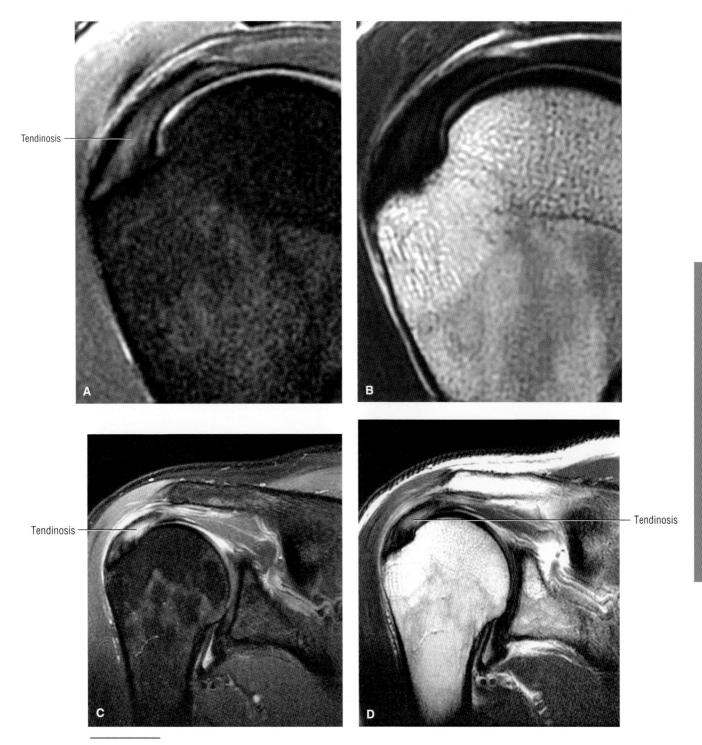

FIGURE 5.22 (**A**) Infraspinatus tendinosis appears hyperintense on this FS PD FSE coronal image. (**B**) Corresponding T2 FSE coronal image shows intact bursal and articular cuff surfaces. Note that cuff degeneration is visualized as intermediate signal intensity, thus increasing the specificity of this imaging sequence. (**C**) A separate area of infraspinatus tendinosis that may be mistaken for a partial articular-side tear is displayed on this FS PD FSE image. (**D**) A coronal T2 FSE image demonstrating tendinosis with no hyperintensity of cuff fibers.

Arthroscopic Classification of Impingement

- Classification system based on arthroscopic findings:

  - Type 1 Impingement

    - Characterized by signs of tendon wear or degeneration on the articular or bursal surface, with associated fraying or irregularity of either articular or bursal structures

    - Subdivided into type 1a (articular) and type 1b (bursal)

    - Intrasubstance degeneration, referred to as type 1c, may be associated with intrasubstance partial tears.

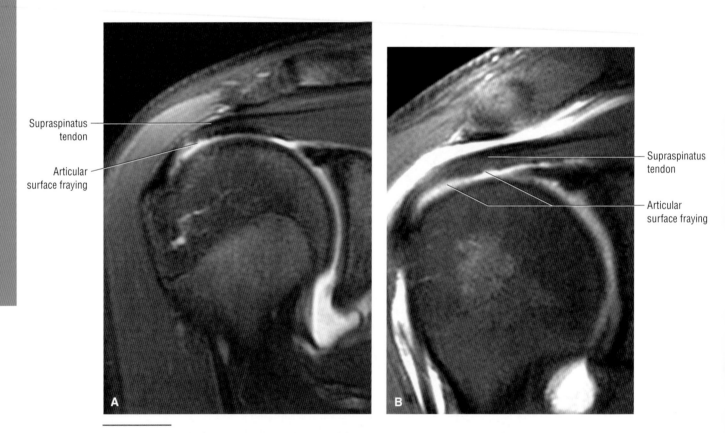

Supraspinatus tendon

Articular surface fraying

Supraspinatus tendon

Articular surface fraying

FIGURE 5.23   (**A**) Articular surface fraying of the supraspinatus in a gymnast. (**B**) Coronal FS PD FSE MR arthrogram in a separate case of articular surface fraying.

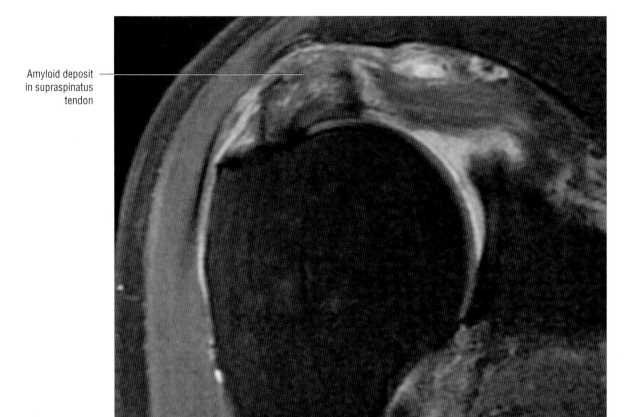

Amyloid deposit in supraspinatus tendon

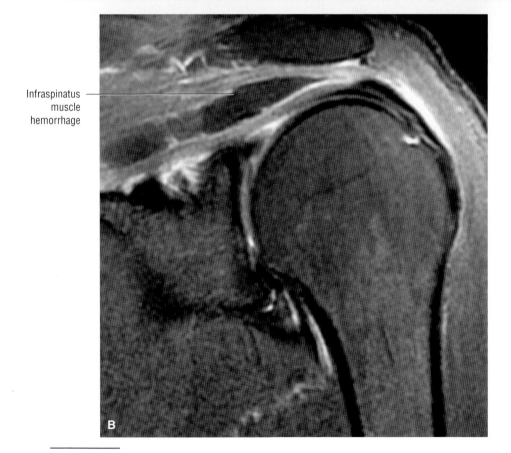

Infraspinatus muscle hemorrhage

FIGURE 5.24 (**A**) Unusual amyloid deposit in the supraspinatus tendon simulating rotator cuff tendinosis with tendon thickening and degeneration. Coronal FS PD FSE. (**B**) Hemorrhagic fluid collection in the infraspinatus muscle without associated tendon tear. Coronal FS PD FSE.

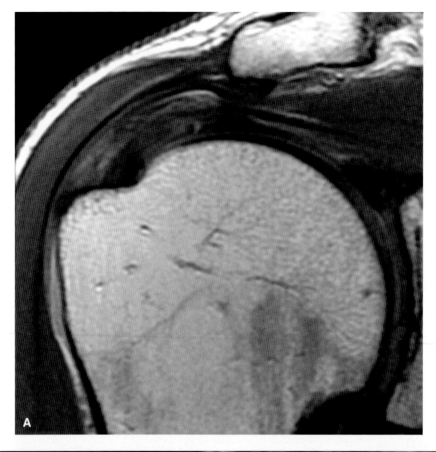

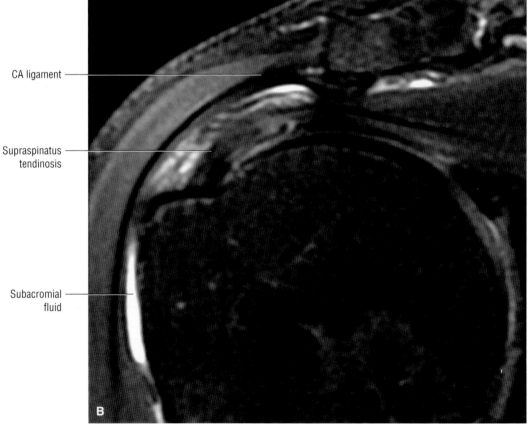

FIGURE 5.25   Severe rotator cuff tendinosis with tendon thickening and increased signal intensity. There is no contour defect in either the bursal or articular surfaces of the supraspinatus. (**A**) Coronal PD FSE image. (**B**) Coronal FS PD FSE image.

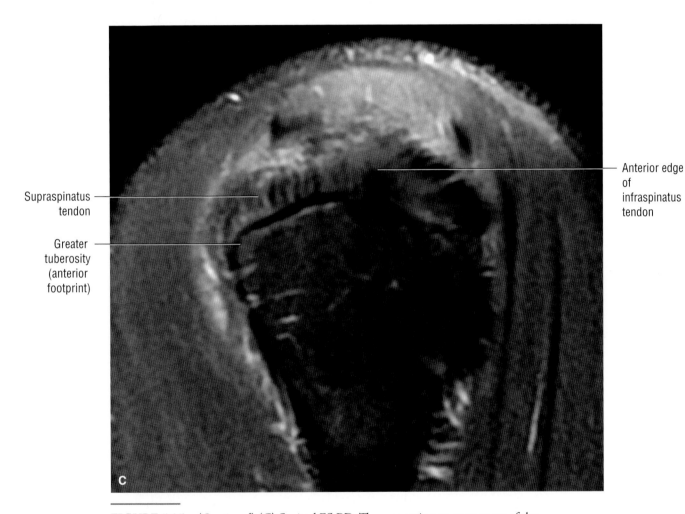

Supraspinatus tendon

Greater tuberosity (anterior footprint)

Anterior edge of infraspinatus tendon

C

FIGURE 5.25   *(Continued)* (**C**) Sagittal FS PD. The supraspinatus component of the rotator cuff is strengthened by the infraspinatus and subscapularis tendons forming a stronger functional unit. The tension on the articular fibers of the supraspinatus is greater than bursal fibers in abduction. The critical zone of the supraspinatus is 1cm proximal to the insertion of its central tendon.[182]

■ Type 2 Impingement

  ▪ In addition to tendon wear or degeneration, there are partial thickness tears of the articular surface in type 2a or the bursal surface in type 2b.

  ▪ Increased-signal-intensity fluid within the bursal or articular surface of the cuff is characteristic of this lesion.

  ▪ Small amounts of fluid may be seen in the subacromial bursa, especially in bursal surface type 2b lesions, in the absence of a full thickness or complete tear.

  ▪ Well-defined, linear high signal intensity on T2-weighted images or an area of increased signal intensity on long-TR/TE images that does not extend to either the articular or bursal surfaces may represent intrasubstance partial tears.

■ Type 3 Impingement

  ▪ Characterized by a full thickness tear of the rotator cuff

  ▪ Without retraction of the cuff, the tear is classified as type 3a.

  ▪ With retraction of the cuff, the tear is classified as type 3b.

  ▪ Without demonstration of a defined defect, retraction of the muscle belly, or extension of fluid across the supraspinatus tendon into the subacromial-subdelotid bursa, a complete tear cannot be unequivocally diagnosed.

  ▪ The presence of small amounts of fluid within the subacromial bursa should not be used as a primary sign of rotator cuff tear, unless associated with a direct communication of fluid from the glenohumeral joint into subacromial-subdeltoid bursa.

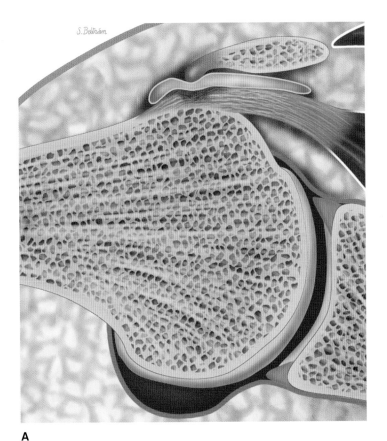

A

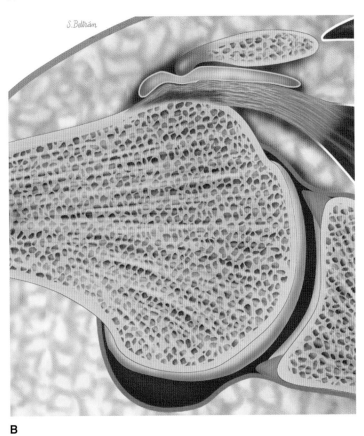

B

FIGURE 5.26   (**A**) Subacromial impingement with subacromial bursal inflammatory changes and development of a bursal-side partial tear of the rotator cuff. (**B**) Articular-side partial tear in subacromial impingement. Bursal inflammatory changes may be present with both bursal and articular side pathology.

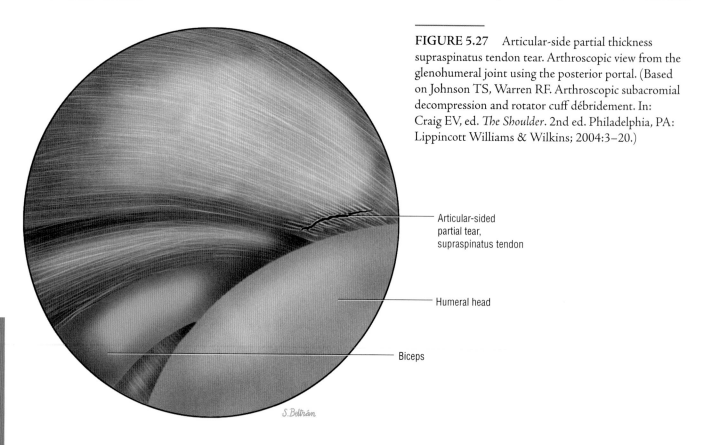

FIGURE 5.27 Articular-side partial thickness supraspinatus tendon tear. Arthroscopic view from the glenohumeral joint using the posterior portal. (Based on Johnson TS, Warren RF. Arthroscopic subacromial decompression and rotator cuff débridement. In: Craig EV, ed. *The Shoulder*. 2nd ed. Philadelphia, PA: Lippincott Williams & Wilkins; 2004:3–20.)

Articular-sided partial tear, supraspinatus tendon

Humeral head

Biceps

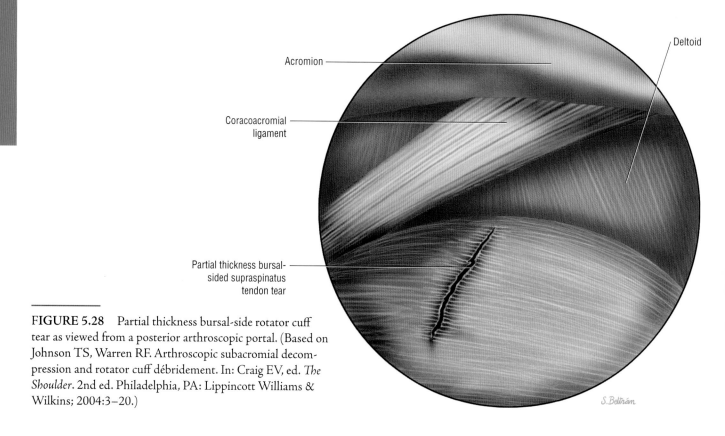

Deltoid

Acromion

Coracoacromial ligament

Partial thickness bursal-sided supraspinatus tendon tear

FIGURE 5.28 Partial thickness bursal-side rotator cuff tear as viewed from a posterior arthroscopic portal. (Based on Johnson TS, Warren RF. Arthroscopic subacromial decompression and rotator cuff débridement. In: Craig EV, ed. *The Shoulder*. 2nd ed. Philadelphia, PA: Lippincott Williams & Wilkins; 2004:3–20.)

MR Appearance of the Acromion in Impingement

- When present, the anterior acromial spur can be identified on MR images and acromial morphology and slope (potential risk factors for anterior acromial impingement) can be characterized.

- An anterior acromial spur (enthesophyte) extends from the anteroinferior surface of the acromion in a medial and inferior direction in the coronal plane.

- Anterior-inferior acromial spurs arise in or adjacent to the attachment of the coracoacromial ligament as a proposed traction osteophyte.

  - The anterior and inferior location of the spur is best shown on sagittal images.

  - Do not misinterpret the normal inferior acromial attachment of the coracoacromial ligament or lateral deltoid attachment as an acromial spur.

- The type 3 or hooked acromion is associated with greater predisposition to rotator cuff tears (i.e., critical zone of supraspinatus tendon).[616]

- A lateral downsloping of the acromion, which narrows the acromiohumeral distance, can be appreciated on coronal oblique images.

  - The inferior surface of the distal acromion is inferior or caudally located relative to the inferior surface of the more proximal aspect of the acromion.

  - Lateral downsloping of the acromion, however, does not correlate with impingement of the supraspinatus tendon.

  - The acromion may appear inferiorly offset relative to the distal clavicle even in the presence of normal acromial slope.

- Anterior downsloping of the acromion is appreciated in the sagittal plane.

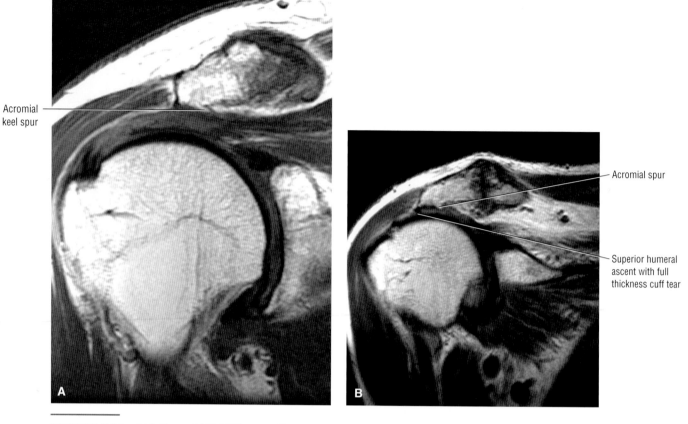

Acromial keel spur

Acromial spur

Superior humeral ascent with full thickness cuff tear

A

B

FIGURE 5.29   (**A**) Coronal PD FSE image illustrates a true acromial "keel" spur associated with cuff impingement. Keel spurs are considered aggressive with respect to their potential to cause damage to the bursal side of the cuff if not removed. (**B**) Complete chronic rotator cuff tear associated with anterior inferior acromial "keel" spur. The associated hypertrophic AC joint is not as important in the pathogenesis or progression of impingement to cuff tear.

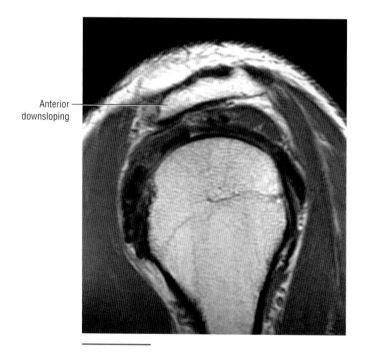

Anterior downsloping

FIGURE 5.30   Anterior downsloping acromion on sagittal PD FSE image.

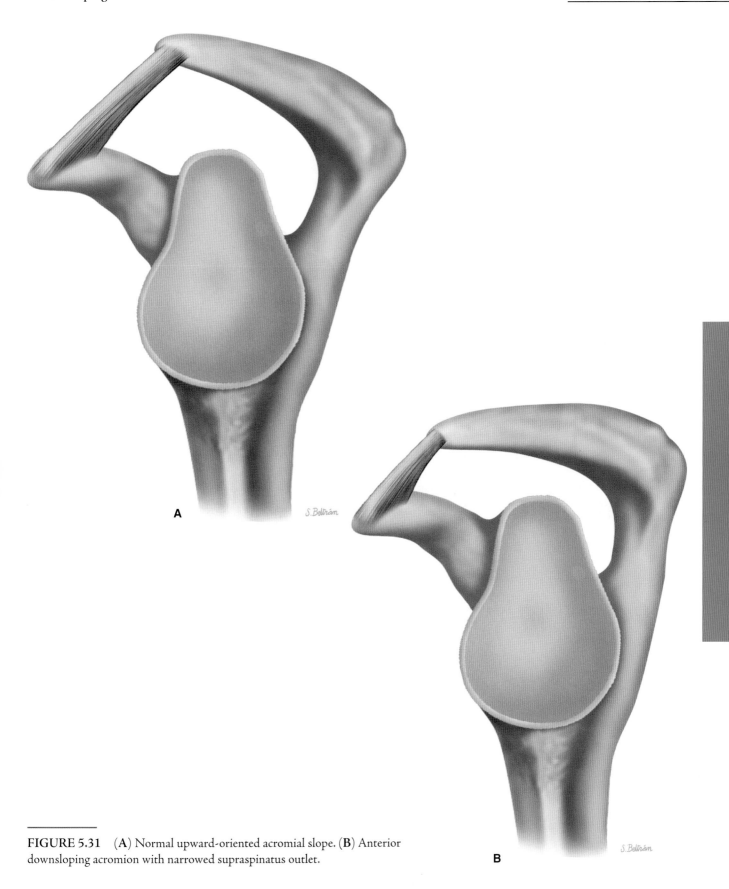

FIGURE 5.31 (**A**) Normal upward-oriented acromial slope. (**B**) Anterior downsloping acromion with narrowed supraspinatus outlet.

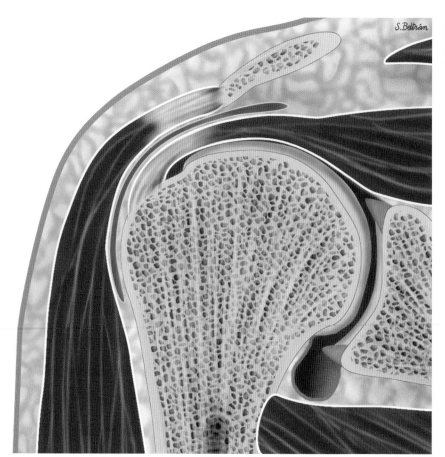

FIGURE 5.32   Lateral downsloping acromion as view on coronal section as a normal variation.

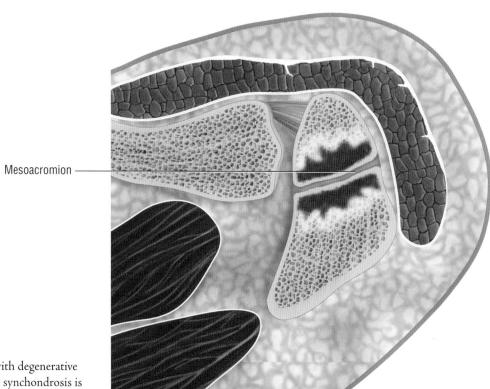

Mesoacromion

FIGURE 5.33   A mesoacromion with degenerative change and osseous edema across the synchondrosis is shown on an axial color illustration.

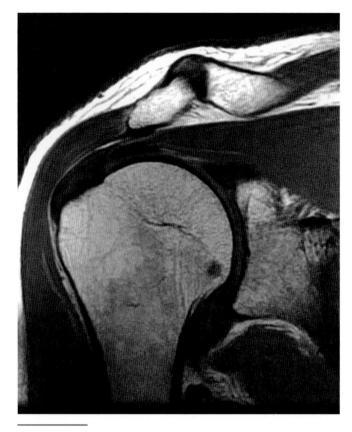

FIGURE 5.34 Lateral downsloping acromion assessed on coronal FSE image.

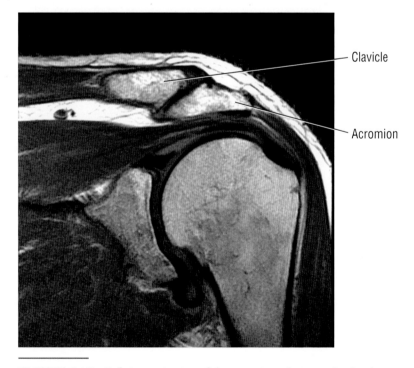

FIGURE 5.35 Inferior projection of the acromion relative to the distal clavicle. Mild arthrosis is also shown on this coronal T2 FSE image.

- Four types of os acromiale have been described:

    - Preacromion

        - In front of the anterior aspect of the AC joint

    - Mesoacromion

        - Extends anteriorly from the posterior aspect of the AC joint and meta-acromion

    - Meta-acromion

        - Extends posterior from the posterior AC joint base of acromion

    - Basiacromion

        - Lateral scapula (root of the acromion)

- Articulation of the synchondrosis is common between the preacromion and mesoacromion or mesoacromion and meta-acromion[665] and a movable unfused segment of the acromion may result in impingement.

    - Axial images best display the morphology and size of the os acromiale unfused segment.

    - Osteophytic lipping at the margins of the acromial gap may cause direct impingement on the rotator cuff and contraction of the deltoid muscle secondary to the downward pull on the os acromiale.

    - Unstable os acromiale is also associated with AC joint degeneration.

- Increased signal intensity on adjacent portions of the acromial marrow on either side of the fusion defect may be present on both STIR and FS PD-weighted FSE sequences in patients with os acromiale.

    - Hyperintensity may correlate with degenerative changes or instability in symptomatic patients.

- The presence of a normal or degenerative os acromiale should be described in both the body and impression of the MRI report.

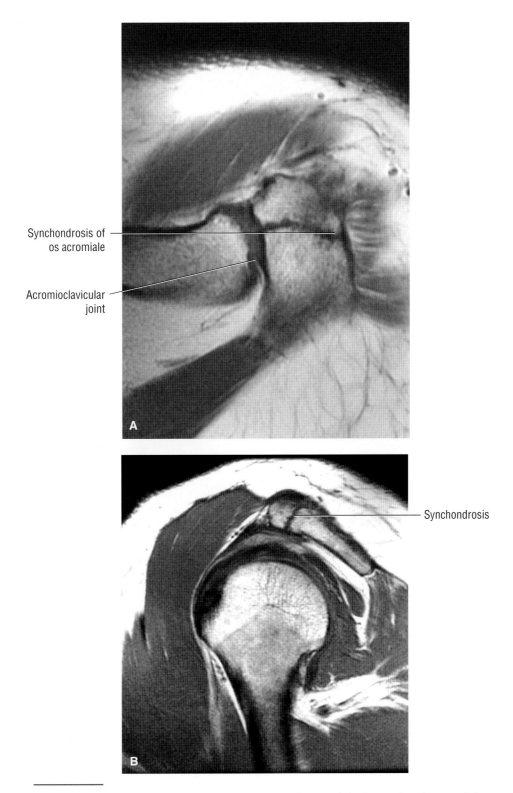

Synchondrosis of
os acromiale

Acromioclavicular
joint

Synchondrosis

FIGURE 5.36 Preacromion without degenerative changes. (**A**) The synchondrosis and the AC joint are shown together on this axial PD FSE image. (**B**) On this sagittal PD FSE image, the synchondrosis could be mistaken for an AC joint.

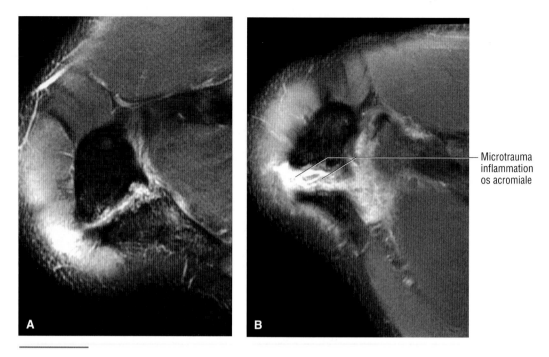

FIGURE 5.37   (**A**) A painful mesoacromion synchondrosis in a basketball player. (**B**) Subsequent severe inflammation of the os acromiale after 6 weeks of intensive weight lifting. Axial FS PD FSE images.

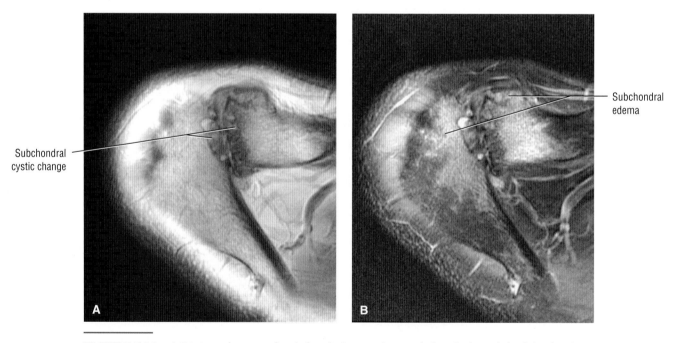

FIGURE 5.38   AC joint arthrosis with subchondral cystic changes (**A**) and edema (**B**) of the distal clavicle and adjacent acromion.

MR Appearance of the Acromioclavicular Joint

■ Arthrosis of the AC joint including callus and osteophytes may contribute to impingement, although less important than inferior acromial spurs.

■ The AC joint may encroach on the supraspinatus outlet and cause an extrinsic indentation on the bursal surface of the musculotendinous junction of the supraspinatus.

■ The portion of the cuff inferior to the AC joint is not as rigidly confined as the critical zone of the supraspinatus, which is more frequently affected by pathologic impingement at the location of the anterior inferior acromion.

■ Even when the contour of the supraspinatus muscle or tendon is deformed by the AC joint, patients may be asymptomatic.

■ Marginal osteophytes of the AC joint may precede the presence of anterior acromial erosion.

■ The coronal oblique and sagittal oblique planes are more useful in showing the relationship of the callus and osteophyte to the subacromial space and bursal cuff surface.

■ Identify edema of the AC joint in the coronal plane and then correlate with superior axial images.[182]

　■ Edema may be asymmetric across the AC joint when viewed in the axial plane.

■ Articular cartilage loss is evident on a fluid sensitive sequence.

■ The intraarticular disc or meniscus of the AC joint is variable in size and shape.

　■ The disc or meniscal homologue degenerates with age.

MR Appearance of Humeral Head Changes

- Humeral head cysts may be present adjacent to an area of rotator cuff tendinosis or tear.

- Greater tuberosity cysts are more common posterior at the greater tuberosity or at its junction with the humeral head adjacent to the capsular insertion.[665]

- Degenerative cysts also occur more superiorly or anteriorly.[665]

- Squaring and sclerosis of the greater tuberosity are best seen on coronal and sagittal oblique images.

- Loss of the acromiohumeral distance is a finding in the later stages of impingement.[46,401]

- Rounding of the greater tuberosity also occurs in advanced impingement and is usually associated with corresponding changes of bone erosion or sclerosis on the inferior acromial surface.

- The posterior aspect of the rotator cuff

    - Attaches adjacent to the bare area of the humeral head

    - Insertion may be fenestrated with arthroscopically visible openings in the superficial layers.

- The bare area of the humeral head

    - Located adjacent to the posterolateral rotator cuff insertion of the infraspinatus

    - Can vary from a few millimeters up to 2 or 3cm in diameter

    - Normal absence of articular cartilage exists in this region

    - Associated with vascular access channels to the subchondral bone

- The Hill-Sachs lesion is located more medially and is surrounded by normal articular cartilage.[554]

- In throwing athletes, subcortical cystic changes occur with the humeral head non-articular contact with the posterior superior glenoid rim.

Coracoacromial Ligament

- The coracoacromial ligament
    - Trapezoid shape to the ligament
    - Attached to the undersurface of the acromion in a broad or wide insertion
    - Varies in thickness from 2 to 5.6mm[174] and twists in a helical orientation inferiorly to its narrow coracoid insertion
- Arthroscopic findings of impingement include erosive changes in the acromial attachment of the coracoacromial ligament.

Imaging of Coracoid Impingement

- Coracoid or subcoracoid impingement related to the entrapment of the subscapularis tendon and muscle between the coracoid process and the lesser tuberosity[182]
- Coracohumeral or subcoracoid impingement occurs secondary to narrowing of the space between the coracoid process and the humeral head.
    - Narrowing most evident in internal rotation[59]
- Coracohumeral impingement is associated with interval measurements less than 8mm (no reproducible cutoff measurement).
    - Pathology is associated with coracohumeral narrowing less than 6mm.
- Developmental enlargement of the coracoid process may contribute to subcoracoid impingement when the humeral head is in forward flexion and internal rotation.

Spectrum of Pathology of Coracoid Impingement

- Partial subscapularis tear

- Synovitis of the rotator interval tissue

- Increased stress on the articular side of the subscapularis with resultant roller-wringer effect on the subscapularis[75]

  - Increase articular surface tensile loads

  - Tensile undersurface failure (TUFF) tears of the deep or articular surface of the subscapularis tendon

- The coracoid tip can impinge on the anterior subscapularis and rotator interval tissue and cause inflammation and articular surface tearing of the distal superior subscapularis tendon.

- Linear longitudinal tears of the superior distal subscapularis are associated with subcoracoid impingement.

  - These linear tears are the result of a repetitive battering-ram effect caused by the coracoid tip.

  - The linear longitudinal splits are caused by both the battering-ram effect and the roller-wringer effect which creates the spreading and compression of the subscapularis tendon against the tip of the coracoid.

- There is repetitive compression of the subscapularis tendon fibers anterior-to-posterior associated with the coracoid tip distracting or spreading subscapularis tendon fibers in the superior-to-inferior direction.

- Subcoracoid stenosis

  - Associated with anterior shoulder pathology as seen with a superior distal subscapularis tendon tear

  - May be seen without an associated subscapularis tendon tear in some patients with anterior shoulder pain

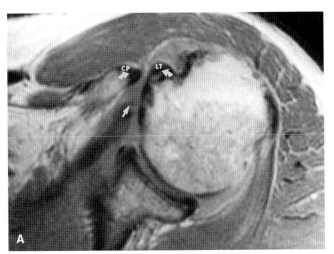
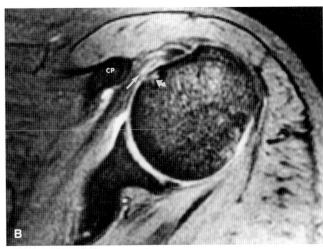

FIGURE 5.39 Coracoid impingement with narrowing (*curved arrows*) between the coracoid process (CP) and humeral head. Associated subscapularis tendon degeneration (*straight arrow*) and subchondral cystic change of the anteromedial humeral head (*curved arrow*) are shown on (**A**) T1 and (**B**) T2*-weighted axial images. LT, lesser tuberosity.

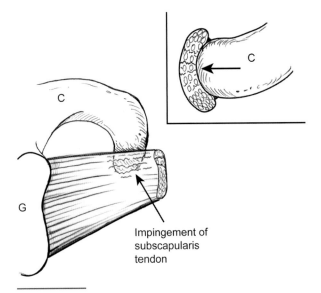

FIGURE 5.40 Schematic of subcoracoid impingement. Repetitive compression of the subscapularis tendon fibers in the anterior-to-posterior direction by the coracoid tip causes spreading of the fibers in the superior-to-inferior direction, with resultant longitudinal splits between subscapularis tendon fiber bundles. C, coracoid; G, glenoid. (Reprinted from Burkhart S, Lo IK, Brady PC, Denard PJ. *The Cowboy's Companion: A Trail Guide for the Arthroscopic Shoulder Surgeon.* Philadelphia, PA: Lippincott Williams & Wilkins; 2012, with permission.)

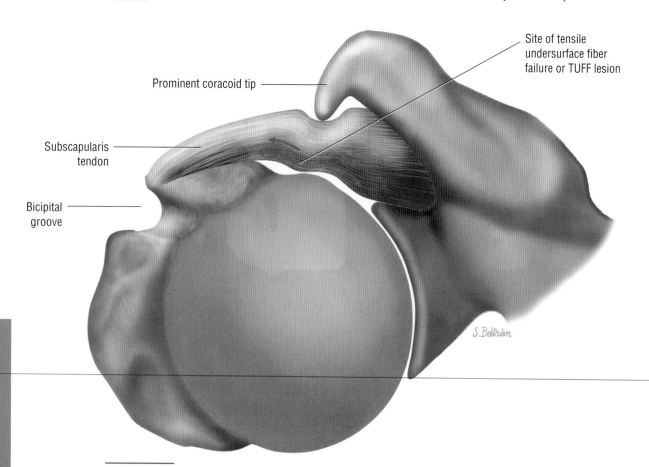

Site of tensile
undersurface fiber
failure or TUFF lesion

Prominent coracoid tip

Subscapularis
tendon

Bicipital
groove

S.Beltrán

FIGURE 5.41   Subcoracoid impingement with tensile forces generated on the convex, articular surface of the subscapularis tendon. (Based on Burkhart SS, Lo IKY, Brady PC. *Burkhart's View of the Shoulder: A Cowboy's Guide to Advanced Shoulder Arthroscopy*. Philadelphia, PA: Lippincott Williams & Wilkins; 2006.)

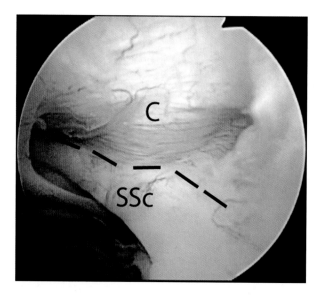

FIGURE 5.42   Right shoulder, posterior glenohumeral viewing portal with a 70° arthroscope demonstrates subcoracoid impingement. With internal and external rotation, the tip of the coracoid creates an indentation (*dashed black lines*) in the subscapularis tendon. C, coracoid; SSc, subscapularis tendon. (Reprinted from Burkhart S, Lo IK, Brady PC, Denard PJ. *The Cowboy's Companion: A Trail Guide for the Arthroscopic Shoulder Surgeon*. Philadelphia, PA: Lippincott Williams & Wilkins; 2012, with permission.)

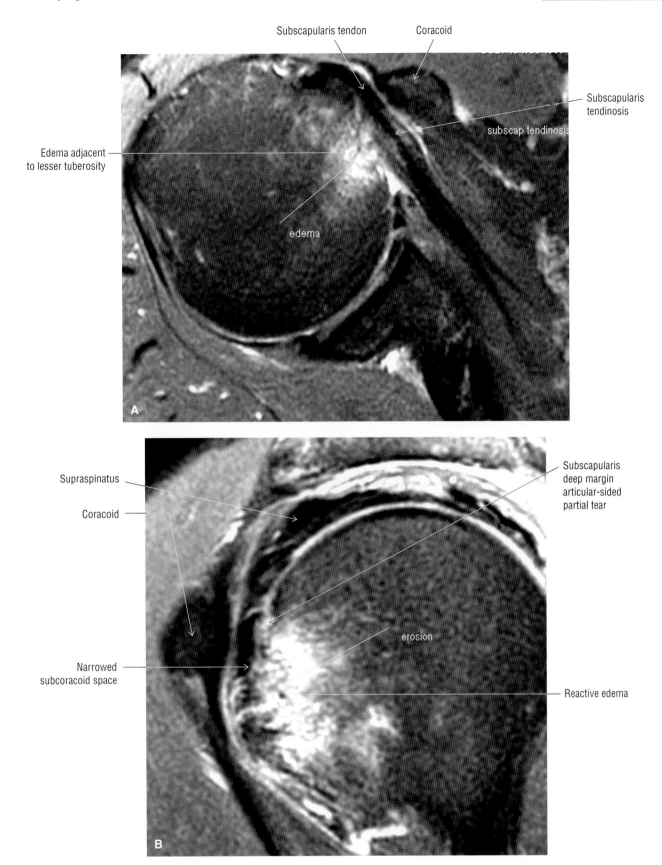

FIGURE 5.43 Subcoracoid impingement is usually characterized by a partial tear of the superior distal subscapularis tendon and synovitis of the rotator interval with impingement between the coracoid and lesser tuberosity. The articular surface of the subscapularis is where abnormal stress develops. Axial FS PD image with edema adjacent to the lesser tuberosity and subscapularis tendinosis with narrowed subcoracoid space. Linear longitudinal tears of the distal subscapularis near its insertion are common. (**A**) Axial FS PD, (**B**) Sagittal FS PD.

Acromioplasty

- Arthroscopic subacromial decompression (ASD) is the method of choice for the treatment of chronic outlet impingement.[46,404]

    - Does not violate the deltoid and overlying deltotrapezial fascia

    - Arthroscopic anterior acromioplasty is indicated for alleviation of pain secondary to the impingement of the anterior inferior surface of the acromion.

    - The coracoacromial ligament is detached from the anterior inferior acromial surface and inflamed or frayed cuff tissue is débrided.

    - Used to treat patients with early impingement, demonstrating degenerative irregularities of the articular bursal surface of the rotator cuff

    - Arthroscopic findings usually include fraying of the articular or bursal surface and evidence of fraying of the coracoacromial ligament as it attaches to the anterior and lateral borders of the anterior inferior surface of the acromion.

    - Kissing lesions are irregularities of the bursal surfaces of the cuff found opposite irregularities or fraying of the coracoacromial ligament.

- Partial thickness tears involving the articular or bursal surfaces of the rotator cuff are treated with subacromial decompression and débridement of the partial thickness tear.

    - The deeper and more extensive the cleavage planes and the larger the flap of cuff produced by the tear, the greater the likelihood that a simple subacromial decompression will be insufficient and either an arthroscopic or an open repair of the more significantly damaged partially torn cuff will be necessary.

Associated Arthroscopic Procedures

- Resection of the coracoacromial ligament is always performed in addition to the acromioplasty.

- If joint pain is associated with impingement, an arthroscopic Mumford procedure (i.e., resection of the distal 2cm of the clavicle) is performed at the same time as ASD.

- If biceps is frayed or attenuated, it is resected from its insertion at the glenohumeral tubercle and a tenodesis is performed.

6

Rotator Cuff Tears, Microinstability, Rotator Cuff Interval/Biceps Pulley, and the Throwing Shoulder

Rotator Cuff Tears, Microinstability, Rotator Cuff Interval/Biceps Pulley, and the Throwing Shoulder

Rotator Cuff Tears

Key Concepts

- Partial thickness rotator cuff tears are articular, bursal, or interstitial (intrasubstance).

- The PASTA lesion
    - Is a type of rim rent tear
    - Definition includes partial articular surface tendon avulsion and not just partial articular-sided supraspinatus tendon avulsion.
    - Articular-sided delamination that extends from the footprint

- The bursal puddle sign of localized fluid correlates with a bursal-sided rotator cuff tear.

- Intrasubstance cysts communicate with partial or full thickness cuff tears.

- Coronal images identify an intact stump of cuff tendon attaching to the greater tuberosity in cuff tears proximal to the tendinous footprint.

- A wavy contour ("cuff wave sign") of the retracted cuff tendon is associated with an easier cuff reattachment as the tissue is more compliant and less scarred.

- Retracted rotator cuff tears are associated with an increase in cross-sectional diameter on sagittal images.

- The normal (without atrophy) supraspinatus muscle nearly occupies the suprascapular fossa as assessed on sagittal images.

- The biceps tendon may be medially subluxed or dislocated anteriorly, deep or within the substance of a torn distal subscapularis tendon.

- Rotator cuff tendon retears may be associated with partial or complete tendon retraction and/or granulation tissue at the tear site simulating apparent cuff continuity.

- Partial tears may involve the articular or bursal surfaces in varying degrees of depth and extension into the tendon.[67,158]

- Intratendinous lesions do not communicate with either the bursal or articular surfaces.

- Complete (full thickness) rotator cuff tears extend through the entire thickness of the rotator cuff, with direct communication between the subacromial bursa and the glenohumeral joint. Full width implies tear extension from anterior to posterior.

- A massive rotator cuff tear involves at least two of the rotator cuff tendons.[384]

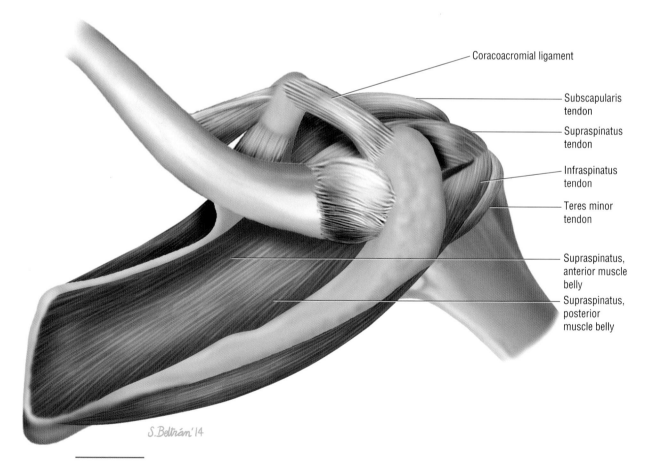

FIGURE 6.1   Rotator cuff and tendons visible in superior view deep to the coracoacromial arch. The four muscles of the rotator cuff include the subscapularis, supraspinatus, infraspinatus, and teres minor. The supraspinatus and infraspinatus tendon join 15mm proximal to their distal insertion on the greater tuberosity.

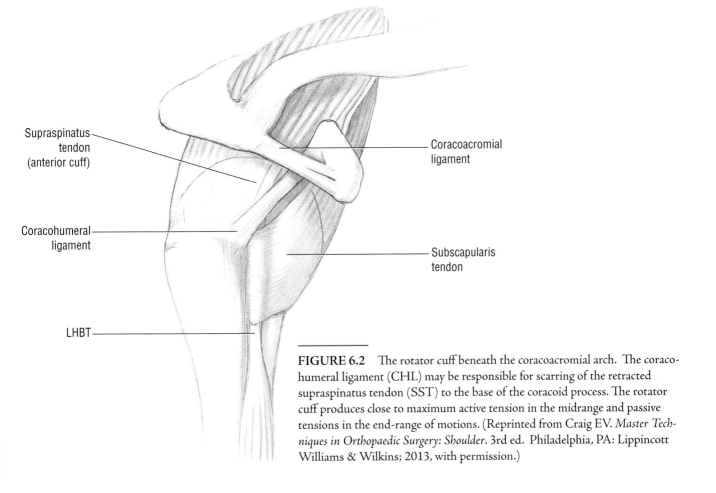

Supraspinatus tendon (anterior cuff)

Coracoacromial ligament

Coracohumeral ligament

Subscapularis tendon

LHBT

FIGURE 6.2 The rotator cuff beneath the coracoacromial arch. The coracohumeral ligament (CHL) may be responsible for scarring of the retracted supraspinatus tendon (SST) to the base of the coracoid process. The rotator cuff produces close to maximum active tension in the midrange and passive tensions in the end-range of motions. (Reprinted from Craig EV. *Master Techniques in Orthopaedic Surgery: Shoulder.* 3rd ed. Philadelphia, PA: Lippincott Williams & Wilkins; 2013, with permission.)

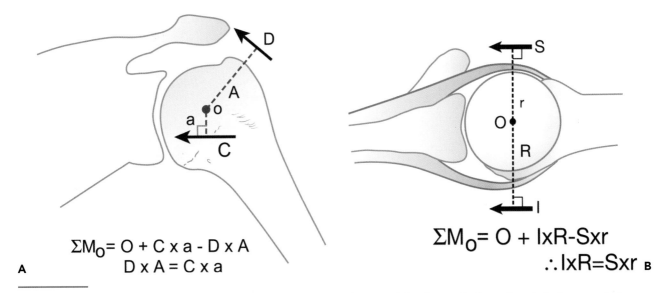

$$\Sigma M_O = O + C \times a - D \times A$$
$$D \times A = C \times a$$

$$\Sigma M_O = O + I \times R - S \times r$$
$$\therefore I \times R = S \times r$$

FIGURE 6.3 (**A**) Balanced force couples are required to maintain the normal glenohumeral relationship. A: In the coronal plane, the combined inferior rotator cuff force (C) is balanced against the deltoid (D). (**B**) In the axial plane, the subscapularis (S) is balanced against the infraspinatus and teres minor (I). The subscapularis has the greatest force-producing capacity of the cuff muscles and contributes passive tension at maximum abduction and lateral rotation. The subscapularis thus plays a key role in providing glenohumeral stability in the position of apprehension. O, center of rotation; A, moment arm of the deltoid; a, moment arm of the inferior rotator cuff; r, moment arm of the subscapularis; R, moment arm of the infraspinatus and teres minor. (Reprinted from Burkhart S, Lo IK, Brady PC, Denard PJ. *The Cowboy's Companion: A Trail Guide for the Arthroscopic Shoulder Surgeon.* Philadelphia, PA: Lippincott Williams & Wilkins; 2012, with permission.)

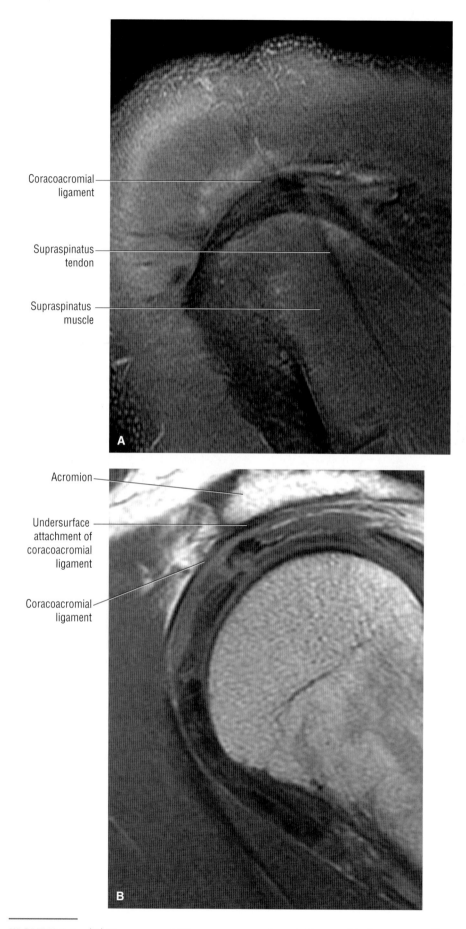

FIGURE 6.4 **(A)** Coracoacromial ligament on superior axial image with the rotator cuff supraspinatus tendon coursing deep to the arch created by the ligament. FS PD axial. **(B)** Sagittal view of the broad attachment of the coracoacromial ligament to the undersurface of the acromion. Sagittal PD image.

Supraspinatus muscle strain

Supraspinatus tendon

Supraspinatus muscle strain

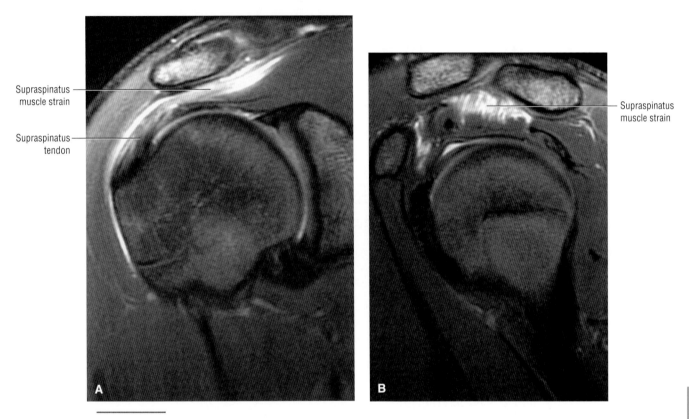

FIGURE 6.5 Superior surface muscle–tendon unit strain of the supraspinatus demonstrates hyperintense muscle edema superior to the tendinous expansion of the cuff on coronal FS PD FSE (**A**) and sagittal FS PD FSE (**B**) images. These muscle–tendon strains occur in younger more athletic patients and usually involve a specific portion of the supraspinatus muscle. This type of muscle strain corresponds to the transition of the supraspinatus intramuscular tendinous core to the more distal tubular extramuscular tendon. In contrast, the posterior muscle belly of the supraspinatus is smaller, unipennate and without an intramuscular tendon. The posterior muscle belly does not generate long contractile forces so muscle strains of these fibers are less common.

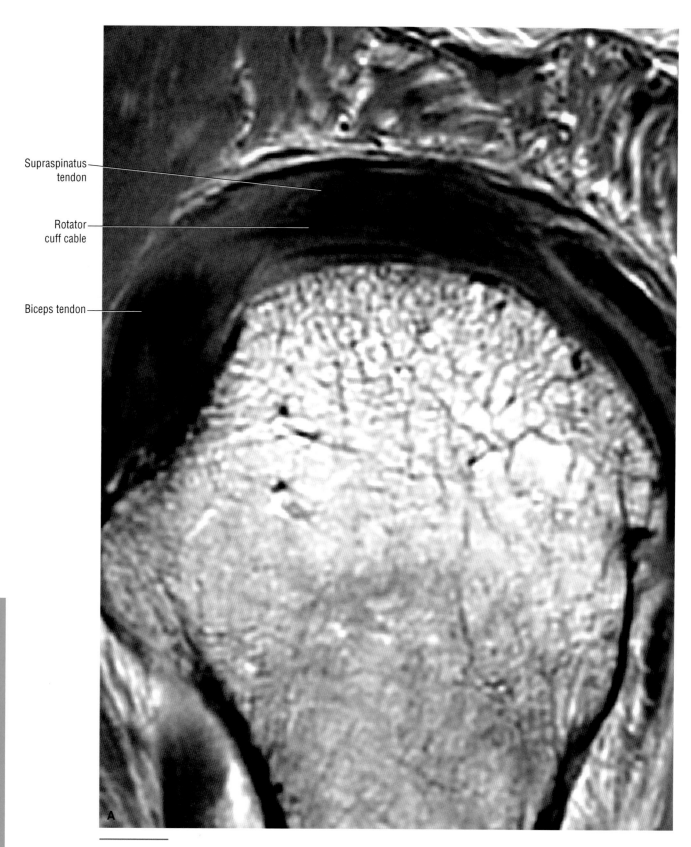

Supraspinatus tendon

Rotator cuff cable

Biceps tendon

FIGURE 6.6   (**A**) Identification of the supraspinatus and rotator cuff cable as an extension of the deep layer of the coracohumeral ligament. T1 sagittal.

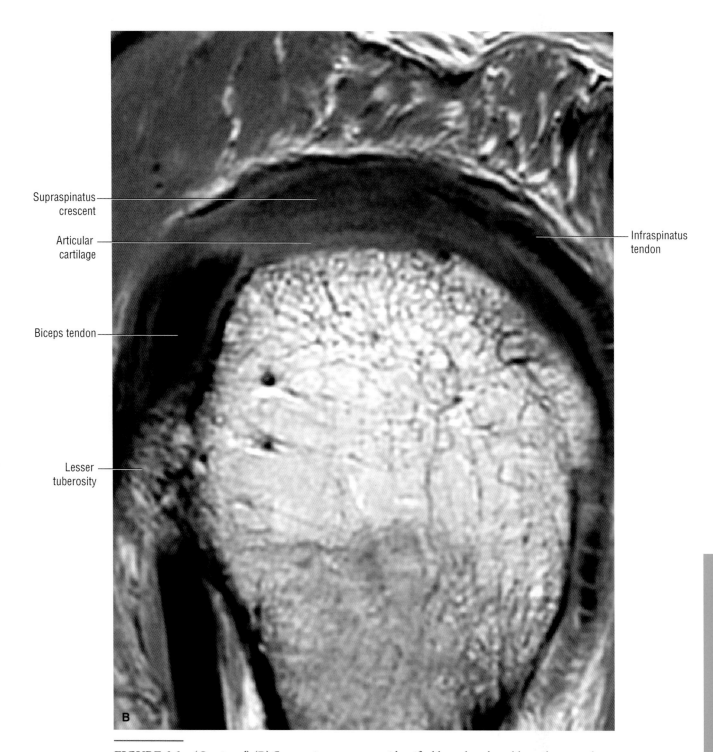

Supraspinatus crescent

Articular cartilage

Biceps tendon

Lesser tuberosity

Infraspinatus tendon

B

FIGURE 6.6   (*Continued*) (**B**) Supraspinatus crescent identified lateral to the cable as shown at the level of the biceps tendon and lesser tuberosity. T1 sagittal.

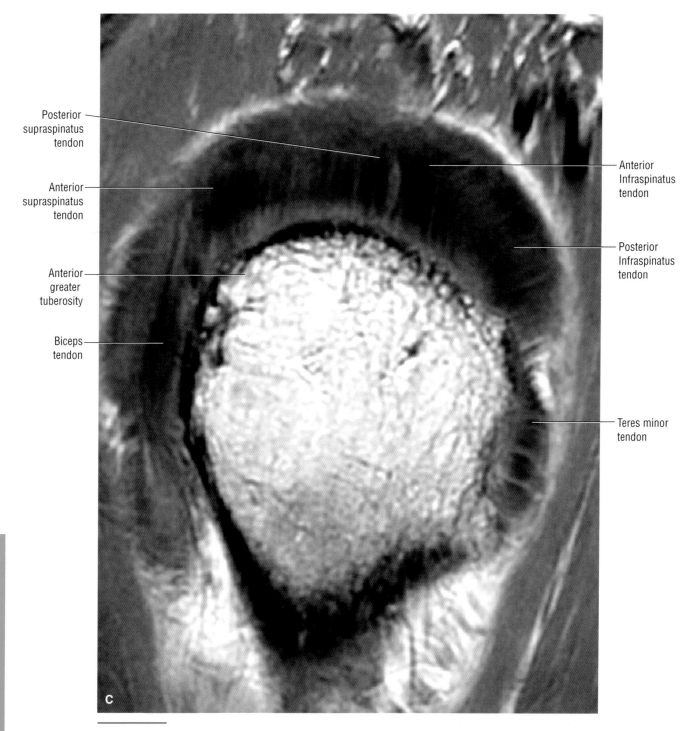

FIGURE 6.6 (*Continued*) (**C**) Peripheral rotator cuff footprint with attachment of the anterior and posterior supraspinatus and the infraspinatus tendon. The anterior external or extramuscular tendon represents approximately 40% of the width of the supraspinatus tendon. The smaller posterior muscle belly of the supraspinatus (without intramuscular tendon) has a flatter, wider posterior tendon which accounts for approximately 60% of the width of the supraspinatus tendon.

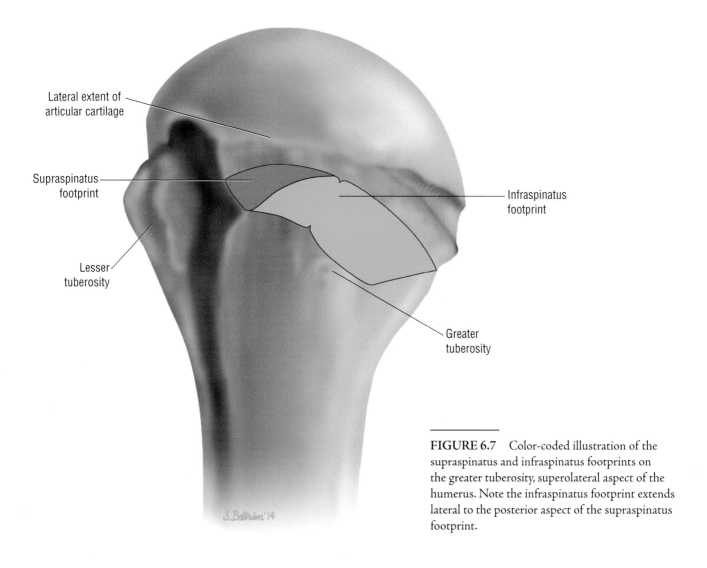

Lateral extent of articular cartilage

Supraspinatus footprint

Lesser tuberosity

Infraspinatus footprint

Greater tuberosity

S.Beltrán '14

FIGURE 6.7 Color-coded illustration of the supraspinatus and infraspinatus footprints on the greater tuberosity, superolateral aspect of the humerus. Note the infraspinatus footprint extends lateral to the posterior aspect of the supraspinatus footprint.

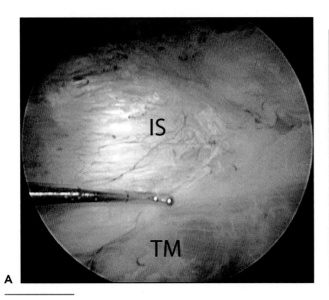

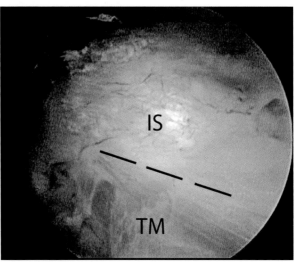

FIGURE 6.8 (**A**) Left shoulder, posterior viewing portal. A probe marks the border between the infraspinatus and teres minor. (**B**) Same shoulder, demonstrates how the muscle belly of the teres minor extends further lateral than that of the infraspinatus. The *dashed lines* outline the interval between the infraspinatus and teres minor. IS, infraspinatus tendon; TM, teres minor tendon. (Reprinted from Burkhart S, Lo IK, Brady PC, Denard PJ. *The Cowboy's Companion: A Trail Guide for the Arthroscopic Shoulder Surgeon*. Philadelphia, PA: Lippincott Williams & Wilkins; 2012, with permission.)

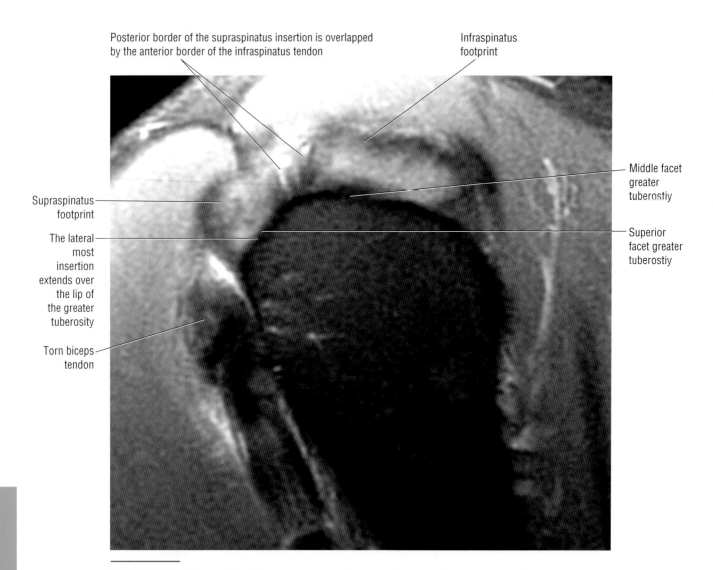

Posterior border of the supraspinatus insertion is overlapped by the anterior border of the infraspinatus tendon

Infraspinatus footprint

Middle facet greater tuberostiy

Superior facet greater tuberostiy

Supraspinatus footprint

The lateral most insertion extends over the lip of the greater tuberosity

Torn biceps tendon

FIGURE 6.9   The width of the supraspinatus footprint from anterior to posterior has an average maximum measurement of 16mm. The average maximum length (as assessed in the coronal plane) of the supraspinatus is 23mm. The supraspinatus tendon usually inserts directly on the lateral humeral head articular cartilage surface throughout the entire anterior to posterior length of the tendon attachment. The supraspinatus tendon anterior edge forms the superior border of the rotator interval.

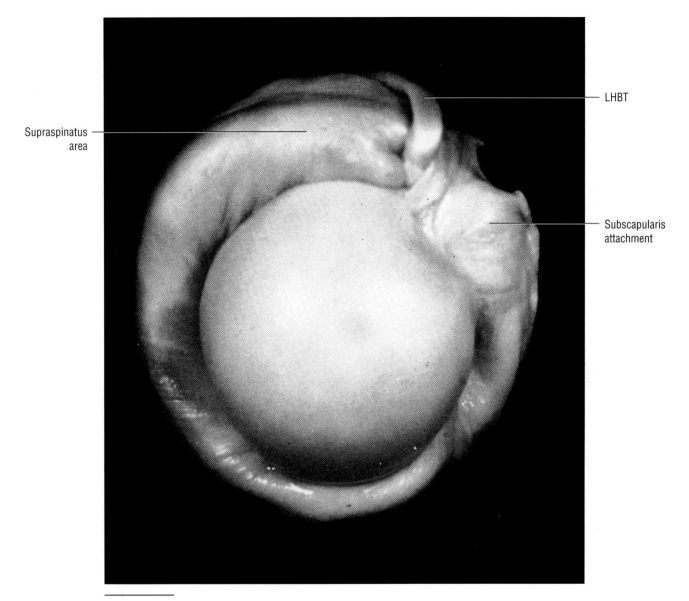

FIGURE 6.10 Left shoulder with intact rotator cuff and normal nondegenerative humeral head articular cartilage. The musculotendinous cuff with its synovial lining is continuous with the articular cartilage. There is no recession of rotator cuff fibers in this 23 yr. old specimen. The sulcus lateral to the peripheral articular cartilage if present would only be visible by the recession of the rotator cuff. (Modified from DePalma AF. *Surgery of the Shoulder*. 3rd ed. Philadelphia, PA: JB Lippincott; 1983.)

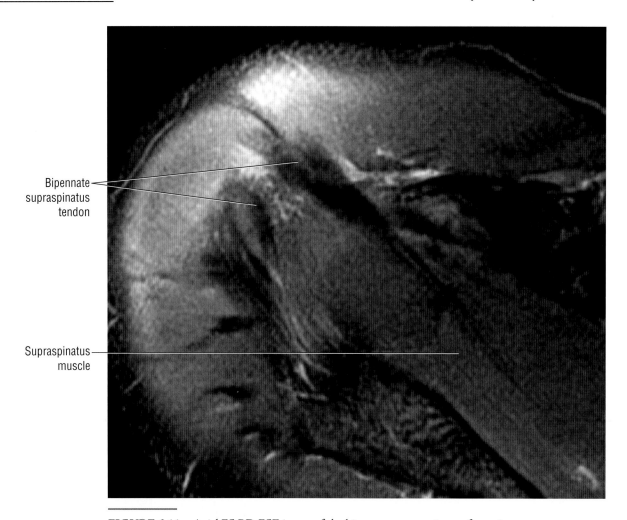

Bipennate
supraspinatus
tendon

Supraspinatus
muscle

FIGURE 6.11 Axial FS PD FSE image of the bipennate supraspinatus footprint.

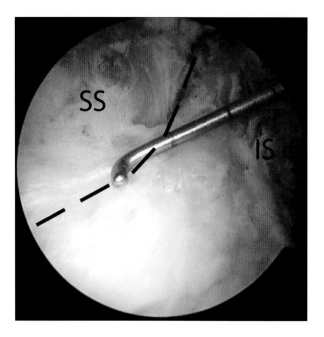

FIGURE 6.12 Left shoulder, lateral subacromial viewing portal, demonstrates the normal infraspinatus tendon insertion. Note that the anterior insertion of the infraspinatus is not directly lateral to the line of its fibers but rather curves anterolaterally to its insertion onto the greater tuberosity (dashed line indicate anterior margin of infraspinatus). IS, infraspinatus; SS, supraspinatus. (Reprinted from Burkhart S, Lo IK, Brady PC, Denard PJ. *The Cowboy's Companion: A Trail Guide for the Arthroscopic Shoulder Surgeon.* Philadelphia, PA: Lippincott Williams & Wilkins; 2012, with permission.)

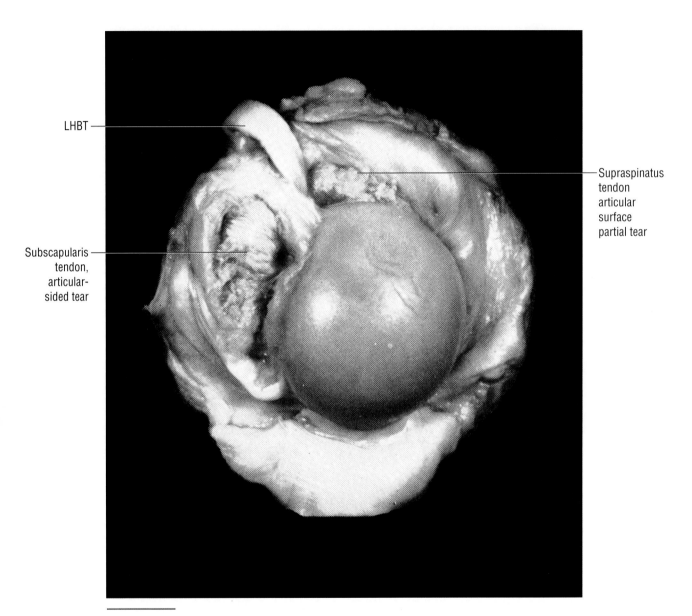

LHBT

Supraspinatus tendon articular surface partial tear

Subscapularis tendon, articular-sided tear

FIGURE 6.13 A 55 yr. old specimen with severe degenerative changes with partial articular-sided tears in the supraspinatus and subscapularis regions of the cuff. The degenerative changes of the articular cartilage in the humeral head are minimal. (Modified from DePalma AF. *Surgery of the Shoulder*. 3rd ed. Philadelphia, PA: JB Lippincott; 1983.)

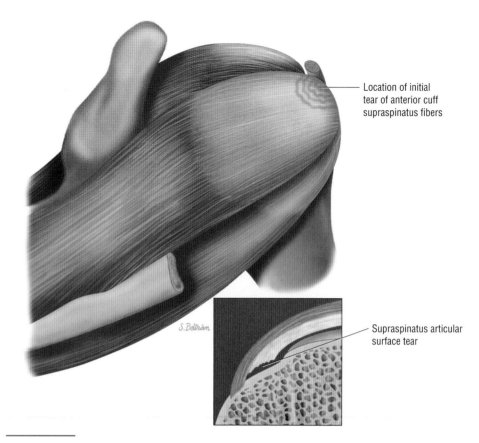

Location of initial tear of anterior cuff supraspinatus fibers

Supraspinatus articular surface tear

FIGURE 6.14   Degenerative cuff pathology with initial failure of the rotator cuff occurring along the articular surface of the supraspinatus adjacent to its greater tuberosity insertion. (Based on Matsen F III, Titelman R, Lippitt S, et al. Rotator cuff. In: Rockwood CA Jr, Matsen FA III, Wirth MA, et al, eds. *The Shoulder*. 3rd ed. Philadelphia, PA: WB Saunders; 2004:791–878.)

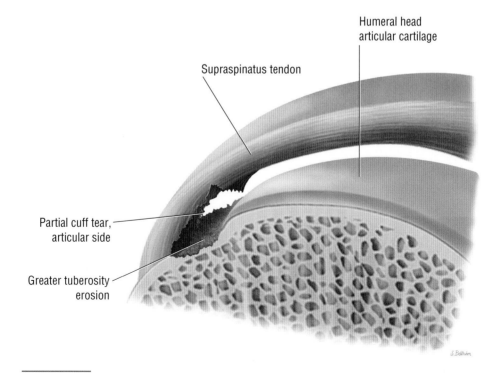

Humeral head articular cartilage

Supraspinatus tendon

Partial cuff tear, articular side

Greater tuberosity erosion

FIGURE 6.15   Rim rent tear of the articular surface of the cuff with erosion of the greater tuberosity.

Partial Tears

- Classified by tendon location
    - Supraspinatus
    - Infraspinatus
    - Subscapularis

- Classified by anatomic location
    - Bursal
    - Articular
    - Interstitial

- Classified by percentage of tendon thickness torn
    - Surgical reattachment of tendon indicated for tears involving 50% or greater of tendon thickness

- Partial thickness bursal-sided rotator cuff tears are most frequently associated with an impingement-type syndrome.[162]
    - Articular-sided cuff tears may be associated with an underlying instability of the shoulder.
    - Partial cuff tears present as fraying without complete disruption of the tendon.
    - Throwers with posterior peel-back lesions have partial thickness articular-sided tears usually located posteriorly at the junction of the supraspinatus and infraspinatus tendons or involving the anterior infraspinatus tendon.
    - Anterior partial cuff articular-sided tears are associated with superior labrum-anterior cuff (SLAC) lesions, which demonstrate the anterior labral components of a type 2 SLAP tear.

- The location of rotator cuff tears is identified as[556]:
    - A: At the articular surface
    - B: At the bursal surface
    - C: A complete tear, connecting articular and bursal tears

- The severity of partial rotator cuff tears (A and B partial tears) has been classified by Snyder[556] as:

    - 0: Normal

    - I: Minimal superficial bursal or synovial irritation or mild capsular fraying in a small localized area (<1cm)

    - II: Fraying and failure of some rotator cuff fibers plus synovial bursal or capsular injury (<2cm)

    - III: Fraying and fragmentation of tendon fibers usually involving the whole surface of a cuff tendon, most commonly the supraspinatus (<3cm)

    - IV: Severe tear with tendon fraying, fragmentation, and sizeable flap tear involving more than a single tendon

- The depth of tendon fiber involvement is also used as a criterion for grading partial tears[157,665]:

    - Grade 1: less than 3mm deep

    - Grade 2: 3 to 6mm deep and less than 50% of the cuff thickness involved

    - Grade 3: A high-grade partial tear more than 6mm deep with more than 50% of the rotator cuff thickness involved

- Non PASTA partial tears: PAINT and STAS lesions

    - Partial thickness articular surface intratendinous (PAINT) tears occur in overhead athletes in which the footprint is intact.

        - Extension of an interstitial component from the articular surface occurs at the posterior supraspinatus or anterior infraspinatus.

    - The supraspinatus tendon articular-side or STAS lesion includes partial thickness cuff tears proximal or exclusive to the footprint without the interstitial delaminating component that is seen with PAINT lesions.

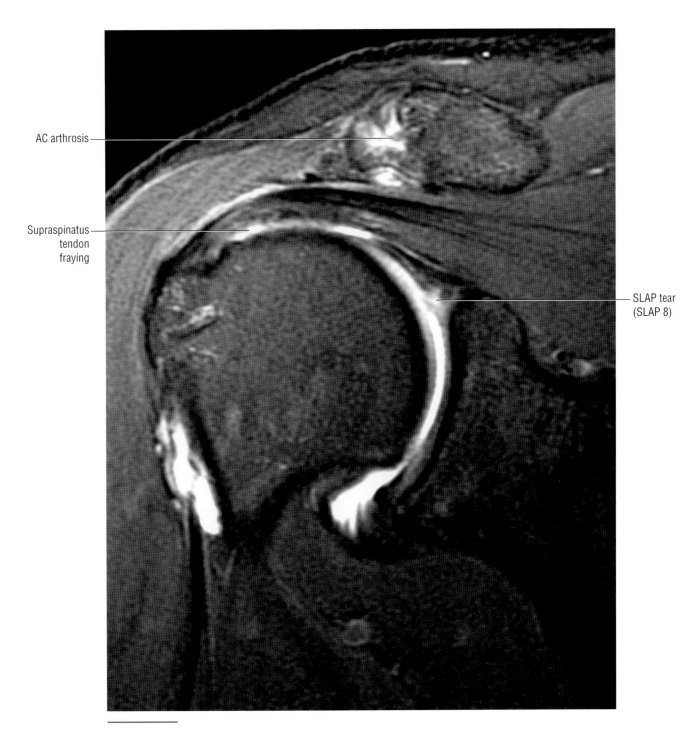

AC arthrosis

Supraspinatus
tendon
fraying

SLAP tear
(SLAP 8)

FIGURE 6.16   FS PD FSE coronal with articular-sided fraying of the supraspinatus tendon.

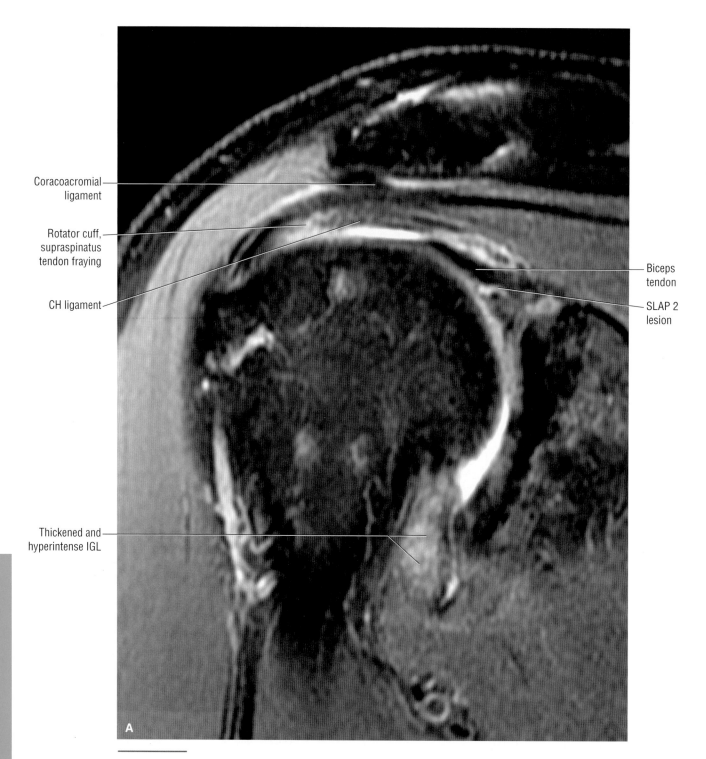

Coracoacromial
ligament

Rotator cuff,
supraspinatus
tendon fraying

CH ligament

Biceps
tendon

SLAP 2
lesion

Thickened and
hyperintense IGL

A

FIGURE 6.17   (**A**) Articular-sided fraying of the supraspinatus in the area of the rotator
cuff crescent lateral to the CH ligament.

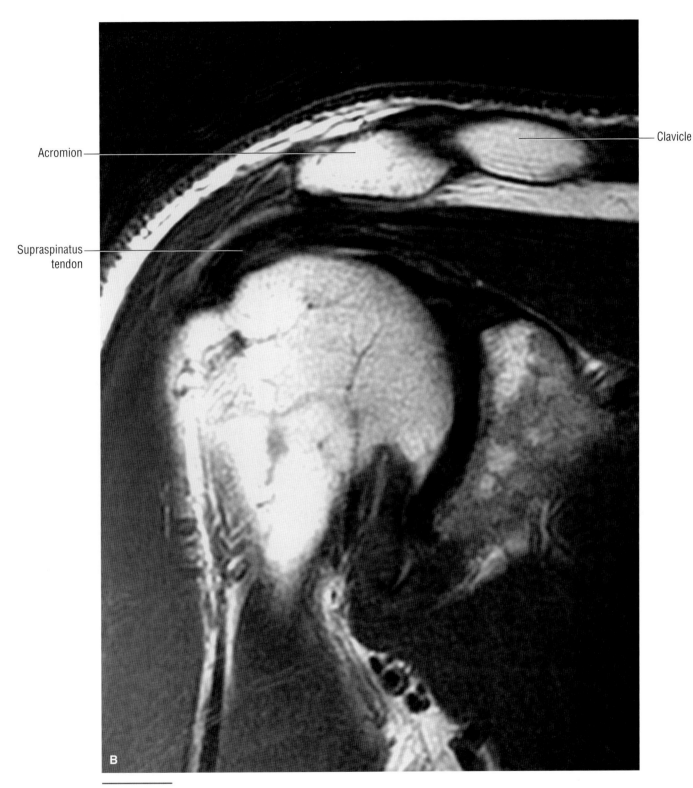

Acromion

Clavicle

Supraspinatus tendon

B

FIGURE 6.17 (*Continued*) (**B**) The articular fraying is not appreciated on the T2 FSE image without the benefit of fat suppression. MR arthrography or careful adjustment of image contrast is required to appreciate the morphology of the articular surface.

Articular surface partial tear

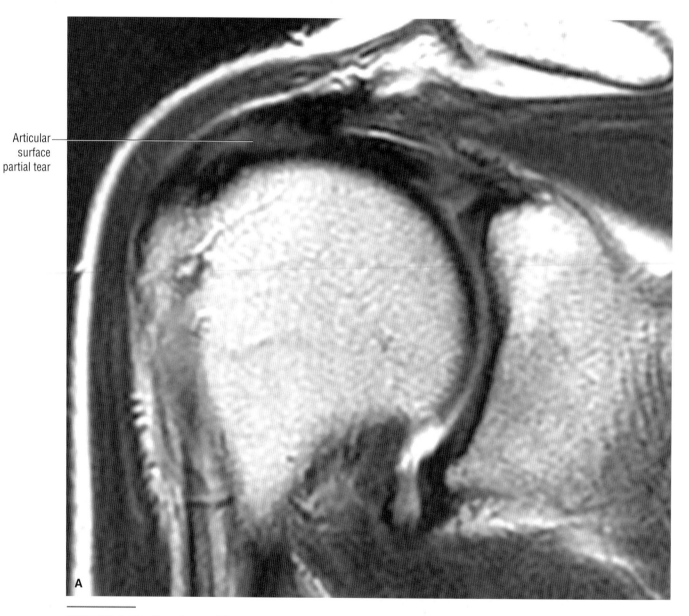

A

FIGURE 6.18 Partial tear of the supraspinatus appreciated best in the FS PD FSE image relative to T2 FSE. The intermediate signal intensity of synovium or granulation tissue may not be appreciated since the role of T2 FSE contrast is to distinguish between tendinosis and partial tear by identifying areas of more mobile protons in discrete regions of fluid signal intensity. Tendinosis or thickened synovium will not become hyperintense on this sequence. (A) Coronal T2 FSE image.

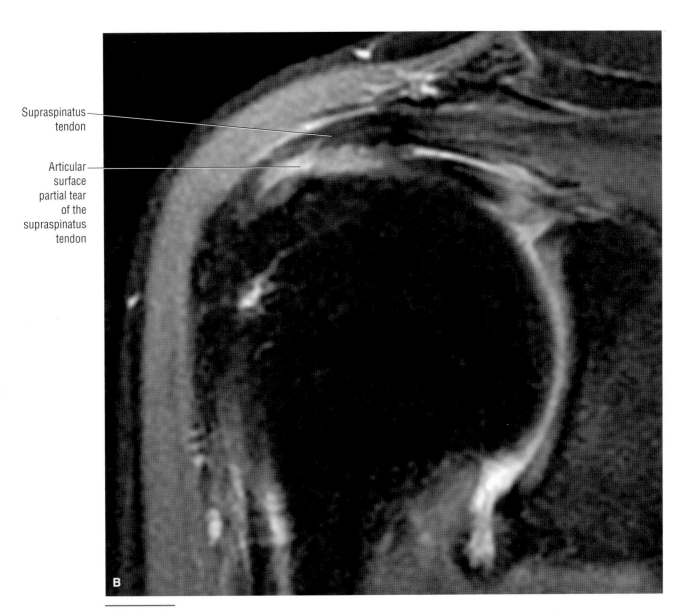

FIGURE 6.18 (*Continued*) (**B**) Coronal FS PD FSE image. This sequence allows the interface between the irregular and attenuated articular surface to be defined in contrast to the intermediate signal of chronically thickened synovium.

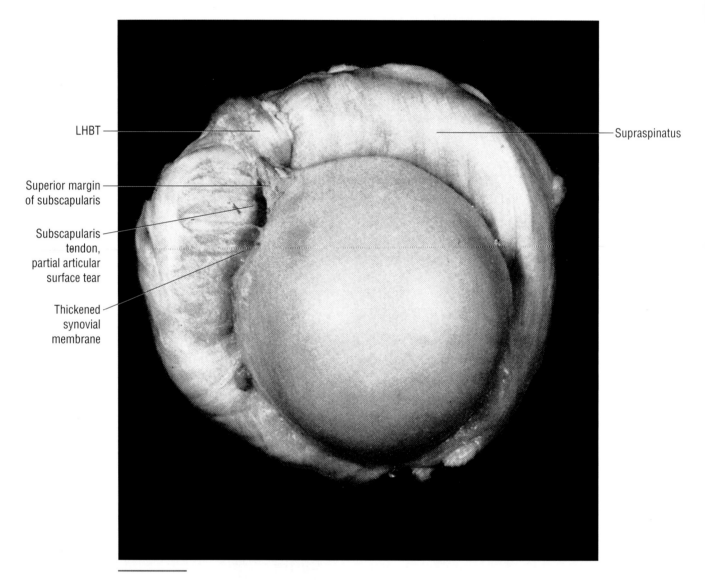

LHBT

Superior margin
of subscapularis

Subscapularis
tendon,
partial articular
surface tear

Thickened
synovial
membrane

Supraspinatus

FIGURE 6.19 Partial tear of the subscapularis tendon. The main tendon of the subscapularis occupies the upper third of the muscle and inserts along the superior aspect of the lesser tuberosity. The subscapularis inserts in a comma-shaped pattern from 7 to 11 o'clock in this right shoulder. The normal subscapularis inserts along the medial aspect of the bicipital groove. (Modified from DePalma AF. *Surgery of the Shoulder*. 3rd ed. Philadelphia, PA: JB Lippincott; 1983.)

Supraspinatus tendon

Bursal irregularity without tear at arthroscopy

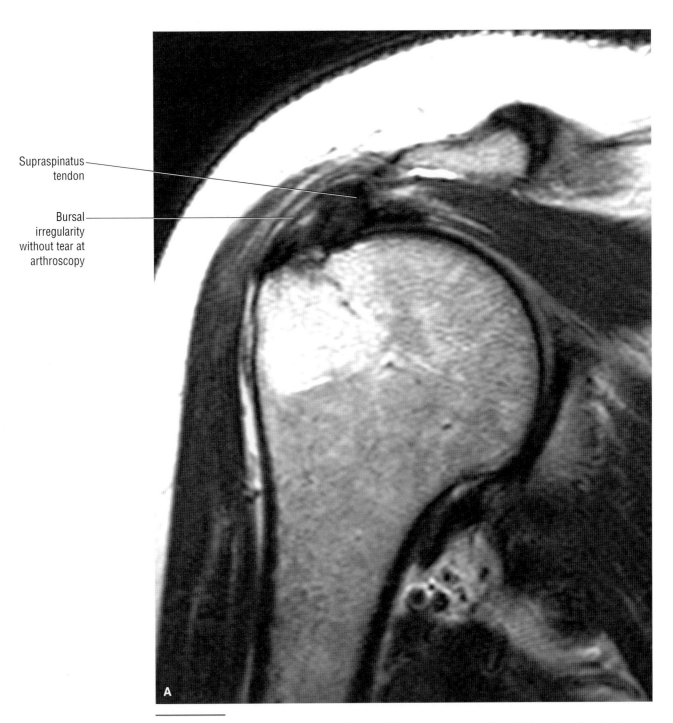

FIGURE 6.20 High-grade interstitial tear of the supraspinatus with a thin bursal roof and an intact articular margin resulting in a negative arthroscopic assessment for cuff tear. (**A**) Coronal T2 FSE.

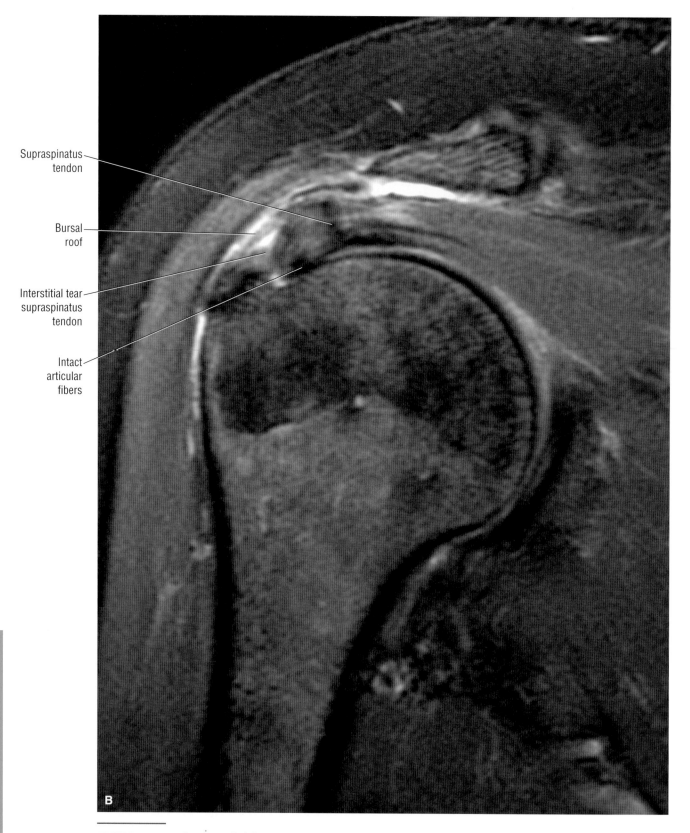

Supraspinatus
tendon

Bursal
roof

Interstitial tear
supraspinatus
tendon

Intact
articular
fibers

FIGURE 6.20 (*Continued*) (**B**) Coronal FS PD FSE image. This high-grade interstitial tear is conspicious on the fluid sensitive sequence. Follow-up MR imaging should be performed to evaluate the integrity of the thin bursal roof or scar in situ of the bursal side of the supraspinatus.

- **Partial Thickness Interstitial (Intrasubstance) Rotator Cuff Tears**
  - Normal rotator cuff tendon composed of parallel layers of collagen fibrils that attach to the greater tuberosity
  - Shear force between layers resulting in tear and partial detachment of tendon from the bone
  - Arthroscopically not visualized
  - Intersititial tear pattern or PITA tear
    - Partial intersitial tendon avulsion (PITA)
    - In arm adduction, cuff collagen layers are more compressed.
  - Arthroscopic signs of an interstitial tear[75]:
    - Dimple sign
      - Supraspinatus insertion between rotator cable and articular margin
      - Dimpling of the tendon represents a positive dimple sign and is associated with an interstitial tear.
    - Sliding layers sign
      - Palpation of rotator cuff from the bursal surface with a probe
        - Intersitital or PITA tear feels like there is a gap between tendon layers or the sliding of one layer of the tendon over the top of another layer.
    - Bubble sign
      - An 18-gauge spinal needle is inserted through intact bursal fibers with attached syringe of fluid.
      - Positive bubble occurs when area of suspected interstitial tear bubbles up with injection of fluid.

- Probe push test
  - Probe pushed on the bursal layer of suspected cuff interstitial tear
  - Probe falls into defect.
- Slit test
  - Slit in bursal fibers of cuff created
  - Arthroscopic grasper inserted into slit to allow visualization of the defect

- Partial rotator cuff tears involving the midsubstance are intrasubstance or interstitial tears.

- Interstitial (intrasubstance) tears do not extend to either the bursal or articular surface; they may not be detected at arthroscopy.

- Interstitial tears may mimic a full thickness tear on clinical assessment.

- With the arm in adduction, there may be minimal joint fluid extravasation between the interstitial layers of the cuff tendon.

- A subset of interstitial tears may have a subtle communication with the articular surface only seen at MR arthrography.

- Intratendinous tears tend not to heal over time.

- PITA Repair[75]
  - Defect opened from bursal side
  - Bone bed prepared laterally to the greater tuberosity
  - Tear repaired
    - Anchors placed in the base of the bone bed

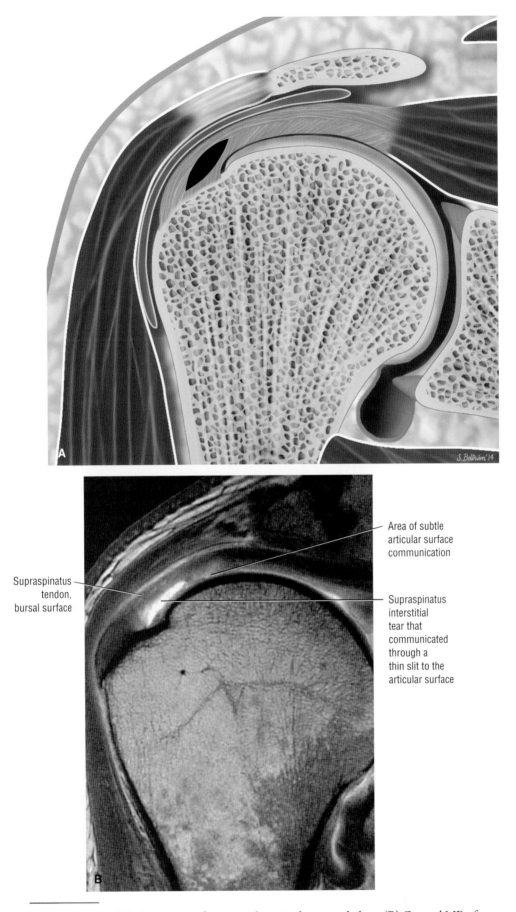

FIGURE 6.21 (**A**) Illustration of interstitial tear in the coronal plane. (**B**) Coronal MR of an apparent supraspinatus interstitial partial tear. A thin slip of frayed articular fibers is seen attaching to the footprint medial to the interstitial tear. Some tears initially assessed as interstitial may in fact have a subtle communication with the articular surface which allows for the influx of joint fluid.

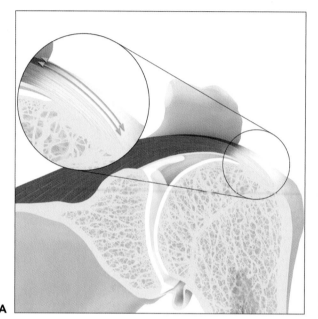

A

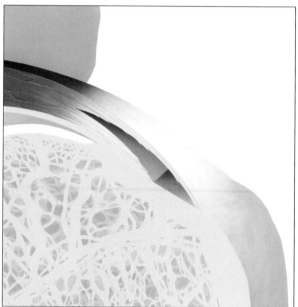

B

C

FIGURE 6.22 Schematic of the supraspinatus attachment. (**A**) The supraspinatus tendon fibers are parallel when they insert onto the greater tuberosity. Interstitial tears can occur as a split between the parallel fibers (**B**) with or (**C**) without avulsion of the tendon from the bone. In either case, the tear will be hidden from view from both the articular and bursal surfaces. (Reprinted from Burkhart S, Lo IK, Brady PC, Denard PJ. *The Cowboy's Companion: A Trail Guide for the Arthroscopic Shoulder Surgeon.* Philadelphia, PA: Lippincott Williams & Wilkins; 2012, with permission.)

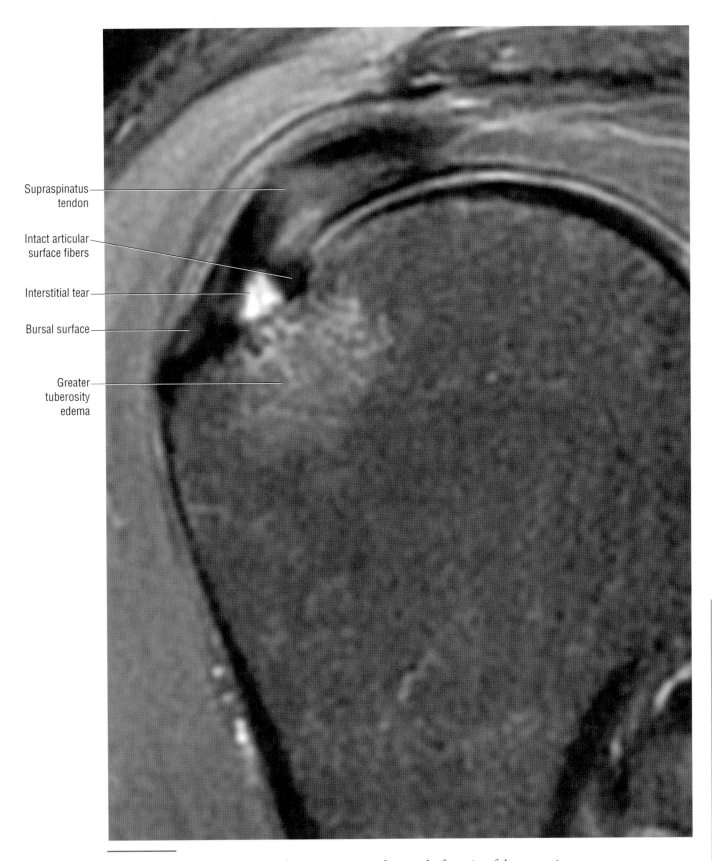

Supraspinatus tendon

Intact articular surface fibers

Interstitial tear

Bursal surface

Greater tuberosity edema

FIGURE 6.23   Interstitial tear with reactive marrow edema at the footprint of the supraspinatus.

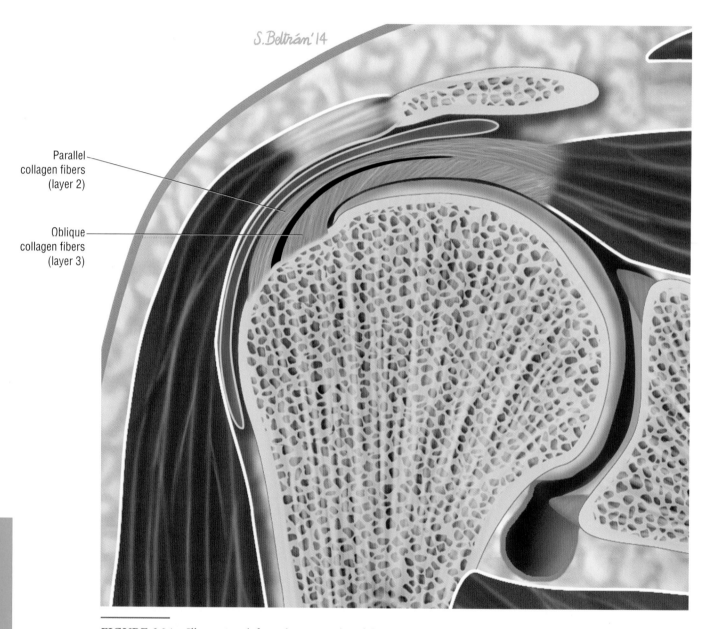

Parallel collagen fibers (layer 2)

Oblique collagen fibers (layer 3)

FIGURE 6.24 Illustration defining layers 2 and 3 of the supraspinatus. The bulk of the thickness of the rotator cuff is formed from layers 2 and 3. Layer 1 is a thin superficial layer of fibers comprising the coracohumeral ligament. Layer 2 is a thicker layer of parallel collagen bundles (parallel tendon fibers). Layers 3 is a deep layer with tendon fibers oriented at 45-degree angle. Layer 4 includes loose connective tissue and is part of the coracohumeral envelope and extends along the bursal and articular surface of the supraspinatus. Layer 5 is the joint capsule.

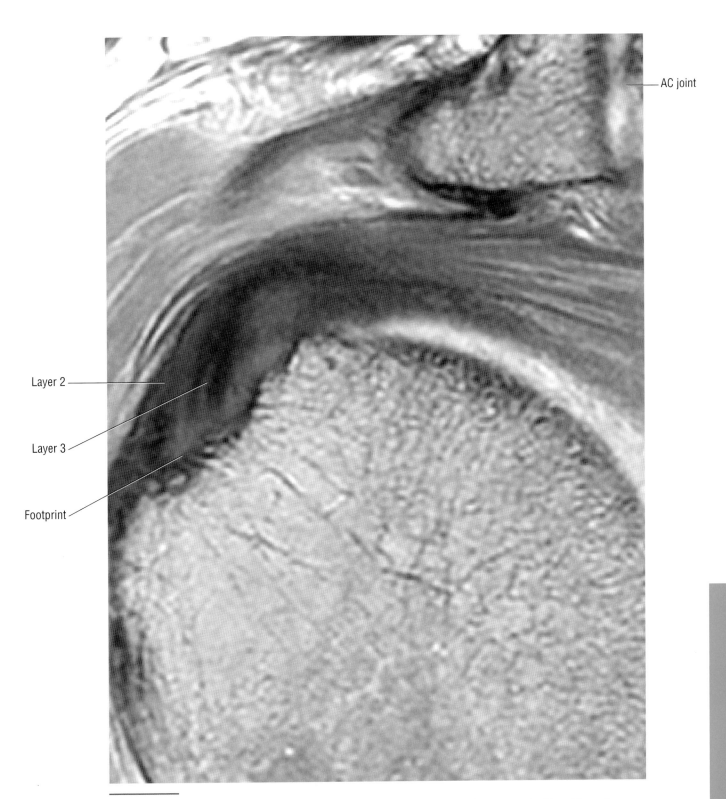

FIGURE 6.25 Intrasubstance or interstitial tears occur between layer 2 (3 to 5mm thick) and layer 3 (3mm thick). The collagen fibers are parallel and densely packed in layer 2. In layer 3, the collagen bundles are smaller and are arranged at a 45-degree orientation. Coronal T1 image.

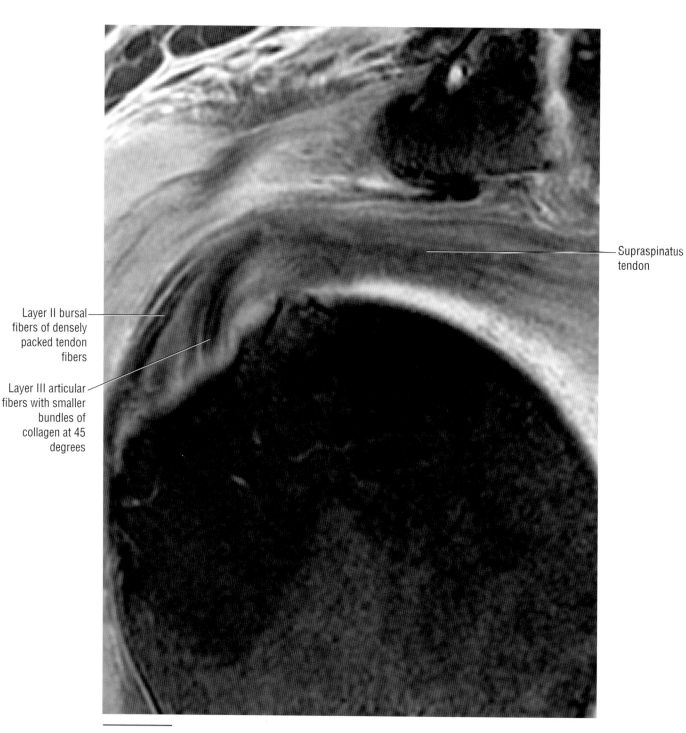

Supraspinatus
tendon

Layer II bursal
fibers of densely
packed tendon
fibers

Layer III articular
fibers with smaller
bundles of
collagen at 45
degrees

FIGURE 6.26   Layer 2 is twice as strong as layer 3 collagen fibers. Delamination or intrasubstance
tears between layers 2 and 3 preferentially occur along this shear plane. Coronal FS PD image.

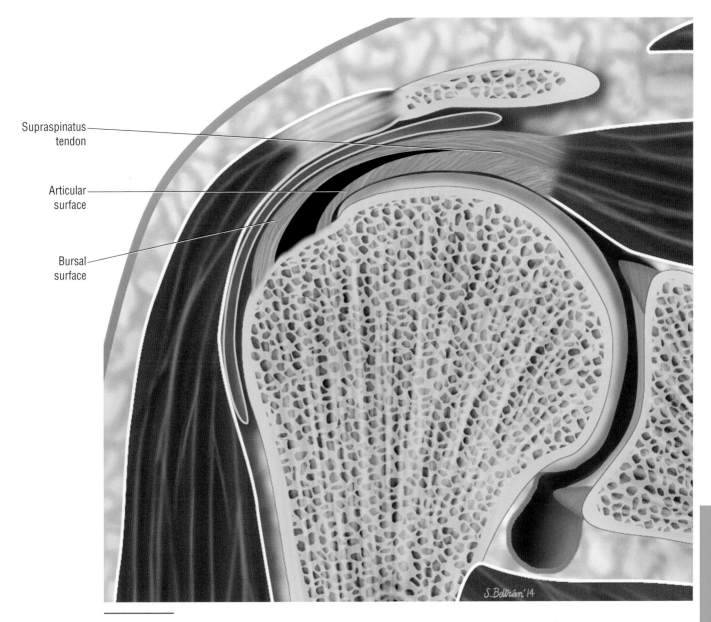

Supraspinatus tendon

Articular surface

Bursal surface

FIGURE 6.27   Interstitial tear extending from the footprint in a medial direction. Idealized interstitial tear plane in which the collagen layers of the rotator cuff tendon are not tensioned, thus improving visualization of fluid signal intensity between tendon layers. In abduction, the tendon layers may separate, and as abnormal force distribution increases, the interstitial tear propagates from the footprint bone bed laterally to an intratendinous horizontal plane medially.

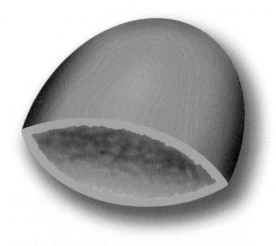

FIGURE 6.28   An interstitial rotator cuff tear can be likened to pita bread in which there is a separation between two intact layers (bursal side and articular side). (Reprinted from Burkhart S, Lo IK, Brady PC, Denard PJ. *The Cowboy's Companion: A Trail Guide for the Arthroscopic Shoulder Surgeon.* Philadelphia, PA: Lippincott Williams & Wilkins; 2012, with permission.)

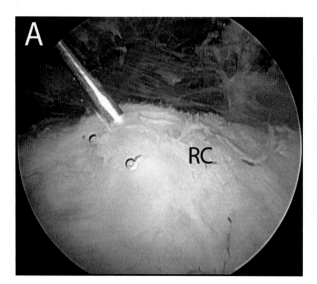
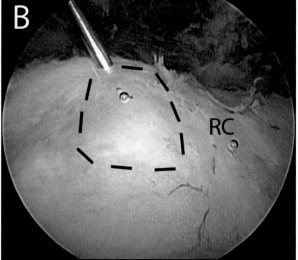

FIGURE 6.29   Bubble sign in left shoulder, viewed from a posterior subacromial portal. (**A**) A spinal needle is inserted into the rotator cuff at the site of a suspected interstitial rotator cuff tear. (**B**) As normal saline is injected, the interstitial defect fills and creates a visible bubble (*dashed black lines*), confirming an interstitial rotator cuff tear. RC, rotator cuff. Reprinted from Burkhart S, Lo IK, Brady PC, Denard PJ. *The Cowboy's Companion: a Trail Guide for the Arthroscopic Shoulder Surgeon.* Philadelphia, PA: Lippincott Williams & Wilkins; 2012, with permission.)

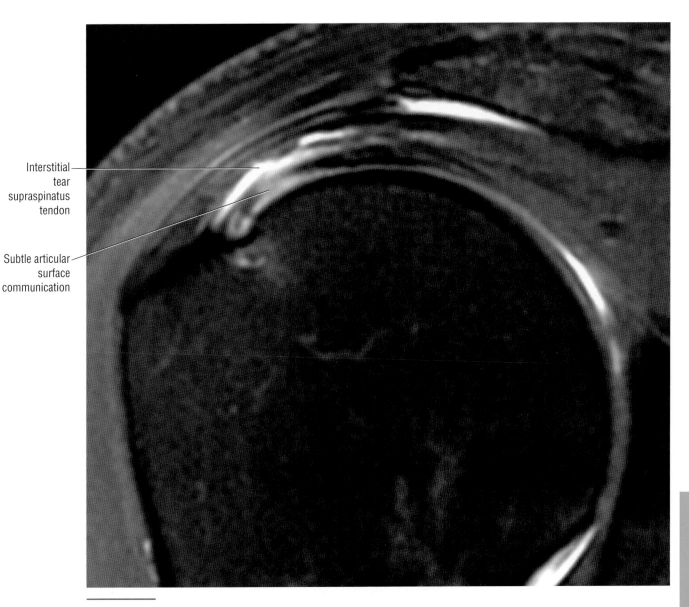

Interstitial tear supraspinatus tendon

Subtle articular surface communication

FIGURE 6.30 Interstitial tear of supraspinatus tendon with hyperintense contrast. Although the articular surface may be evaluated as intact on non-contrast MRI or arthroscopy, MRI arthrography reveals the communication of this apparent interstitial tear with the articular surface. Hyperintense signal, however, can be present in an interstitial tear without articular surface communication.

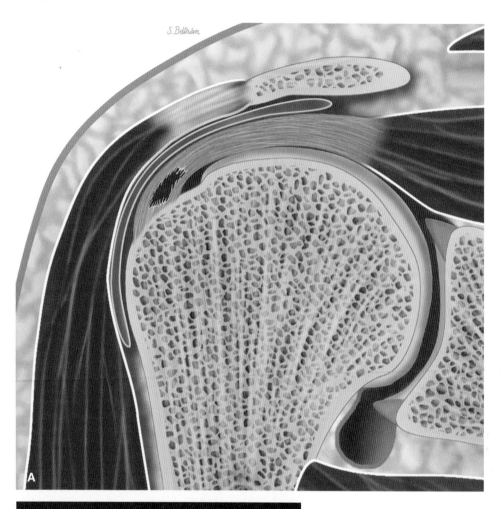

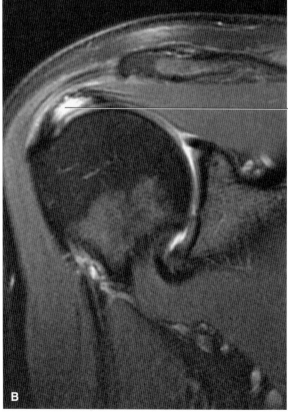

Interstitial tear,
supraspinatus
tendon

FIGURE 6.31 (**A**) Intrasubstance or interstitial tear of the supraspinatus without bursal or articular surface extension. (**B**) Coronal FS PD FSE image demonstrates the hyperintense interstitial tear without loss of continuity of the corresponding bursal or articular surfaces. In this example, the interstitial tear is located between the tendon layers without detachment from bone at the cuff footprint.

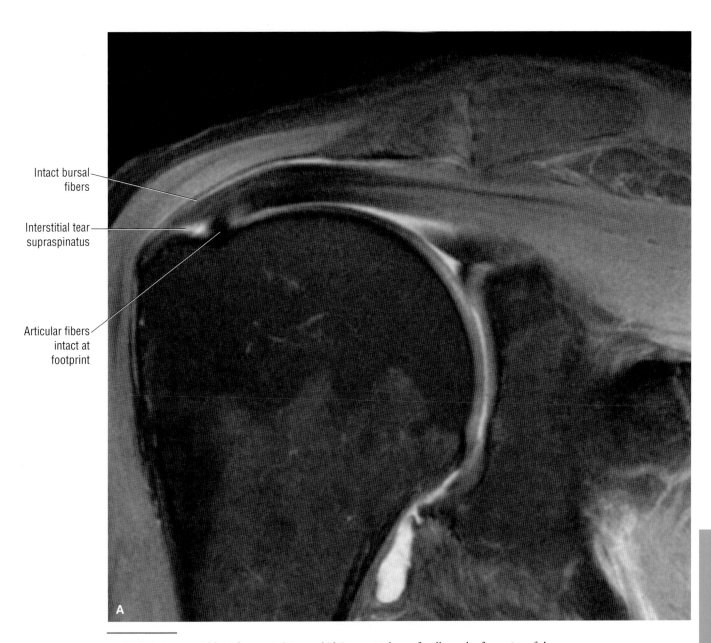

Intact bursal fibers

Interstitial tear supraspinatus

Articular fibers intact at footprint

FIGURE 6.32   Mild Arthrosis AC Joint: (**A**) Interstitial tear focally at the footprint of the supraspinatus without a delamination component on a FS PD FSE coronal image. The majority of interstitial tears occur at the footprint or tendinous attachment to bone. The addition of a shear force between collagen layers of the tendon result in the propagation of the tear in a medial direction between tendon layers. The detachment of the footprint fibers is hidden between the articular and bursal layers of the cuff.

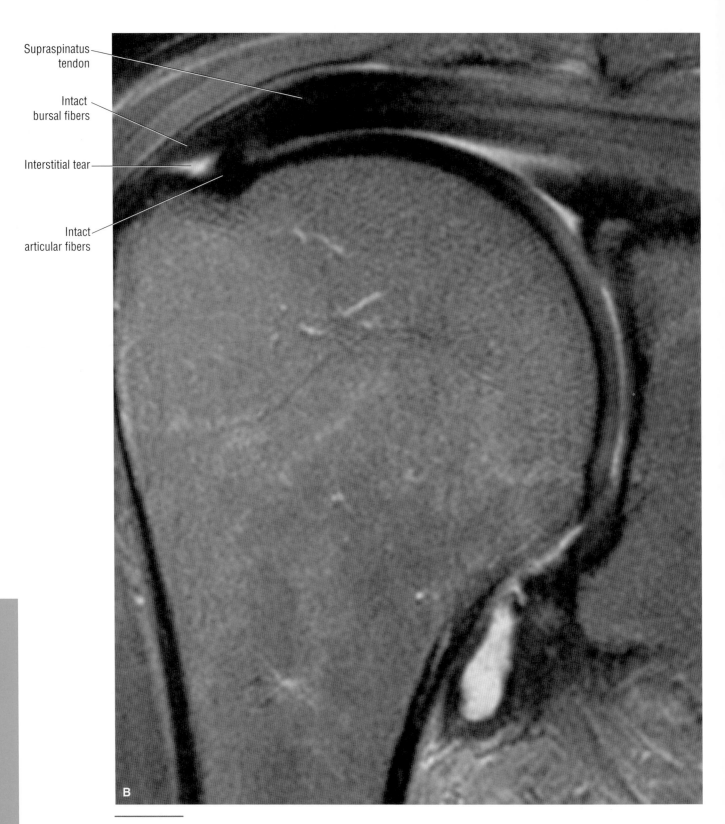

Supraspinatus tendon

Intact bursal fibers

Interstitial tear

Intact articular fibers

FIGURE 6.32   (*Continued*) (**B**) Corresponding non-fat suppressed T2 FSE coronal image. The hyperintense signal on the T2 FSE is characteristic of a tear. Tendon degeneration in tendinosis would not generate this degree of fluid hyperintensity.

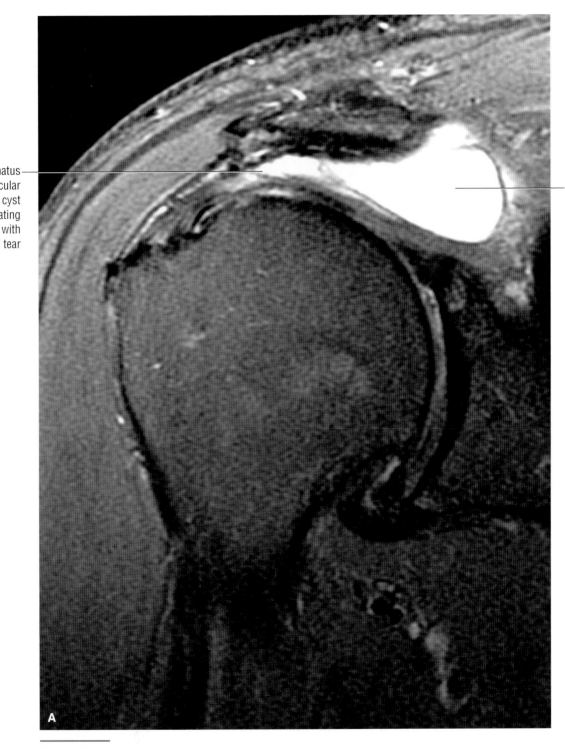

Supraspinatus intramuscular cyst communicating with interstitial tear

Intramuscular cyst

FIGURE 6.33 Intramuscular cyst of the supraspinatus as a marker of an adjacent interstitial tear. (**A**) Coronal FS PD. Intramuscular cysts are associated with rotator cuff tendon tears especially the supraspinatus. Approximately half of the intramuscular cysts are associated with partial thickness tears.

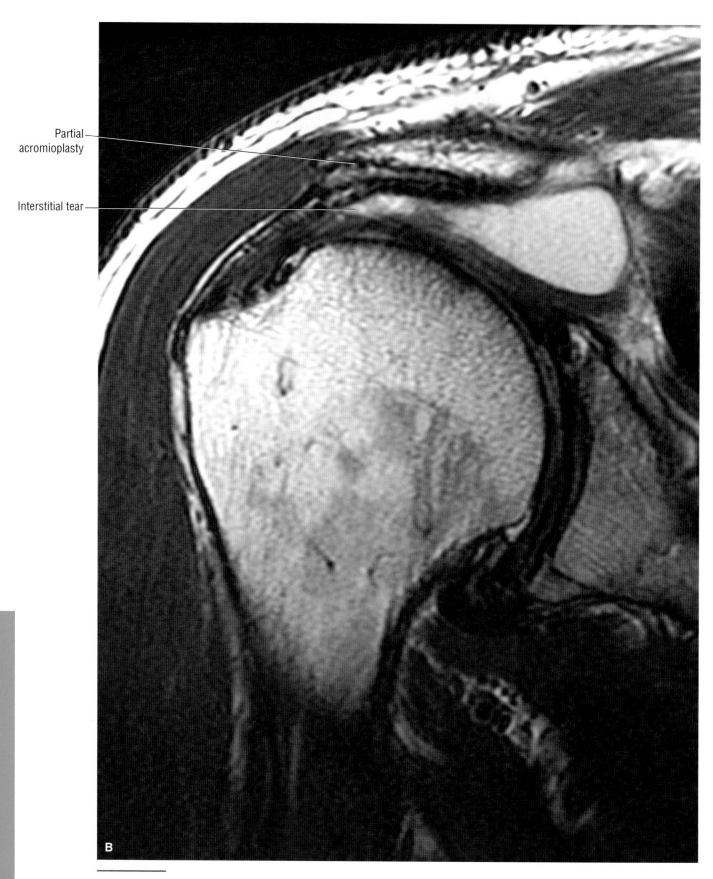

Partial
acromioplasty

Interstitial tear

FIGURE 6.33   *(Continued)* **(B)** Coronal T2 FSE. Intramuscular cysts may be associated with rotator cuff tears of adjacent tendons in addition to the cyst containing muscle

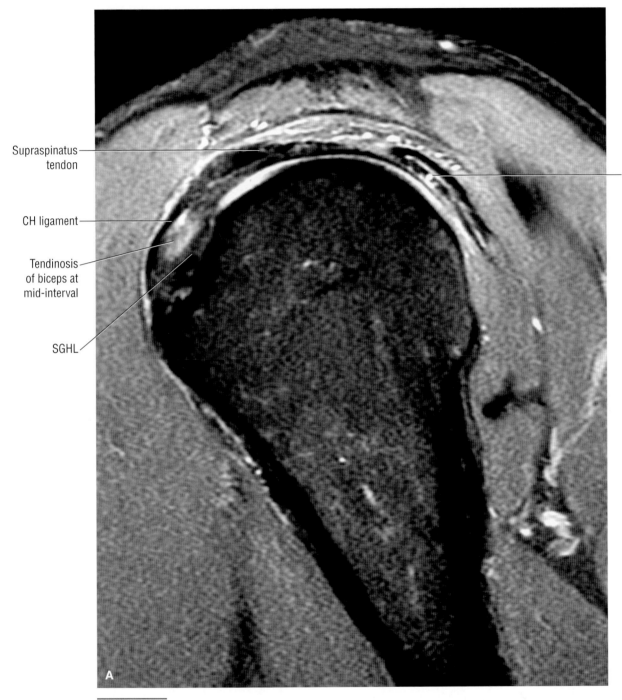

Supraspinatus tendon

CH ligament

Tendinosis of biceps at mid-interval

SGHL

Infraspinatus interstitial tear as nidus for generating communicating intramuscular cyst

FIGURE 6.34   Interstitial tear of the infraspinatus with linear hyperintense signal of the tendon communicating with an infraspinatus intramuscular cyst. The resultant cyst is multilobulated and multiseptated. (**A**) Sagittal FS PD. The interstitial tear propagates from the anterior to posterior aspect of the infraspinatus tendon in a horizontal or delaminating tear pattern.

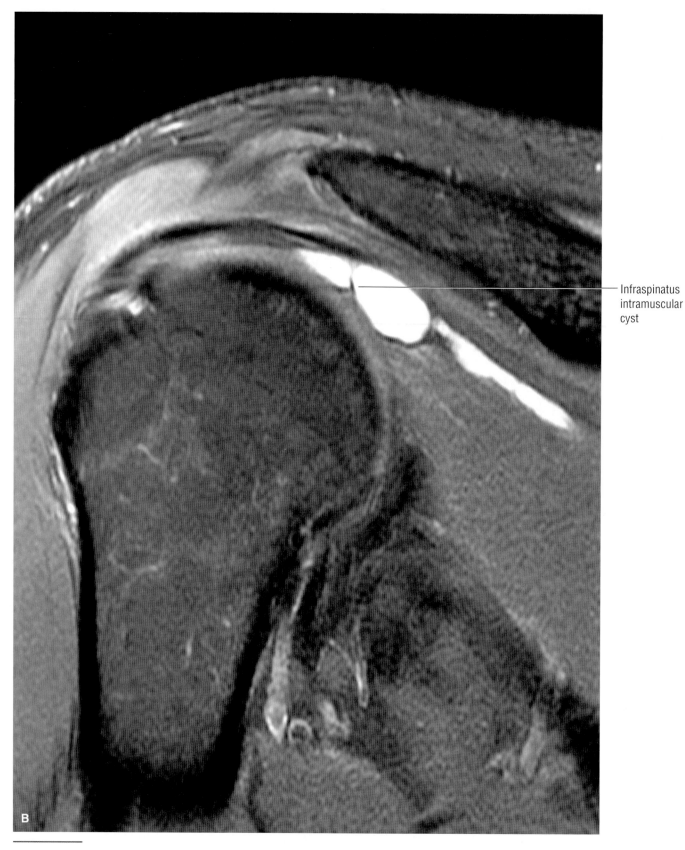

Infraspinatus
intramuscular
cyst

FIGURE 6.34   (*Continued*) (**B**) Coronal FS PD. The interstitial or delaminating component of
the infraspinatus tendon corresponds to the infraspinatus intramuscular cyst. Propagation of the
intrasubstance tear to an adjacent tendon, however, may result in an intramuscular cyst associated
with an intact tendon.

- **Bursal Surface Tears**
  - Less common than PASTA lesions
  - Bursal-sided tears may be associated with a localized fluid collection within the subacromial bursa located adjacent to the bursal-sided tear site.
    - The puddle sign represents hyperintense fluid in the subacromial bursa as a marker for adjacent bursal-sided cuff pathology.
  - Coronal MR images are used to identify which rotator cuff tendon is involved and the percent thickness of the affected tendon. Sagittal images cannot be used as a primary interpretation plane for cuff tears (especially bursal-sided tears) since a sagittal image obtained lateral to intact articular fibers may give the false impression that there is a full thickness cuff tear present. Only when viewing consecutive sagittal images would it be appreciated that the more medially located articular surface fibers of the cuff were in fact intact. Thus, the primary interpretation plane for cuff tears including bursal-sided tears should be the coronal plane with the secondary reading plane represented by sagittal images.
  - Inferior acromial osteophytes will preferentially abrade the bursal surface of the rotator cuff (normally, tensile undersurface forces that result in collagen fiber failure are greater on the articular surface in the absence of keel osteophytes).
  - Association with extrinsic impingement
    - Acromioplasty usually required
  - Arthroscopic repair
    - Small bursal tears with repair in situ[619]
      - Confirm medial wall (articular side) of the rotator cuff is intact.
      - Torn bursal margins débrided to healthy tissue
      - Lateral greater tuberosity bone bed is prepared.
    - Completion of the tear
      - High-grade bursal-sided partial tears with significant delamination and flap formation can be treated similar to full thickness cuff tears.
    - Double-row repair for high-grade lesions with poor tissue quality
      - Multiple knots tied medially to resist tendon pull out in poor-quality tissue

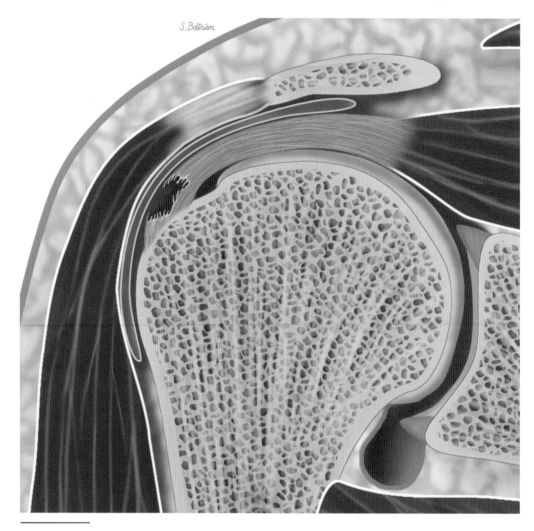

S. Beltrán

FIGURE 6.35   Bursal surface partial thickness rotator cuff tear.

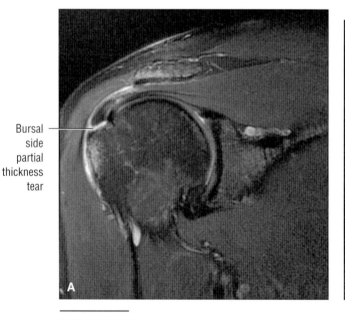

Bursal
side
partial
thickness
tear

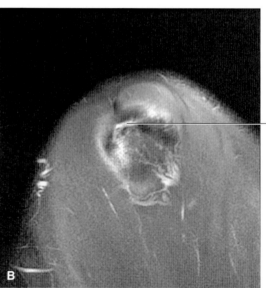

Bursal surface
tear lateral to
intact articular
fibers

FIGURE 6.36   (**A**) High-grade or severe partial rotator cuff tear of the bursal surface. A sizable flap tear involving both the supraspinatus and conjoined portions of the cuff is demonstrated. (**B**) This sagittal image lateral to the articular fibers demonstrates fluid between torn bursal fibers and the greater tuberosity. Associated subacromial impingement requires repair accompanied by arthroscopic decompression, with recessing and smoothing of the undersurface of the acromion and the inferior surface of the AC joint.

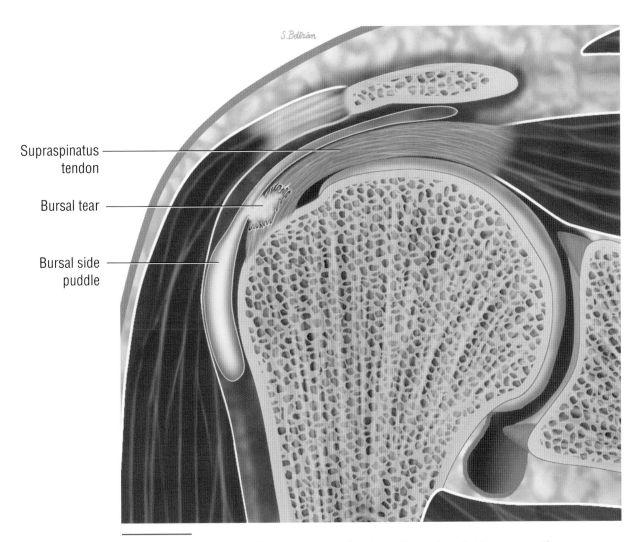

Supraspinatus tendon

Bursal tear

Bursal side puddle

FIGURE 6.37   Bursal puddle sign associated with an adjacent bursal-side rotator cuff tear as seen on a color coronal section. If this localized collection of subacromial fluid is identified without a full thickness tear, then the diagnosis of bursal-side fraying or partial thickness tear must be assumed. It is the preferential collection of localized fluid within the confines of the subacromial bursa that correlates with bursal-sided pathology. The torn edges of the tendon and bursa can catch under the subacromial osteophyte when the arm is elevated and produce severe preoperative pain and disability. Bursal tears are thus associated with extrinsic impingement and usually require treatment with an acromioplasty with repair. Repair is performed in situ or with completion of the tear for high-grade lesions.

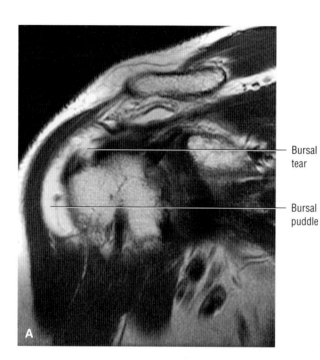

Bursal
tear

Bursal
puddle

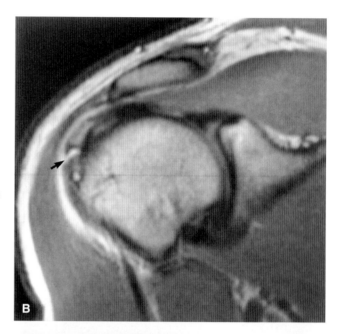

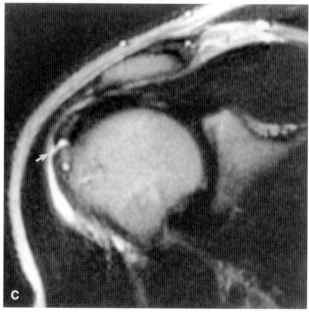

FIGURE 6.38   Bursal puddle sign associated with an adjacent bursal-side rotator cuff tear. (**A**) Bursal-sided tear on a coronal T2 FSE image. (**B,C**) Partial thickness bursal surface tear (*arrows*) in communication with the subacromial-subdeltoid bursa. Fluid is hyperintense on intermediate weighted and T2-weighted FSE coronal oblique mages. As a subtype of partial thickness rotator cuff tears, bursal surface tears are less common than their PASTA counterparts. In high-grade bursal-sided partial tears, the aim is to repair the tendon back to bone without sacrificing the intact articular-sided remaining tendon. Rehabilitation after repair is faster than for full thickness tears as there is minimal tension on the repair since the articular footprint is intact.

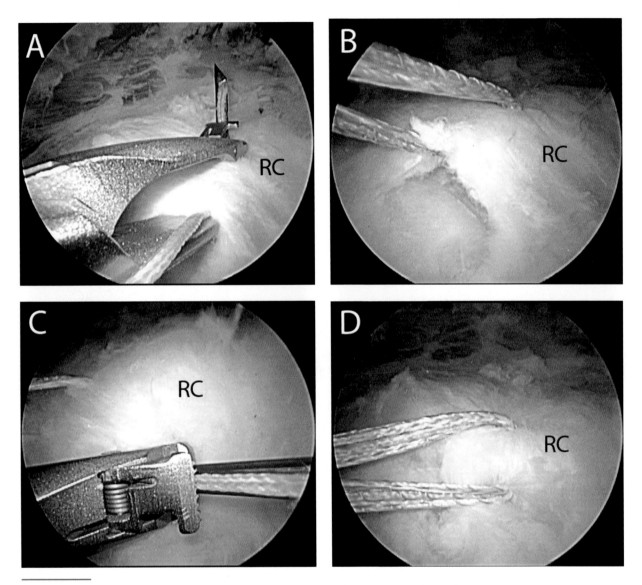

FIGURE 6.39   Mattress stitch placement for SpeedFix (Arthrex, Inc., Naples, FL) repair of a bursal surface rotator cuff tear in a left shoulder viewed from a posterior subsacromial portal. (**A**) A #2 Fiber-Wire leader of a FiberTape suture is passed with a Scorpion FastPass through the anterior aspect of the tear and (**B**) retrieved out the lateral portal. (**C**) The FiberWire leader of the suture that exits the rotator cuff inferiorly is loaded onto the Scorpion and passed through the posterior aspect of the tear. (**D**) View after placement of an inverted mattress stitch. RC, rotator cuff. (Reprinted from Burkhart S, Lo IK, Brady PC, Denard PJ. *The Cowboy's Companion: A Trail Guide for the Arthroscopic Shoulder Surgeon*. Philadelphia, PA: Lippincott Williams & Wilkins; 2012, with permission.)

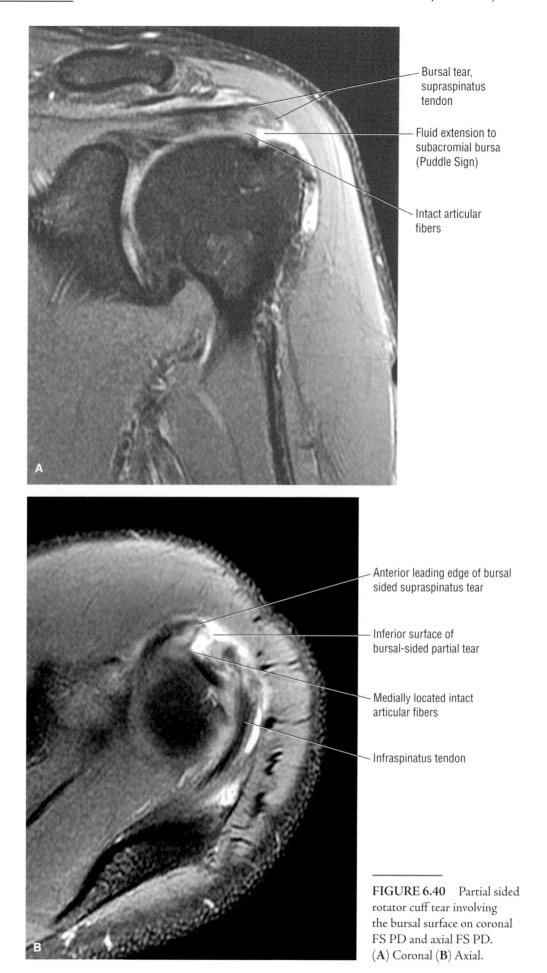

Bursal tear, supraspinatus tendon

Fluid extension to subacromial bursa (Puddle Sign)

Intact articular fibers

Anterior leading edge of bursal sided supraspinatus tear

Inferior surface of bursal-sided partial tear

Medially located intact articular fibers

Infraspinatus tendon

FIGURE 6.40   Partial sided rotator cuff tear involving the bursal surface on coronal FS PD and axial FS PD. (**A**) Coronal (**B**) Axial.

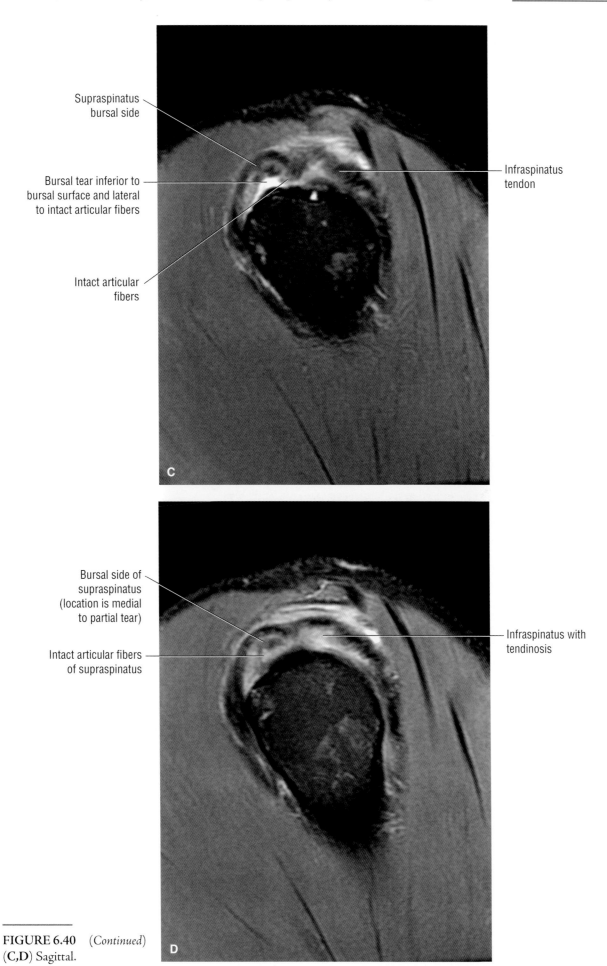

FIGURE 6.40 (*Continued*) (**C,D**) Sagittal.

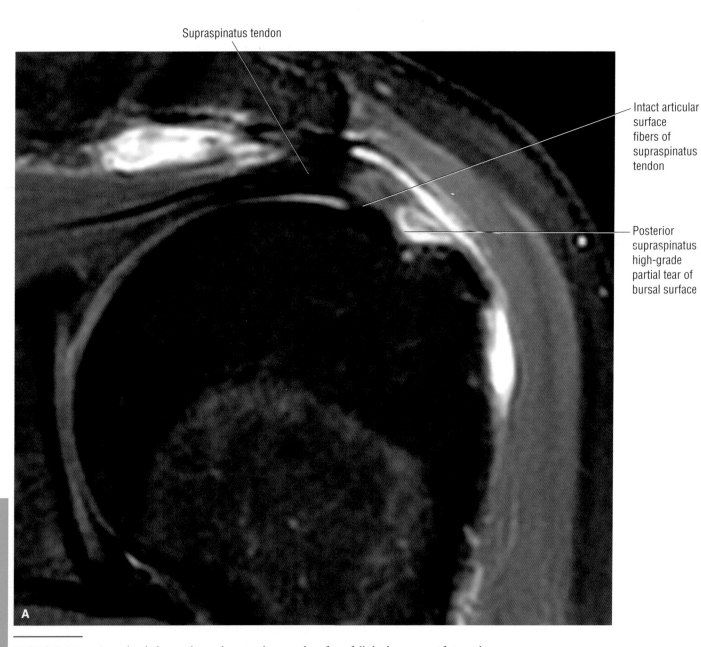

Supraspinatus tendon

Intact articular
surface
fibers of
supraspinatus
tendon

Posterior
supraspinatus
high-grade
partial tear of
bursal surface

FIGURE 6.41   Bursal-sided partial tear that may be mistaken for a full thickness tear if viewed on a
sagittal image lateral to the intact articular fibers. (**A**) Coronal FS PD.

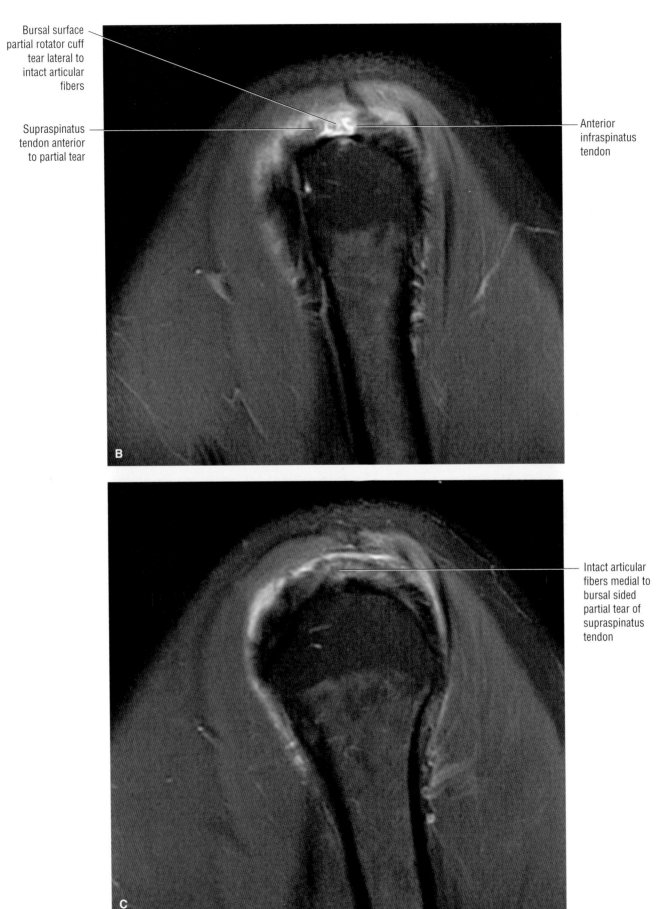

FIGURE 6.41   (*Continued*) (**B,C**) Sagittal FS PD. Without the benefit of the more medial sagittal image, the tear pattern may be mistakened for a full thickness tear on lateral sagittal images through the rotator cuff.

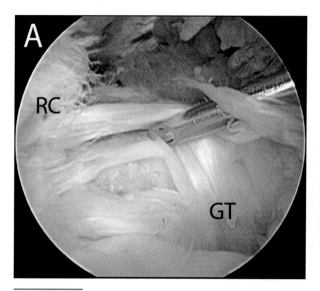
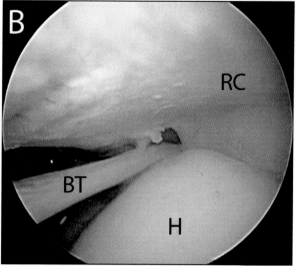

FIGURE 6.42   (**A**) Right shoulder, posterior subacromial viewing portal demonstrates a large
bursal surface rotator cuff tear with poor-quality remaining rotator cuff tissue. (**B**) Intraarticular
view from a posterior view in the same shoulder demonstrates an intact medial footprint. BT, biceps
tendon; GT, greater tuberosity; H, humerus; RC, rotator cuff. (Reprinted from Burkhart S, Lo IK,
Brady PC, Denard PJ. *The Cowboy's Companion: A Trail Guide for the Arthroscopic Shoulder Surgeon.*
Philadelphia, PA: Lippincott Williams & Wilkins; 2012, with permission.)

■ Rim Rent Tears

- ■ Rim rent tear as a partial thickness articular-sided tear
  (All PASTA lesions are considered rim rent tears, but not all rim
  rent tears are PASTA tears because not all rim rent tears have an
  interstitial delamination component.)

- ■ The *rim rent tear* describes a partial thickness articular or deep
  surface tear of the rotator cuff at its attachment to the greater
  tuberosity.

- ■ Includes supraspinatus and infraspinatus articular-sided footprint
  tears

    - ▨ Rotator cuff lesions start where loads are greatest, at the
      articular surface of the anterior insertion of the supraspi-
      natus adjacent to the LHBT.

- ■ Cuff tendon fibers fail when applied load exceeds their strength.

■ PASTA Lesions

- ■ Partial Articular Surface Tendon Avulsion (PASTA)

    - ▨ Term is used in same context as a rim rent except for the
      additional finding of an articular flap component.

- ■ Includes delamination tears of the articular surface of the
  supraspinatus tendon

- Preservation of intact rotator cuff
  - Maintenance of normal length-tendon relationship
- The term "PASTA lesion" is used to describe partial tears as a III or a IV using the Snyder classification.[146]
- Demonstrate significant tendon fragmentation or have a flap component that can be arthroscopically repaired provided the retracted and thickened rotator cable is not mistaken for articular fibers of the supraspinatus tendon
  - Cable preservation describes the cable in anatomic position.
  - Cable restoration used when the cable has shifted medially
  - The goal is to mobilize the medial footprint assuming the remaining bursal fibers are strong.
  - In an older patient without good-quality bursal tissue, the partial articular-sided tear may require tear completion and then repair.
- More common in repetitive overhead sports and in patients less than 45 years of age
  - High-level throwing athletes respond better to débridement and rehabilitation than repair.
- Selective delamination of the opposite or bursal surface of the cuff is also possible ("reverse PASTA").
  - In cases of bursal surface tearing, continuity of articular fibers is maintained in an attenuated peripheral cuff.
- Intraarticular repair of PASTA lesions
  - Younger patients benefit from repair in contrast to the degenerative PASTA lesions in older patients which are best treated with débridement alone.
  - Reduces the articular flap to the footprint
    - Caution recommended so as not to mistake the retracted rotator cable for an articular flap. This aggressive repair would overtension the PASTA repair if the cable was moved laterally toward the footprint.
  - PASTA lesions greater than 50% (defect of 6 to 8mm) have improved outcomes with repair.
  - Maintains tension of bursal surface of the rotator cuff
  - Repair of PASTA lesions is performed with at least 25% good-quality bursal tendon remaining.[75]

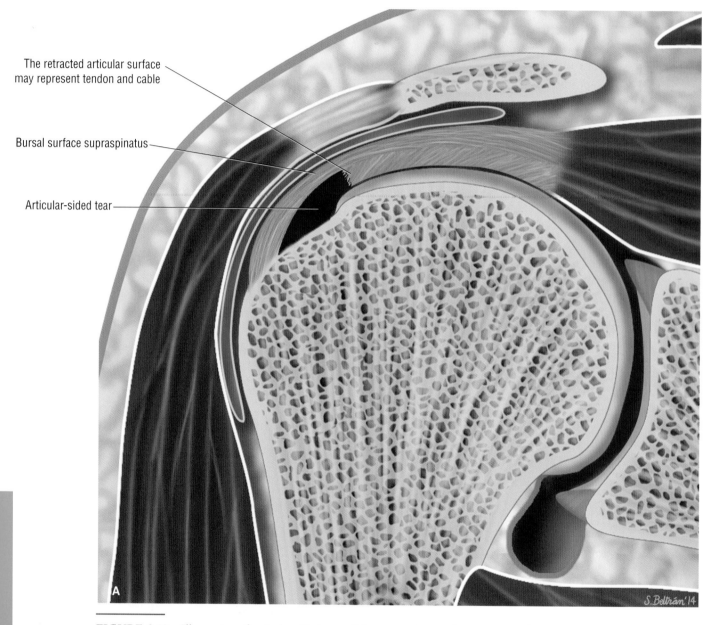

The retracted articular surface
may represent tendon and cable

Bursal surface supraspinatus

Articular-sided tear

FIGURE 6.43 Illustration of articular-sided tear of the supraspinatus. Rim rent tear of
the articular side of the supraspinatus footprint attachment. (**A**) Coronal color illustration. The retracted articular-sided fibers frequently represent the cable which may also be
retracted and appear thicker and can easily be mistakened for the retracted tendon.

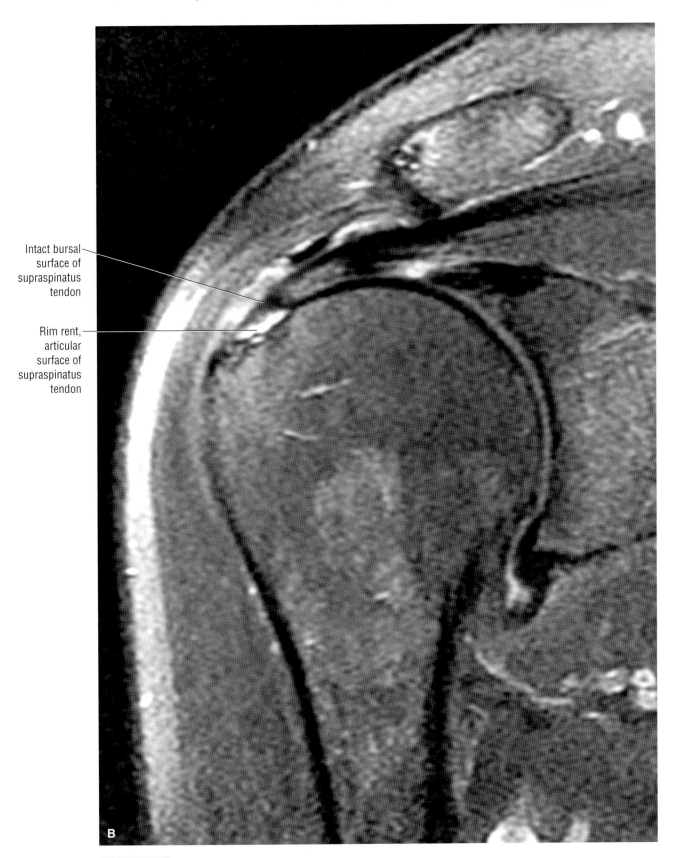

Intact bursal surface of supraspinatus tendon

Rim rent, articular surface of supraspinatus tendon

FIGURE 6.43   *(Continued)* **(B)** Coronal FS PD.

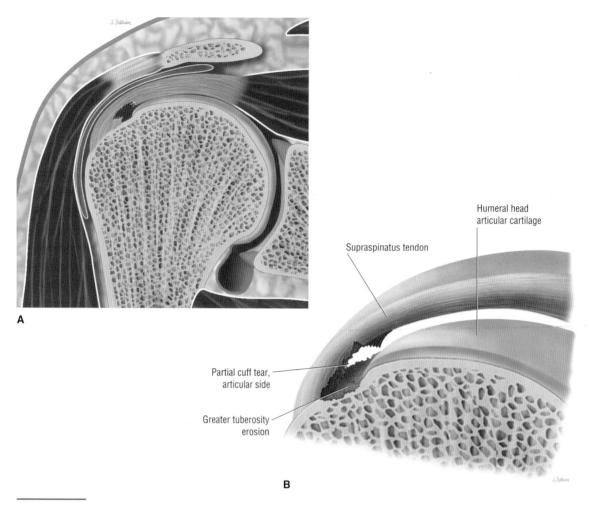

FIGURE 6.44   (**A**) Partial thickness articular-side tear of the rotator cuff. (**B**) Rim rent tear of the articular surface of the cuff with erosion of the greater tuberosity.

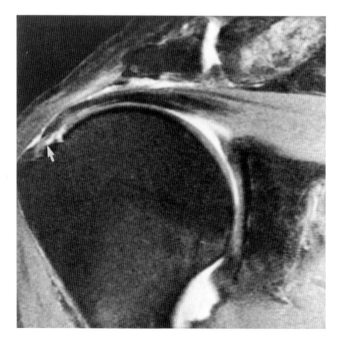

FIGURE 6.45   Partial tear with abnormal attenuation (*arrow*) of the distal conjoined supraspinatus and infraspinatus cuff tendons. Fluid is hyperintense and cuff degeneration is intermediate in signal intensity. There is no direct communication of fluid between the glenohumeral joint and subacromial-subdeltoid bursa on this FS PD-weighted FSE coronal oblique image.

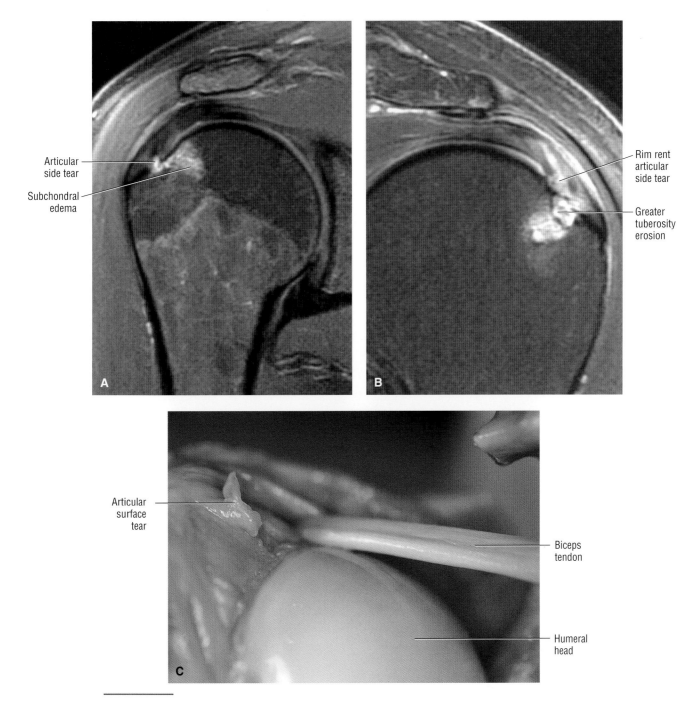

FIGURE 6.46 (**A**) Partial thickness articular-side tear with adjacent osseous reaction on coronal FS PD FSE image. (**B**) Coronal FS PD FSE image illustrating a separate case of a rim rent partial articular-side cuff tear with adjacent greater tuberosity edema and erosion. (**C**) Articular surface irregularity on the undersurface of the cuff. The LHBT is intact.

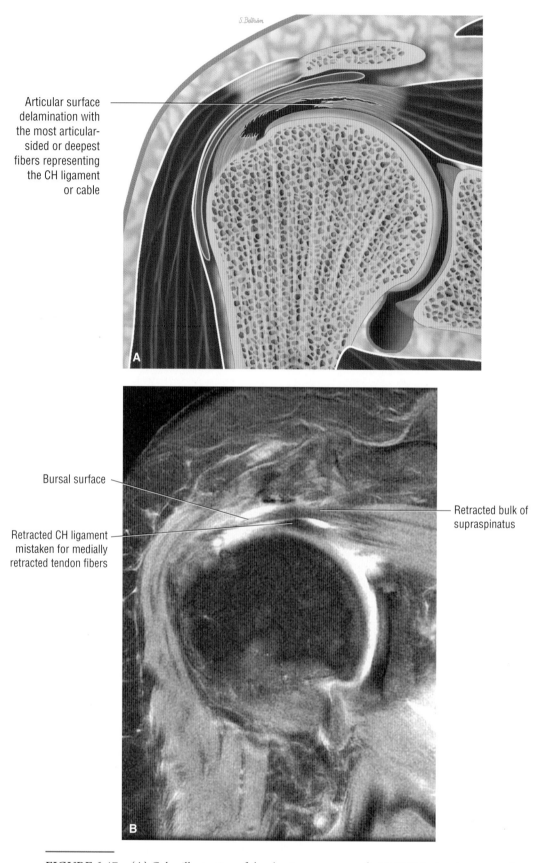

Articular surface delamination with the most articular-sided or deepest fibers representing the CH ligament or cable

Bursal surface

Retracted CH ligament mistaken for medially retracted tendon fibers

Retracted bulk of supraspinatus

FIGURE 6.47 (**A**) Color illustration of the classic appearance of a PASTA lesion; however, what has been thought to represent the retracted articular surface of the supraspinatus is in fact in most cases the retracted cable or coracohumeral ligament. This has important implications in the PASTA repair because if the articular-sided coracohumeral ligament is anchored laterally, it will overtension the cuff repair. (**B**) Accurate depiction of the PASTA type tear showing the attenuated bursal surface intact with the retracted supraspinatus and retracted cable. The retracted articular supraspinatus tendon fibers will retract over the cable (CH ligament). Coronal FS PD image.

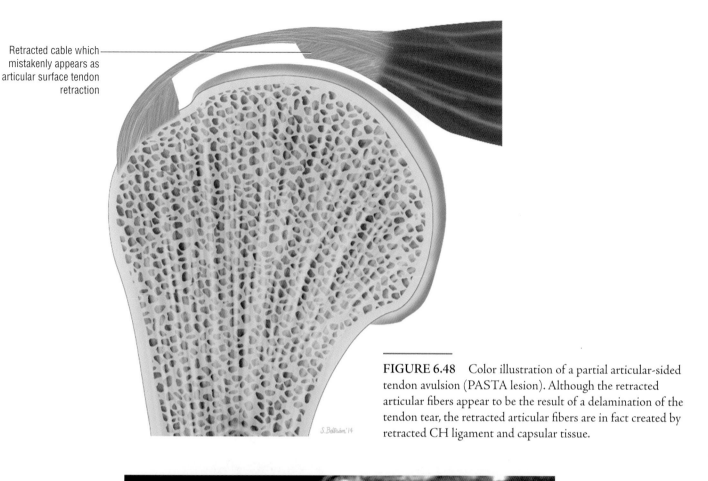

Retracted cable which mistakenly appears as articular surface tendon retraction

S.Beltrán'14

FIGURE 6.48   Color illustration of a partial articular-sided tendon avulsion (PASTA lesion). Although the retracted articular fibers appear to be the result of a delamination of the tendon tear, the retracted articular fibers are in fact created by retracted CH ligament and capsular tissue.

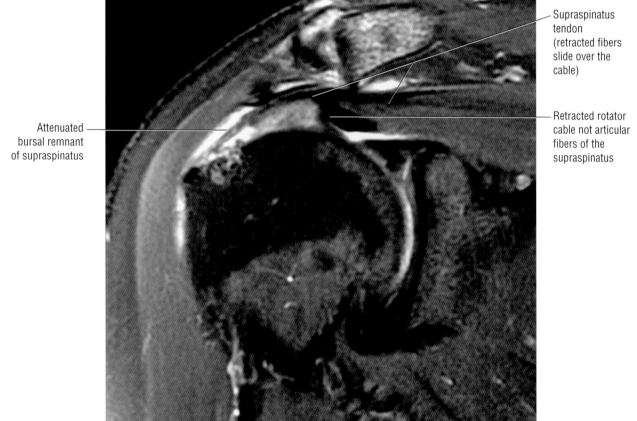

Supraspinatus tendon (retracted fibers slide over the cable)

Retracted rotator cable not articular fibers of the supraspinatus

Attenuated bursal remnant of supraspinatus

FIGURE 6.49   Coronal FS PD image where the articular side is the retracted rotator cuff cable. The supraspinatus tendon avulsion is retracted superior to the cable. There is an attenuated bursal remnant of the supraspinatus that extends to the footprint.

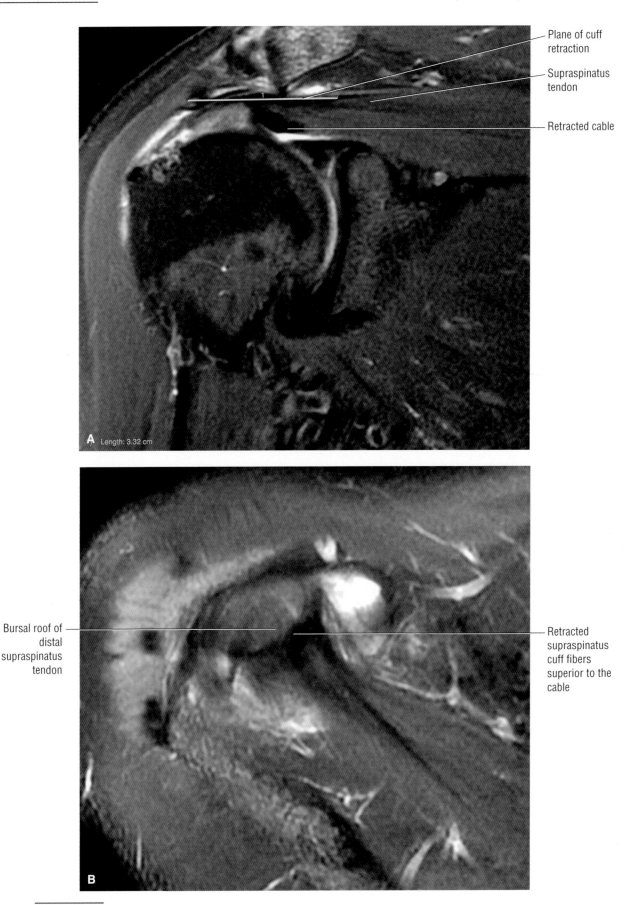

FIGURE 6.50 (**A**) Coronal image location corresponding to the retracted fibers 0f the supraspinatus ten-don. Coronal FS PD. (**B**) Axial view of the retracted supraspinatus fibers above the rotator cuff cable. Axial FS PD image. Cable preservation implies the CH ligament is in anatomic position while cable restoration indicates the cable is medially displaced and needs to be restored to a functional location.

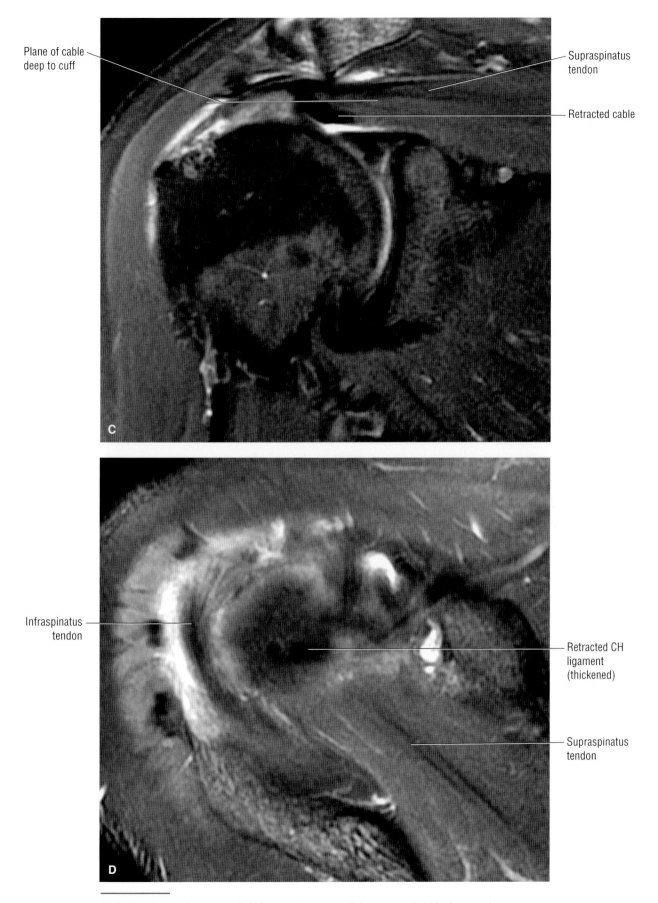

FIGURE 6.50 (*Continued*) (**C**) Image location of the retracted cable deep to the articular side of the supraspinatus tendon tear. Coronal FS PD image. (**D**) Axial view of retracted coracohumeral ligament deep to the retracted supraspinatus component of the PASTA lesion. Axial FS PD image.

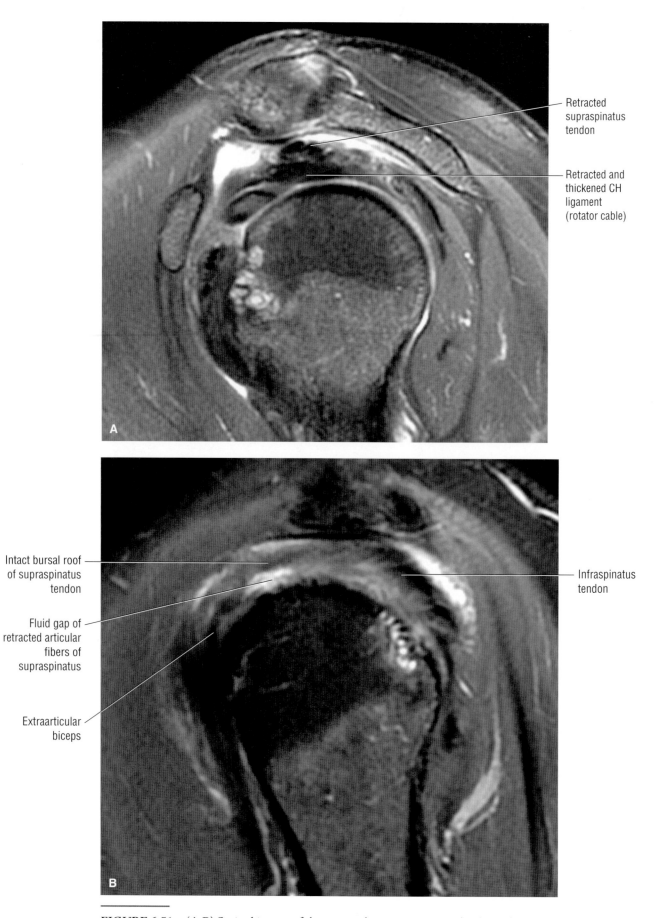

FIGURE 6.51   (**A,B**) Sagittal images of the retracted supraspinatus tendon lying directly on top of the thickened coracohumeral ligament which represents the retracted cable. Peripherally (image B is lateral to image A), the fluid gap from the retracted articular fibers of the supraspinatus tendon are defined.

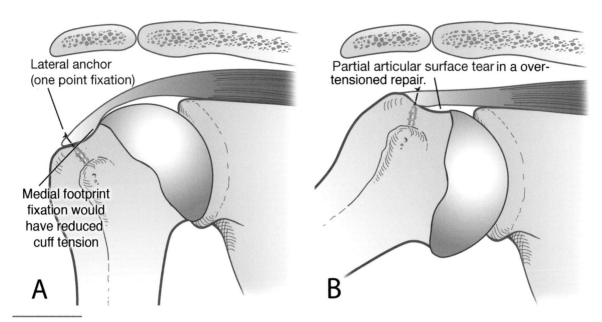

FIGURE 6.52 Schematic drawing of a single-row suture anchor repair for a partial thickness articular surface rotator cuff tear (PASTA). (**A**) Point fixation is potentially overtensioned with a lateral row repair. (**B**) When the shoulder is abducted, a similar overtensioned PASTA lesion demonstrates lifting of the medial footprint. If the coracohumeral ligament or cable represents the articular side of the PASTA lesion, then it would be preferable not to anchor the cable laterally because this would result in overtensioning of the cable. Articular-sided cuff fibers once identified should be mobilized to the medial footprint in a functional repair. This concept of repair with minimal tension of cuff fibers will allow for healing assuming secure fixation. (Reprinted from Burkhart S, Lo IK, Brady PC, Denard PJ. *The Cowboy's Companion: A Trail Guide for the Arthroscopic Shoulder Surgeon*. Philadelphia, PA: Lippincott Williams & Wilkins; 2012, with permission.)

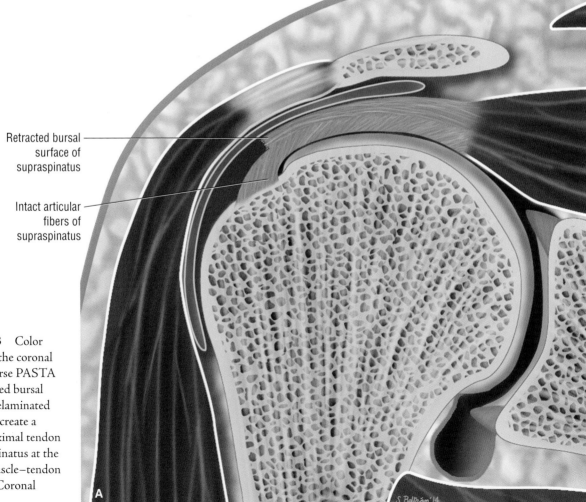

FIGURE 6.53 Color illustration in the coronal plane of a reverse PASTA lesion. Retracted bursal fibers of the delaminated supraspinatus create a thickened proximal tendon of the supraspinatus at the level of the muscle–tendon junction. (**A**) Coronal illustration.

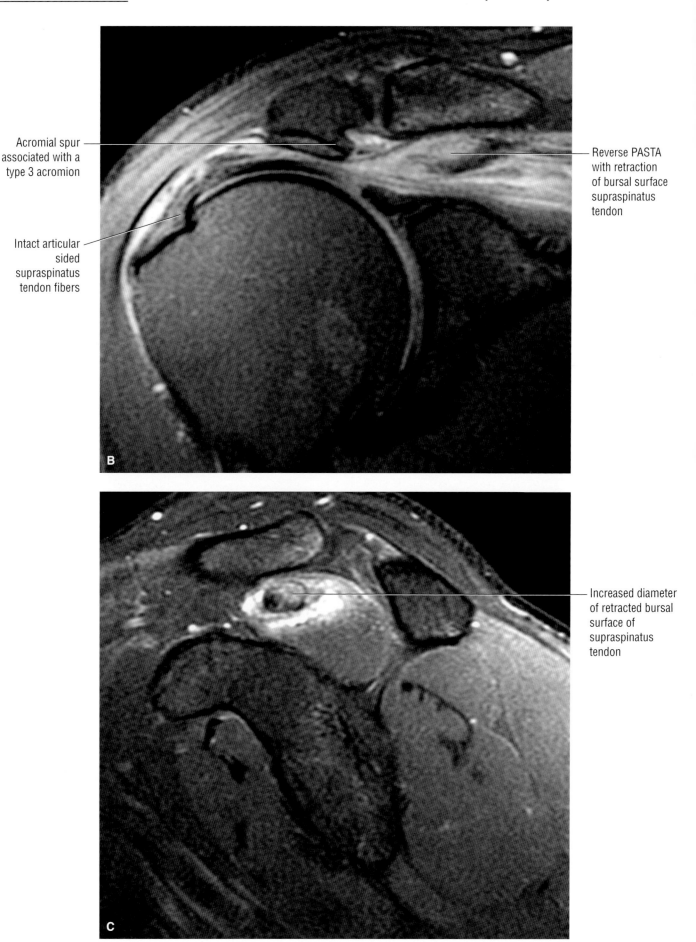

Acromial spur associated with a type 3 acromion

Intact articular sided supraspinatus tendon fibers

Reverse PASTA with retraction of bursal surface supraspinatus tendon

Increased diameter of retracted bursal surface of supraspinatus tendon

FIGURE 6.53   (*Continued*) (**B**) Coronal FS PD. (**C**) Sagittal FS PD.

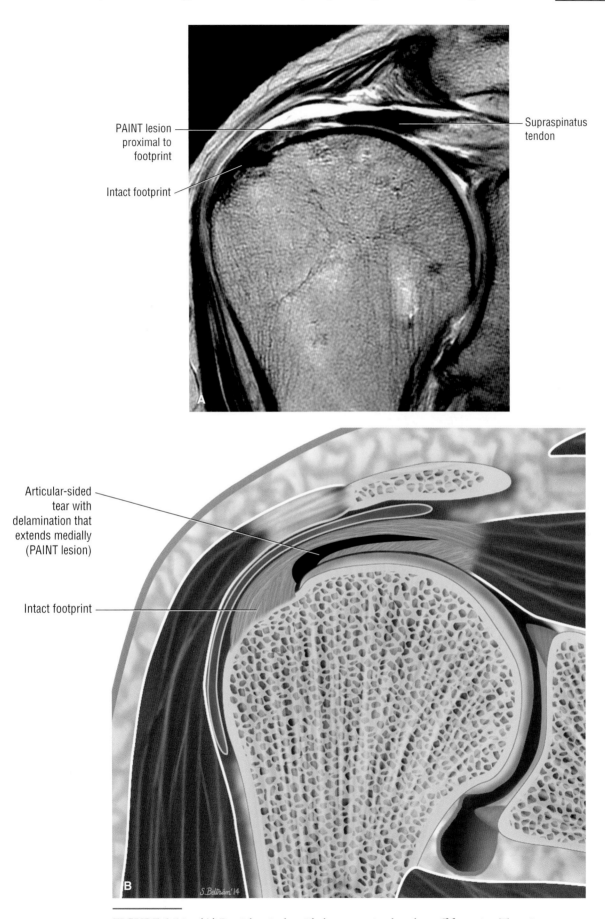

FIGURE 6.54 (**A**) Partial articular-sided tear proximal to the cuff footprint. There is a secondary interstitial component. This has been referred to as the PAINT lesion or a Partial Articular Surface and Intratendinous rotator cuff tear. (**B**) PAINT Lesion—articular-sided tear with secondary interstitial component. (**A**) Coronal MR arthrogram. (**B**) Color illustration.

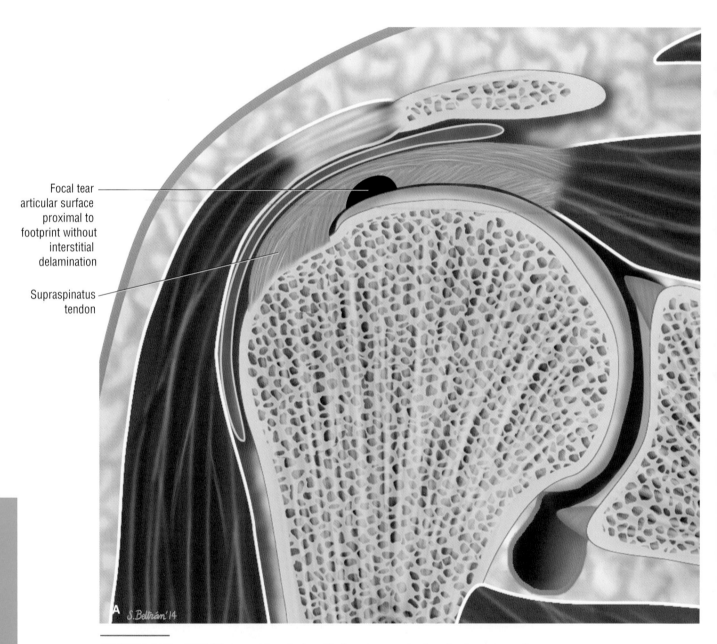

Focal tear
articular surface
proximal to
footprint without
interstitial
delamination

Supraspinatus
tendon

FIGURE 6.55 STAS lesion with articular-sided tearing proximal to the footprint and without a delamination or intratendinous component. (**A**) Coronal color illustration.

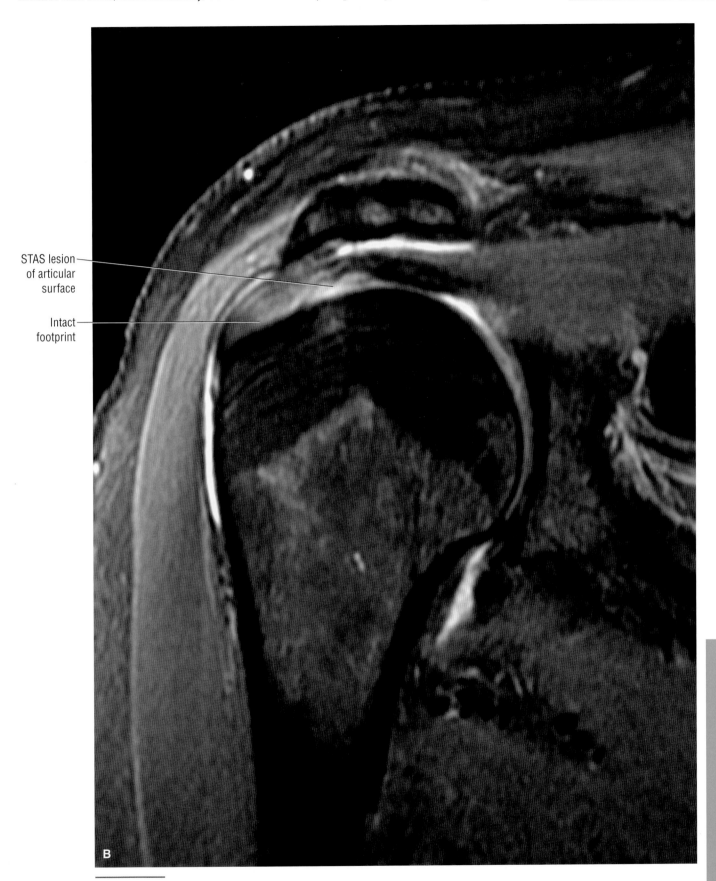

STAS lesion
of articular
surface

Intact
footprint

FIGURE 6.55   (*Continued*) (**B**) Coronal FS PD. The STAS lesion or Supraspinatus Tendon Articular
Side lesion is proximal or exclusive to the supraspinatus footprint.

MR Appearance of Partial Tears

■ Small amounts of fluid may be seen in the subacromial bursa, especially in bursal surface lesions, in the absence of a full thickness or complete tear.

■ In addition to a partial thickness tear, there may be associated tendon thinning and fraying.

■ On FS PD FSE or T2-weighted FSE images, well-defined linear high-signal-intensity changes that do not extend to either the articular or bursal surfaces are associated with an intrasubstance partial tear.

■ Because of the T1 shortening effects of gadolinium, MR arthrography with intraarticular Gd-DTPA administration is useful in highlighting small, partial tears involving the articular surface.

■ Partial articular surface tears not seen on conventional arthrograms may be identified using MR arthrography, especially in areas of granulation tissue in chronic tears.

    ■ Tears are bright on T1-weighted postinjection images.[167]

■ In patients with tendinosis or tendon degeneration alone, there is no extension of contrast on postinjection images, and the supraspinatus tendon can be seen to be intact.

■ Intraarticular contrast is not helpful in the identification of partial bursal surface tears and does not enhance intrasubstance tears.

■ Identify MR findings of extrinsic impingement which may be associated with bursal surface tears.

■ MR images can be used to identify partial thickness cuff tears that involve greater than 25% of the tendon width.

    ■ Require acromioplasty and repair

■ PASTA lesions involving over 50% of the footprint require repair.

    ■ A defect of over 6 to 8mm is also repaired

    ■ Subacromial decompression not indicated in younger patients with a PASTA lesion

    ■ Subacromial decompression is used in older ortinpaedts with bursitis and mechanical fraying on the undersurface of the acromion and the CA ligament.

Full Thickness Rotator Cuff Tears

- Bursal cuff (layer 2) and articular cuff (layer 3) are characterized by differences in the orientation of collagen bundles and thus create a shear plane susceptible to cuff delamination.

- Rotator cuff disruption may be characterized as[339]:
  - Partial or full thickness
  - Acute or chronic
  - Traumatic or degenerative
  - Contributing factors include trauma, attrition, ischemia, and subacromial abrasion.

- The mechanism of cuff tears usually involves an attritional tear of the rotator cuff tendons with or without subacromial impingement.

- A cuff tear as a result of a traumatic injury occurs in the setting of preexisting tendon degeneration.

- Partial thickness tears progress to full thickness lesions.

- The rotator cuff is subjected to traction, compression, contusion, subacromial abrasion, inflammation, and, most importantly, age-related degeneration.

- Rotator cuff tendon fibers may fail a few at a time or en masse.

- Torn tendon fibers retract because they are under load even with the arm at rest.

- Healing cuff scar tissue lacks normal tendon resilience and may be at an increased risk of failure with subsequent loading.

- Because of the marked ability of the cuff to repair itself, the degeneration process continues and propagates until a full thickness anterior supraspinatus tendon defect is produced.

- Because the full thickness tendon defect concentrates loads at its margin, additional tendon fiber failure may subsequently occur with even smaller applied loads.

- A supraspinatus defect will propagate posteriorly through the remainder of the supraspinatus and may then involve the infraspinatus.

- Intramuscular cysts[262] may dissect along the path of the torn rotator cuff tendon.

- AC joint cysts may communicate with an extensive rotator cuff tear and present as a superior pseudotumor of the shoulder.[598]

  - Once the apron effect of the rotator cuff is lost, the humeral head displaces superiorly, placing increased loads on the biceps tendon.

- The LHBT is frequently ruptured in chronic rotator cuff deficiency.

  - As the rotator cuff defect propagates, the tear may destabilize the LHBT and involve the subscapularis tendon.

- Biceps pulley lesions are associated with medial displacement of the biceps tendon.

Chronicity of Full Thickness Tears

- Rotator cuff arthropathy develops with failure and abrasive contact between the chondral surface of the humeral head and the coracoacromial arch, causing degenerative joint disease.

- After minimal débridement, chronic complete rotator cuff tears are assessed at their greatest point of retraction for muscle changes, including:

  - Atrophy[350]

  - Fatty degeneration

  - Retraction

  - Loss of excursion[75,124]

Size of Full Thickness Tears

- Tear size is assessed on MR examination as the size of the fluid-filled gap or retraction from medial to lateral in the coronal plane and anterior to posterior in the sagittal plane.

- Cuff size and quality of muscle and tendon, including atrophy, rupture of the biceps tendon, and shoulder weakness, are important prognostic factors in determining surgical outcome.

- Cuff tendon retraction can be staged in the coronal plane.

  - Stage 1 (adjacent to the tendon insertion)

  - Stage 2 (retraction superior to the humeral head)

  - Stage 3 (proximal retraction to the glenoid margin)[75,124]

Geometry of Full Thickness Tears

- Type 1 Crescent Tears
  - Treated with end-to bone repair
- Type 2 Longitudinal
  - Treated with margin convergence
- Type 3 Massive and Contracted
  - Treated with interval slide or partial repair
- Type 4 Tear
  - Arthropathy treated with arthroplasty[75]

Infraspinatus and Teres Minor Involvement

- Isolated infraspinatus full thickness tears are uncommon.[664]
  - May be found in the throwing athlete with involvement of the articular surface of the supraspinatus–infraspinatus junction or anterior infraspinatus articular surface
- Tears of the teres minor are unusual, but the superior fibers of the teres minor may be involved with a massive rotator cuff tear.

Quality of Muscle and Tendon in Full Thickness Tears

- The rotator cuff tendon edges may be good, fair, or poor.
- Atrophy is also graded in a similar fashion as mild, moderate, or severe.
- Snyder[544] classified complete rotator cuff tears based on size and complexity into the following categories:
  - 0: Tear lacks full thickness communication between the bursal and articular surfaces, even if partial tears exist on both.
  - I: A small complete tear (puncture)
  - II: A moderate (<2cm) tear involving one tendon without retraction
  - III: A large (3 to 4cm) complete tear involving an entire tendon with minimal retraction of the torn edge
  - IV: A massive cuff tear involving two or more cuff tendons, usually with associated retraction and scarring of the remaining tendon ends. Tears in this group may be subclassified or determined to be irreparable.[75,124]

Specific Rotator Cuff Patterns

- **Crescent Tears**
  - Avascular region (supraspinatus and anterior half of the infraspinatus)
  - May be minimally symptomatic because of the torn rotator cuff's ability to transmit load to the humeral head by utilizing the cable region[446]
  - Double-row repair versus single-row repair
    - Single row triple loaded anchors near the medial edge of the footprint to minimize suture-cuff tension.
    - Most double row repairs will lateralize the cable and overtension it.

- **L-Shaped and U-Shaped Tears**
  - Tear mobility must be understood for tension-free repair to bone.
  - Identify apex of the tear and the corner of the L to ensure correct closure of the cuff defect.[446]

- **Large and Massive Rotator Cuff Tears**
  - A biomechanically sound repair without complete closure of the defect may suffice if anatomic repair is not possible.

- **Rotator Cable**
  - Anatomic thickening of collagen fibers within rotator cuff
    - The rotator cable should not be mistaken for retracted fibers of the articular surface of the cuff; otherwise, the attempted cuff repair may result in overtensioning of cuff fibers by inadvertently attempting to advance cable tissue with retracted cuff fibers to the cuff footprint (which would not be anatomic for the cable).
  - Extension of coracohumeral ligament along the articular surface of the cuff which is located medial to the rotator cuff crescent tissue
  - The rotator cable extends from a bifurcated insertion on both sides of the long head of the biceps to across the supraspinatus to the inferior margin of the infraspinatus.
  - Classic crescent region of the rotator cuff enclosed within the arc of the rotator cuff
  - Most tears within the rotator cable region will have a stable fulcrum of motion, preserved clinical motion, and minimal strength deficit.

- Tears that extend through the rotator cable attachments result in an unstable fulcrum, loss of motion, and significant strength deficit.
  - The goal in rotator cable assessment is to attempt to return the cable to a functional location corresponding to the previous location of the functioning cable assuming the rotator cuff tendon footprint has been restored.[75,124]

- Massive rotator cuff tears alternative technique of not completely closing the defect
  - Tears that extend into a second tendon do not maintain preserved function.
  - If a complete repair is not possible, a partial repair attempting to reattach the subscapularis and infraspinatus tendons can restore cable attachment and thus cuff function, balance cuff force couples, and create a stable fulcrum of motion.

- Complete rotator cuff repair is more desirable than partial rotator cuff repair.

- Complete cuff repair that respects natural cuff footprint and functional cable location will result in a low-tension anatomic repair.
  - Requires evaluation of the medial-to-lateral and anterior-to-posterior mobility of the tear margins[75,124,446,528]

Rotator Cuff Repair Techniques

- Medial-to-lateral direction
  - Crescent-shaped tear
- Anterior-to-posterior convergence
  - U-shaped or reverse L-shaped tears
- Interval slide technique
  - Used in severe chronic causes when margins of the rotator cuff are scarred to internal deltoid fascia or when there is no mobility from a medial-to-lateral and an anterior-to-posterior direction
  - Massive rotator cuff tears require interval slide technique because of scarring or lack of mobility.[75,124,141,182,234,559]

Rotator Cuff Releases in Large and Massive Tears with Decreased Mobility

- Rotator cuff tears anatomically reduced to the footprint do not require any advanced release.

■ Releases are performed based on inherent mobility of the rotator cuff tissue and thus are usually described in the setting of massive rotator cuff tears. The size of the cuff tear alone, however, does not directly determine cuff mobility or the necessity for a complex release.

■ Releases may also be required in the presence of adhesive capsulitis or revision of a previous scarred cuff with loss of mobility.

■ Bursal-sided releases
   ■ If the cuff is adhesed and scarred to the undersurface of the acromion and internal deltoid fascia[182,559]

■ Articular-sided releases
   ■ Capsular release
      ■ Used in crescent type tears where the direction of the repair is generally from a medial-to-lateral direction
      ■ Capsular release provides 1 to 1.5cm additional mobility.
      ■ If mobility of cuff margin post-release is sufficient, then tendon repair to bone is performed.
      ■ If cuff mobility is inadequate post-release, then interval slide is employed.

■ Interval slides
   ■ Most U-shaped and L-shaped have adequate mobility and can be repaired by principles of margin convergence.
   ■ Irreparable cuff tears post-standard capsular releases can benefit from an interval slide to improve mobility versus older patients with poor tissue quality may be candidates for partial repair or débridement alone.

Partial Rotator Cuff Repair Concept

■ Seventy percent of massive immobile cuff tears can be repaired following single or double interval slide repairs.

■ Thirty percent of massive immobile cuff tears require a partial balanced rotator cuff repair because a complete cuff repair is not possible even with the use of releases.

■ Restore anterior and posterior rotator cable attachments to include the upper subscapularis and the infraspinatus tendons.[106]

■ Most common partial repair scenario is for combined subscapularis, supraspinatus, and infraspinatus tendon tears.[75,124]

MR Appearance of Full Thickness Tears

■ Complete (full thickness) tears of the rotator cuff, with or without proximal retraction[440,481,489]

■ The combination of FS PD-weighted FSE and T2-weighted FSE sequences improves the characterization of tear morphology.

■ In patients older than 40 years of age, rotator cuff tendon tears are frequently associated with acute glenohumeral dislocations.

■ Infrequent traumatic tears in younger individuals may avulse a segment of the greater tuberosity.

■ The size of a rotator cuff tear can be determined by measuring its long diameter in centimeters.

   ■ Small cuff tear = <1cm

   ■ Medium cuff tear = 1 to 3cm

   ■ Large cuff tear = 3 to 5cm

   ■ Massive tear = >5cm

■ However, the number of tendons involved, and their level of retraction, is of more clinical significance than size.

Primary Signs of Full Thickness Tears

■ Visualization of a tendon defect or tendinous gap

■ Tendon retraction assessed in the coronal plane for medial to lateral extent and sagittal plane for anterior to posterior extent

■ Joint fluid or granulation tissue at the cuff tear site, which is seen as areas of intermediate to increased signal intensity on T1-weighted and PD-weighted images

■ Depending on the complexity of the tear and the degree of retraction of the supraspinatus, a large fluid-filled gap may not be seen on sagittal images, especially if there is a delamination component to the cuff tear.

■ Fluid signal appearing superior, anterior, and inferior along the undersurface of the supraspinatus tendon is characteristic of a complete tear.

■ Acute rotator cuff tears are often associated with muscle and MTU edema in addition to retraction of the involved tendons of the rotator cuff.

■ Superior ascent of the humeral head occurs with loss of the depressor action of the torn cuff and may occur with acute multitendon (massive) cuff tears.

■ Massive cuff tears may involve the supraspinatus, the infraspinatus, and the subscapularis tendons.

　■ The LHBT is also frequently disrupted in massive cuff tears.

■ Nonacute cuff tears require evaluation of the integrity and loss of continuity of torn tendon edges.

■ In subacute tears, FS PD FSE images may be more useful than T2 FSE studies because the relative hyperintensity of granulation tissue and synovium helps to define the tendon edges.

■ Isolated infraspinatus tears are identified on posterior coronal and sagittal images.

■ The increased cross-sectional diameter sign of the retracted tendon may be helpful in more subtle cases of subacute supraspinatus or infraspinatus tendon tears.

■ The retracted cuff tendon may be seen as far medially as the level of the bony glenoid rim.

　■ Tendon retraction even to the glenoid should be measured in medial to lateral extent.

　　■ Uninvolved areas of the tendon adjacent to the tear site may demonstrate degenerative changes or partial thickness tear.

　　■ Less frequently, the remaining tendon demonstrates normal signal intensity or morphology.

　■ Margins may be thickened in response to healing or attenuated in more chronic tears.

　　■ Fluid sensitive sagittal oblique images are used to identify the anteroposterior extent of the cuff tear.

Secondary Signs of Full Thickness Tears

■ Supplanted by identification of the primary diagnostic criteria of tendon signal and morphology depicted by using higher resolution images, the combination of FS PD FSE and T2 FSE coronal images, and MR arthrography when indicated

■ Subacromial-subdeltoid bursal fluid, which should be readily identifiable, especially when there is a large volume of articular and bursal fluid associated with a complete tear

　■ Fluid in the subacromial bursa may also be present in impingement or in a partial bursal surface tear without communication with the glenohumeral joint.[484]

- Rarely, a massive synovial reaction (hyperintense on FS PD FSE) may develop and fill the gap of a rotator cuff tear.
  - The biceps tendon may be difficult to find at surgery if it is encased in concentric layers of hypertrophied gelatinous synovium.
  - Inflammatory arthropathy and even infection may present with similar imaging characteristics.
  - Rice bodies (discrete synovial fronds) or subcutaneous edema, however, is not associated with this type of synovial response.
- Subacromial and subdeltoid peribursal fat changes may also be considered secondary signs of cuff pathology.

Appearance of Massive Cuff Tears

- Supraspinatus, infraspinatus, and subscapularis tendon retraction to the glenoid
- Combined tear length >2cm on coronal and width >2cm on sagittal images requires interval slide or partial repair in 75% of cases.
- Combined length and width >3cm requires treatment with an interval slide or partial repair in all cases.
- More than 75% fatty infiltration of the infraspinatus is a poor prognostic sign for functional improvement following repair.
- Secondary Changes in Massive Cuff Tears
  - Glenohumeral chondral degeneration
  - Eburnation of the inferior acromion
- Massive rotator cuff tears with significant retraction can result in traction of the suprascapular nerve at the suprascapular notch.[75,124,141,182,234,559]
- Arthroscopic Revision Rotator Cuff Repair
  - Most recurrent tears requiring revision were initially massive rotator cuff tears.
  - Revision repair done arthroscopically produces excellent functional outcome in the majority of cases.
- Revision Surgery Categories
  - Missed pathology such as an overlooked subscapularis tear
  - Postoperative stiffness
    - Require capsular release and subacromial lysis of adhesions

- ■ Structural failure of the repair
    - ■ Biomechanical failure of repair, biologic failure, or structural failure of repair construct secondary to aggressive postoperative rehabilitation
- ■ The biceps in revision rotator cuff repair
    - ■ Biceps tenodesis at the superior aspect of the bicipital groove performed in the younger, high-demand patient and where cosmesis is important
    - ■ Tenotomy—low-demand patient
        - • Popeye deformity may be noticeable.
- ■ Suture anchors have transferred the weak link in rotator cuff repair from the bone to the rotator cuff tendon.

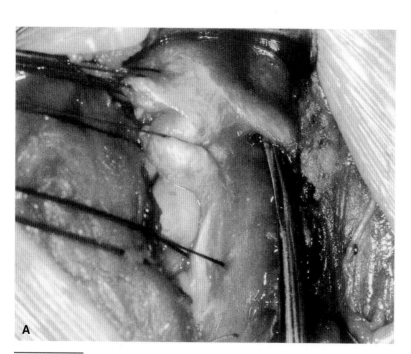
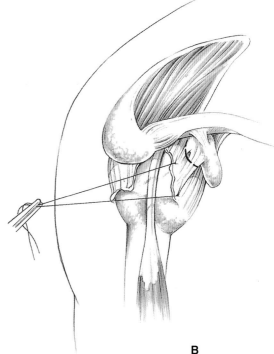

FIGURE 6.56 (**A**) The coracohumeral ligament (at end of instrument) is contracted, tethering the retracted tear edge to the coracoid. (**B**) This ligament must be divided (*dashed line*) and the coracoid base freed to mobilize the tendon. The coracohumeral ligament can be identified at arthroscopy and should be assessed as either in anatomic position (cable preservation) or shifted medially with the associated cuff tear (cable restoration). (Reprinted from Miniaci A, Iannotti JP, Williams GR, Zuckerman, JD. *Disorders of the Shoulder: Sports Injuries.* 3rd ed. Philadelphia, PA: Lippincott Williams and Wilkins; 2014, with permission.)

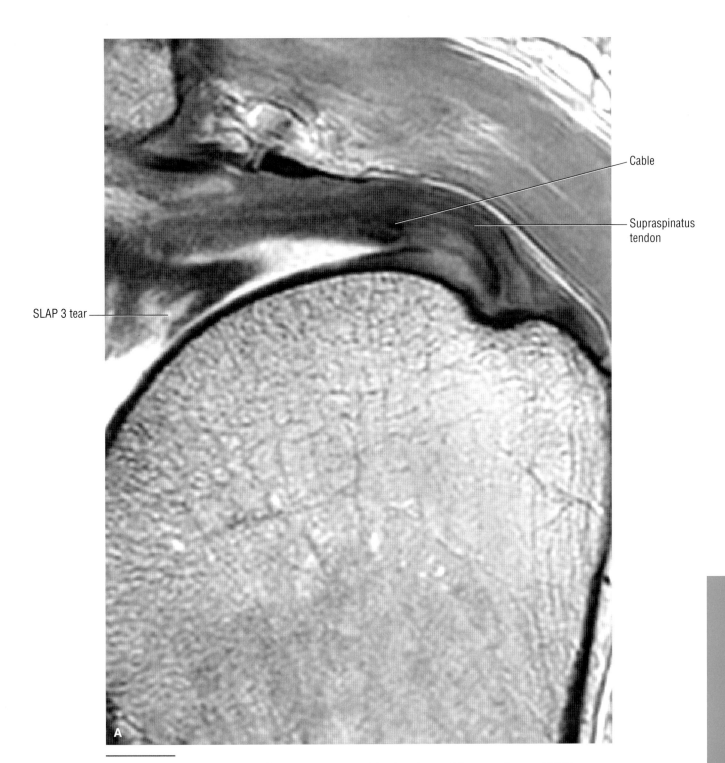

FIGURE 6.57 Rotator cuff cable as an extension of the deep layer of the coracohumeral (CH) ligament. The supraspinatus tendon inserts 1 mm lateral from the articular margin of the humeral head. The CH ligament is in its correct anatomic position medial to the articular margin of the humerus. (**A**) Coronal T1 image.

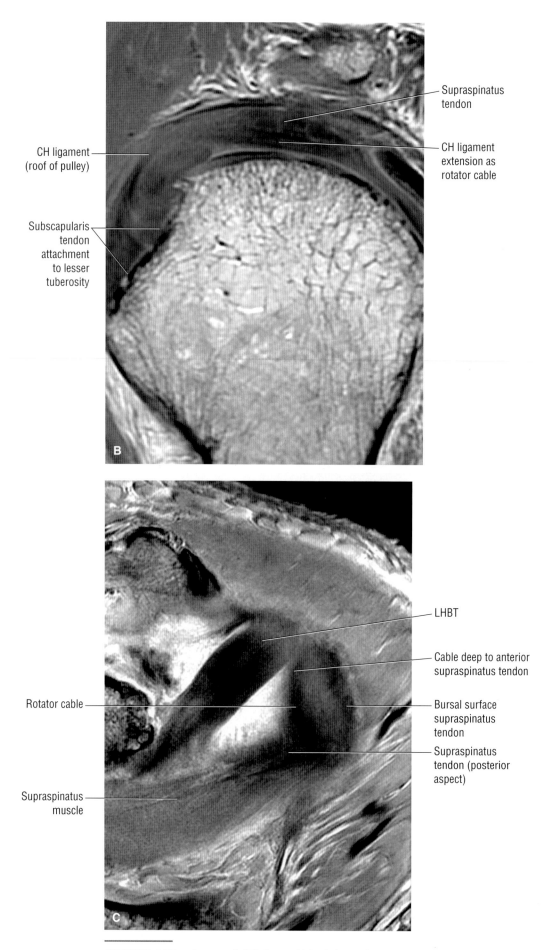

FIGURE 6.57 *Continued.* (**B**) Sagittal T1. (**C**) Axial FS PD.

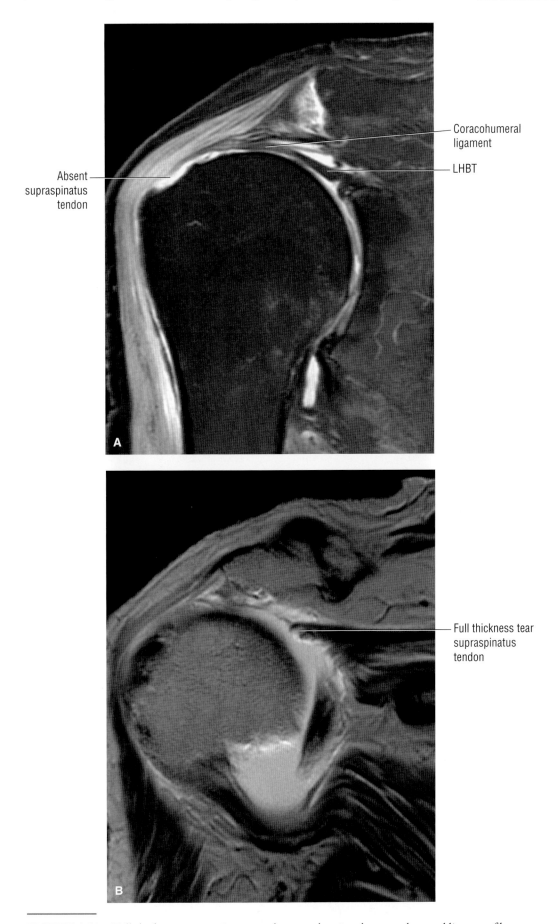

FIGURE 6.58 Full thickness supraspinatus tendon tear showing the coracohumeral ligament fibers without the adjacent supraspinatus tendon. There is adhesion of the retracted CH ligament to the supraspinatus tendon tear. (**A**) Coronal FS PD. (**B**) Coronal T2 FSE.

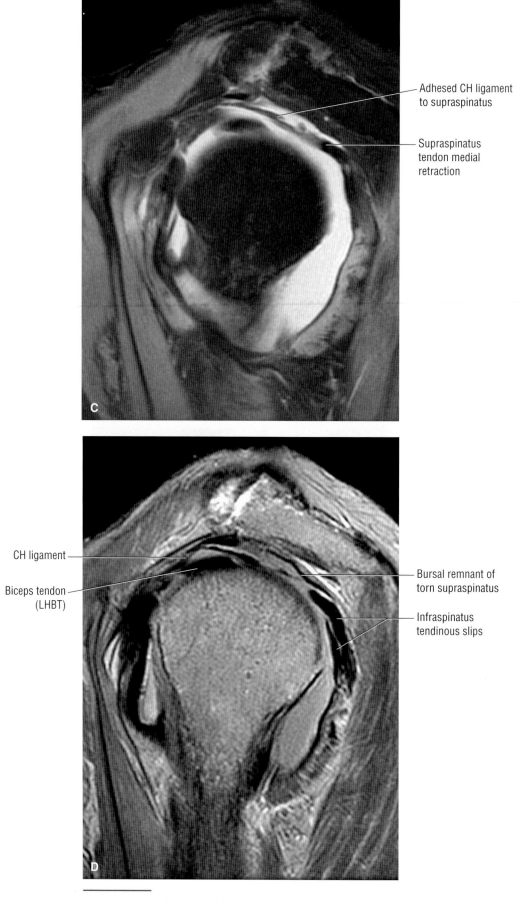

FIGURE 6.58 (*Continued*) (**C**) Sagittal FS PD. (**D**) Sagittal T2 FSE.

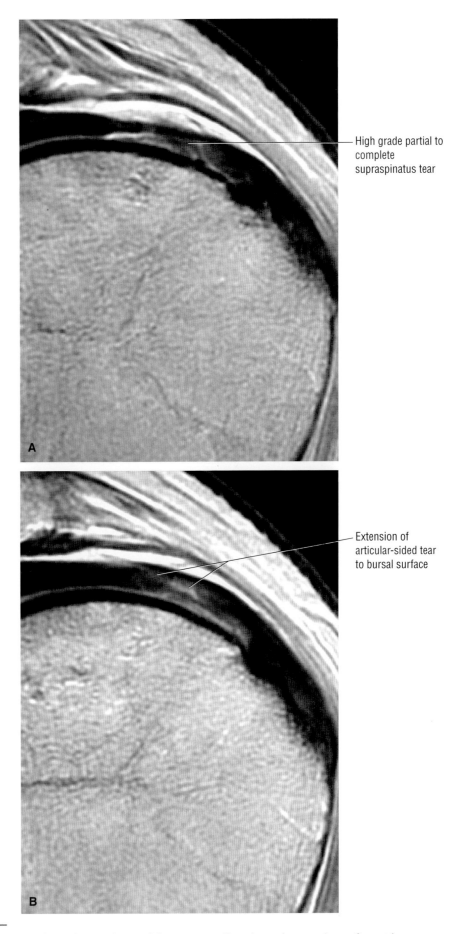

High grade partial to complete supraspinatus tear

Extension of articular-sided tear to bursal surface

FIGURE 6.59 High-grade partial tear of the rotator cuff involving the articular surface with secondary bursal surface communication. This creates a full thickness extension. (**A**) Coronal FS PD. (**B**) Coronal FS PD.

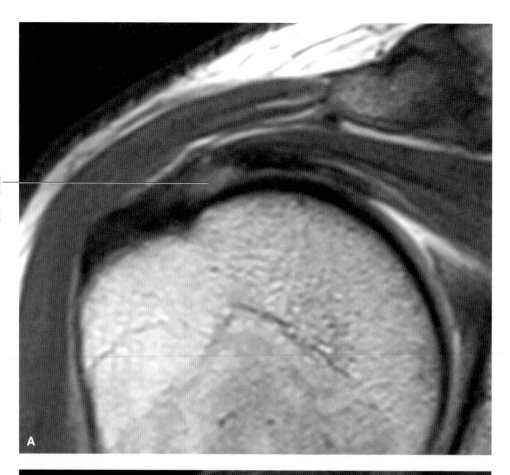

Articular-sided
component of
supraspinatus
tendon tear

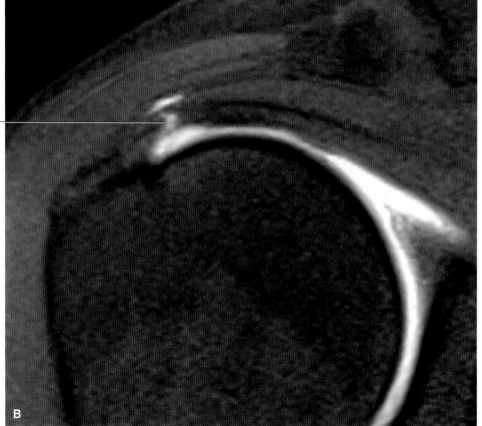

Contrast
communication
from articular to
bursal surface

FIGURE 6.60   Focal full thickness perforation of the supraspinatus appreciated only on MR arthrography. Without arthrography, the cuff pathology has the appearance of an articular-sided tear. (**A**) Coronal T2. (**B**) Coronal fat suppressed T1 MR arthrogram.

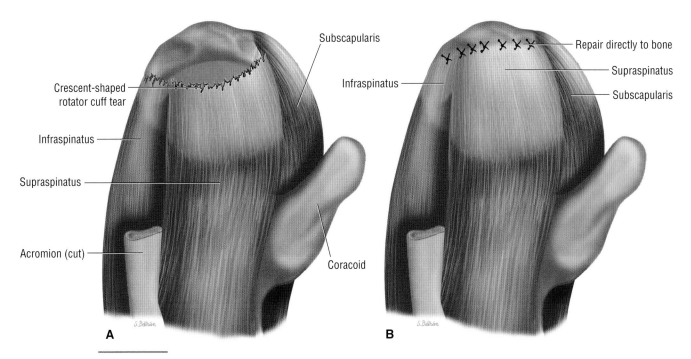

FIGURE 6.61 Crescent-shaped rotator cuff tear (**A**) and repair directly to bone (**B**). Rotator cuff tears can be classified as crescent-shaped tears, U-shaped tears, L-shaped and reverse L-shaped tears, and massive contracted immobile tears. (Based on Burkhart SS, Lo IKY, Brady PC. *Burkhart's View of the Shoulder: A Cowboy's Guide to Advanced Shoulder Arthroscopy.* Philadelphia, PA: Lippincott Williams & Wilkins; 2006.)

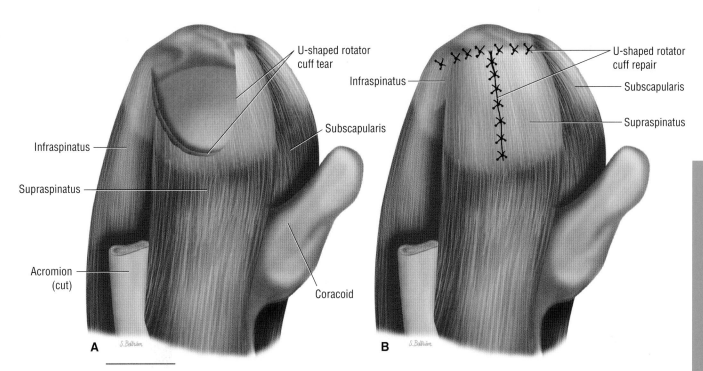

FIGURE 6.62 (**A**) U-shaped rotator cuff tear involving the supraspinatus and infraspinatus tendons. (**B**) Repaired U-shaped tear using a side to side repair and attachment of margin to bone. (Based on Burkhart SS, Lo IKY, Brady PC. *Burkhart's View of the Shoulder: A Cowboy's Guide to Advanced Shoulder Arthroscopy.* Philadelphia, PA: Lippincott Williams & Wilkins; 2006.)

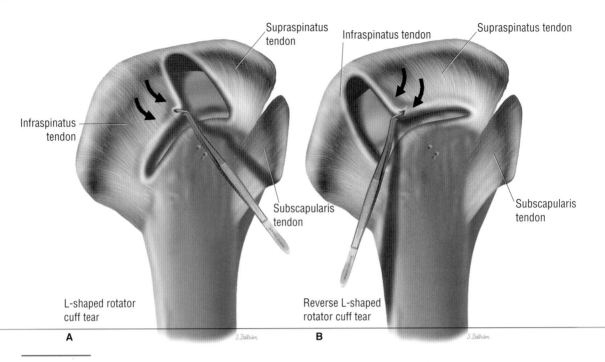

FIGURE 6.63   L-shaped (**A**) and reverse L-shaped (**B**) rotator cuff tendon tears. (Based on Burkhart SS, Lo IKY, Brady PC. *Burkhart's View of the Shoulder: A Cowboy's Guide to Advanced Shoulder Arthroscopy.* Philadelphia, PA: Lippincott Williams & Wilkins; 2006.)

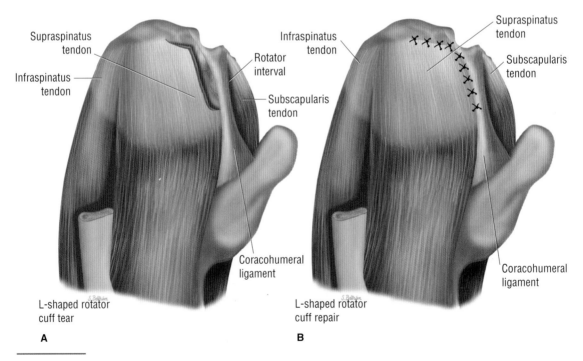

FIGURE 6.64   (**A**) Superior view of an L-shaped rotator cuff tear. (**B**) Repair of an L-shaped tear along its longitudinal split and margin. (Based on Burkhart SS, Lo IKY, Brady PC. *Burkhart's View of the Shoulder: A Cowboy's Guide to Advanced Shoulder Arthroscopy.* Philadelphia, PA: Lippincott Williams & Wilkins; 2006.)

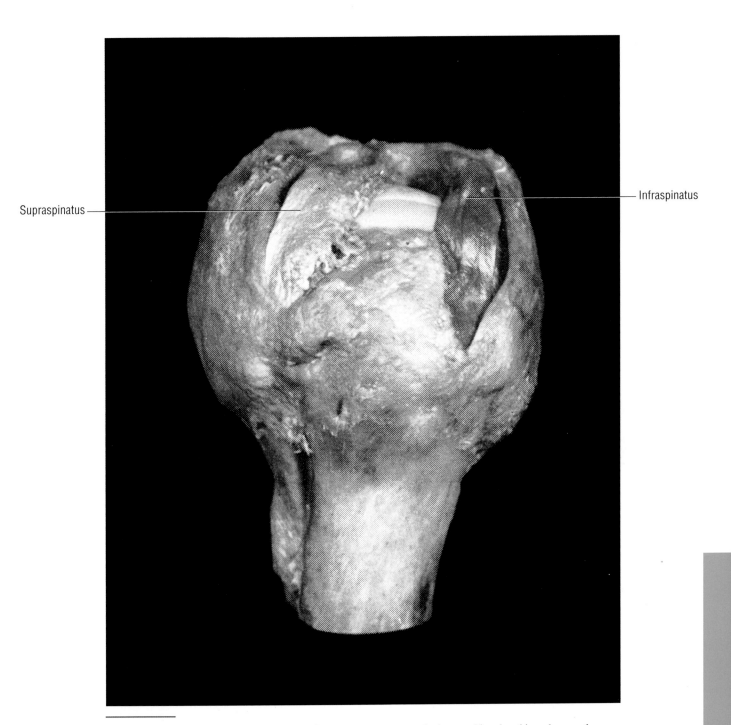

Supraspinatus

Infraspinatus

FIGURE 6.65   The cuff has pulled away from its insertion into the humeral head and has elongated proximally, creating a triangular defect in the supraspinatus and infraspinatus regions. The edges of the defect are thin and smooth; the tuberosities are atrophic and exhibit considerable roughening. (Modified from DePalma AF. *Surgery of the Shoulder*. 3rd ed. Philadelphia, PA: JB Lippincott; 1983.)

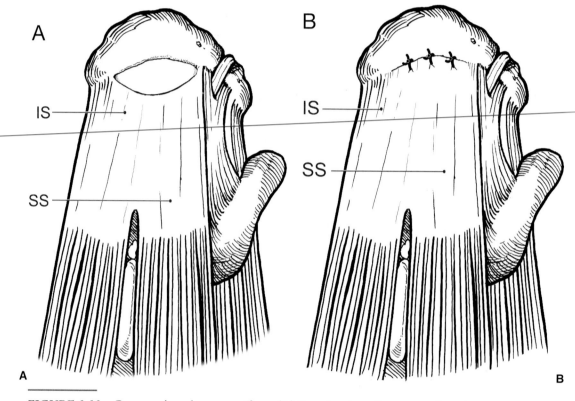

FIGURE 6.66 Crescent-shaped rotator cuff tear. (**A**) Superior view of a crescent-shaped rotator cuff tear involving the supraspinatus and infraspinatus tendons. (**B**) Crescent-shaped tears demonstrate excellent mobility from a medial-to-lateral direction and can be repaired directly to bone. Anchors (triple-loaded) are placed 1 to 1.2cm apart and 5mm lateral to the articular cartilage. This technique minimizes the tension in the rotator cuff repair and creates a strong tendon-to-bone construct avoiding excess cuff tension. SS, supraspinatus; IS, infraspinatus. (Reproduced with permission from Burkhart SS, Lo IK, Brady PC. *Burkhart's View of the Shoulder: A Cowboy's Guide to Advanced Shoulder Arthroscopy*. Philadelphia, PA: Lippincott Williams & Williams; 2006.)

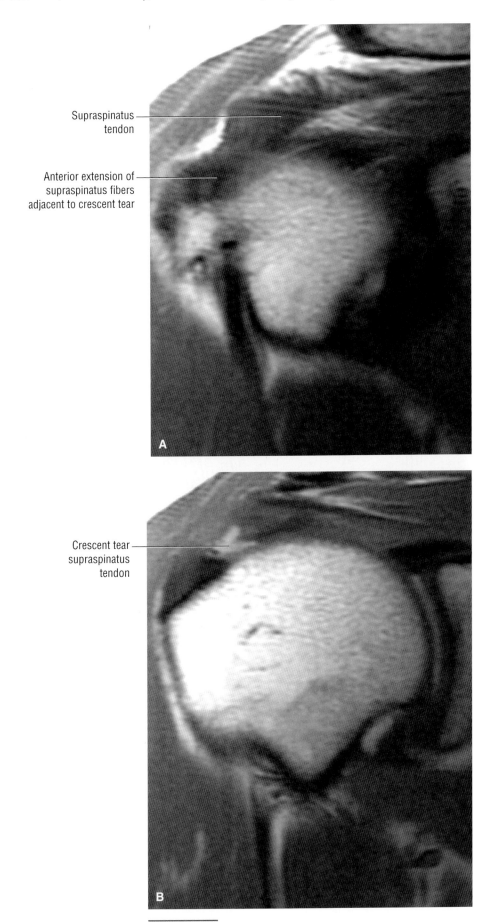

FIGURE 6.67 Crescent tear lateral to the rotator cuff cable involving the supraspinatus tendon. (**A**) PD coronal. (**B**) Coronal T2.

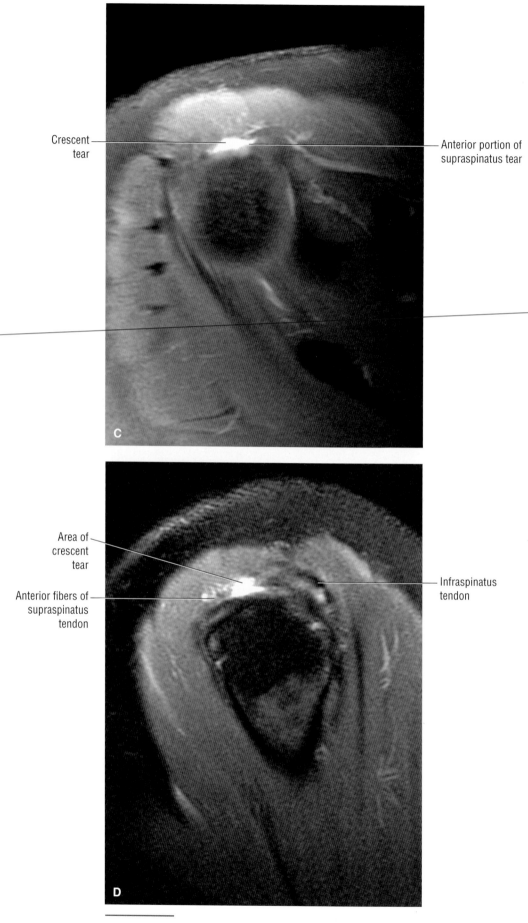

Crescent tear

Anterior portion of supraspinatus tear

Area of crescent tear

Anterior fibers of supraspinatus tendon

Infraspinatus tendon

FIGURE 6.67 (*Continued*) (**C**) Axial FS PD. (**D**) Sagittal FS PD.

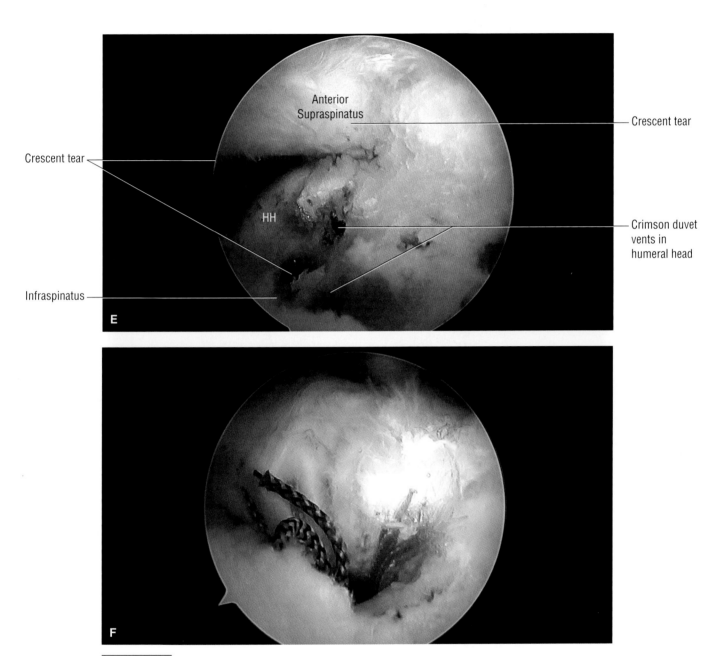

FIGURE 6.67 *(Continued)* (**E,F**) Arthroscopic views of the crescent tear before and after repair. Posterolateral portal, 70-degree scope. Typical crescent tear with intact cable in (**E**). The multiple bone marrow vents enable the formation of a Crimson Duvet to supply blood flow, platelets (with growth factors), and mesenchymal stem cells to promote healing and footprint regeneration. Posterolateral portal 70-degree scope view of crescent repair (**F**). Versalok suture anchor using Orthocord high-strength suture in a single anchor shown at the medial footprint. Inverted mattress suture technique used.

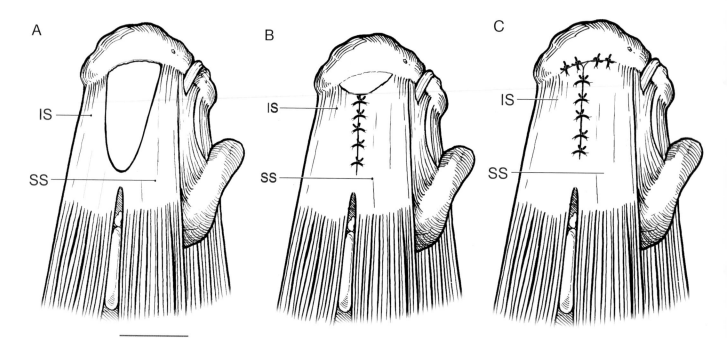

FIGURE 6.68 U-shaped rotator cuff tear. (**A**) Superior view of a U-shaped rotator cuff tear involving the supraspinatus and infraspinatus tendons. (**B**) U-shaped tears demonstrate excellent mobility from an anterior-to-posterior direction and are initially repaired with side-to-side sutures using the principle of margin convergence. (**C**) The repaired margin is then repaired to bone in a tension-free manner. SS, supraspinatus; IS, infraspinatus. In rotator cuff repairs, side-to-side repairs are performed before inserting suture anchors. Suture anchors are inserted near the medial edge of the anatomic neck and not lateral on the greater tuberosity. Anchors enter the bone at a 45-degree angle under strong subchondral bone, a few millimeters lateral to the humeral head articular cartilage on the debrided cortex. (Reproduced with permission from Burkhart SS, Lo IK, Brady PC. *Burkhart's View of the Shoulder: A Cowboy's Guide to Advanced Shoulder Arthroscopy*. Philadelphia, PA: Lippincott Williams & Williams; 2006.)

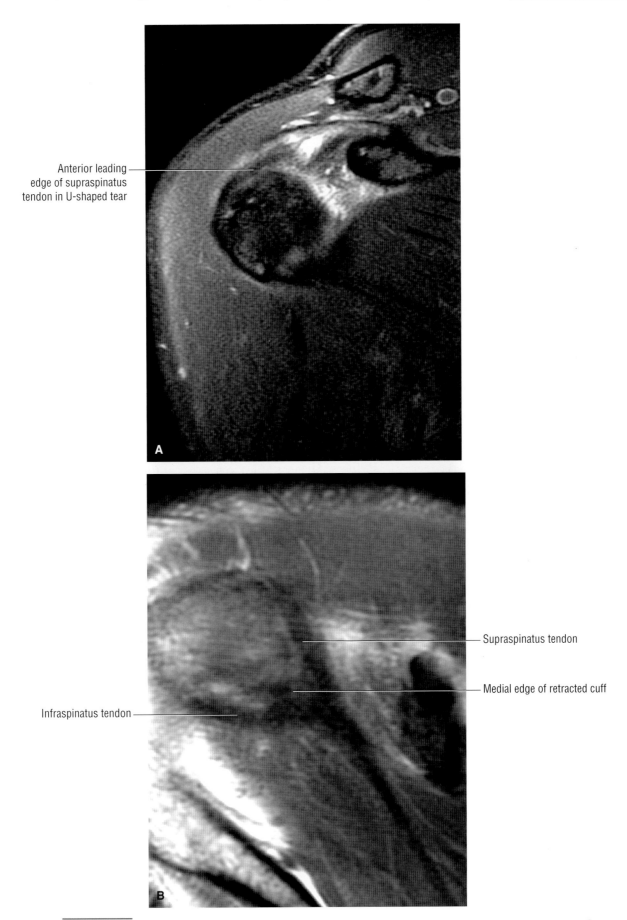

FIGURE 6.69 U-shaped tear of the supraspinatus tendon as created by the retracted medial edge of the cuff. (**A**) Coronal FS PD. (**B**) Axial PD. A U-shaped tear can be thought of as an extension of an enlarged crescent tear.

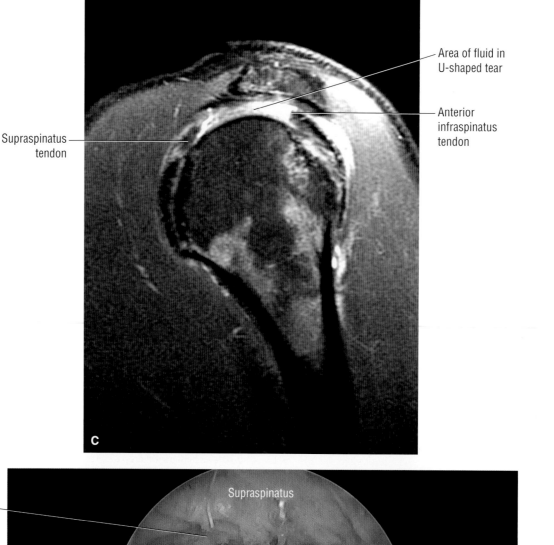

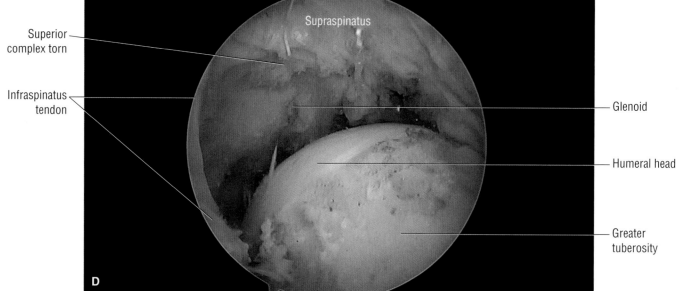

FIGURE 6.69 *(Continued)* (**C**) Sagittal FS PD. (**D**) Arthroscopic view (70-degree scope, posterolateral, portal).

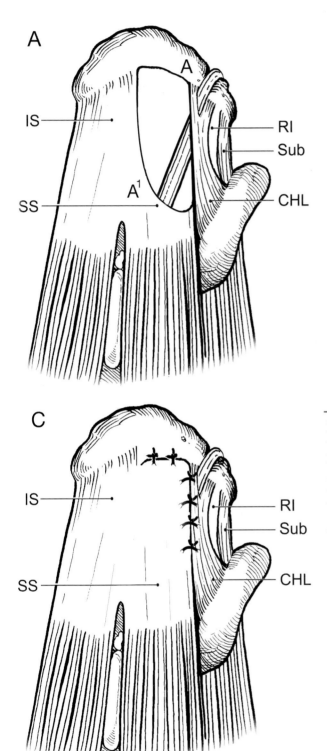

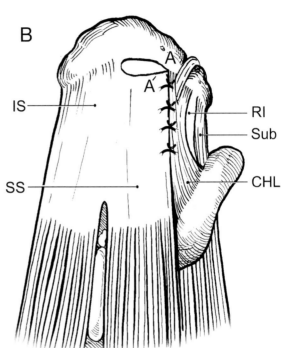

FIGURE 6.70   Schematic of a repair of an L-shaped rotator cuff tear. (**A**) Superior view of a chronic L-shaped rotator cuff tear, which has assumed a U-shaped configuration. (**B**) L-shaped tears demonstrate excellent mobility from an anterior to posterior direction. One of the tear margins (usually the posterior leaf) is more mobile. These tears may be repaired initially by side-to-side sutures using the principle of margin convergence so that the anterolateral corner of the supraspinatus (A) converges to meet its anatomic insertion point (A). (**C**) The converged margin is then repaired to bone in a tension-free manner. Alternatively, the corner of the L may first be repaired with a suture anchor, followed by additional tendon-to-bone repair with suture anchors (if needed), and then side-to-side closure of the remaining defect. L-shaped tears sometimes benefit from a bridging repair with a medial anchor strapping the tendon down by sutures going to a lateral anchor. The key in any type of cuff pattern repair is to respect, preserve, and protect cable function realizing that most double-row repairs will lateralize the cable and overtension the repair. CHL, coracohumeral ligament; IS, infraspinatus tendon; RI, rotator interval; SS, supraspinatus tendon; Sub, subscapularis tendon. (Reprinted from Burkhart S, Lo IK, Brady PC, Denard PJ. *The Cowboy's Companion: A Trail Guide for the Arthroscopic Shoulder Surgeon*. Philadelphia, PA: Lippincott Williams & Wilkins; 2012, with permission.)

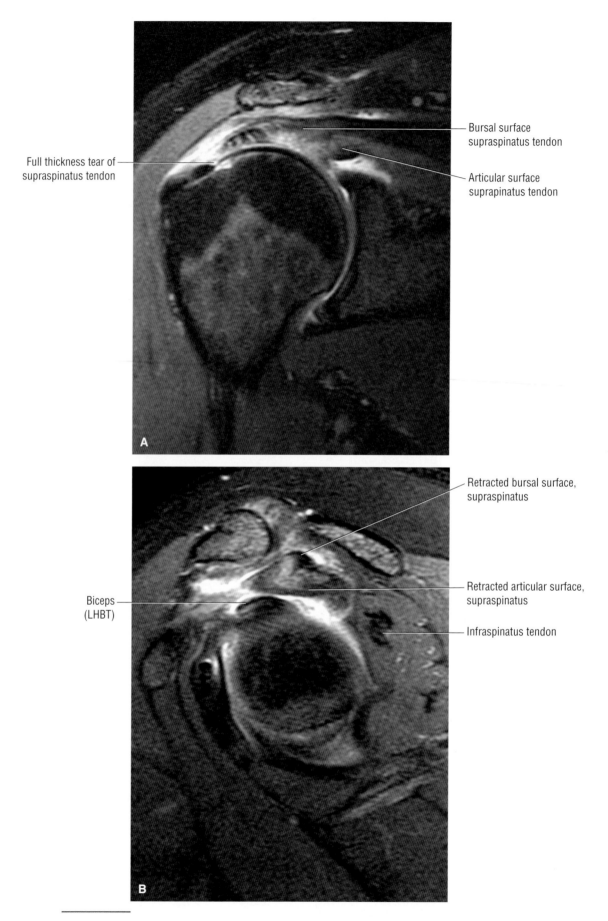

FIGURE 6.71 L-shaped tear with full thickness retraction of the supraspinatus component of the rotator cuff. The infraspinatus contribution is intact, thus contributing to the L morphology. (**A**) FS PD coronal. (**B**) FS PD sagittal.

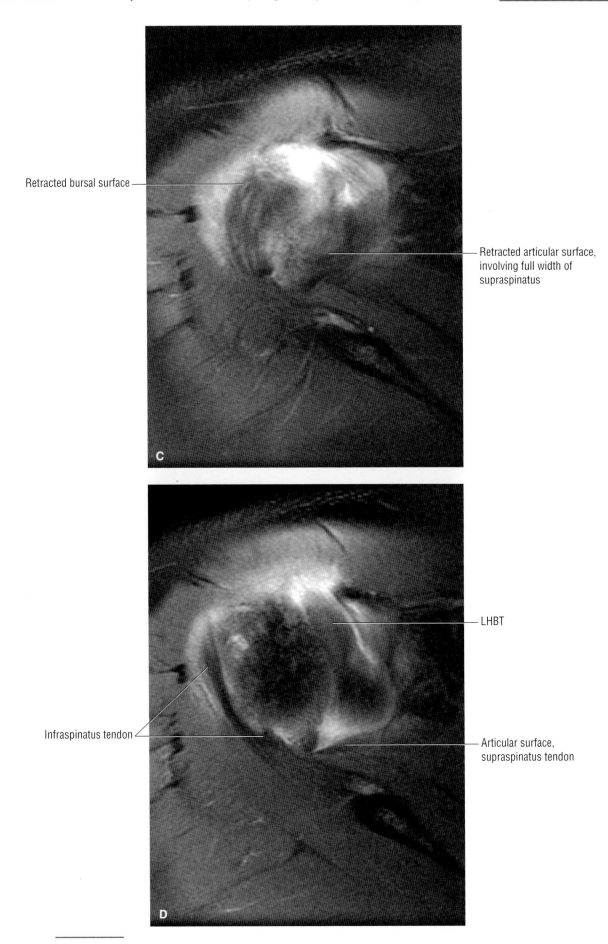

FIGURE 6.71 (*Continued*) (**C,D**) Axial FS PD images. The direct axial images confirm the L-shaped tear pattern with apex anterior (the direction of restoration required in approximating the cuff repair).

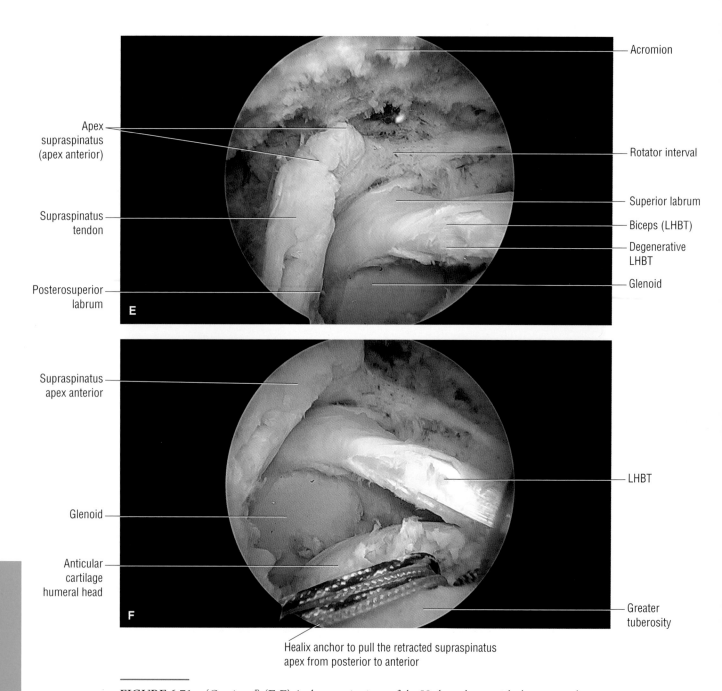

Acromion

Apex
supraspinatus
(apex anterior)

Rotator interval

Superior labrum

Supraspinatus
tendon

Biceps (LHBT)

Degenerative
LHBT

Posterosuperior
labrum

Glenoid

E

Supraspinatus
apex anterior

LHBT

Glenoid

Anticular
cartilage
humeral head

Greater
tuberosity

F

Healix anchor to pull the retracted supraspinatus
apex from posterior to anterior

FIGURE 6.71   (*Continued*) (**E,F**) Arthroscopic views of the U-shaped tear with the retracted apex of the supraspinatus. Posterolateral portal 70-degree scope. Healix knotless anchor uses a dual-thread technology to maximize fixation and pull-out strength. Suture anchors when located in the ideal position are on the edge of the articular cartilage and directed medially under the subchondral bone. Anchors are positioned to slightly angle away from each other (1 to 1.2cm apart and 5mm lateral to the articular cartilage). Sutures are passed 1 to 1.5cm medial to the edge of the cuff with an angle of 25 to 30 degrees between each suture to create a fan-shaped pattern.

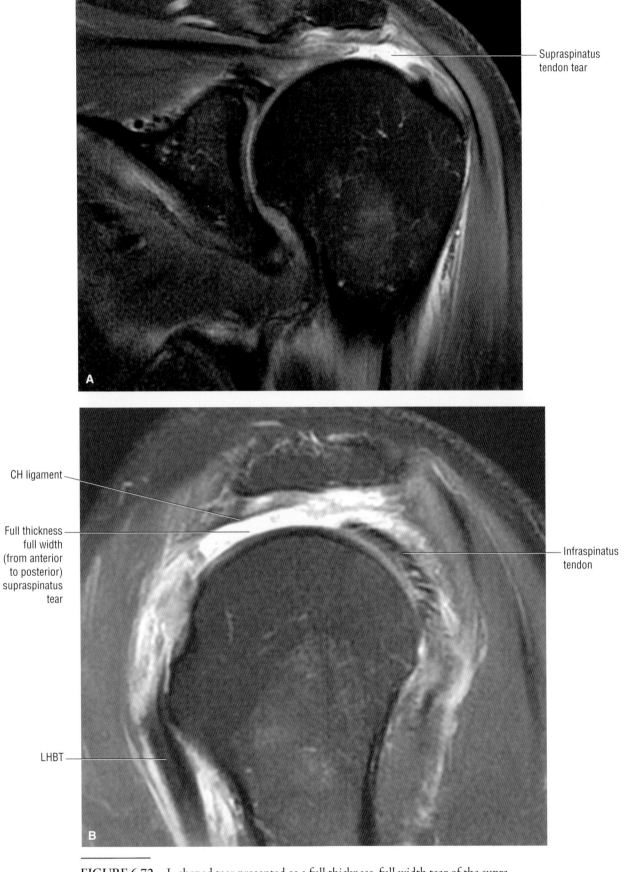

Supraspinatus
tendon tear

CH ligament

Full thickness
full width
(from anterior
to posterior)
supraspinatus
tear

Infraspinatus
tendon

LHBT

FIGURE 6.72   L-shaped tear presented as a full thickness, full width tear of the supraspinatus from anterior to posterior. (**A**) Coronal FS PD. (**B**) Sagittal FS PD.

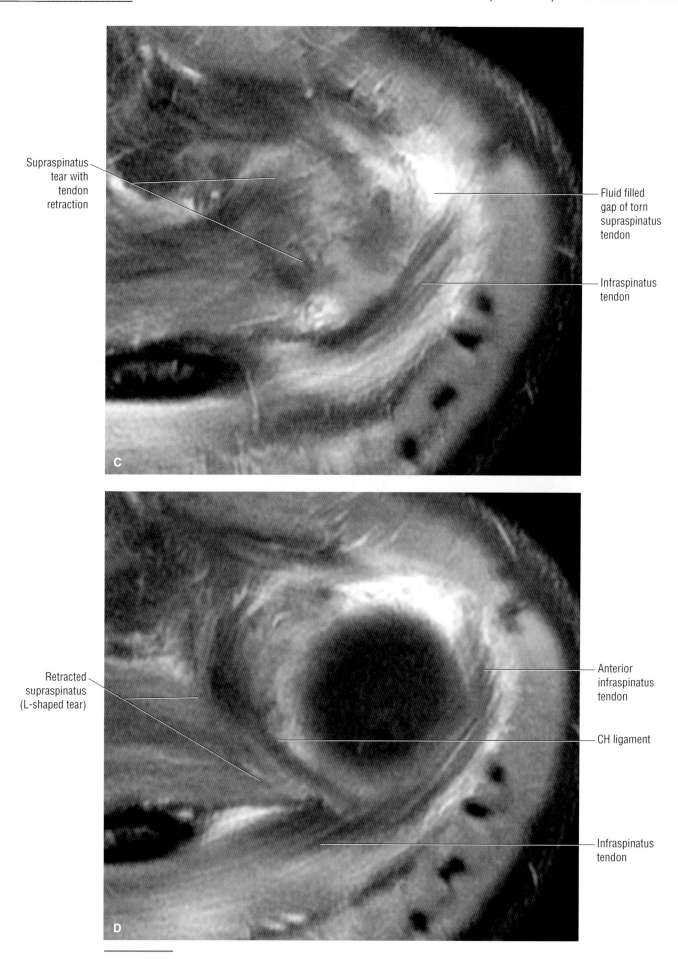

FIGURE 6.72 *(Continued)* (**C,D**) Axial FS PD.

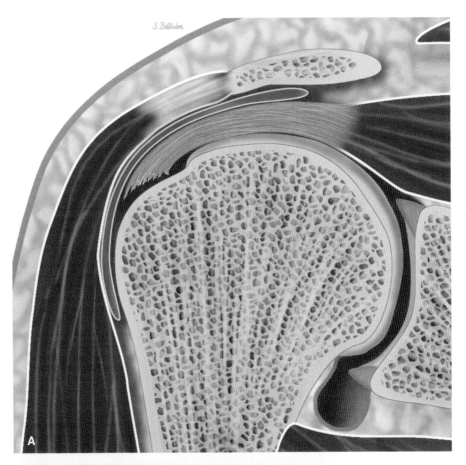

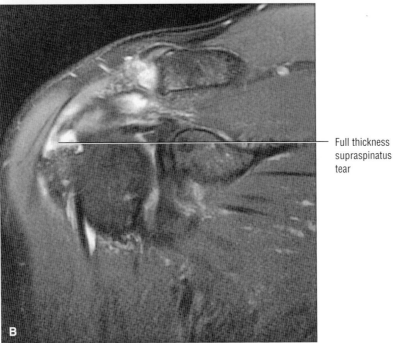

Full thickness
supraspinatus
tear

FIGURE 6.73 (**A**) Coronal section showing a stage 1 full thickness tear with the torn edge adjacent to the greater tuberosity. (**B**) Coronal FS PD FSE image shows a stage 1 full thickness cuff tear with the torn cuff edge adjacent to the greater tuberosity. MR image with fluid-filled gap at the anterior supraspinatus footprint.

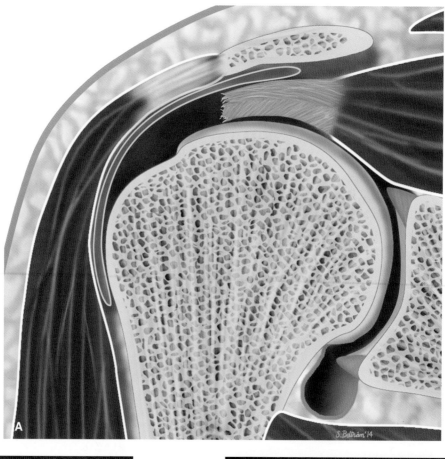

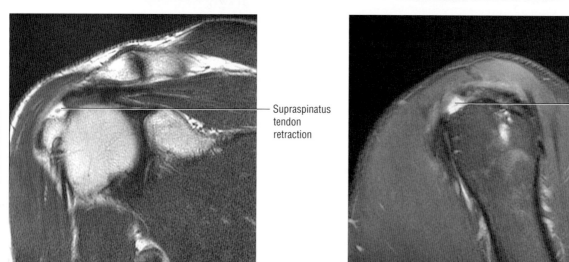

Supraspinatus
tendon
retraction

Supraspinatus
tendon
tear

FIGURE 6.74 **(A)** Coronal color section, **(B)** coronal T2 FSE image, and **(C)** sagittal FS PD FSE image of a stage 2 full thickness rotator cuff tear with supraspinatus tendon retraction superior to the humeral head. The extent of the cuff tear is measured medial to lateral in the coronal plane and anterior to posterior in the sagittal plane.

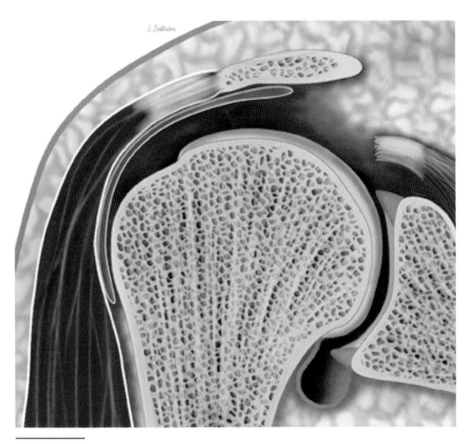

FIGURE 6.75   Stage 3 full thickness rotator cuff tear with tendon retraction to the level of the glenoid.

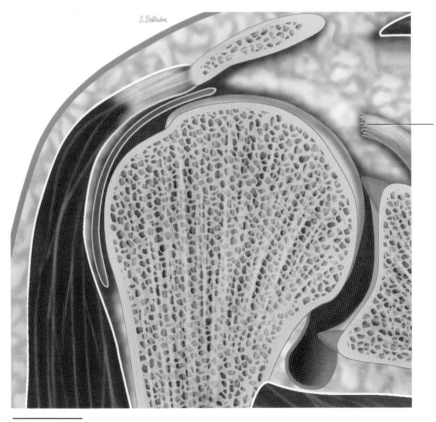

Retracted cuff with atrophy

FIGURE 6.76   Chronic rotator cuff fatty atrophy associated with proximal retraction.

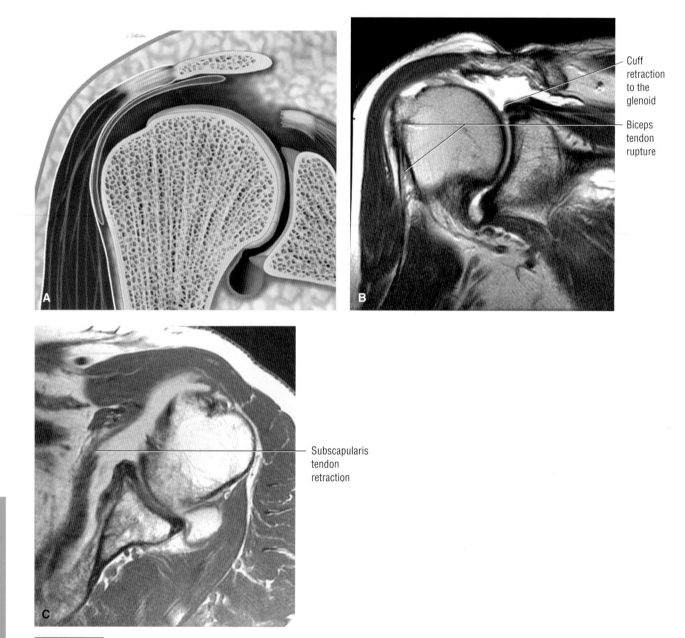

FIGURE 6.77   (**A**) Coronal color section, (**B**) coronal T2 FSE image, and (**C**) axial PD FSE image show a stage 3 full thickness rotator cuff tear with tendon retraction to the level of the glenoid. Medial retraction is shown in the associated subscapularis tendon tear.

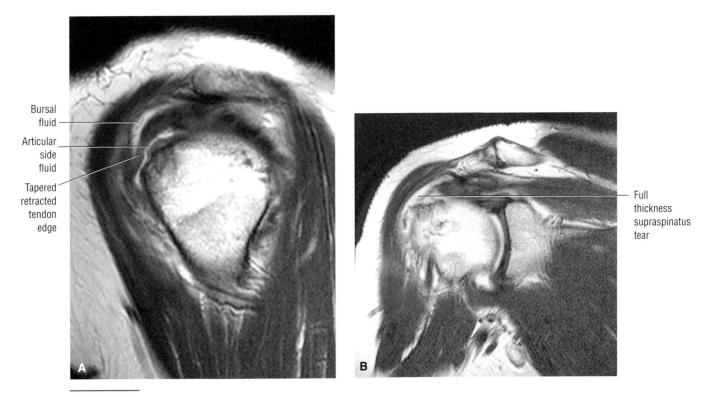

Bursal fluid

Articular side fluid

Tapered retracted tendon edge

Full thickness supraspinatus tear

FIGURE 6.78 (**A**) Sagittal T2 FSE and (**B**) coronal FSE images display hyperintense fluid signal intensity surrounding the anterior, bursal, and articular surfaces of the anterior cuff.

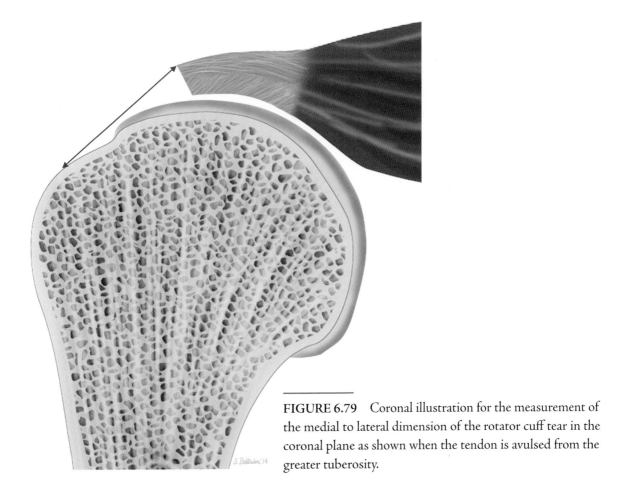

FIGURE 6.79 Coronal illustration for the measurement of the medial to lateral dimension of the rotator cuff tear in the coronal plane as shown when the tendon is avulsed from the greater tuberosity.

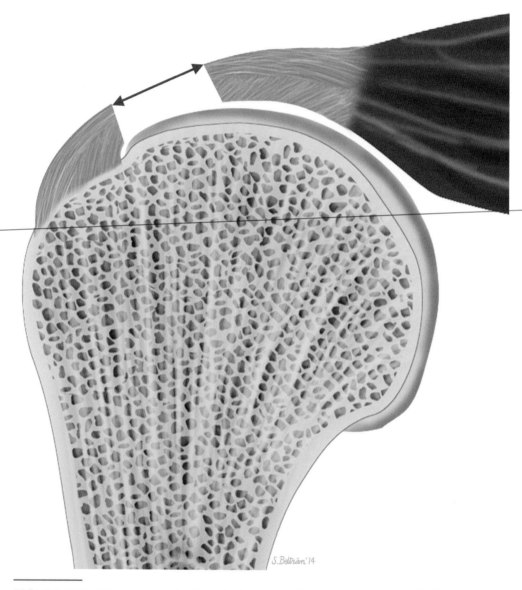

FIGURE 6.80 Measurement of cuff size in the coronal plane when there is a residual stump of tendon attached to the greater tuberosity. Measurement of cuff size can be made from anterior to posterior in a similar fashion in the sagittal plane. The presence of a stump of cuff tendon lateral to a full thickness tear indicates that there exists a more complex tear, with an additional side-to-side component to the defect.

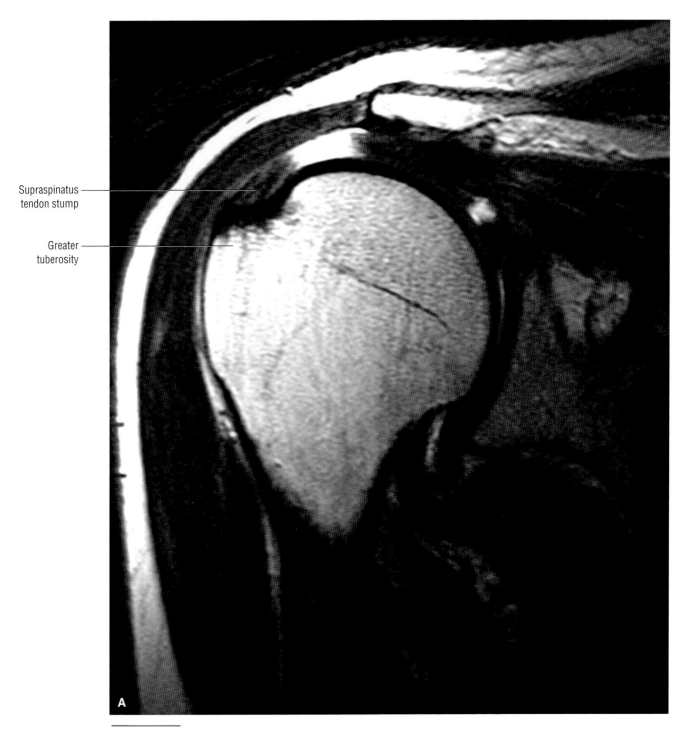

Supraspinatus
tendon stump

Greater
tuberosity

FIGURE 6.81   Full thickness supraspinatus tear adjacent to greater tuberosity tendinous stump. (**A**) Coronal T2. The remaining stump of the supraspinatus tedon will require a side-to-side repair. Cuff tears with a residual stump are more time sensitive and should be evaluated for more urgent repair to ensure complete repair.

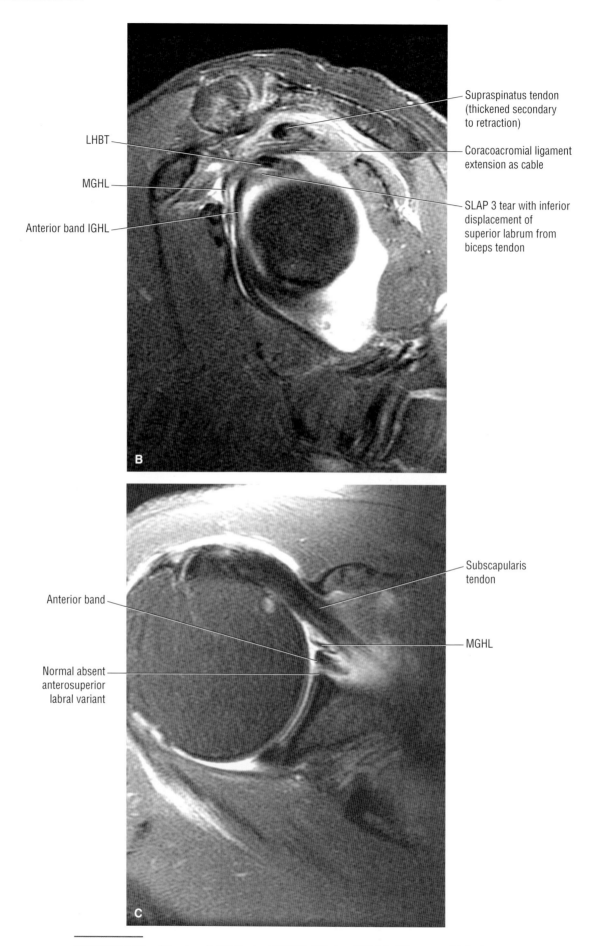

FIGURE 6.81 (*Continued*) (**B**) Sagittal FS PD. (**C**) Axial FS PD. There is mild thickening of the retracted supraspinatus tendon in the sagittal plane.

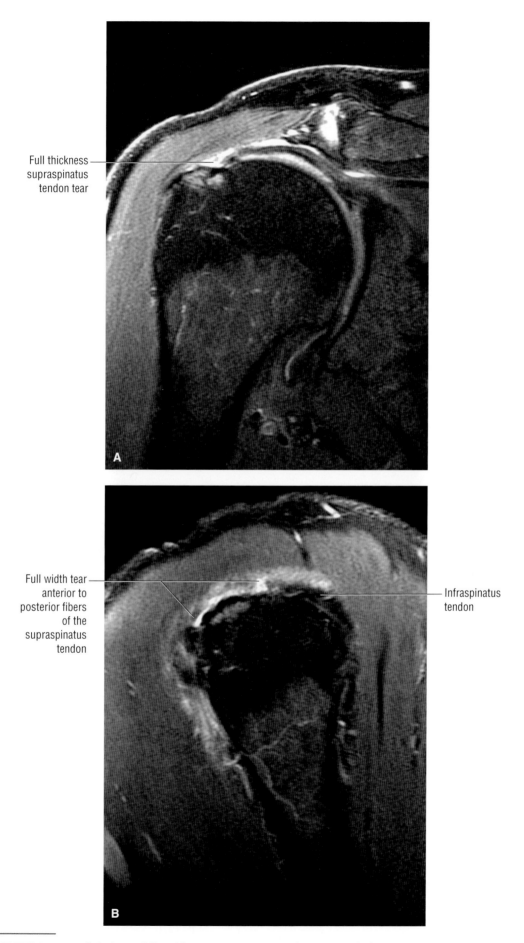

FIGURE 6.82   Full thickness full width tear supraspinatus with retraction. (**A**) Coronal FS PD. (**B**) Sagittal FS PD.

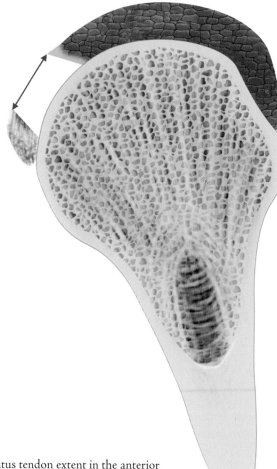

FIGURE 6.83   Measurement of supraspinatus tendon extent in the anterior to posterior direction with residual stump anteriorly at the footprint.

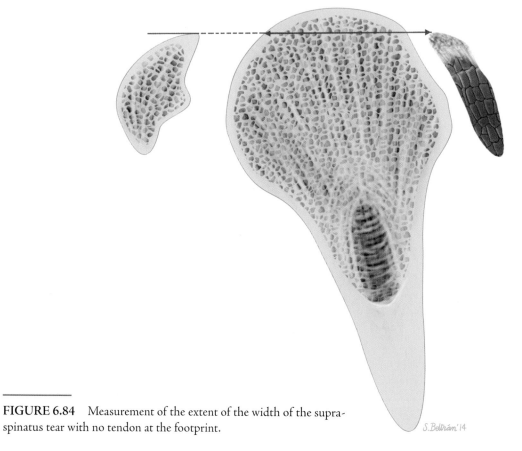

FIGURE 6.84   Measurement of the extent of the width of the supra-spinatus tear with no tendon at the footprint.

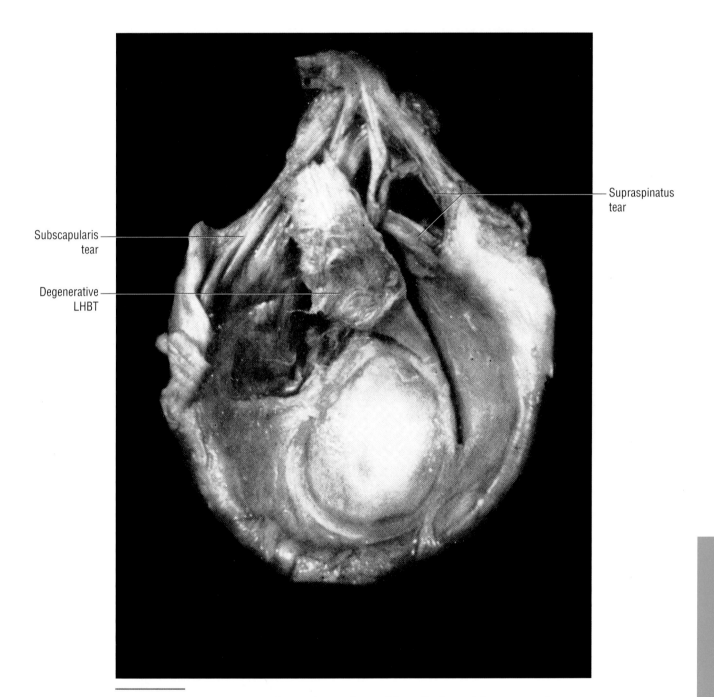

Subscapularis tear

Degenerative LHBT

Supraspinatus tear

FIGURE 6.85   A specimen with complete avulsion of the cuff, advanced degenerative changes, and hypertrophy and fraying of the biceps tendon. (Modified from DePalma AF. *Surgery of the Shoulder*. 3rd ed. Philadelphia, PA: JB Lippincott; 1983.)

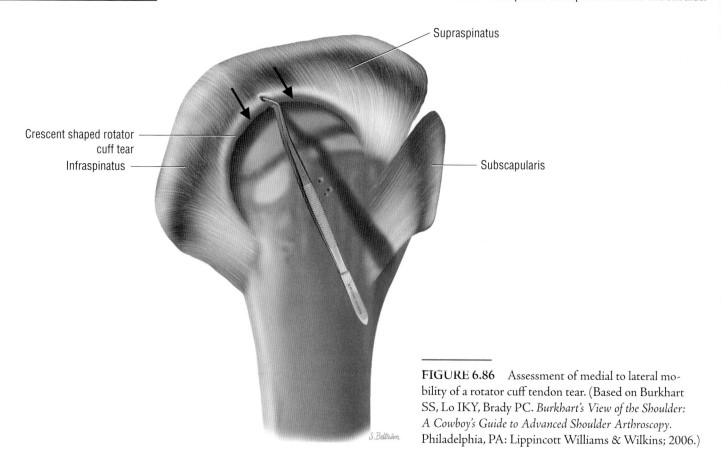

FIGURE 6.86 Assessment of medial to lateral mobility of a rotator cuff tendon tear. (Based on Burkhart SS, Lo IKY, Brady PC. *Burkhart's View of the Shoulder: A Cowboy's Guide to Advanced Shoulder Arthroscopy.* Philadelphia, PA: Lippincott Williams & Wilkins; 2006.)

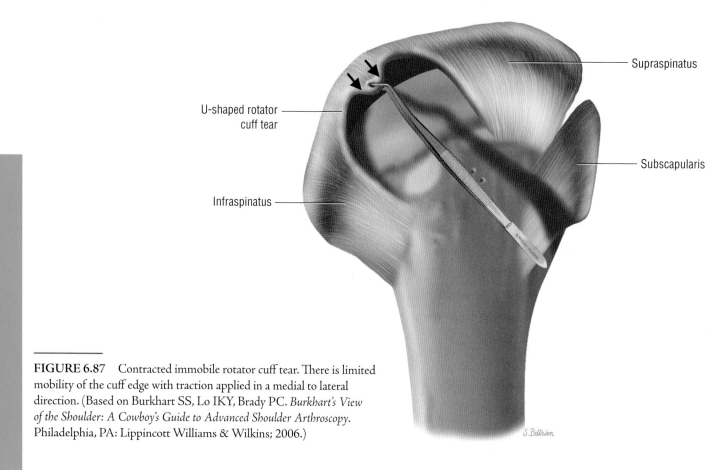

FIGURE 6.87 Contracted immobile rotator cuff tear. There is limited mobility of the cuff edge with traction applied in a medial to lateral direction. (Based on Burkhart SS, Lo IKY, Brady PC. *Burkhart's View of the Shoulder: A Cowboy's Guide to Advanced Shoulder Arthroscopy.* Philadelphia, PA: Lippincott Williams & Wilkins; 2006.)

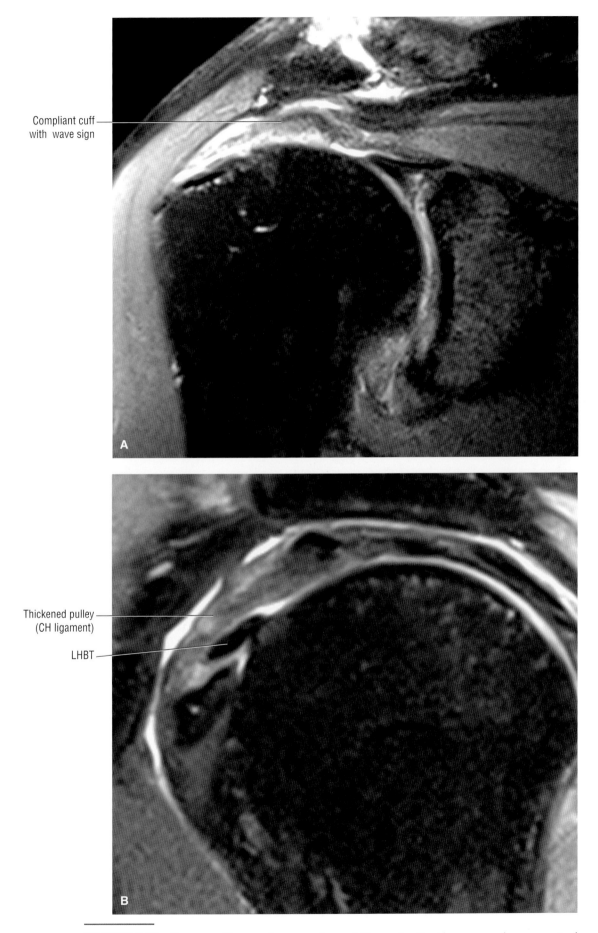

Compliant cuff with wave sign

Thickened pulley (CH ligament)

LHBT

FIGURE 6.88   Rotator cuff supraspinatus tendon mobility as visualized by a wave or lax contour in the coronal plane. Associated thickening of the biceps pulley is present. (**A**) Coronal FS PD. (**B**) Sagittal FS PD.

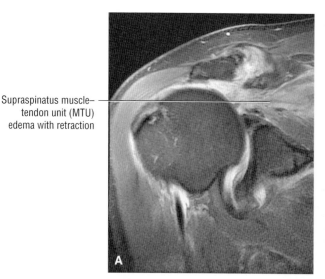

Supraspinatus muscle–
tendon unit (MTU)
edema with retraction

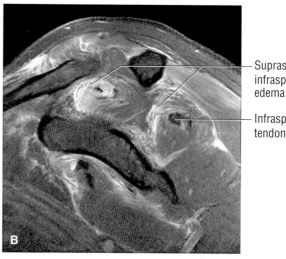

Supraspinatus and
infraspinatus MTU
edema

Infraspinatus
tendon retraction

FIGURE 6.89   (**A**) Coronal FS PD FSE and (**B**) sagittal FS PD FSE images of hyperintense muscle–tendon signal intensity associated with a large full thickness acute rotator cuff tear. There is secondary superior ascent of the humeral head.

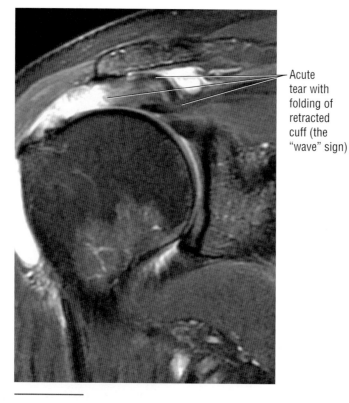

Acute
tear with
folding of
retracted
cuff (the
"wave" sign)

FIGURE 6.90   Coronal FS PD FSE image showing the wave sign of a retracted supraspinatus tendon as a sign of a reparable acute cuff tear without associated scarring.

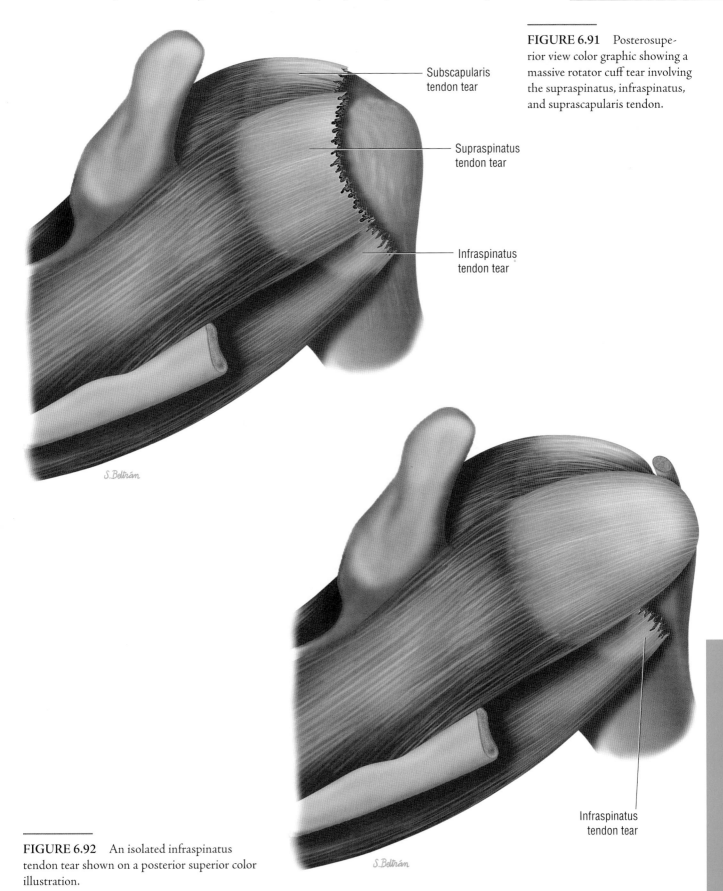

FIGURE 6.91 Posterosuperior view color graphic showing a massive rotator cuff tear involving the supraspinatus, infraspinatus, and suprascapularis tendon.

Subscapularis tendon tear

Supraspinatus tendon tear

Infraspinatus tendon tear

Infraspinatus tendon tear

FIGURE 6.92 An isolated infraspinatus tendon tear shown on a posterior superior color illustration.

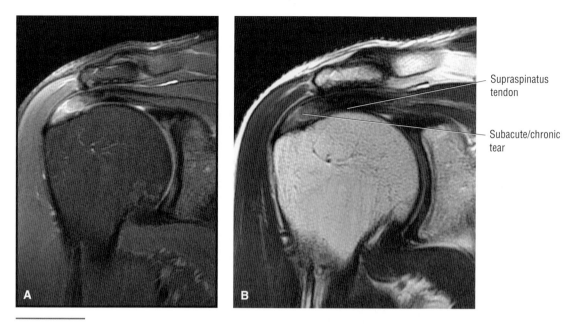

Supraspinatus
tendon

Subacute/chronic
tear

FIGURE 6.93   Coronal images depicting a nonacute supraspinatus tendon tear. The supraspinatus tendon shows residual hyperintensity at the tear site on FS PD FSE images (**A**) and intermediate signal intensity on T2 FSE images (**B**).

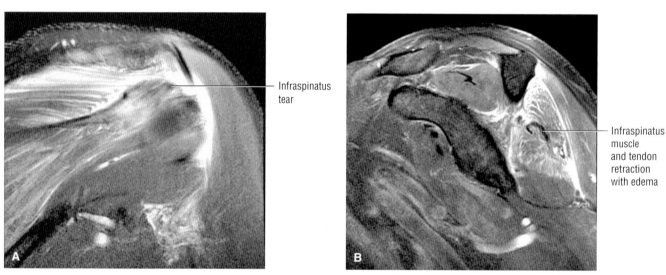

Infraspinatus
tear

Infraspinatus
muscle
and tendon
retraction
with edema

FIGURE 6.94   An isolated infraspinatus tendon tear shown on (**A**) a posterior coronal FS PD FSE image and (**B**) a sagittal FS PD FSE image. The normal infraspinatus usually has three pennate origins. The fibers converge into a tendon which passes posterior to the capsule of the shoulder joint to attach to the middle facet of the greater tuberosity.

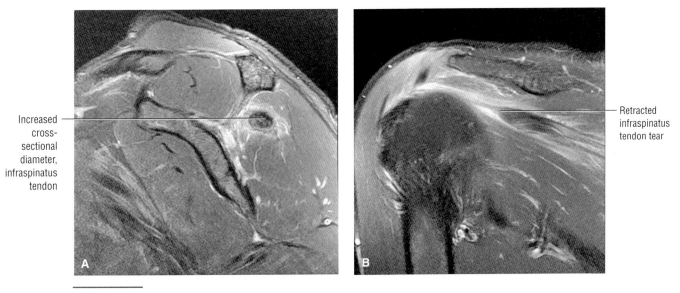

FIGURE 6.95   Increased cross-sectional diameter "sign" of a retracted infraspinatus tendon in an isolated tendon tear of the rotator cuff is seen on (**A**) sagittal FS PD FSE and (**B**) coronal FS PD FSE images. Increased tendon diameter is useful as a secondary sign of supraspinatus or infraspinatus tendon retraction. External rotation of the shoulder can also result in an increase cross-sectional diameter of the tendon.

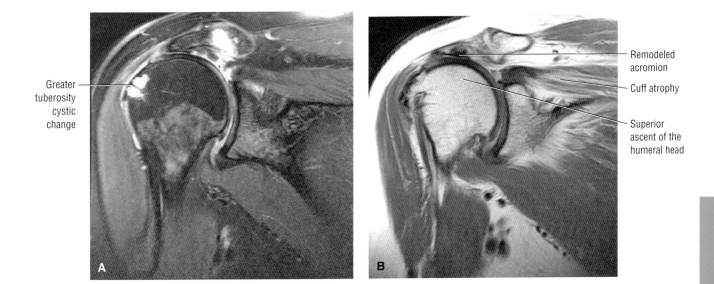

FIGURE 6.96   Coronal FS PD FSE (**A**) and T2 FSE (**B**) images showing chronic cuff arthropathy with superior ascent of the humeral head, contact and remodeling of the undersurface of the acromion, greater tuberosity cystic change, and fatty atrophy of the supraspinatus. The atrophic cuff is associated with a decrease cross-sectional diameter and internal fatty change of the muscle.

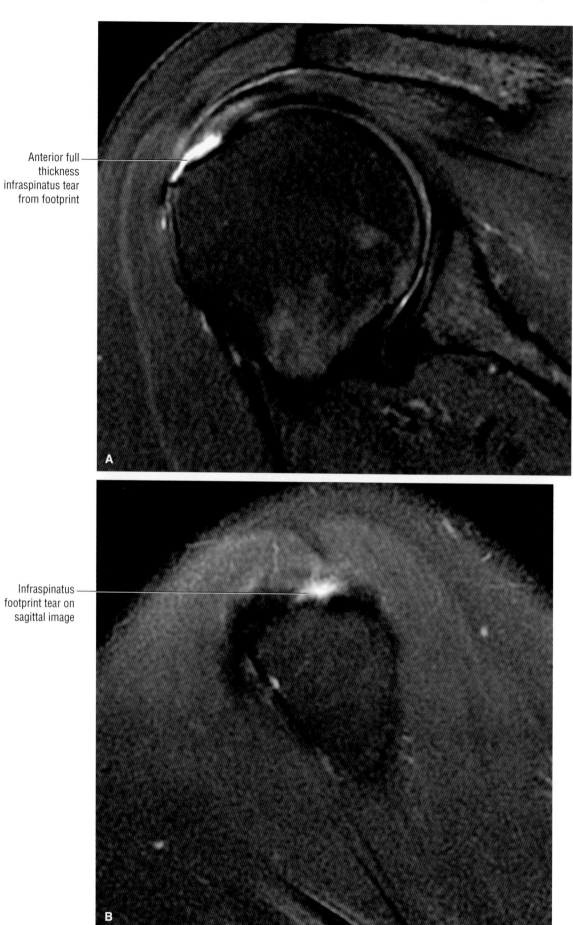

Anterior full thickness infraspinatus tear from footprint

Infraspinatus footprint tear on sagittal image

FIGURE 6.97 Anterior infraspinatus full thickness tendon tear. (**A**) FS PD coronal. (**B**) FS PD sagittal.

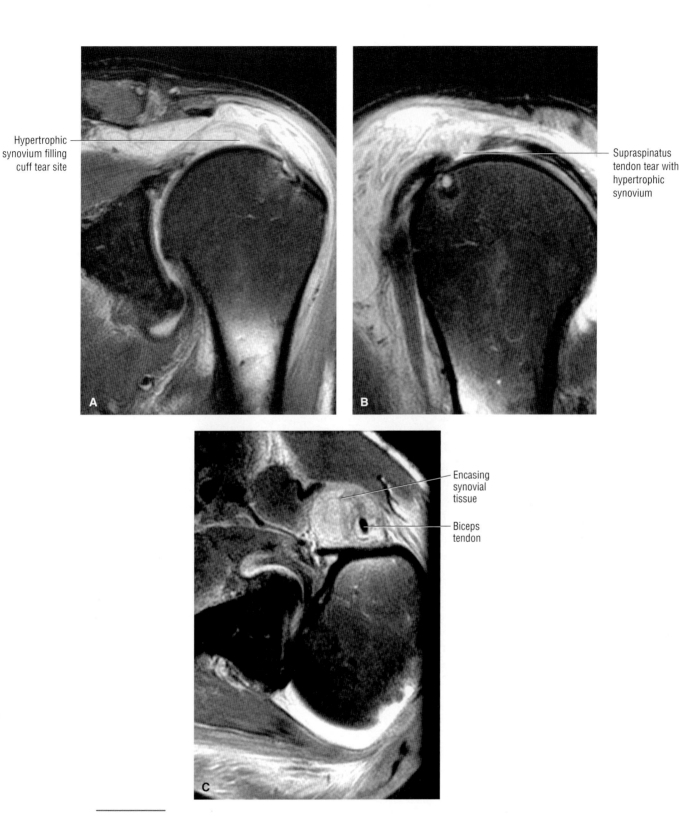

Hypertrophic synovium filling cuff tear site

Supraspinatus tendon tear with hypertrophic synovium

Encasing synovial tissue

Biceps tendon

FIGURE 6.98 Hyperintense hypertrophic synovium occupying the tendinous gap of a full thickness rotator cuff tear on a coronal FS PD FSE image (**A**) and sagittal FS PD FSE image (**B**). (**C**) The biceps tendon is encased in a massive thickened synovial envelope on this axial FS PD FSE image. This degree of synovial reaction may be mistakened for severe cuff tendinosis instead of space occuring synovial hypertrophy.

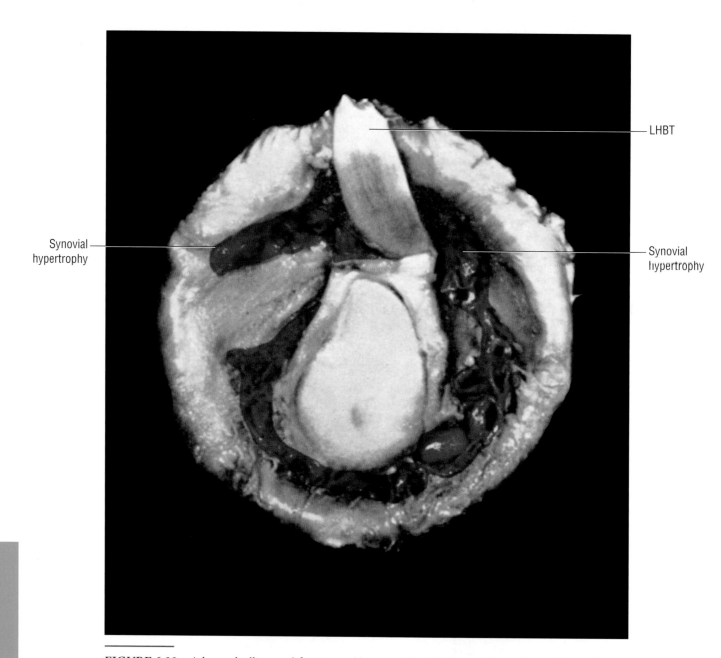

Synovial hypertrophy

LHBT

Synovial hypertrophy

FIGURE 6.99   Advanced villous proliferation and hypertrophy of the synovial membrane. Synovial proliferation (as seen in adhesive capsulitis) usually involves the axillary pouch on coronal images and subscapularis recess and rotator interval on sagital images. (Modified from DePalma AF. *Surgery of the Shoulder*. 3rd ed. Philadelphia, PA: JB Lippincott; 1983.)

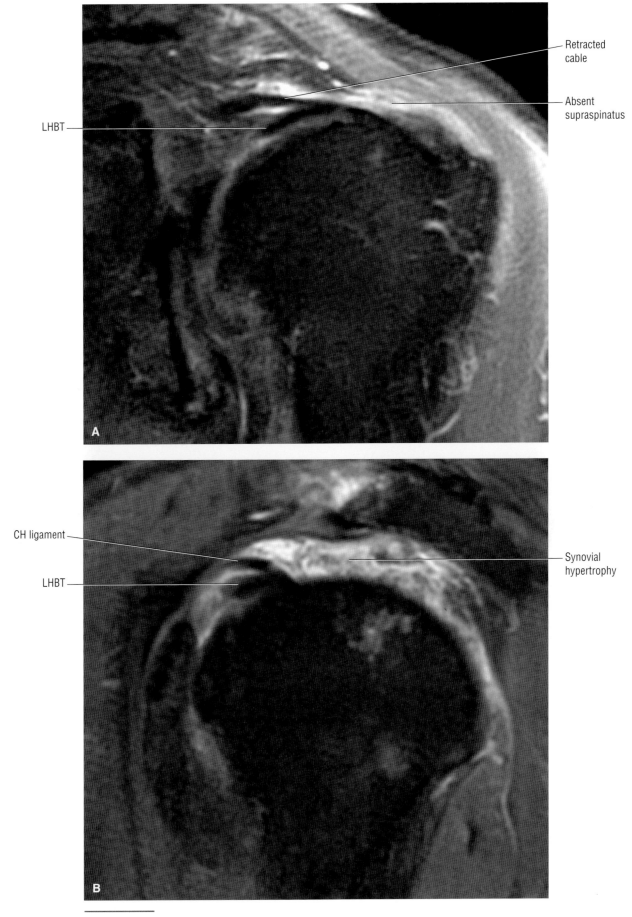

FIGURE 6.100 Rotator cuff full thickness tear associated with synovial hypertrophic reaction. (**A**) Coronal FS PD. (**B**) Sagittal FS PD.

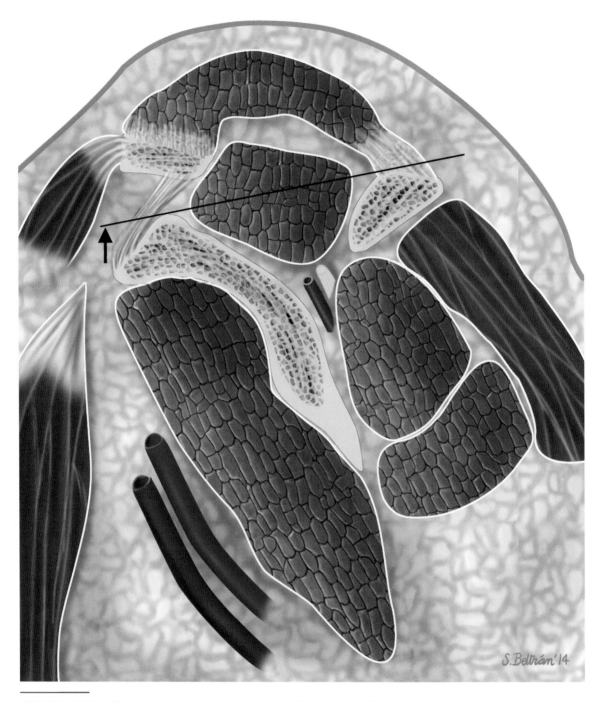

FIGURE 6.101　Tangent sign as viewed in the sagittal plane from a reference line between the cora-coid and scapular spine to assess supraspinatus muscle bulk. The supraspinatus muscle is above the tangent line indicating normal muscle bulk. In the Goutallier atrophy classification, the supraspinatus is classified from stage 0 (normal) to stage 4 (more fat than muscle). The classification is used to as-sess the reparability of large rotator cuff tears. Stage 0—normal muscle; stage 1—some fatty streaks; stage 2—less than 50% fatty muscle athropy; stage 3—fat is equal to muscle; and stage 4—greater than 50% fatty muscle atrophy. In this illustration, the supraspinatus projects above the line between the coracoid and scapular spine.

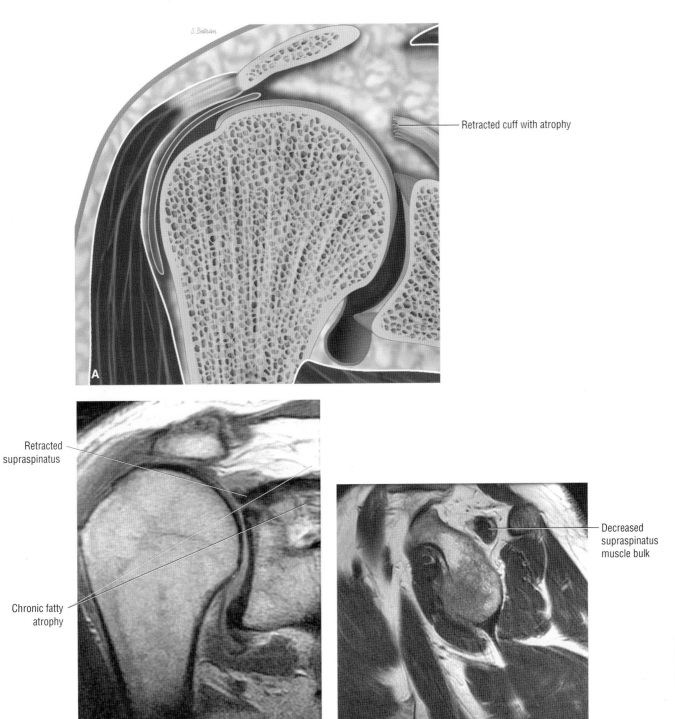

FIGURE 6.102   (A) Chronic rotator cuff fatty atrophy associated with proximal retraction. (B) Coronal PD FSE image showing supraspinatus atrophy with increased fat signal intensity superior to the retracted rotator cuff tendon. (C) Sagittal PD FSE image showing decreased supraspinatus muscle bulk with circumferential fat signal intensity extending from the supraspinatus fossa to the supraspinatus outlet. (Goutallier stage 4).

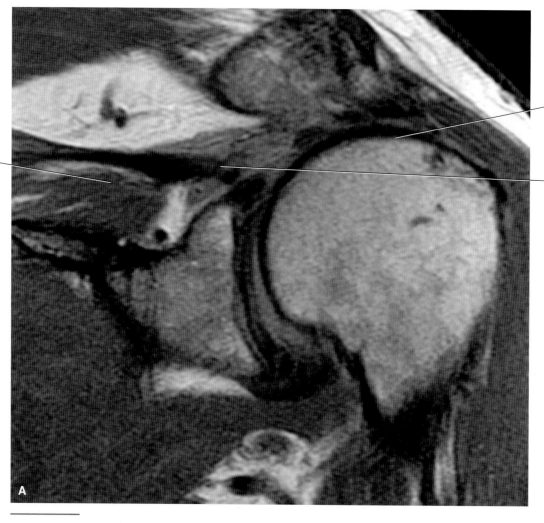

FIGURE 6.103   Severe cuff atrophy with muscle–tendon retraction of the supraspinatus and infraspinatus (**A**) Coronal PD. Muscle atrophy is associated with full thickness, full-width tears. Rotator cuff muscles with fatty atrophy (supraspinatus and infraspinatus) do less well subsequent to rotator cuff repair. Quantitative grading of supraspinatus atrophy and fatty replacement can be evaluated by the occupation ratio (measure of muscle atrophy) or the Goutallier system using a ratio of muscle to fat.

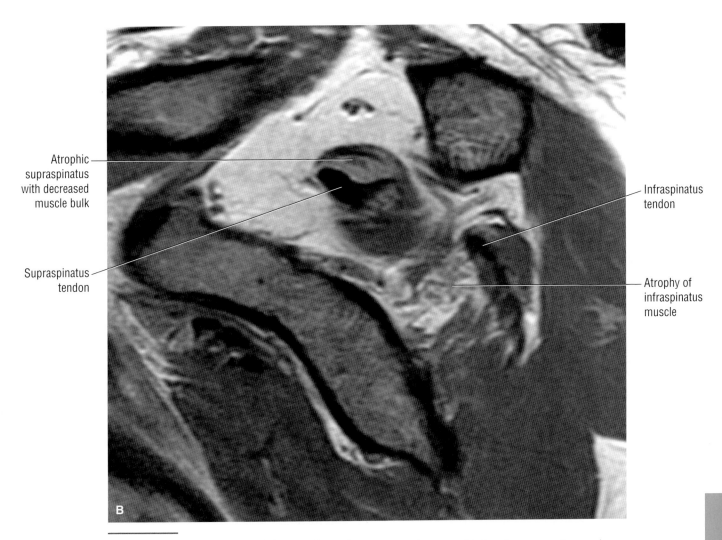

Atrophic suprapinatus with decreased muscle bulk

Suprapinatus tendon

Infraspinatus tendon

Atrophy of infraspinatus muscle

B

FIGURE 6.103 (*Continued*) (**B**) Sagittal PD. Severe supraspinatus and infraspinatus muscle atrophy with decrease muscle bulk leaving the hypointense tendon to occupy a greater percentage of the tendon muscle unit. The sagittal image shown would be the equivalent of the scapular "Y" view.

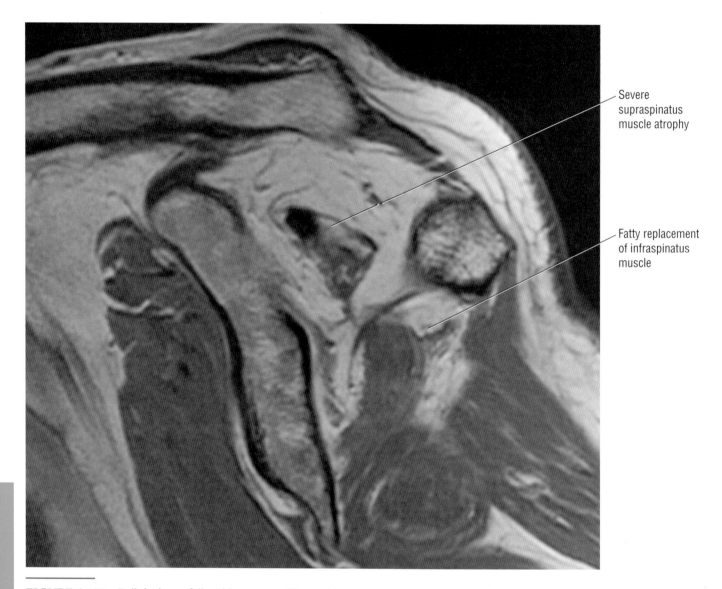

Severe
supraspinatus
muscle atrophy

Fatty replacement
of infraspinatus
muscle

FIGURE 6.104 Full thickness full width rotator cuff tear with tendon retraction to the glenoid
and severe atrophy of the supraspinatus. The occupation ratio is less than 0.4 for the supraspinatus.
There is additional atrophy of the infraspinatus muscle. There is a decreased cross-sectional area of
the supraspinatus muscle relative to the supraspinatus fossa. Sagittal PD FSE.

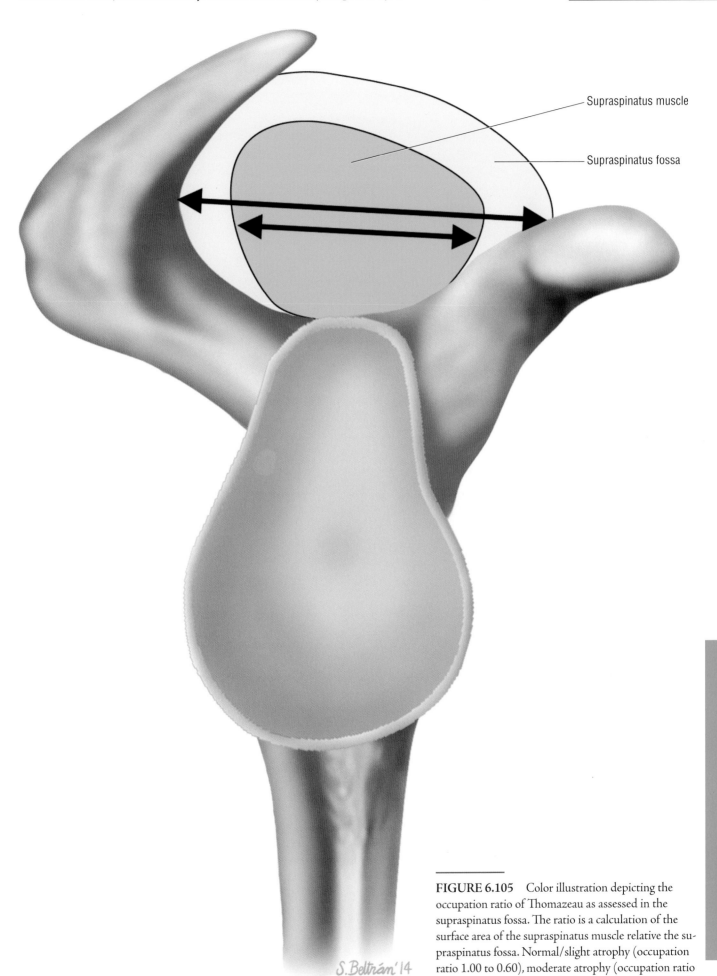

Supraspinatus muscle

Supraspinatus fossa

FIGURE 6.105 Color illustration depicting the occupation ratio of Thomazeau as assessed in the supraspinatus fossa. The ratio is a calculation of the surface area of the supraspinatus muscle relative the supraspinatus fossa. Normal/slight atrophy (occupation ratio 1.00 to 0.60), moderate atrophy (occupation ratio 0.60 to 0.40), severe atrophy (occupation ratio <0.40).

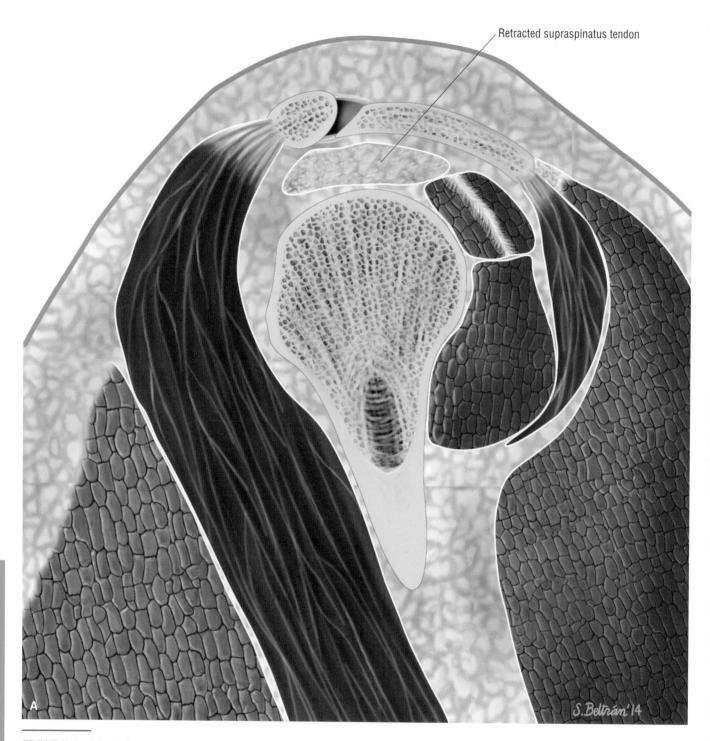

Retracted supraspinatus tendon

FIGURE 6.106   False assessment of rotator cuff atrophy as a result of medial tendon retraction. The coronal image correctly shows relative preservation of muscle bulk medial to the sagittal plane used to evaluate atrophy. A more medial sagittal image proximal to the retracted muscle–tendon junction would give a more accurate assessment of the degree of supraspinatus muscle atrophy. (**A**) Sagittal illustration.

FIGURE 6.106   *(Continued)*
(**B**) Coronal illustration showing that a sagittal assessment lateral to the retracted supraspinatus muscle may overestimate fatty atrophy.

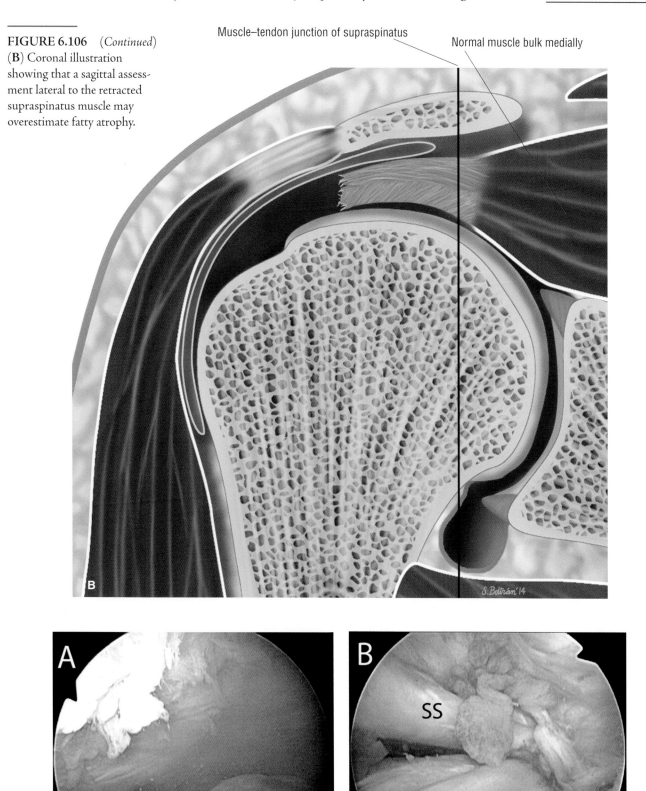

Muscle–tendon junction of supraspinatus

Normal muscle bulk medially

FIGURE 6.107   Right shoulder, posterior viewing portal demonstrating a massive rotator cuff tear.
(**A**) The greater tuberosity footprint is bare. (**B**) There is retraction of the rotator cuff medial to the glenoid. Arthroscopic example of significant medial cuff retraction. G, glenoid; H, humerus; SS, supraspinatus tendon. (Reprinted from Burkhart S, Lo IK, Brady PC, Denard PJ. *The Cowboy's Companion: A Trail Guide for the Arthroscopic Shoulder Surgeon.* Philadelphia, PA: Lippincott Williams & Wilkins; 2012, with permission.)

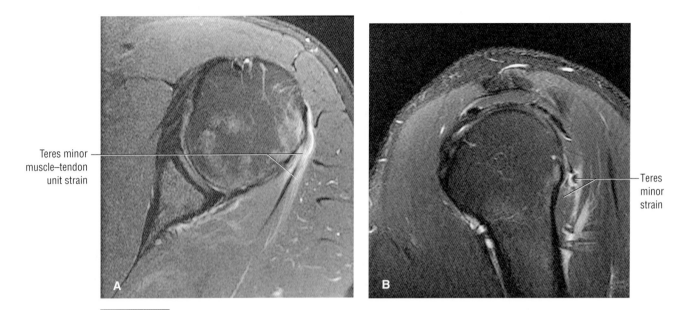

Teres minor
muscle–tendon
unit strain

Teres
minor
strain

FIGURE 6.108   Isolated teres minor muscle–tendon unit overload/strain on (**A**) axial and (**B**) sagittal FS PD FSE images.

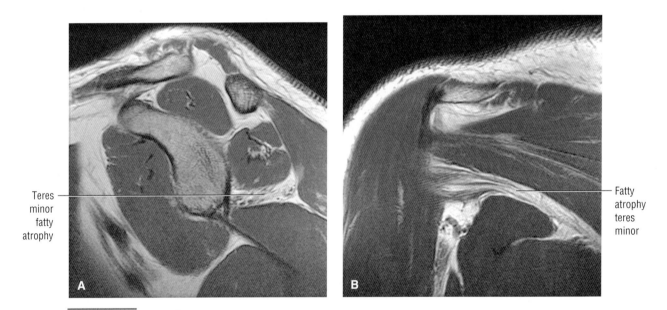

Teres
minor
fatty
atrophy

Fatty
atrophy
teres
minor

FIGURE 6.109   Isolated fatty atrophy of the teres minor muscle in quadrilateral space syndrome on (**A**) sagittal and (**B**) coronal PD FSE images. Quadrilateral space syndrome may actually be an unusual cause of isolated teres minor atrophy. Humeral decentering relative to the teres minor nerve branch, in close proximity to the joint capsule may represent a stronger association.

Subscapularis

Subscapularis-Biceps-Subcoracoid Space

- Normally, there is a 2- to 3-mm bare strip devoid of articular cartilage located medial to the subscapularis footprint.

- The intact subscapularis tendon does not have any linear longitudinal splits.

- The tip of the coracoid is identified anterior to the upper border of the subscapularis.

- The "rolling wave" is an indentation of the subscapularis/rotator interval junction seen with internal and external rotation of the humerus.
    - The indentation is a result of the coracoid tip.

Subscapularis Tendon Tears

- The subscapularis muscle forms the anterior cuff.

- The inferior third of the subscapularis insertion of the humerus is primarily muscular with minimal intervening tendinous tissue.[362]

- The subscapularis is multipennate and is dually innervated by the upper and lower subscapular nerves.

- The axillary neurovascular bundle, including the axillary nerve, is located in proximity to the anterior inferior surface of the muscle as it passes around the inferior border of the subscapularis to enter the quadrilateral space.
    - The axillary nerve is at risk in operative repair of subscapularis tendon avulsions if the retracted tendon and localized hemorrhage obscure the course of the nerve.
    - The axillary nerve may be incarcerated in scar tissue with the subscapularis tendon stump.

- Isolated avulsion of the subscapularis is associated with severe external rotation or hyperextension of the shoulder.[316]
    - Repair of isolated subscapularis tears is often performed with tenodesis or tenotomy of the biceps tendon to improve shoulder function.[151]

- Anterior dislocation of the shoulder may be associated with subscapularis avulsion in patients over 30 years of age.
    - Anterior shoulder pain and pain with forward flexion and external rotation may accompany weakness.

- Anterior instability may also coexist with subscapularis rupture.

- Increased passive external rotation of the affected shoulder and a positive lift-off test are observed on physical examination.

Arthroscopic Assessment of the Subscapularis Tendon

- Viewing with a 70° arthroscope gives a more complete view of the inferior footprint of the subscapularis.[75,124,141,182,234,559]

- The medial sling (pulley) is composed of a deep layer made up of the medial head of the coracohumeral ligament and a thin superficial layer composed of the superior glenohumeral ligament.

- The insertional footprint of the medial sling is at the superior aspect of the lesser tuberosity adjacent to the footprint of the superolateral subscapularis on the lesser tuberosity.

- In the location where the superior subscapularis tears from the lesser tuberosity, the adjacent medial sling also tears and disrupts the biceps pulley.

- The torn medial sling (or biceps pulley) forms a comma-shaped arc of tissue at arthroscopy referred to as the comma sign at the superolateral corner of the subscapularis tendon.

- At arthroscopy, even the retracted subscapularis tendon is associated with the comma sign at the lateral border of the subscapularis.

- Nonretracted subscapularis tears may be associated with full thickness or partial thickness articular surface tendon (PASTA) lesions.

- A biceps tenodesis is usually performed in cases of subscapularis repair since tears of the upper subscapularis tendon are associated with a tear of the medial sling of the biceps and thus biceps instability.

- The bicipital groove marks the lateral border of the lesser tuberosity and the normal lateral insertion of the subscapularis tendon.

- Fatty infiltration of the subscapularis muscle does not prevent improvement postsurgical repair.
  - This unique property of the subscapularis is related to its function as an anterior restraint whether the muscle is functional or not.

- Thus, the subscapularis tendon should be repaired regardless of chronicity or the degree of fatty degeneration.

- The normal subscapularis footprint is associated with a medial border of a 2- to 3-mm strip of bare bone or bone strip. (Insertion is 2 to 3mm lateral to the articular margin).

- A PASTA lesion of the subscapularis tendon involves tendon disruption from the lesser tuberosity lateral to the strip of bare bone.

  - A subscapularis PASTA lesion may be associated with partial avulsion of the medial sling or biceps pulley.

- Full thickness tears of the subscapularis are associated with a disruption of the medial sling.

  - This rupture of the biceps pulley results in an unstable biceps tendon.

- The biceps is addressed by tenotomy or tenodesis.

- The arthroscopic comma sign is used to identify the superolateral subscapularis.

- Occult tears of the subscapularis:

  - There are two occult tear patterns that require careful inspection by the 70° arthroscope for proper visualization:
    - Distal bursal surface tear
    - Variant of a short PASTA lesion at the upper subscapularis tendon combined with an intact biceps pulley (medial sling)

  - Most articular-sided or deep margin partial articular-sided tears of the subscapularis are associated with medial sling disruptions.[75,124,141,182,234,559]

MR Appearance of Subscapularis Tendon Tears

- Most subscapularis tendon tears occur in association with tears of the supraspinatus and infraspinatus tendons.

  - However, injury to the subscapularis may occur as an isolated partial tear independent of any other cuff pathology.[451]

- Subscapularis tendon injuries range from small corner tears at the superior edge, adjacent to the bone tendon junction, to chronic massive retracted tears with fatty atrophy of the muscle.

  - Partial tears may be associated with thickening of the subscapularis tendon in conjunction with regions of fiber discontinuity.

- Increased signal intensity on fluid sensitive images can be observed on coronal oblique and sagittal oblique images through the subscapularis; however, it is the axial plane that is most important and specific for the evaluation of subscapularis tendon tears.

- A partial tear of the attachment of the subscapularis to the lesser tuberosity is associated with a deficiency in the superior aspect of the tendon insertion onto the lesser tuberosity just inferior to the coracoid process.

- Complete detachment from the lesser tuberosity is associated with fluid signal intensity extending anterior to the retracted tendon.

- Avulsion fractures of the lesser tuberosity are uncommon and usually occur in younger patients.[515]

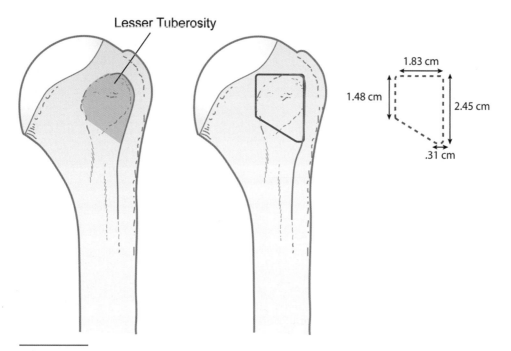

FIGURE 6.110   Schematic of the normal subscapularis tendon footprint. Since the average subscapularis footprint is approximately 2.5cm from top to bottom, two to three anchors are needed to repair a completely retracted subscapularis tendon tear. Note that the footprint is wider proximally than distally, indicating a relatively more important force-generating function for the upper subscapularis than for the lower. The subscapularis functions as an internal rotator and anterior stabilizer of the glenohumeral joint. The subscapularis in conjunction with the infraspinatus and teres minor keeps the humeral head centered on the glenoid fossa. (From Burkhart S, Lo IK, Brady PC, Denard PJ. *The Cowboy's Companion. A Trail Guide for the Arthroscopic Shoulder Surgeon.* Philadelphia, PA: Lippincott Williams & Wilkins; 2012.)

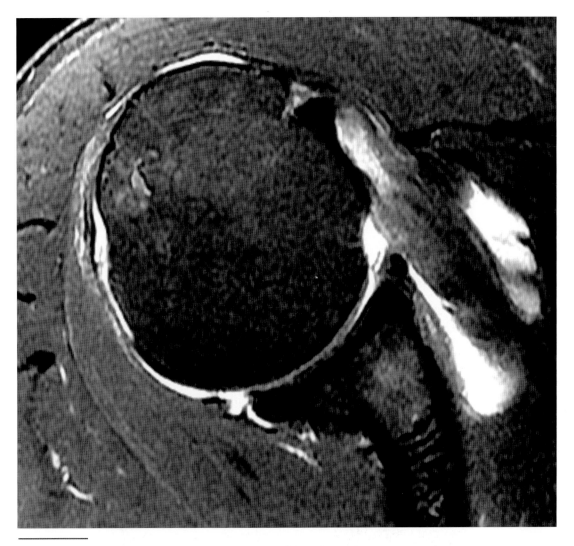

FIGURE 6.111   Partial longitudinal tear footprint of the subscapularis. FSPD axial image.

- Associated biceps tendon abnormalities, including medial dislocation

- A full thickness tear of the subscapularis tendon may be retracted, with the torn anterior capsule proximal to the lesser tuberosity to the level of the anterior glenoid rim.[557]

- The location of the biceps relative to the intertubercular groove, the status of the remaining rotator cuff tendons, and the finding of degenerative joint changes are assessed prior to surgery.

- Partial tears may show fraying at the attachment site of the tendon to the lesser tuberosity.

- Splitting along the superior rolled border of the tendon edge is also seen with partial tears.

- Interstitial tears may extend along a segment of the distal subscapularis.

■ FUSSI (Fraying of the Upper border of the Subscapularis tendon often associated with Subacromial Impingement) lesion of the subscapularis tendon

- ■ Represents subscapularis tendon degeneration and intrasubstance longitudinal splits of tendon fibers

- ■ Identify localized or focal nodular enlargement on sagittal or axial images

- ■ Occurs on the upper border of the subscapularis tendon medial to the edge of the glenoid

- ■ Spares the lateral subscapularis tendon and its attachment to the lesser tuberosity

- ■ A focal nodule (the Conrad lesion) if present may contain a hidden longitudinal split and granulation tissue (and tendon synovitis).

- ■ Concurrent subacromial impingement (cuff and CA ligament fraying)[559]

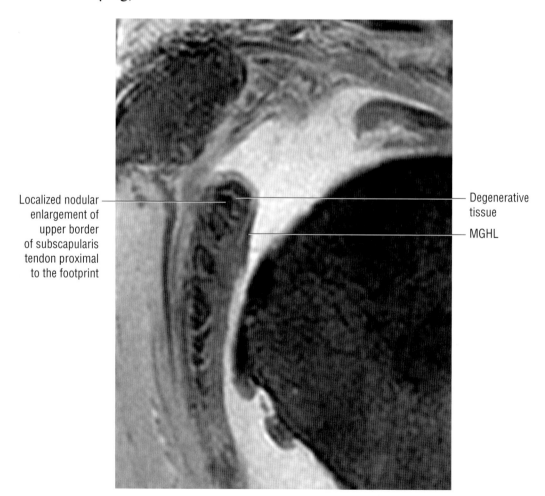

Localized nodular enlargement of upper border of subscapularis tendon proximal to the footprint

Degenerative tissue

MGHL

FIGURE 6.112   FUSSI (Fraying of the Upper border of the Subscapularis tendon associated with Subacromial Impingement) lesion involving the upper subscapularis with localized subscapularis tendon degeneration and enlargement medial to the edge of the glenoid. Sagittal FS PD FSE image.

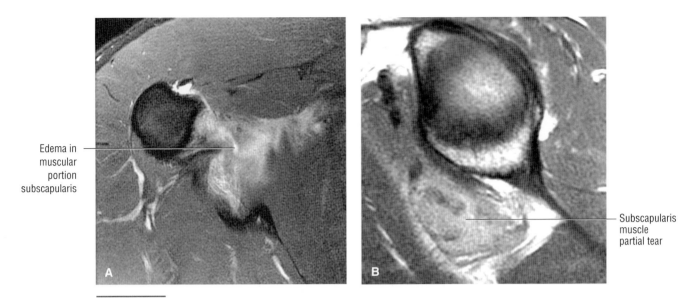

FIGURE 6.113 Inferior muscle belly partial tear of the subscapularis on (**A**) axial FS PD FSE and (**B**) sagittal PD FSE images.

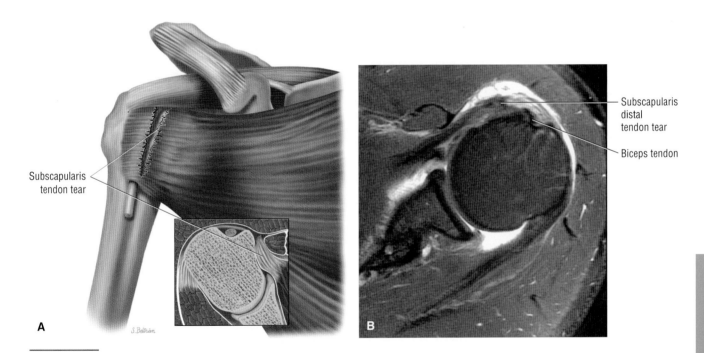

FIGURE 6.114 (**A**) Isolated subscapularis tendon tear without associated biceps tendon dislocation. (**B**) Subscapularis tendon tear with involvement of anterior or superficial fibers. Subscapularis tendon tears are associated with biceps tendon instability with laxity or disruption of the CHL–SGHL sling. SGHL tears are frequently associated with superior distal subscapularis tendon disruptions. Axial FS PD FSE image. The biceps pulley or medial sling is abnormal even if the biceps is not dislocated if there is an associated subscapularis tendon tear. Identify a thickened CH ligament on sagittal images regardless if the biceps tendon is situated within the groove.

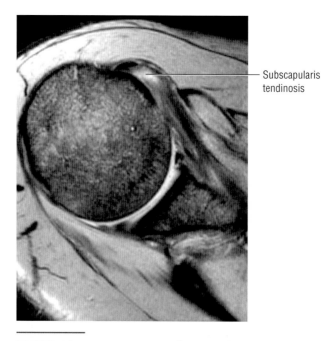

Subscapularis
tendinosis

FIGURE 6.115 Degenerative fraying and
tendinosis of the distal leading edge of the
subscapularis tendon.

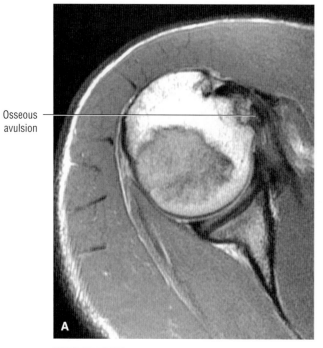

Osseous
avulsion

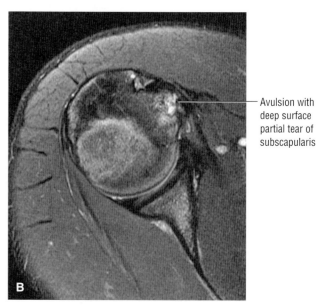

Avulsion with
deep surface
partial tear of
subscapularis

FIGURE 6.116 Axial PD FSE (**A**) and FS PD FSE (**B**) images showing a subscapularis tendon
tear with deep fiber osseous avulsion from the lesser tuberosity in a wrestler. Longitudinal split
tears may occur with footprint disruptions. Nonretracted subscapularis tendon tears are either full
thickness or partial articular surface tendon (PASTA) lesions.

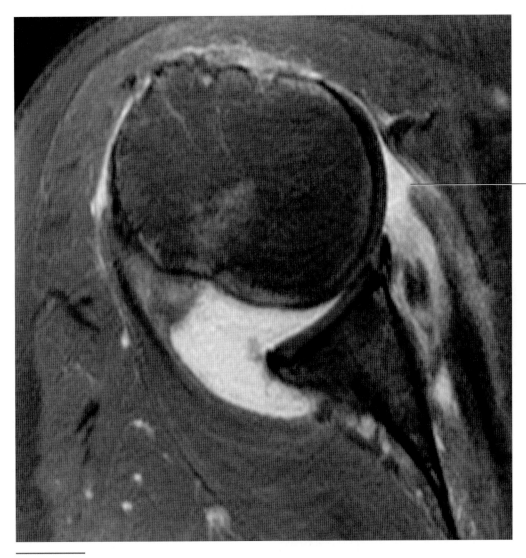

Retracted
subscapularis
tendon

FIGURE 6.117   Complete rupture of the subscapularis tendon with retraction to the glenoid rim on an axial FS PD. The humeral head is no longer centered on the glenoid fossa. Complete tears can be classified as involving the superior one-third or two-thirds versus upper 25% or upper 50%. A complete rupture will show retraction of upper and lower tendon fibers.

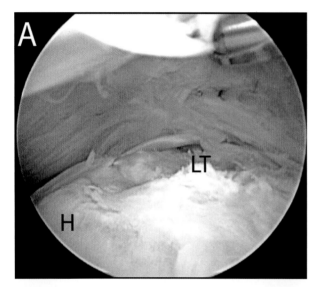

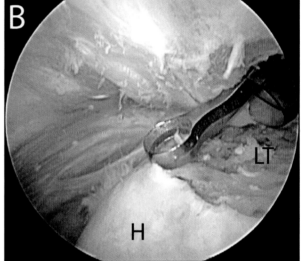

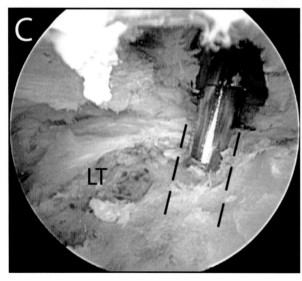

FIGURE 6.118 (**A**) Right shoulder, posterior viewing portal with a 70° arthroscope, demonstrates a bare lesser tuberosity in an individual with a retracted subscapularis tendon tear and a chronically retracted long head of the biceps, with an "empty" bicipital groove. Restoration of the footprint depends upon defining the margins of the lesser tuberosity. (**B**) The medial margin of the lesser tuberosity is easily defined adjacent to the articular margin. (**C**) Defining the lateral margin of the lesser tuberosity requires identification of the bicipital groove (outlined by *dashed black lines*). H, humerus; LT, lesser tuberosity. (Reprinted from Burkhart S, Lo IK, Brady PC, Denard PJ. *The Cowboy's Companion: A Trail Guide for the Arthroscopic Shoulder Surgeon.* Philadelphia, PA: Lippincott Williams & Wilkins; 2012, with permission.)

FIGURE 6.119   Isolated subscapularis tendon tear without associated biceps tendon dislocation. Subscapularis tendon tears are associated with biceps tendon instability with laxity or disruption of the CHL–SGHL sling. SHGL tears are frequently associated with superior distal subscapularis tendon disruptions.

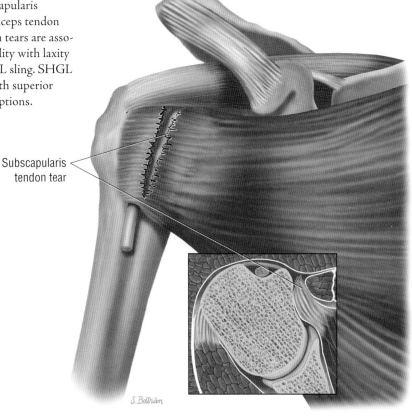

Subscapularis tendon tear

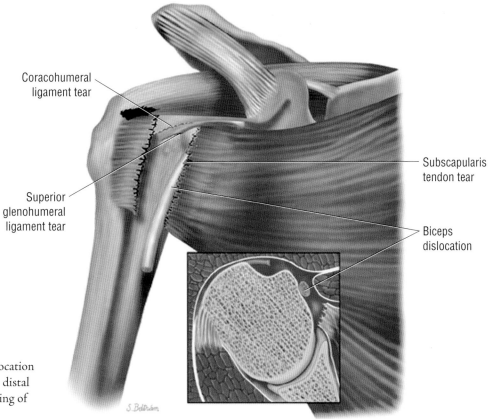

Coracohumeral ligament tear

Superior glenohumeral ligament tear

Subscapularis tendon tear

Biceps dislocation

FIGURE 6.120   Biceps dislocation associated with rupture of the distal subscapularis tendon and tearing of CHL–SGHL sling.

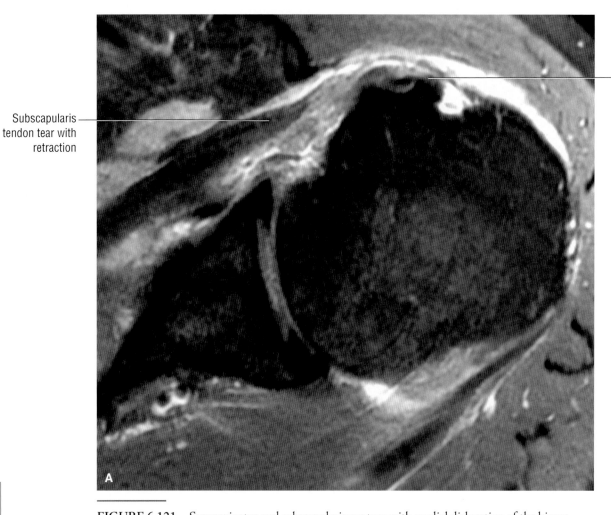

Subscapularis tendon tear with retraction

Biceps tendon instability

FIGURE 6.121   Supraspinatus and subscapularis rupture with medial dislocation of the biceps tendon anterior to the lesser tuberosity. The biceps pulley must be ruptured (secondary to the dislocation) and there is both medial dislocation of the biceps in the axial plane and inferior displacement of the biceps in the sagittal plane. In cases of subscapularis retraction, the subscapularis tendon must be fully mobilized to facilitate the repair. The biceps pulley can be used to identify the torn end of the subscapularis tendon at arthroscopy. (**A**) Axial FS PD.

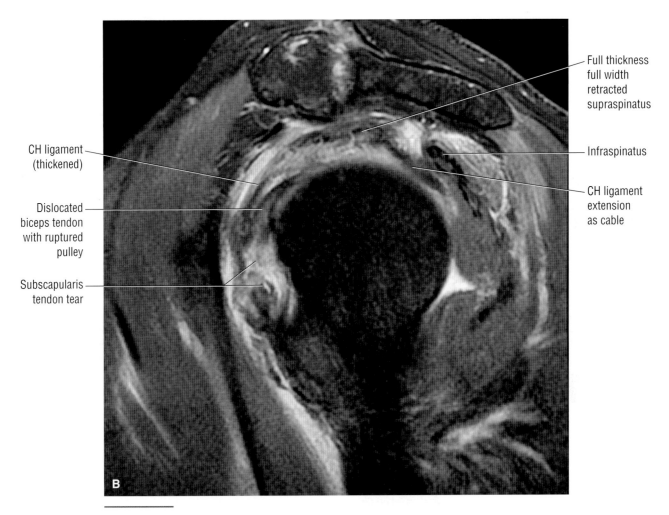

CH ligament (thickened)

Dislocated biceps tendon with ruptured pulley

Subscapularis tendon tear

Full thickness full width retracted supraspinatus

Infraspinatus

CH ligament extension as cable

FIGURE 6.121 *(Continued)* (**B**) Sagittal FS PD. The coracohumeral ligament is thickened and the superior glenohumeral ligament is disrupted (absent). The delamination with greater retraction of deep articular fibers is evident in the sagittal plane. In full thickness tears of the subscapularis tendon associated with biceps dislocation, the LHBT is treated with either tenodesis or tenotomy prior to repairing the subscapularis.

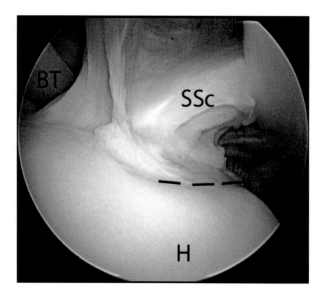

FIGURE 6.122 Left shoulder, posterior glenohumeral viewing portal with a 70° arthroscope, demonstrates the normal medial footprint of the subscapularis tendon. As shown in this image, there is normally a 2- to 3-mm bare strip just medial to the subscapularis tendon. The *dashed lines* outline the anterior articular margin of the humeral head. BT, biceps tendon; H, humerus; SSc, subscapularis tendon. (Reprinted from Burkhart S, Lo IK, Brady PC, Denard PJ. *The Cowboy's Companion: A Trail Guide for the Arthroscopic Shoulder Surgeon.* Philadelphia, PA: Lippincott Williams & Wilkins; 2012, with permission.)

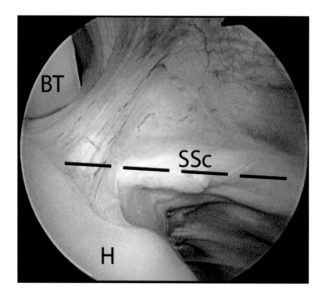

FIGURE 6.123 Left shoulder, posterior viewing portal. When viewed with a 70° arthroscope, the biceps tendon should lie anterior to the plane of the subscapularis tendon (*dashed black lines*). BT, biceps tendon; H, humerus; SSc, subscapularis tendon. (Reprinted from Burkhart S, Lo IK, Brady PC, Denard PJ. *The Cowboy's Companion: A Trail Guide for the Arthroscopic Shoulder Surgeon.* Philadelphia, PA: Lippincott Williams & Wilkins; 2012, with permission.)

Postoperative Cuff

Issues of the Postoperative Rotator Cuff

- Rotator cuff repair goal is to provide for secure fixation of the tendon with a tension-free technique.
    - This may be best accomplished using a single row of medial anchors.
        - There is too much tension required to reduce a cuff tendon laterally as opposed to medial footprint restoration.
        - Three sutures per anchor in a single row technique also minimizes tendon gap formation.
- Three months postoperatively on MRI, the rotator cuff tendons are undergoing revascularization and the intermediate intensity of the repair site may mimic the appearance of a recurrent tear.
- Intact cuff morphology requires contrast adjustment (contrast on monitor) to appreciate continuity of cuff surfaces.
- High-strength sutures can produce significant artifact that can generate localized hyperintense signal and mimic a recurrent tear.
- T1 or intermediate weighted MR sagittal oblique images must be extended medially enough to section the cuff muscle belly located medial to the muscle-tendon junction.
- If the sagittal images are located lateral to the muscle, then cuff atrophy will be overestimated.
- Fatty infiltration of the rotator cuff muscle (supraspinatus or infraspinatus) up to 75% does not preclude cuff repair.
- The subscapularis is unique as complete healing and reversal of pseudoparalysis may occur in patients with 100% fatty infiltration.
    - The subscapularis derives much of its function from a tenodesis effect and thus the subscapularis responds to fatty infiltration differently than the supraspinatus or infraspinatus.
- Available bone bed of the greater tuberosity is a consideration for preoperative planning, otherwise bone graft must be considered.
- Rotator Cuff Adhesion
    - Supraspinatus and infraspinatus may be adhesed to the inferior surface of the infraspinatus.
    - Requires modified double interval slide to increase lateral excursion of the rotator cuff tendons to reach the bone bed[75,124,141,182,234,559]

Surgical Management

■ The repair procedure of choice begins with an arthroscopic subacromial decompression, followed by a deltoid-splitting approach to gain access to the torn cuff.[67]

■ The supraspinatus most commonly tears at its insertion on the greater tuberosity.

■ Primary repairs are fixed directly to the bone with drill holes or suture anchors.

■ A Mumford procedure may be performed when AC degeneration is evident.

■ The rotator cuff is usually repaired with nonabsorbable sutures or suture anchors (used in arthroscopic repairs) to reattach the avulsed tendon to a denuded bed of bone.

■ Suture anchors can be used to repair more massive cuff tears as well as isolated supraspinatus injuries.

    ■ The suture anchors should be located lateral to the edge of the humeral head articular cartilage and directed medial and inferiorly into subchondral bone (45 degrees or tent peg angle).

■ The deltoid-sparing aspect of the arthroscopic repair represents an advantage over open procedures.

    ■ Postoperative inflammation usually resolves by 6 weeks.

■ Postoperative MR examination should document healing of the repaired cuff with a reestablished supraspinatus tendon footprint over the greater tuberosity.

■ Arthroscopic repair of an isolated supraspinatus full thickness tear usually results in complete tendon healing.

■ Superior ascent of the humeral head, remodeling of the undersurface of the acromion, and fatty atrophy of the rotator cuff are all indicators of a difficult direct cuff repair.[53]

■ A soft tissue grasper may be used at arthroscopy to test the mobility of the cuff and to assess the need for a capsule release or interval slide.

■ Scar tissue is removed to expose a retracted supraspinatus.

■ Rotator cuff may adhere to or retract from the undersurface of the acromion with no tendinous attachment to the humeral head.

    ■ Cuff atrophy may be minimal in this scenario since there is a fixation point to bone by scar tissue.

- Suture anchors should be evaluated for retraction (superior displacement relative to the humeral head contour).[330]

  - Titanium suture anchors can be seen on postoperative radiographs if the anchor fails and pulls out.

  - Plastic or polymer radiolucent anchors may be difficult to locate even on an MR study.

MR Appearance of the Postoperative Rotator Cuff

- MR imaging has also been used for postoperative evaluation of rotator cuff repairs.[371,528]

- Changes caused by acromioplasty, resection of the distal end of the clavicle, and division of the coracoacromial ligament are also displayed on MR images and include:

  - Persistent changes from impingement (including tendon degeneration, partial tear, and retear; a rough undersurface of the acromion; or residual AC joint callus or osteophytes)

  - Deltoid attachment instability

  - Nerve damage

- The rotator cuff interval between the supraspinatus and subscapularis tendons may be interrupted at surgery, allowing communication of contrast with the subacromial-subdeltoid bursa, even though the rotator cuff repair is intact.

- The isolated finding of subacromial-subdeltoid fluid is not sufficient to diagnose a failed repair or retear of the rotator cuff.

- Relative increased cuff signal intensity on FS PD FSE images may also be seen in the postoperative cuff repair without retear.

- Some retears may be associated with granulation tissue and adhesions and may appear as a low signal intensity tear on T2-weighted images without associated fluid signal intensity at the tear site or in the subacromial-subdeltoid bursa.

- The presence of a gap or defined defect in the cuff associated with extension of fluid signal intensity on T2-weighted or FS PD-weighted FSE sequences is diagnostic for a retorn repair.

■ Optimal placement of suture anchors are 5mm lateral to the humeral head articular cartilage at a 45-degree angle.[559]

   ■ Anchors are properly placed near the medial edge of the anatomic neck rather than laterally on the greater tuberosity.

■ The microfracture site of punctures may be seen on coronal images. The Crimson Duvet technique creates vents lateral to the anchors. The resultant superclot overlies the surface of the greater tuberosity and the cuff following repair.

■ Intact rotator cuff repairs may demonstrate intermediate signal at the repair site without loss of repair continuity.

■ If a partial cuff repair is indicated in the management of a massive or large rotator cuff tear, there may be portions of the rotator cuff tendons that are not in continuity on sequential MR coronal images. The description of the intact tendon should be made and the area of discontinuity should be described as this may represent the desired functional outcome in this situation.[559]

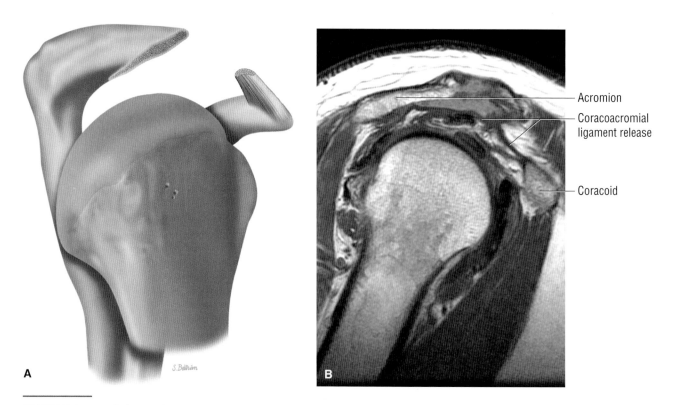

FIGURE 6.124 (**A**) Partial anterior acromioplasty. The coracoacromial ligament (CA) should be released from the acromion and not resected from under the deltoid to allow the ligament to reattach to the acromion and reconstitute the anterior arch. (**B**) Subacromial decompression performed for a partial thickness rotator cuff tear. In cuff impingement, the coracoacromial ligament is frayed and fragmented and associated with synovitis. Decompression results in a flat undersurface of the acromion and release of the CA ligament. The inferior lip of the distal clavicle is also removed if it extends inferior to the flattened acromion. Coplaning the distal clavicle avoids a step-off between the acromion and clavicle.

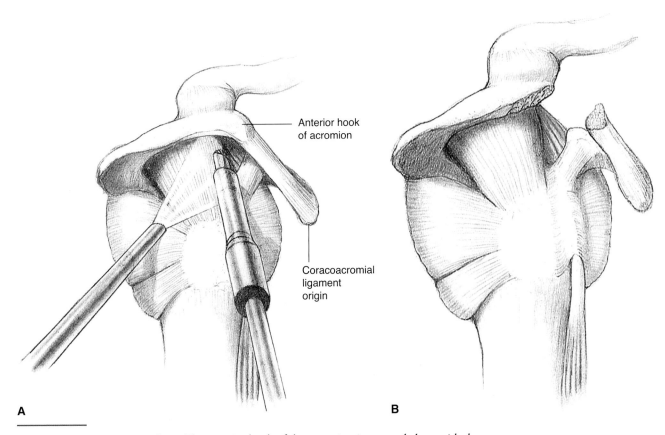

Anterior hook
of acromion

Coracoacromial
ligament
origin

A

B

FIGURE 6.125 Acromioplasty. The anterior hook of the acromion is resected along with the origin of the CA ligament, leaving a flat acromial undersurface. (**A**) Prior to resection. (**B**) After arthroscopic acromioplasty. The arthroscopic shaver is first used to resect the soft tissue from the inferior surface of the acromion before performing a subacromial decompression. A hooked-tipped electrode completes the resection of the coracoacromial ligament off the anterior and lateral aspects of the acromion. A 4-mm burr is used to measure the amount of anterior acromial resection which is initiated at the anterolateral corner of the acromion. During subacromial decompression, any prominence identified along the undersurface of the distal clavicle can be resected back. (Reprinted from Craig EV. *Master Techniques in Orthopaedic Surgery: Shoulder.* 3rd ed. Philadelphia, PA: Lippincott Williams & Wilkins; 2013, with permission.)

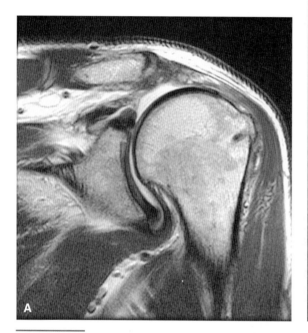

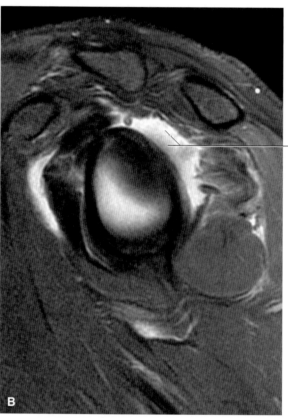

Postoperative
retear

FIGURE 6.126   Massive retear of the rotator cuff tendons after repair. The retracted supraspinatus and infraspinatus tendons are shown on coronal PD FSE (**A**) and sagittal FS PD FSE (**B**) images. Large and massive rotator cuff tears usually extend through the rotator cable attachments and result in an unstable fulcrum of glenohumeral rotation. Included are tears that extend anteriorly into the upper half of the subscapularis tendon or posterior cuff tears that extend through the inferior half of the infraspinatus tendon. Unlike single-tendon cuff tears which may have preserved function or be asymptomatic, massive tears that involve a second tendon are not as well tolerated.[75]

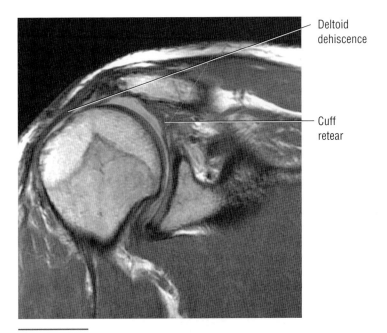

FIGURE 6.127 Postoperative deltoid avulsion. In the presence of a symptomatic AC joint, an undersurface claviculoplasty is performed, which protects and preserves the deltoid origin. Although these avulsions may not be painful, they can be repaired along with a re-repair of the cuff to allow the patient to lift the arm with a functioning deltoid.

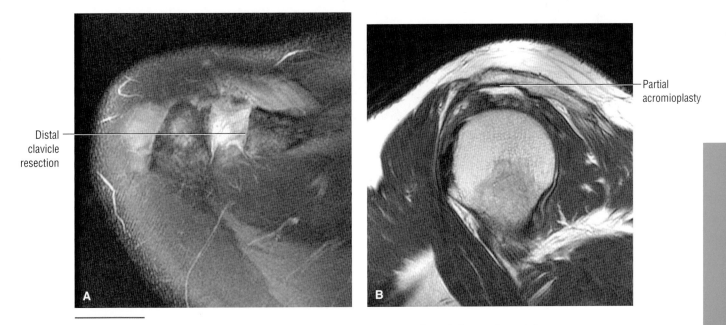

FIGURE 6.128 A Mumford or arthroscopic distal clavicle resection (ADCR) is performed for symptomatic AC joints. Coplaning or the "mini-Mumford" is also an option to remove inferior AC joint spurs. (A) Axial FS PD FSE and (B) sagittal T2 FSE images. Distal clavicle excision starts with resection of the anterosuperior clavicle progressing posterior and then inferior. 10mm of bone is removed (twice the diameter of a 5.5-mm shaver). The AC ligaments are left intact if possible.

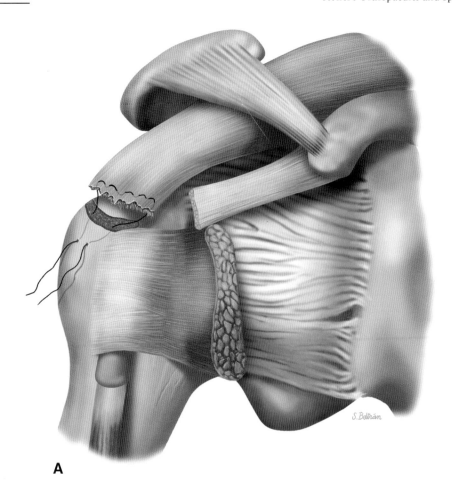

A

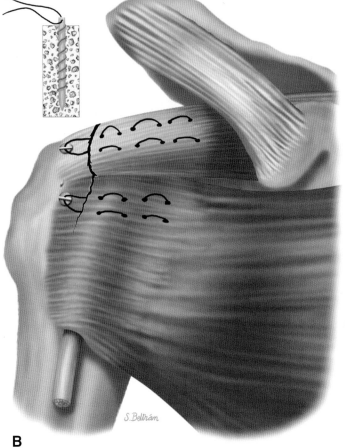

B

FIGURE 6.129 (**A**) Tendon-to-bone rotator cuff repair with suturing of the edge of the distal cuff into a prepared humeral head trough. (**B**) Suture anchor repair of the supraspinatus and subscapularis tendons. Suture anchors do not preclude postoperative MR assessment. Arthroscopy spares damage to the deltoid and allows an ideal subacromial decompression. A torn rotator cuff is shorter and does not have the length of the original tendon. This understanding has led to the concept of using a single row (of medial suture anchors) repair directed to the medial footprint adjacent to the humeral head articular cartilage. Overtensioning of the supraspinatus will occur if the tendon is pulled laterally over the footprint. The cable must not be overtensioned as well by mistakenly shifting its position laterally.

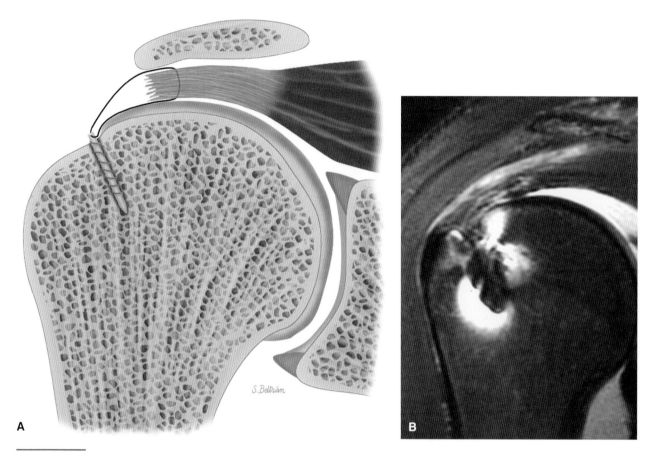

FIGURE 6.130   (**A**) The majority of torn rotator cuffs can be repaired arthroscopically. Suture anchor fixation of the rotator cuff tear to bone is shown. Anchors are placed adjacent to the articular cartilage. The anchors are inserted near the medial edge of the anatomic neck entering the subchondral bone at a 45-degree angle. Triple-loaded anchors maximizes the number of passes through each centimeter of the tear. The goal is to create a secure fixation of the tendon and minimize tension on the repair. (**B**) Coronal FS PD FSE image showing the suture anchors (two or three anchors may be needed) located lateral to the edge of the articular cartilage and directly obliquely and medial into subchondral bone. There is residual cuff tendinosis and subacromial bursal fluid.

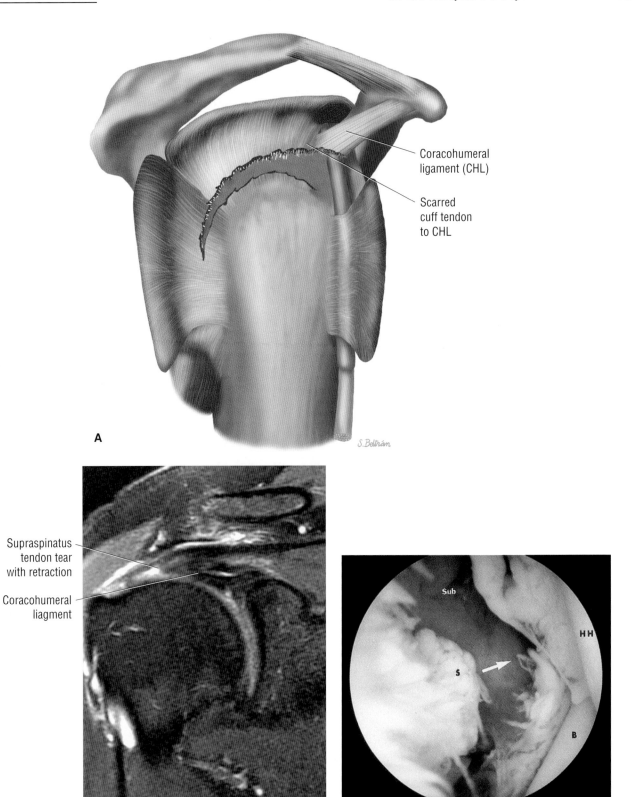

FIGURE 6.131   (**A**) Adherence of the retracted rotator cuff to the coracohumeral ligament. (**B**) Coronal FS PD FSE image showing the thickened coracohumeral ligament associated with torn and retracted supraspinatus. (**C**) A corresponding arthroscopic view shows the articular surface of the avulsed supraspinatus tendon (S; *arrow*). B, biceps tendon; HH, humeral head; Sub, subacromial space.

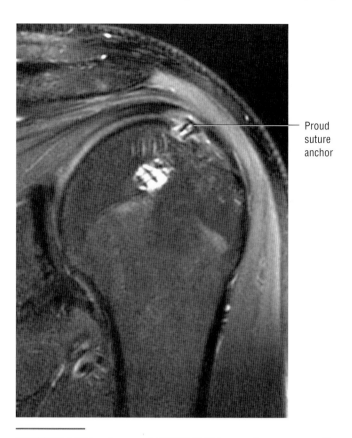

FIGURE 6.132 A coronal FS PD FSE image after rotator cuff repair shows a proud suture anchor superficial to the humeral head contour.

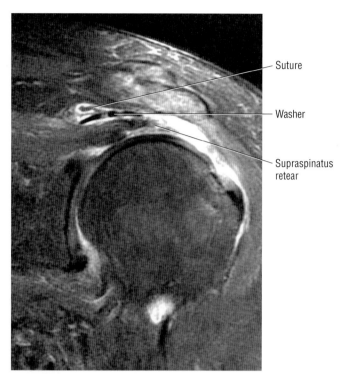

FIGURE 6.133 Coronal FS PD FSE image showing a cuff retear with subacromial displacement of a linear cuff washer with attached suture. The washer was used to gain greater cuff surface purchase.

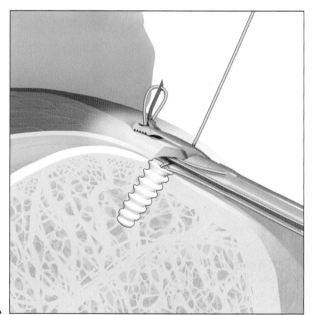

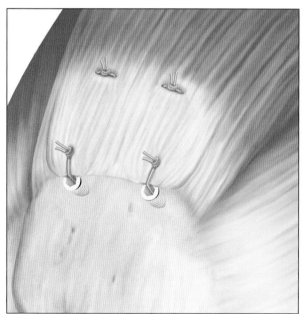

FIGURE 6.134 Schematic of correct placement of medial sutures. (**A**) Medial sutures have been properly placed 2 to 3mm lateral to the musculotendinous junction. (**B**) View following knot tying. (Reprinted from Burkhart S, Lo IK, Brady PC, Denard PJ. *The Cowboy's Companion: A Trail Guide for the Arthroscopic Shoulder Surgeon*. Philadelphia, PA: Lippincott Williams & Wilkins; 2012, with permission.)

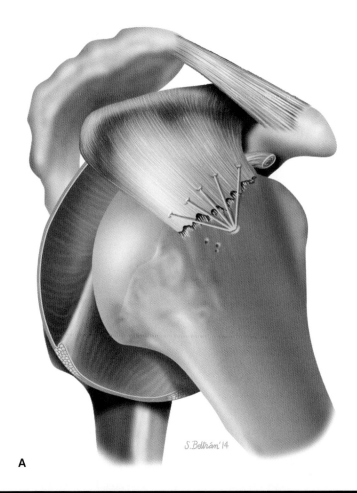

A

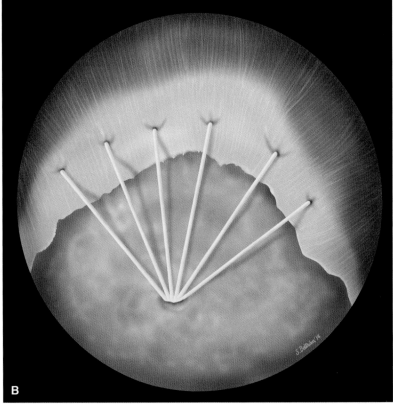

B

FIGURE 6.135 Double row parachute. Parachute repair technique as a novel approach to bring all of the components of the retracted cuff to an anatomic footprint. (**A**) 3D color illustration. (**B**) Superior view color illustration.

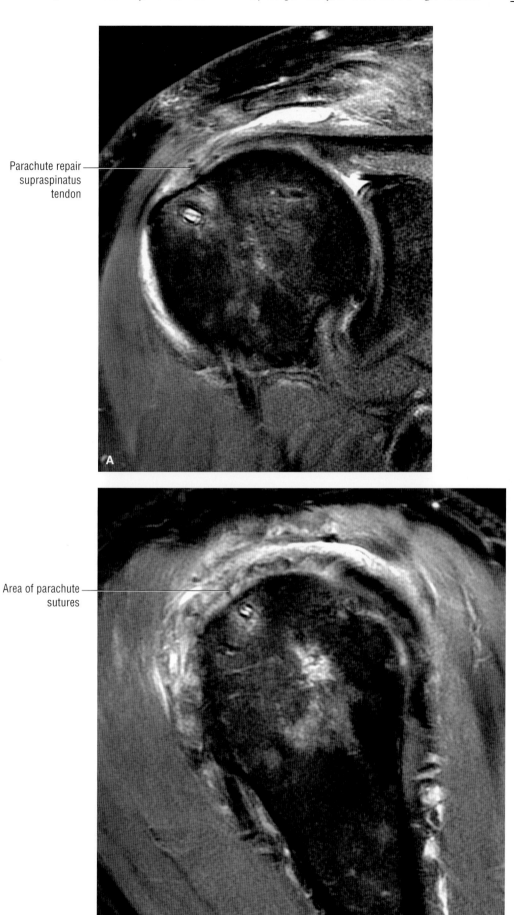

FIGURE 6.136 Parachute repair with cuff continuity of supraspinatus (**A**) FS PD coronal. (**B**) FS PD sagittal.

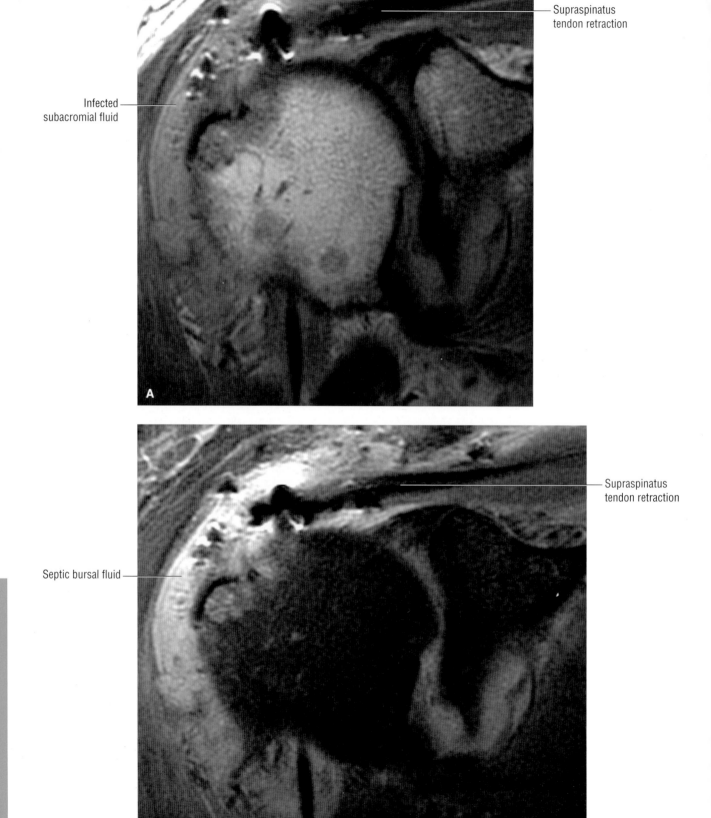

FIGURE 6.137   Retear of rotator cuff repair associated with joint sepsis. (**A**) PD coronal.
(**B**) FS PD coronal.

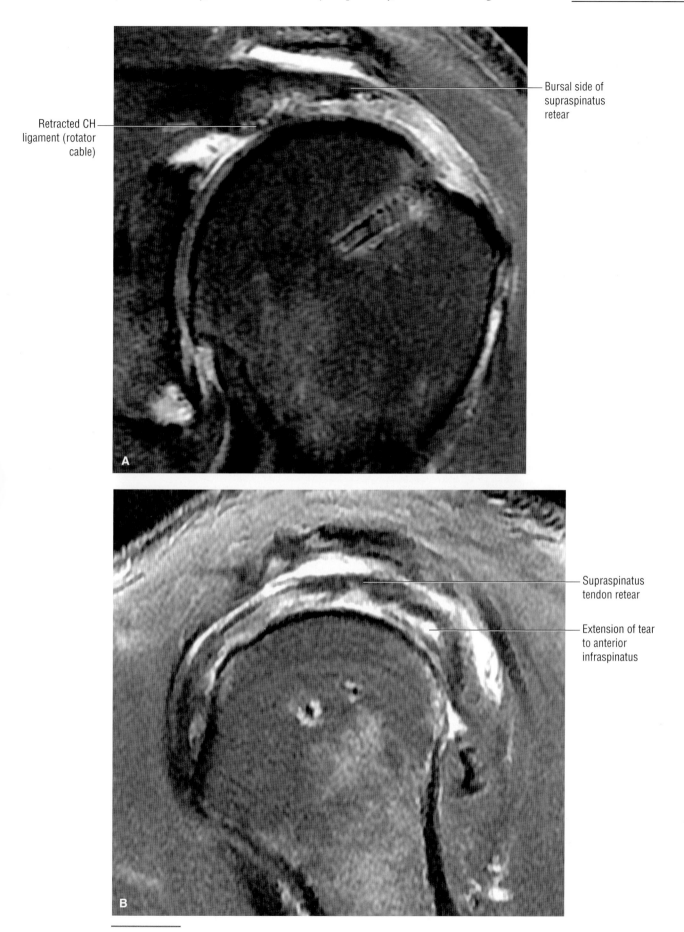

FIGURE 6.138   Full thickness rotator cuff tear with retracted rotator cable along the articular side of the cuff. This represents a recurrent tear post-anchor. (**A**) FS PD coronal. (**B**) FS PD sagittal.

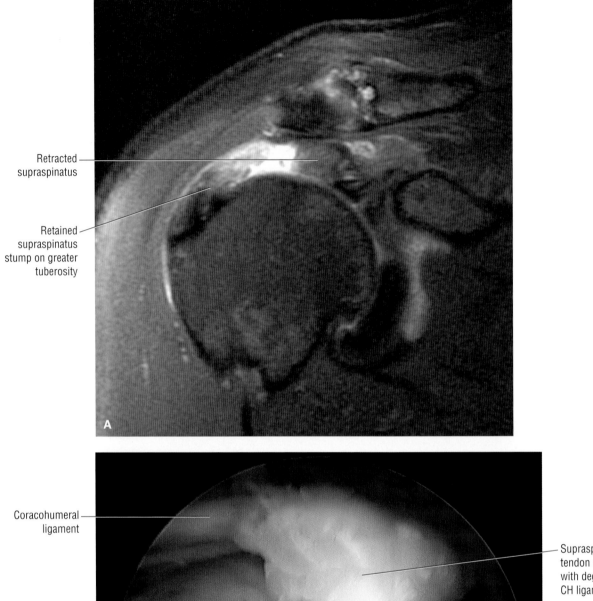

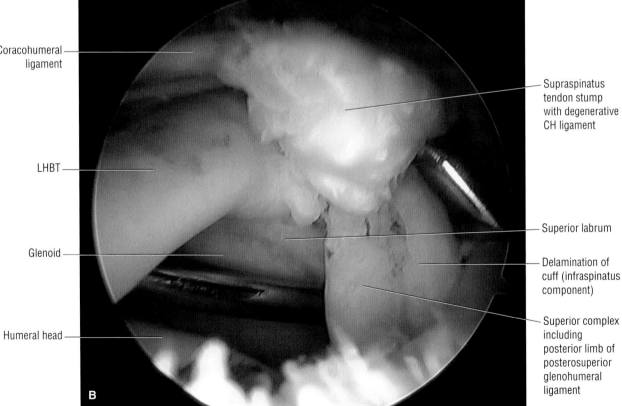

FIGURE 6.139   Preoperative full thickness cuff tear with retracted supraspinatus tendon. (**A**) Coronal FS PD. (**B,C**) Arthroscopic images with 30-degree scope. (**D–F**) Post-repair Healix and Versalok anchors. (**D**) Coronal FS PD. (**E**) Sagittal FS PD. (**F**) Arthroscopic view with 70-degree scope.

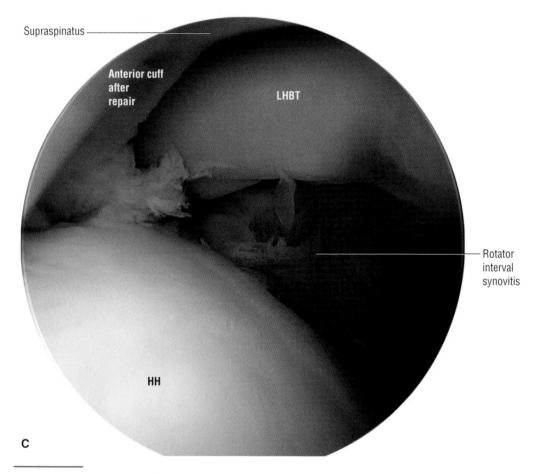

FIGURE 6.139 (*Continued*) Posterolateral portal, 30-degree scope from bursal surface.

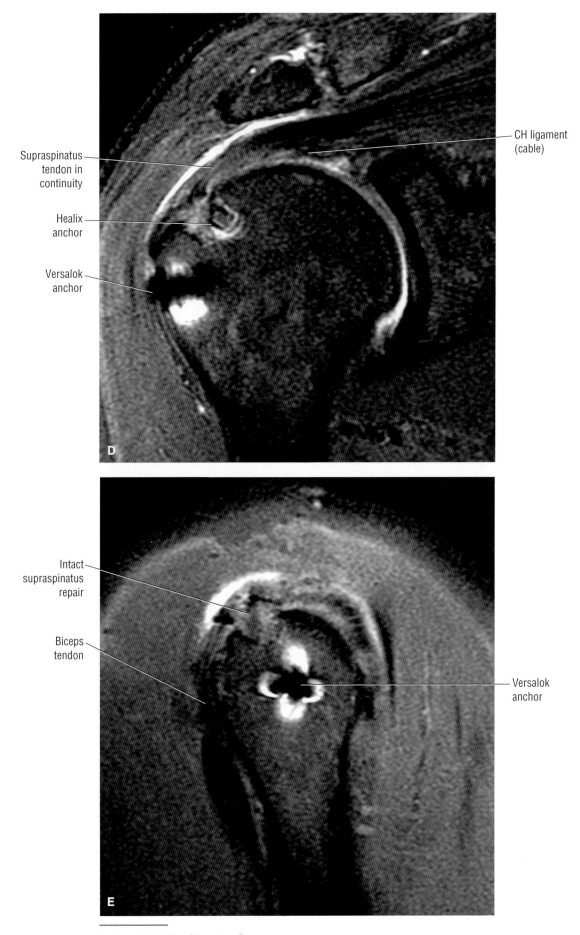

FIGURE 6.139   (*Continued*)

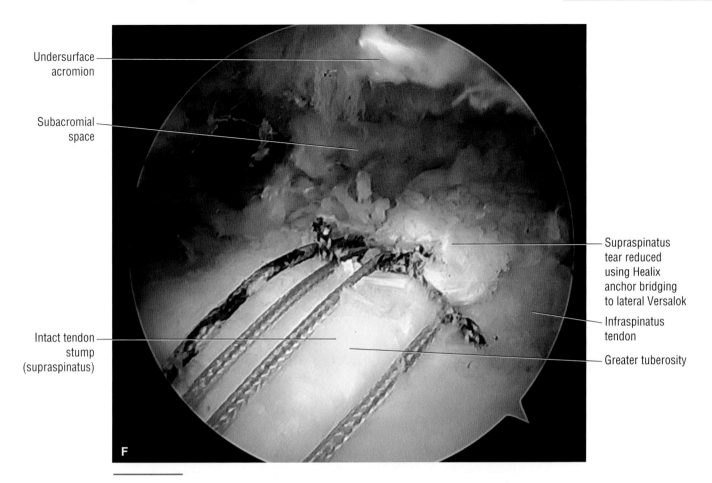

Undersurface acromion

Subacromial space

Supraspinatus tear reduced using Healix anchor bridging to lateral Versalok

Infraspinatus tendon

Intact tendon stump (supraspinatus)

Greater tuberosity

FIGURE 6.139 (*Continued*) (**F**) Posterolateral portal, 70-degree scope. Since the quality of the retracted supraspinatus tendon was poor, the medially placed Healix anchor permitted a more secure repair without being dependent on the quality of the greater tuberosity stump. The tendon edge was repaired to both tendon stump and bony bed. The lateral Versalok secured the repair independent of the strength of the stump.

- The three components of an ideal cuff repair should use:
  - Single row of strong suture anchors loaded with three strands of high strength suture
  - Medial edge insertion of anchors on anatomic neck, a few millimeters lateral to the humeral head cartilage
  - Microfracture vents (Crimson Duvet)[75,559]

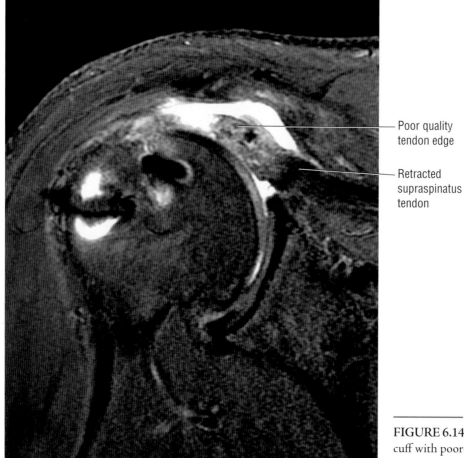

Poor quality
tendon edge

Retracted
supraspinatus
tendon

FIGURE 6.140 Failed repair of the rotator
cuff with poor-quality tendon edge of the
retracted supraspinatus.

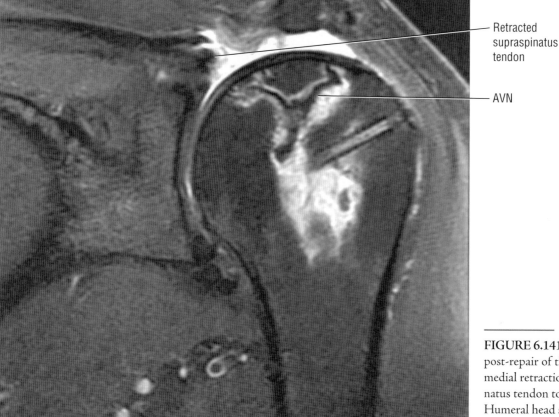

Retracted
supraspinatus
tendon

AVN

FIGURE 6.141 Recurrent tear
post-repair of the supraspinatus with
medial retraction of the supraspinatus tendon to the glenoid fossa.
Humeral head shows characteristic
changes of AVN.

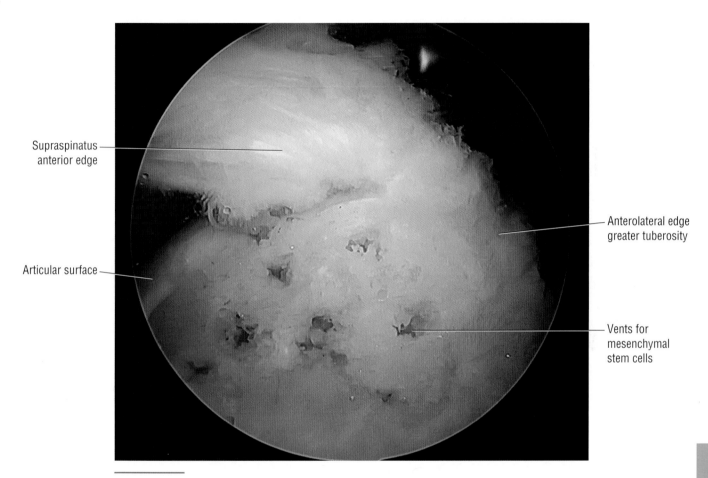

Supraspinatus anterior edge

Articular surface

Anterolateral edge greater tuberosity

Vents for mesenchymal stem cells

FIGURE 6.142 Arthroscopic view of Crimson Duvet with subchondral vents created for the influx of mesenchymal stem cells. Posterolateral portal with a 70-degree scope. These microfracture punctures are placed in the greater tuberosity lateral to the anchors. The vents enter the bone marrow directed toward the humeral shaft to avoid compromising the fixation of the anchors. The Crimson Duvet superclot is created for growth factors and to establish a new blood supply for the rotator cuff repair (crescent tear repair).

Microinstability

Key Concepts

■ The term microinstability was developed to characterize the spectrum of pathologic processes that occur in the upper half of the shoulder joint.

■ The structures involved in microinstability include the biceps, the biceps pulley, the biceps root attachment, the rotator cuff, and the rotator cuff interval.

■ Microinstability does not refer to anteroinferior instability but instead denotes pathologic conditions in the superior half of the shoulder.

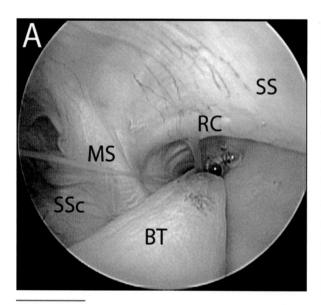
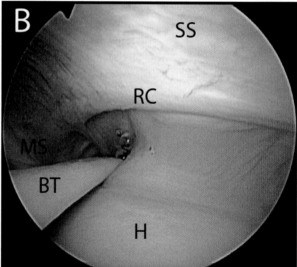

FIGURE 6.143   Right shoulder, posterior viewing portal, demonstrating the connection between the subscapularis (SSc) and the supraspinatus (SS) via the medial sling (MS). **(A)** The rotator cable (RC) of the rotator cuff merges with the medial sling anteriorly. As such, when the medial sling detaches during a subscapularis tear, the comma sign may be followed to locate the anterolateral corner of the supraspinatus tendon. **(B)** A profile view of the rotator cable further shows this constant relationship. BT, biceps tendon; G, glenoid; H, humerus. (Reprinted from Burkhart S, Lo IK, Brady PC, Denard PJ. *The Cowboy's Companion: A Trail Guide for the Arthroscopic Shoulder Surgeon.* Philadelphia, PA: Lippincott Williams & Wilkins; 2012, with permission.) The medial sling is the biceps pulley which is a stabilizing sling for the long head of the biceps tendon. The pulley is a tendoligamentous sling within the rotator interval . The pulley system consists of the coracohumeral ligament, the superior glenohumeral ligament, fibers of a supraspinatus tendon slip, and fibers of the subscapularis tendon.

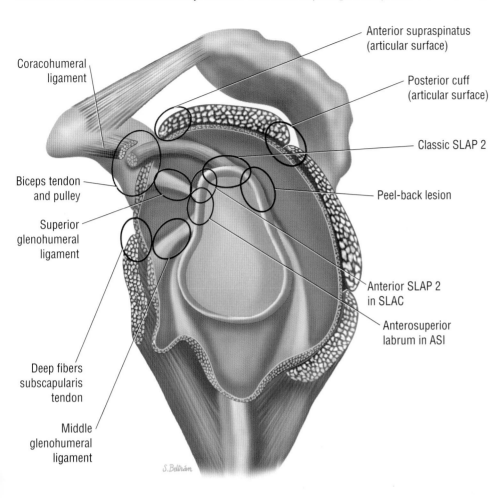

Coracohumeral ligament

Anterior supraspinatus (articular surface)

Posterior cuff (articular surface)

Classic SLAP 2

Biceps tendon and pulley

Peel-back lesion

Superior glenohumeral ligament

Anterior SLAP 2 in SLAC

Anterosuperior labrum in ASI

Deep fibers subscapularis tendon

Middle glenohumeral ligament

S.Beltrán

FIGURE 6.144 Potential sites of involvement in microinstability, including the anterior supraspinatus and anterior component of a SLAP 2 in the SLAC lesion; the posterior cuff and posterior component of a SLAP 2 in the posterior peel-back lesion; the classic anterior-to-posterior SLAP 2 lesion; anterosuperior impingement (ASI) involving the superior subscapularis, CHL–SGHL complex, the anterior supraspinatus, and anterosuperior labrum; and the middle glenohumeral ligament (MGL) in anterior laxity.

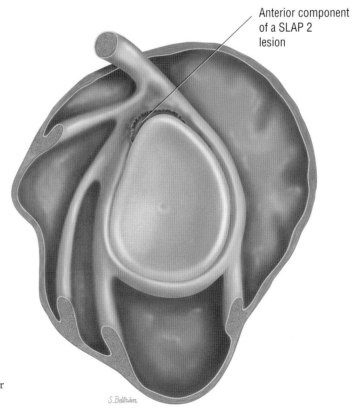

Anterior component of a SLAP 2 lesion

FIGURE 6.145 SLAC lesion with partial articular-side supraspinatus tendon tear and anterior SLAP lesion.

S.Beltrán

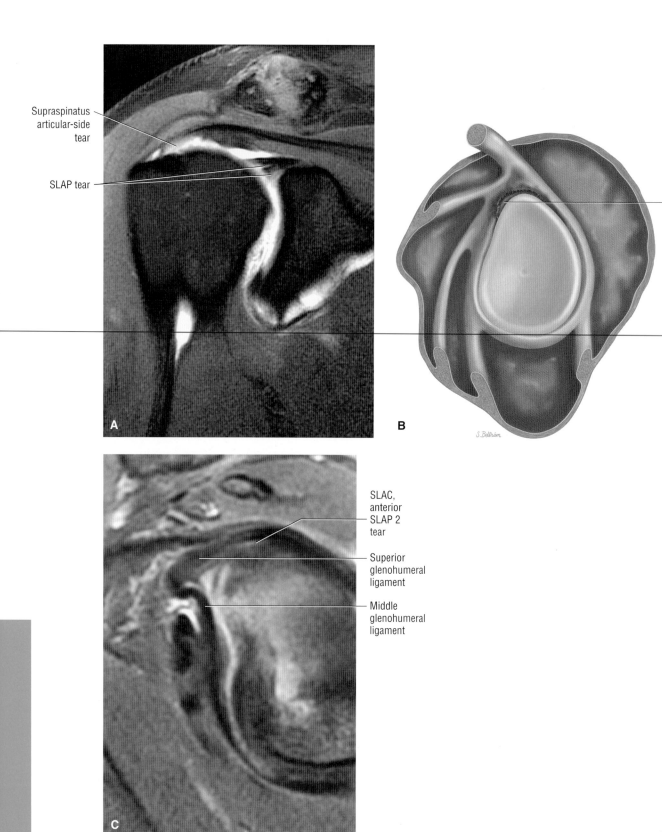

FIGURE 6.146   (A) Coronal FS PD FSE image of an SLAC lesion with partial articular-side supraspinatus tendon tear and anterior SLAP lesion. Sagittal color section (B) and FS PD FSE image (C) demonstrate labral separation of the anterior component of a SLAP 2 lesion.

Structures Involved in Microinstability Lesions

- Superior structures:
    - The biceps and its associated pulley (CHL and SGHL)
    - The biceps root attachment/superior labrum (SLAP lesions)
    - The rotator cuff
- Anterior structures:
    - Rotator interval, including the SGHL in the anterior superior portion and the MGHL inferior to the SGHL
- At arthroscopy, the rotator interval is directly visualized between the intraarticular biceps, superior labrum, MGHL, and humeral head.
- Sectioning of the rotator interval has been demonstrated to produce increased inferior and posterior humeral head translation.
    - There is increased anterior translation of the humeral head at 60° of flexion characterized as microinstability.[208]

Pathologic Changes in Microinstability Pathology

- The spectrum of pathologic changes in microinstability pathology includes:
    - SGHL avulsion or laxity
    - MGHL avulsion producing straight anterior laxity
    - SLAP lesions (types 1 to 10)
        - A type 10 SLAP lesion is a type 2 SLAP tear with extension into the rotator interval (alternate definition with extension to the posteroinferior labrum).
    - Posterior peel-back SLAP tears
    - Interval defects or biceps pulley lesions
    - Articular-side cuff lesions (partial thickness and typically non-crescentic in location)
        - These articular-side tears may occur from abrasion of the rotator cuff on the glenoid either anteriorly or posteriorly.
- The estimated incidence of microinstability is 6%.
- The etiology is repetitive stress or acute injury.
- The clinical diagnosis of microinstability is made based on findings from the history and physical examination.
    - MR and arthroscopic findings confirm the diagnosis.

Clinical Symptoms of Microinstability

- Rotator cuff tendinosis or pain

- A subjective feeling of slipping of the shoulder when not abducted and externally rotated (This slipping is perceived by the patient as an abnormal or uncomfortable motion or laxity between the glenoid and humeral head.)

- Easy fatigue of the shoulder muscles or parascapular pain

- Impingement-like pain, which may mimic rotator cuff disease

- The various mechanisms of injury in microinstability determine the location of the involved structures as indicated:

  - The application of traction forces in the overhead position may produce a SLAP or SLAC lesion.

  - A seat belt across the involved shoulder (roll-around seat belt on impact) is associated with SLAC lesions.

  - A fall on the abducted arm is associated with the classic and SLAP variants.

  - "Throwing out" of the shoulder may produce an MGHL injury.

  - Overhead repetitive work or sports activity and professional throwing athletes may present with posterior peel-back SLAP with posterior superior instability due to glenohumeral internal rotation deficit (GIRD).

  - No trauma history may be associated with biceps pulley lesions.

- There is no one specific clinical test (Jobe's, load and shift, O'Brien's, or Speed's test) that is reliably positive for confirmation of the diagnosis of instability.

MR Examinations in Microinstability

- Posterior coronal images and sagittal and axial images display peel-back lesions with posterosuperior labral tears. Axial and sagittal images may further show an early pattern of eccentric sclerosis or wear as a pre-posterior peel-back lesion.

- Coronal plane images are used to distinguish a type 2 or 3 BLC with a normal biceps labral sulcus from a SLAP lesion.

- MR arthrography optimizes depiction of biceps pulley lesions, with improved appreciation of the degree of injury to the CHL and SGHL.

- Partial thickness articular surface tears are seen as a detachment of cuff fibers at their footprint attachment to the greater tuberosity both on ABER MR arthrograms and routine phased-array coil imaging of the shoulder.

Arthroscopic Findings in Microinstability

- Superior labral detachment and extensions (synovial reaction and chondral erosions may be associated findings)
- Capsular (SGHL and MGHL) tears and laxity
- Laxity of the rotator interval
- Non-crescentic articular-side partial thickness rotator cuff lesions
- The attachment of the CHL at the bicipital groove (lateral lip or greater tuberosity side)
  - The CHL is a bursal structure and cannot be visualized from the articular surface.
- Biceps pulley lesions with either biceps subluxation on dislocation

Surgical Options for Microinstability

- Imbrication of capsular laxity in the rotator interval if laxity is present
- If detached, the anterior superior labrum is reattached.
- The anatomic attachment of the SGHL and/or MGHL is repaired if displaced, especially if these structures are scarred and in an abnormal position.
- SLAP tears are repaired, as is the biceps anchor if detached.
- Tenotomy/tenodesis is performed if there is a severe disruption of the biceps pulley.
- The subscapularis or supraspinatus tendons are also repaired along with the biceps pulley.

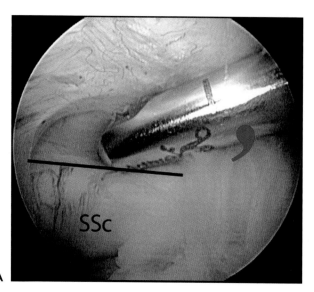

A

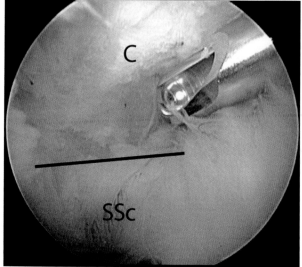

B

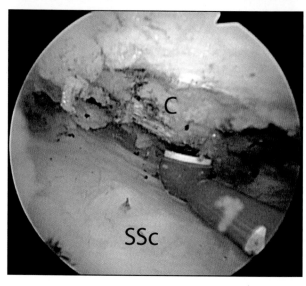

C

FIGURE 6.147   Creating a window in the rotator interval. (**A**) Right shoulder, posterior viewing portal with a 30° arthroscope, demonstrates use of a shaver to create a window in the rotator interval medial to the comma tissue (*blue comma symbol*) and above the superior border of the subscapularis tendon (*black line*). The medial sling or pulley is composed of the medial fibers of the coracohumeral ligament and the superior glenohumeral ligament. A torn medial sling forms a distinctive comma-shaped arc of soft tissue (*comma sign*) at the superolateral corner of the subscapularis (**B**) The tip of the coracoid is identified. (**C**) After the tip of the coracoid is identified, a 70° arthroscope is inserted, and the coracoid tip is skeletonized with an electrocautery. C, coracoid; SSc, subscapularis tendon. (Reprinted from Burkhart S, Lo IK, Brady PC, Denard PJ. *The Cowboy's Companion: A Trail Guide for the Arthroscopic Shoulder Surgeon*. Philadelphia, PA: Lippincott Williams & Wilkins; 2012, with permission.)

SLAC Lesions

Key Concepts

- The SLAC lesion is associated with an articular-side partial thickness anterior supraspinatus tendon lesion.

- The SLAC lesion is combined with the anterior component of a SLAP 2 tear.

- The SLAC lesion is a type of instability and not an impingement lesion.

- The SLAC lesion represents an injury to the anterior-superior glenoid labrum that involves the insertion of the SGHL and the anterior portion of the biceps tendon.[542]

  - The term "SLAC lesion" refers to the combination of the labral and cuff injuries.

- Because of the resultant anterosuperior instability, the articular surface of the anterior supraspinatus tendon contacts the anterior superior labrum (the anterior component of a type 2 SLAP lesion) and glenoid.

- Severe contact can result in a partial thickness rotator cuff tear on the articular side of the supraspinatus tendon.

- The mechanism of injury represents either a repetitive overhead activity or a traumatic event.

  - The trauma, including falls and motor vehicle accidents, involves an anterior superior subluxation episode.

  - In overhead activity, the patient's dominant arm is commonly affected.

  - In motor vehicle accidents, the arm on the side of the shoulder strap is frequently involved.

- The SLAC lesion is primarily an instability problem.

- The anterior rotator cuff component is different from the lesion that impingement or traumatic injury causes.

  - Contact between the cuff and the anterior superior glenoid labrum results from increased anterior-superior translation.

- Corrective treatment addresses the underlying instability and not just the rotator cuff.

Rotator Cuff Interval

Key Concepts

- The rotator interval is contained between the supraspinatus and sub-scapularis tendons.

- The CHL is a bursal structure and the SGHL is an articular structure.

- The confluence of the medial CHL and SGHL is an articular structure.

- The confluence of the medial CHL and SGHL forms the biceps pulley within the rotator cuff interval.

- Failure of the biceps pulley or sling is associated with medial sublux-ations and dislocations of the biceps tendon.

The Rotator Interval

- Is a triangular area of tissue that functions to allow rotational motion around the coracoid process[301]

- Is defined by the supraspinatus tendon above, the leading edge of the subscapularis tendon below, the base of the coracoid process medially, and the transverse humeral ligament (overlying the intertubercular groove) laterally[380]

- Biceps pulley is composed of both the medial portion (limb) of the coracohumeral ligament and the SGHL.

- Contains a bursal layer and an articular layer:
    - The bursal layer of the interval is the CHL.
    - The articular layer of the interval is the SGHL.
    - The CHL and SGHL become confluent at their attachment to the greater and lesser tuberosities.
    - Boundaries of the rotator interval are:
        - The anterior edge of the supraspinatus tendon at the superior edge
        - The superior edge of the subscapularis tendon at the inferior edge
        - The transverse ligament over bicipital groove at the apex

- The humeral head cartilage at the floor
- The capsule of the rotator interval at the roof

- At the level of the coracoid and BLC, the origin of the coracohumeral ligament can be seen on the lateral aspect of the base of the coracoid.
  - In this proximal portion of the rotator cuff interval, the SGHL is anterior to the biceps tendon.
  - The CHL forms a roof over both the SGHL and proximal biceps tendon in this location.

- At the midportion of the rotator cuff interval, the T-shaped link or junction is formed when the SGHL changes direction to create an anterior floor for the biceps pulley and intersects the undersurface of the overlying CHL.[301]

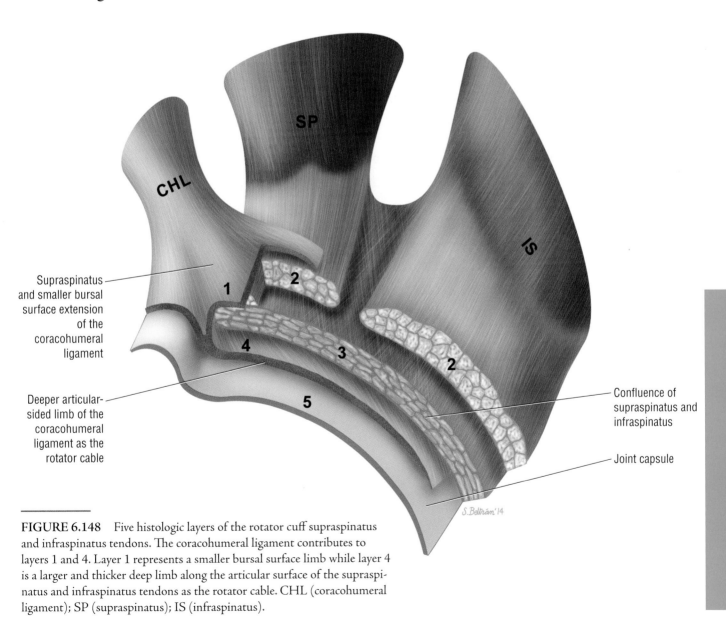

FIGURE 6.148 Five histologic layers of the rotator cuff supraspinatus and infraspinatus tendons. The coracohumeral ligament contributes to layers 1 and 4. Layer 1 represents a smaller bursal surface limb while layer 4 is a larger and thicker deep limb along the articular surface of the supraspinatus and infraspinatus tendons as the rotator cable. CHL (coracohumeral ligament); SP (supraspinatus); IS (infraspinatus).

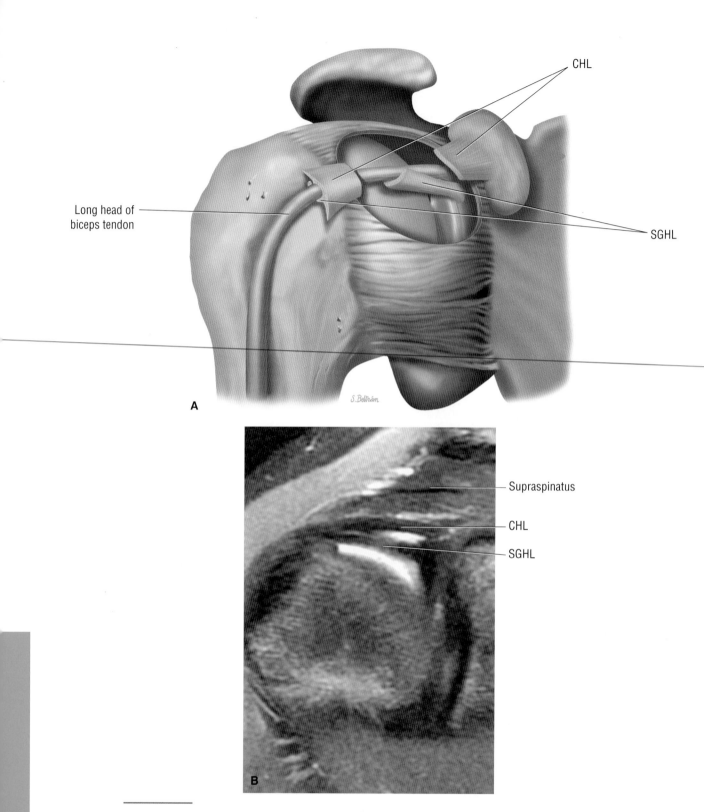

Long head of biceps tendon

CHL

SGHL

A

S.Beltrán

Supraspinatus

CHL

SGHL

B

FIGURE 6.149   The rotator cuff interval, demonstrating the confluence of CHL and SGHL (SGL) to form the biceps pulley or sling at the entrance of the intertubercular groove. (**A**) The superior aspect of the glenohumeral joint capsule is windowed to reveal the contribution of the CHL to the roof and the SGHL to the floor of the biceps pulley. (Based on Habermeyer P, Magosch P, Pritsch M, et al. Anterosuperior impingement of the shoulder as a result of pulley lesions: a prospective arthroscopic study. *J Shoulder Elbow Surg* 2004;13[1]:5.) Consecutive coronal oblique FS PD FSE images show the transition from the CHL and SGHL anteriorly (**B**).

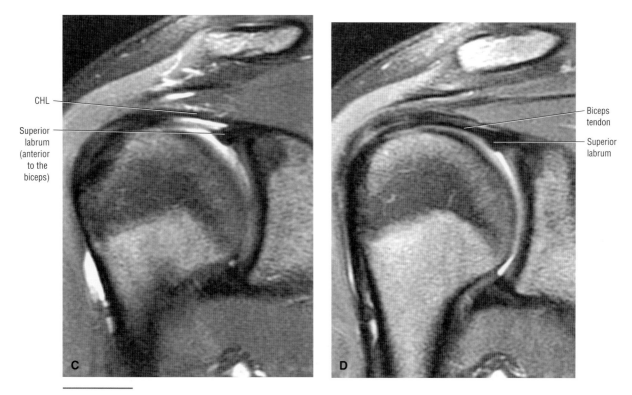

FIGURE 6.149 (*Continued*) To the CHL one image posteriorly (**C**) and to the intraarticular biceps one more image posterior (**D**). The CHL (which forms the roof of the biceps pulley) and the SGHL (which forms the floor of the biceps pulley) are visualized anterior to the biceps in their proximal course through the rotator cuff interval.

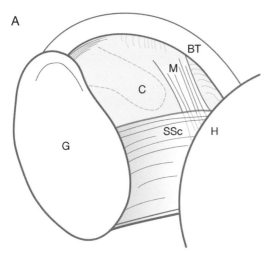

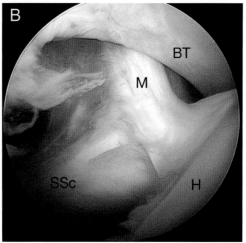

FIGURE 6.150 This drawing (**A**) and corresponding arthroscopic photo (**B**) represent the view of the anterior structures from a posterior viewing portal of a right shoulder. An axial schematic drawing (**C**) further clarifies the normal anatomy. The medial sling (M) of the biceps tendon (BT) inserts onto the lesser tuberosity of the humerus (H) adjacent to the superolateral margin of the subscapularis (SSc). C, coracoid; G, glenoid. (Reprinted from Burkhart S, Lo IK, Brady PC, Denard PJ. *The Cowboy's Companion: A Trail Guide for the Arthroscopic Shoulder Surgeon.* Philadelphia, PA: Lippincott Williams & Wilkins; 2012, with permission.)

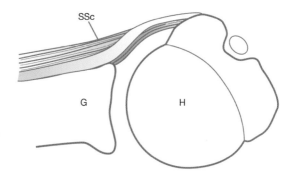

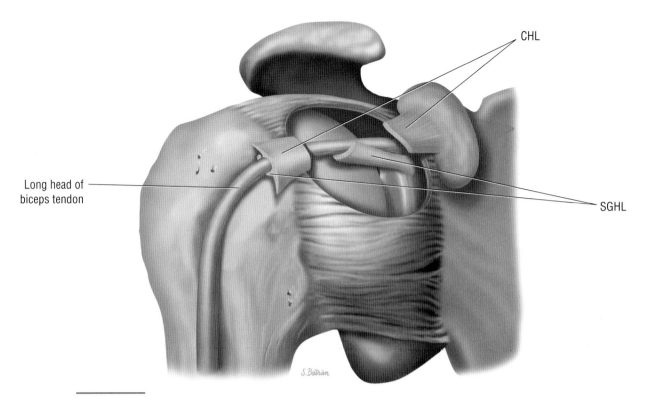

FIGURE 6.151   The rotator cuff interval, demonstrating the confluence of CHL and SGHL (SHL) to form the biceps pulley or sling at the entrance of the intertubercular groove. The superior aspect of the glenohumeral joint capsule is windowed to reveal the contribution of the CHL to the roof and the SGHL to the floor of the biceps pulley. (Based on Habermeyer P, Magosch P, Pritsch M, et al. Anterosuperior impingement of the shoulder as a result of pulley lesions: a prospective arthroscopic study. *J Shoulder Elbow Surg* 2004;13[1]:5).

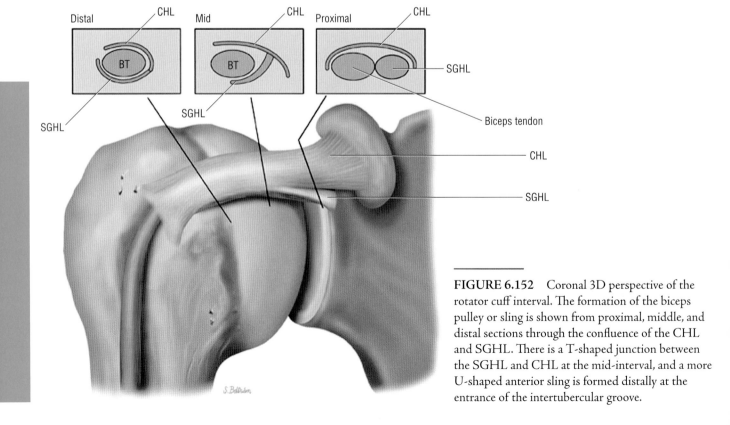

FIGURE 6.152   Coronal 3D perspective of the rotator cuff interval. The formation of the biceps pulley or sling is shown from proximal, middle, and distal sections through the confluence of the CHL and SGHL. There is a T-shaped junction between the SGHL and CHL at the mid-interval, and a more U-shaped anterior sling is formed distally at the entrance of the intertubercular groove.

- The SGHL can be seen between the biceps and subscapularis tendons.
  - The CHL bridges the gap between the supraspinatus and subscapularis tendons.
  - The SGHL courses lateral to the MGHL to contact the inferior surface of the CHL, forming the biceps pulley.

- In the distal portion of the rotator cuff interval, the anterior confluence of the CHL and SGHL form a U-shaped sling.[301]
  - The SGHL inserts onto the lesser tuberosity in the distal portion of the rotator cuff interval at the entrance of the intertubercular groove.

- The lateral band of the CHL inserts on both the greater tuberosity and on the anterior border of the supraspinatus.[380]

- The smaller medial portion crosses anteriorly, over the intraarticular biceps, to insert on the lesser tuberosity, the superior fibers of the subscapularis, and the transverse ligament.
  - Tears of the anterior supraspinatus may involve the lateral band of the CHL, whereas tears of the superior distal fibers of the subscapularis tendon may involve both the SGHL and the medial band of the CHL.

- The formation of the biceps pulley by the medial portion of the CHL and the SGHL and the superior fibers of the subscapularis prevents medial subluxations and dislocations by stabilizing the biceps tendon in a sling.

- The rotator cuff interval capsule provides stability, resisting inferior and posterior glenohumeral translation through the direct contribution of the CHL and secondarily by the negative pressure that it maintains in the glenohumeral joint.[301,380]

- The LHBT functions as an anterior stabilizer of the glenohumeral joint by increasing resistance to torsional forces in abduction and external rotation and by reducing stress on the IGHL.

- In the acute setting, a rotator interval tear associated with trauma may be the result of either extension of the anterior supraspinatus tearing to involve the lateral CHL or extension of the superior subscapularis tendon tearing to involve the SGHL and medial CHL.

- A pulley tear may occur initially as an isolated lesion prior to secondary involvement of the rotator cuff.[380]

- Approximately half of subscapularis tendon tears involve both the SGHL and CHL.

- In chronic lesions, the rotator interval capsule and ligaments may become thickened and scarred.

- Intermediate signal intensity is visualized with synovial hypertrophy or granulation tissue.

- There is an association between adhesive capsulitis, synovitis of the axillary pouch, subscapularis recess, and rotator interval.

- In shoulders with multidirectional instability, the rotator interval may be larger than would normally be found.

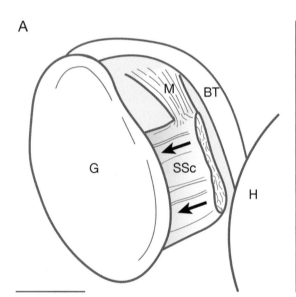

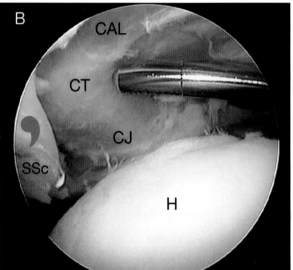

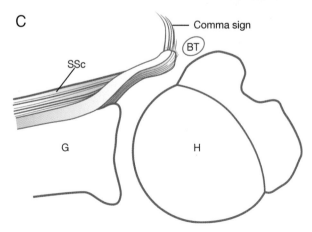

FIGURE 6.153 This drawing (**A**) and corresponding arthroscopic photo (**B**) represent a complete subscapularis tendon (SSc) tear with medial retraction (*black arrows*) almost to the level of the glenoid (G) in association with a medially dislocated biceps tendon (BT). An axial projection is also shown in (**C**). In this situation, the comma sign (*blue comma symbol*) leads to the superolateral border of the subscapularis tendon. CAL, coracoacromial ligament; CJ, conjoined tendon; CT, coracoid tip; G, humerus; M, medial sling. (Reprinted from Burkhart S, Lo IK, Brady PC, Denard PJ. *The Cowboy's Companion: A Trail Guide for the Arthroscopic Shoulder Surgeon.* Philadelphia, PA: Lippincott Williams & Wilkins; 2012, with permission.)

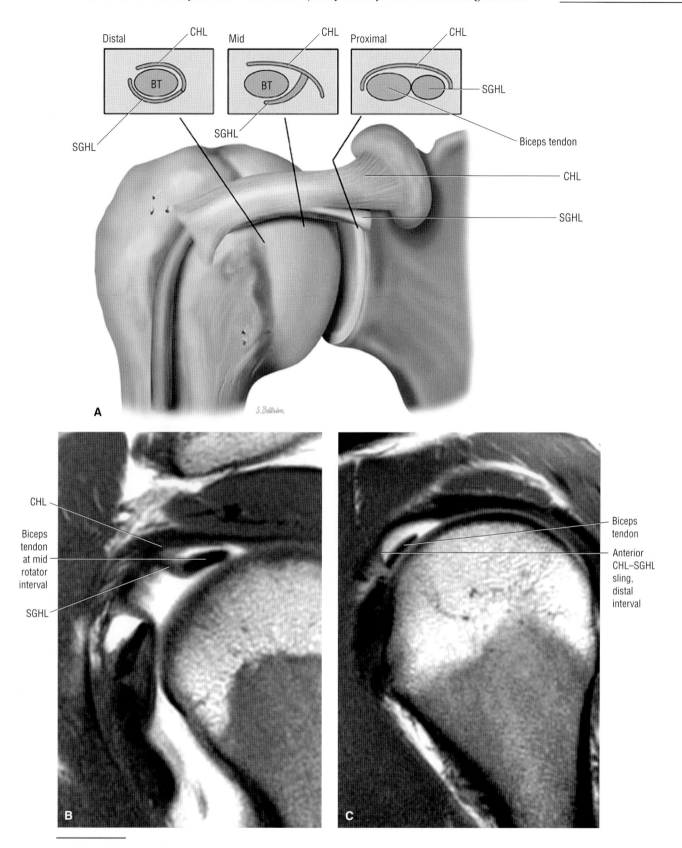

FIGURE 6.154 (**A**) Coronal 3D perspective of the rotator cuff interval. The formation of the biceps pulley or sling is shown from proximal, middle, and distal sections through the confluence of the CHL and SGHL. There is a T-shaped junction between the SGHL and CHL at the mid-interval, and a more U-shaped anterior sling is formed distally at the entrance of the intertubercular groove. A perpendicular junction between the SGHL and CHL medial to the formation of the more U-shaped biceps pulley developed in the distal portion of the rotator cuff interval. Corresponding sagittal PD FSE MR arthrograms, mid-interval (**B**) and distal interval (**C**).

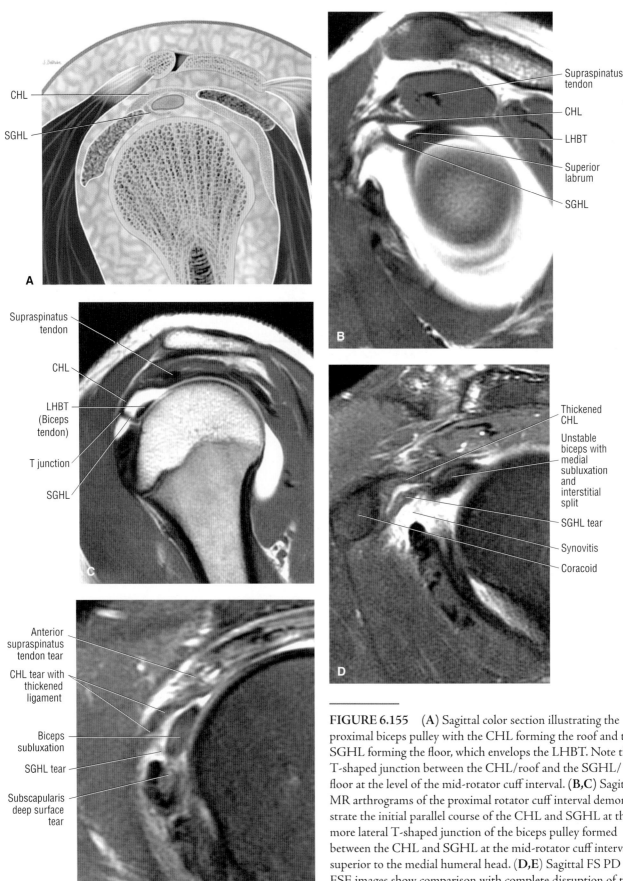

FIGURE 6.155 **(A)** Sagittal color section illustrating the proximal biceps pulley with the CHL forming the roof and the SGHL forming the floor, which envelops the LHBT. Note the T-shaped junction between the CHL/roof and the SGHL/floor at the level of the mid-rotator cuff interval. **(B,C)** Sagittal MR arthrograms of the proximal rotator cuff interval demonstrate the initial parallel course of the CHL and SGHL at the more lateral T-shaped junction of the biceps pulley formed between the CHL and SGHL at the mid-rotator cuff interval, superior to the medial humeral head. **(D,E)** Sagittal FS PD FSE images show comparison with complete disruption of the biceps pulley with abnormal laxity and thickening of the CHL–SGHL complex medially **(D)** and complete absence of the SGHL at the mid-rotator cuff interval in the expected location of the T junction between the CHL and SGHL **(E)**.

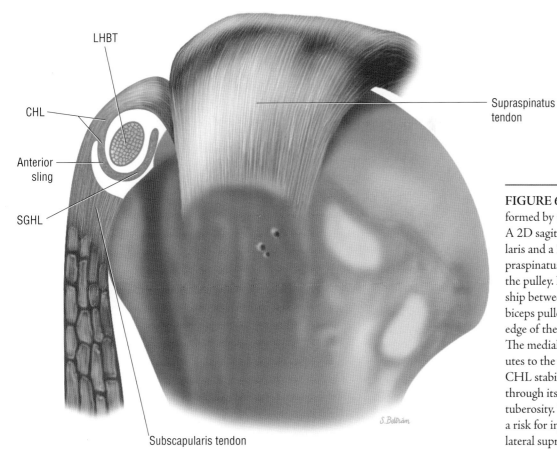

LHBT

CHL

Anterior sling

SGHL

Subscapularis tendon

Supraspinatus tendon

FIGURE 6.156 Biceps pulley formed by the CHL and SGHL. A 2D sagittal section of the subscapularis and a 3D perspective of the supraspinatus are shown in proximity to the pulley. Note the intimate relationship between the CHL (roof of the biceps pulley) and the anterior leading edge of the supraspinatus tendon. The medial CHL primarily contributes to the pulley, whereas the lateral CHL stabilizes the biceps (LHBT) through its attachment to the greater tuberosity. These lateral fibers are at a risk for injury with anterior and far lateral supraspinatus tears.

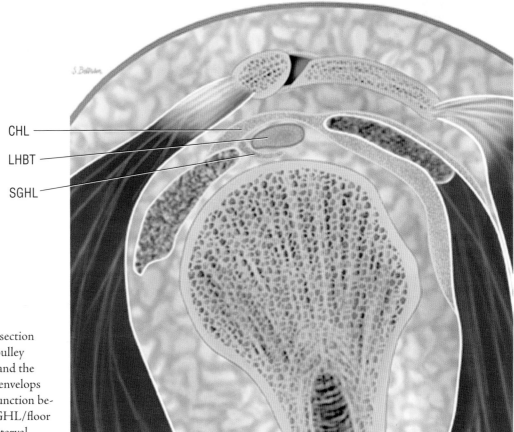

CHL

LHBT

SGHL

FIGURE 6.157 Sagittal color section illustrating the proximal biceps pulley with the CHL forming the roof and the SGHL forming the floor, which envelops the LHBT. Note the T-shaped junction between the CHL/roof and the SGHL/floor at the level of mid-rotator cuff interval.

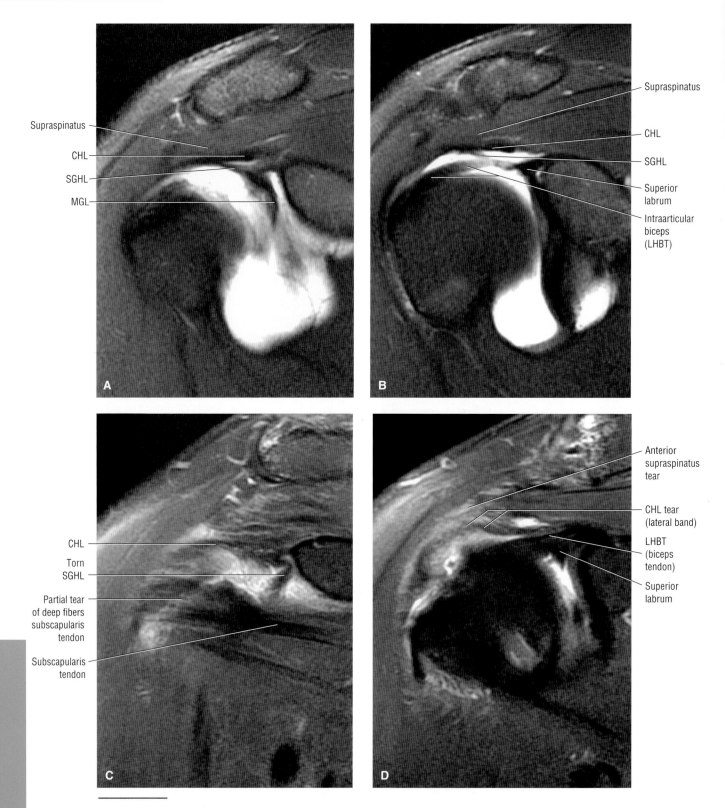

Supraspinatus

CHL

SGHL

MGL

Supraspinatus

CHL

SGHL

Superior
labrum

Intraarticular
biceps
(LHBT)

CHL

Torn
SGHL

Partial tear
of deep fibers
subscapularis
tendon

Subscapularis
tendon

Anterior
supraspinatus
tear

CHL tear
(lateral band)

LHBT
(biceps
tendon)

Superior
labrum

FIGURE 6.158 (**A**) The proximity of the CHL to the anterior border of the supraspinatus and its relationship to the SGHL and MGHL (MGL) are shown on this anterior coronal MR arthrogram. (**B**) CHL, SGHL, and intraarticular biceps are visualized on one image posterior to (**A**). (**C**) Coronal FS PD FSE image shows comparison in a separate case with a torn and medially retracted SGHL in the rotator cuff interval in a case of biceps instability and medial subluxation. (**D**) Coronal FS PD FSE image demonstrates discontinuity of the CHL in conjunction with an anterior supraspinatus.

Biceps Pulley Lesions

Key Concepts

- Biceps pulley lesions are associated with tearing of the deep fibers of the distal subscapularis and articular surface of the distal supraspinatus tendon.

- The medially dislocated biceps tendon is displaced either intraarticularly, between the coracohumeral ligament and the subscapularis tendon, or extra-articularly.

- Intraarticular dislocation is associated with disruption of both the lesser tuberosity attachment of the subscapularis tendon and the SGHL–CHL complex.

- Extra-articular subluxation is associated with an anterolateral supraspinatus tendon tear with extension into the lateral coracohumeral ligament.

- A biceps pulley lesion is an interruption of the surrounding sheath of the LHBT with an intact rotator cuff.

- The SGHL and the CHL blend together at the entrance of the sulcus to form the U-shaped section of the biceps pulley or sling.

- Biceps tendon instability is associated with abnormalities of the rotator cuff (the subscapularis and supraspinatus components).[31]

- The superior insertion fibers of the subscapularis tendon are intimately associated with the proximal opening to the bicipital groove.

- The medial wall of the bicipital sheath is composed of the SGHL–medial CHL complex.

- Tears of this complex may occur with or without associated tearing of the distal subscapularis tendon fibers and result in biceps tendon subluxation.
    - Occult bicipital instability represents the hidden lesion.[619]

- The CHL normally inserts with the fibers of the subscapularis and traverses the intertubercular groove to contribute to the lateral aspect of the biceps sheath and supraspinatus.

- The medial CHL prevents medial subluxation of the biceps and contributes directly to the roof and anterior superior aspect of the biceps tendon.

- The lateral CHL attaches more posteriorly to the greater tuberosity.

- The arthroscopic findings of biceps pulley lesions are based on a combination of findings in lesions of the subscapularis tendon, the SGHL–medial CHL complex, and the lateral CHL.

Habermayer Classification of Biceps Pulley Lesions[76,199]

- Type 1 Pulley Lesion

  - Restricted or limited to an isolated surface of the pulley without involvement of the supraspinatus or subscapularis tendons

- Type 2 Pulley Lesion

  - Involves articular-side tearing of the supraspinatus tendon in association with pulley failure and mild medial subluxation of the biceps tendon

- Type 3 Pulley Lesion

  - Demonstrates partial deep surface tearing of distal subscapularis tendon fibers

  - The biceps undergoes medial subluxation, partially extending beyond the containment of the CHL–SGHL sling.

- Type 4 Pulley Lesion

  - Represents a dislocation of the biceps tendon

  - There is partial tearing of both the supraspinatus and subscapularis tendons in association with the medially displaced biceps tendon, which is located anterior to the lesser tuberosity.

  - The supraspinatus and subscapularis tears are more extensive than those observed in types 2 and 3 lesions, respectively.

- Although this classification addresses only partial tears of the supraspinatus and subscapularis tendons, complete tears are also associated with biceps subluxations and dislocations.

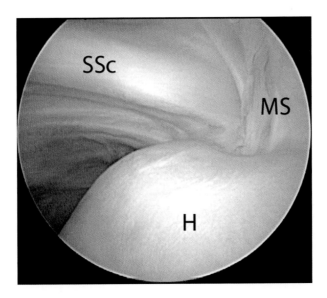

FIGURE 6.159 Right shoulder, posterior viewing portal with a 70° arthroscope, demonstrates a normal subscapularis tendon. Note: A normal subscapularis tendon does not display any linear longitudinal splits. H, humerus; MS, medial sling of the bicep tendon; SSc, subscapularis tendon. (Reprinted from Burkhart S, Lo IK, Brady PC, Denard PJ. *The Cowboy's Companion: A Trail Guide for the Arthroscopic Shoulder Surgeon.* Philadelphia, PA: Lippincott Williams & Wilkins; 2012, with permission.)

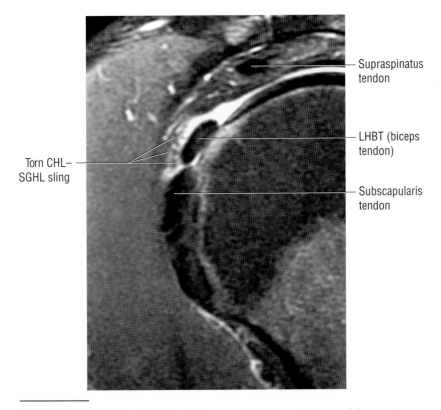

FIGURE 6.160 Type 1 (isolated) biceps pulley lesion with tear of the anterior CHL–SGHL sling shown on a sagittal FS PD FSE image. The articular surface of the supraspinatus and deep fibers of the subscapularis are intact.

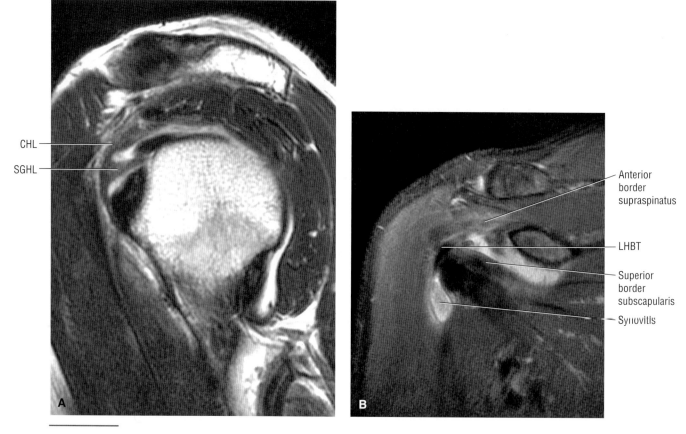

FIGURE 6.161 Thickened SGHL and CHL components of the biceps pulley seen at the mid-rotator interval on sagittal T2 FSE (**A**) and coronal FS PD FSE (**B**) images.

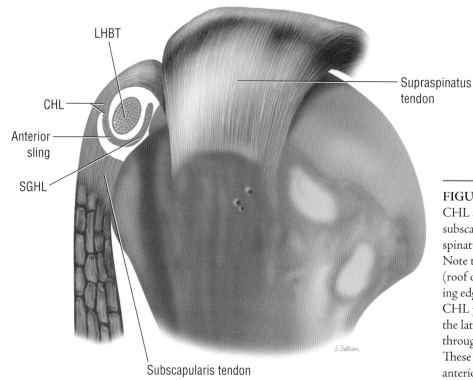

FIGURE 6.162 Biceps pulley formed by the CHL and SGHL. A 2D sagittal section of the subscapularis and a 3D perspective of the supraspinatus are shown in proximity to the pulley. Note the intimate relationship between the CHL (roof of the biceps pulley) and the anterior leading edge of the supraspinatus tendon. The medial CHL primarily contributes to the pulley, whereas the lateral CHL stabilizes the biceps (LHBT) through its attachment to the greater tuberosity. These lateral fibers are at a risk for injury with anterior and far lateral supraspinatus tears.

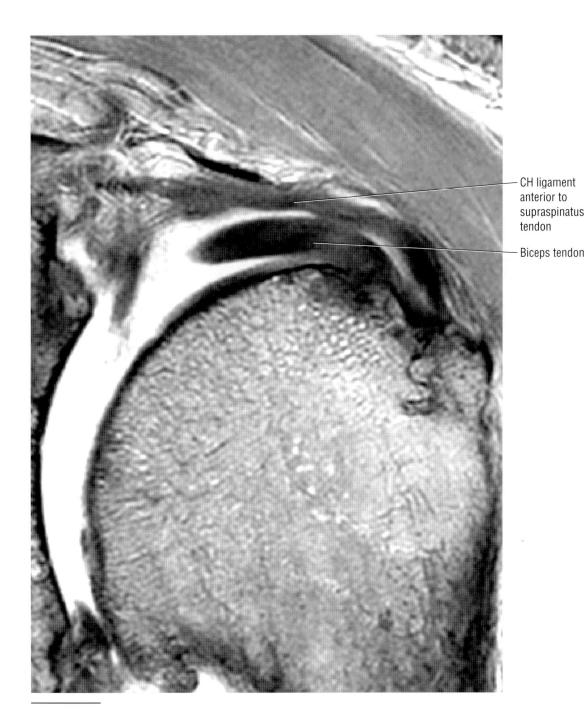

CH ligament anterior to supraspinatus tendon

Biceps tendon

FIGURE 6.163 The coracohumeral ligament viewed anterior to the supraspinatus in the coronal plane represents the deeper extension of this ligament, which forms the rotator cable along the articular surface of the supraspinatus and infraspinatus tendons. Coronal T1 MR arthrogram image.

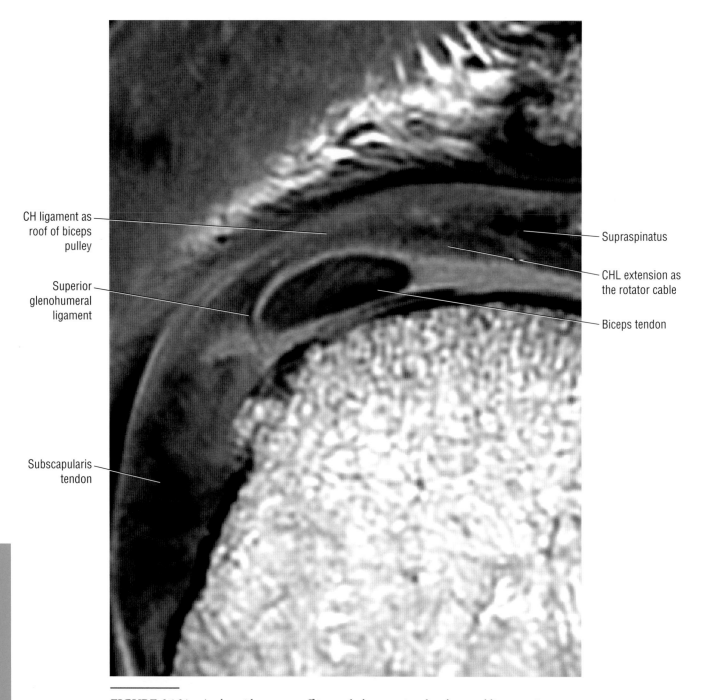

FIGURE 6.164   At the mid-rotator cuff interval, the superior glenohumeral ligament is perpendicular to the coracohumeral ligament. The coracohumeral ligament forms the roof over the biceps tendon. There are two extensions of the CH ligament. The deeper more substantial extension courses along the articular surface of the supraspinatus and infraspinatus tendons and constitutes the rotator cuff cable.

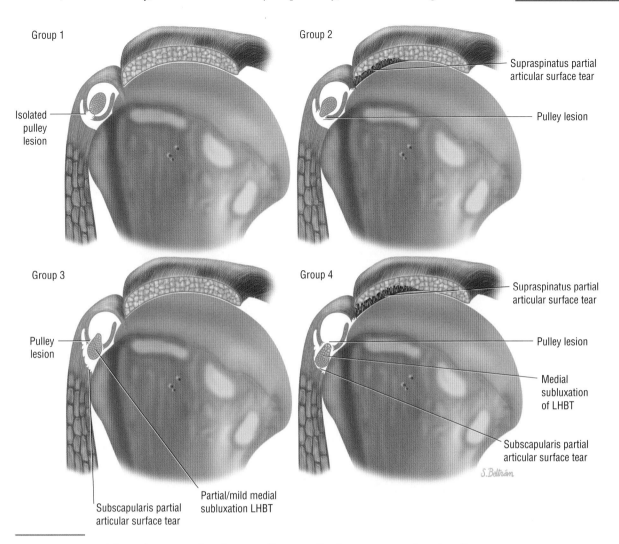

FIGURE 6.165 The Habermeyer classification of biceps pulley lesions groups them into four subtypes. Type 1 lesions are isolated pulley lesions with an intact supraspinatus and subscapularis tendon. Type 2 represents a pulley lesion and a partial articular surface supraspinatus tendon tear. Type 3 is a pulley lesion with partial medial subluxation of the biceps tendon associated with a partial articular or deep surface tear of the superior distal fibers of the subscapularis tendon. Type 4 combines the pulley lesion with partial articular surface tears of both the supraspinatus and subscapularis tendons. There is frank medial subluxation of the LHBT as the contributions of the CHL (roof of the sling) and SGHL (floor of the sling) are affected.

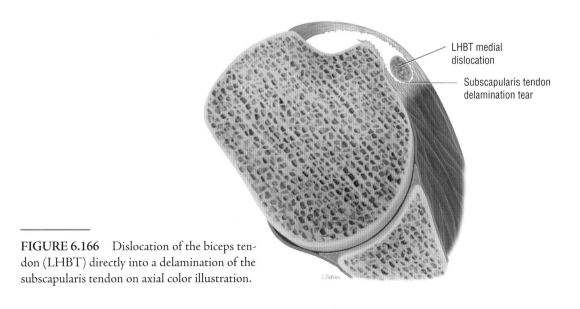

FIGURE 6.166 Dislocation of the biceps tendon (LHBT) directly into a delamination of the subscapularis tendon on axial color illustration.

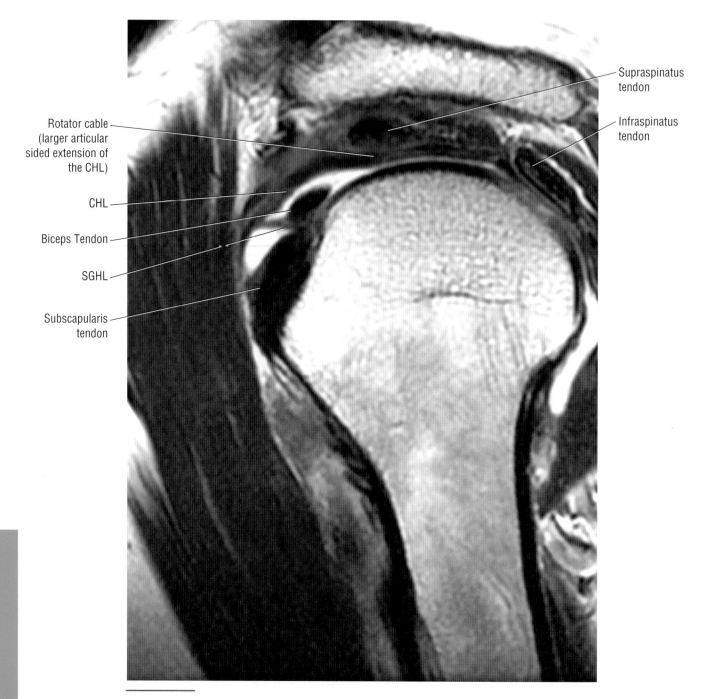

FIGURE 6.167   Normal coracohumeral ligament with deep cable extension along the articular surface of the supraspinatus. The superior glenohumeral ligament (SGHL) is perpendicular to the CHL at the midinterval.

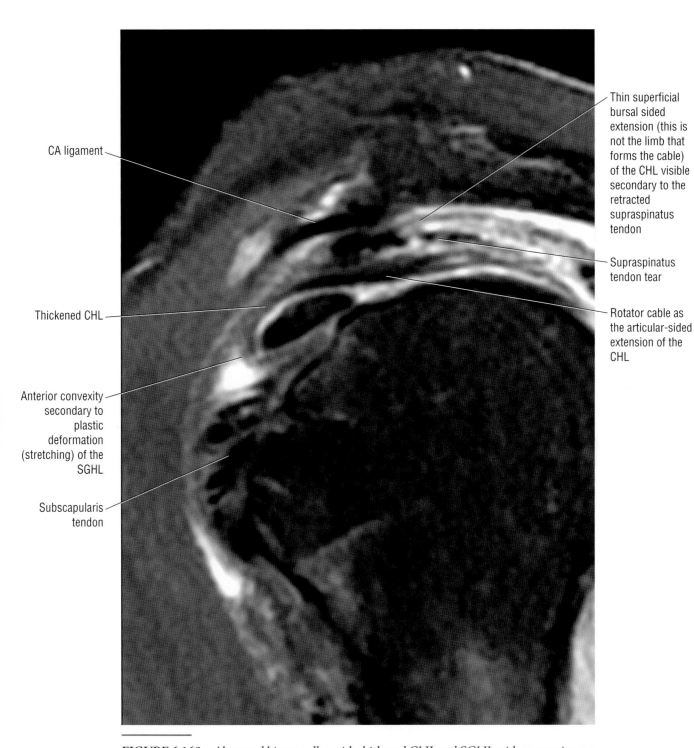

CA ligament

Thickened CHL

Anterior convexity secondary to plastic deformation (stretching) of the SGHL

Subscapularis tendon

Thin superficial bursal sided extension (this is not the limb that forms the cable) of the CHL visible secondary to the retracted supraspinatus tendon

Supraspinatus tendon tear

Rotator cable as the articular-sided extension of the CHL

FIGURE 6.168   Abnormal biceps pulley with thickened CHL and SGHL with an anterior convex or bowing contour of the deformed SGHL. This represents a plastic deformation or stretching of the pulley without rupture.

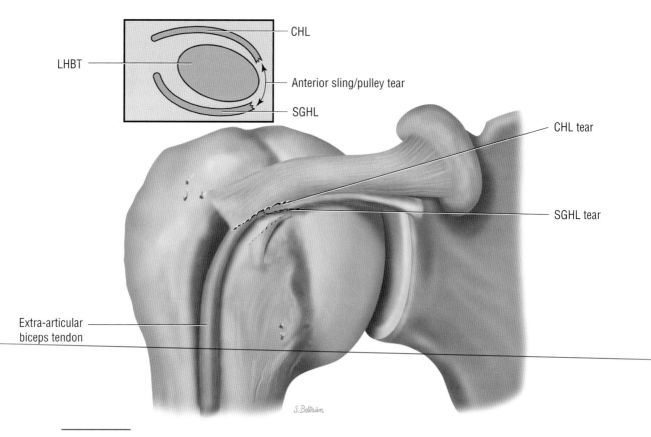

FIGURE 6.169   A type 1 biceps pulley lesion with a torn anterior CHL–SGHL sling. The biceps tendon (LHBT), although unstable, has not undergone subluxation.

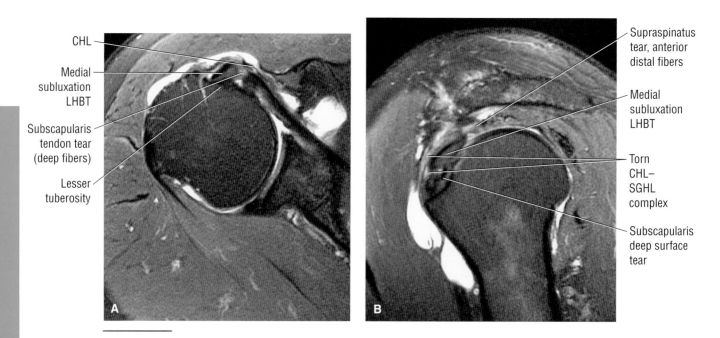

FIGURE 6.170   A type 4 biceps pulley disruption with biceps tendon medial subluxation anterior to the lesser tuberosity is shown on an axial FS PD FSE image (**A**) and sagittal FS PD FSE image from lateral to medial (**B**). Associated tears of both the supraspinatus and subscapularis are present.

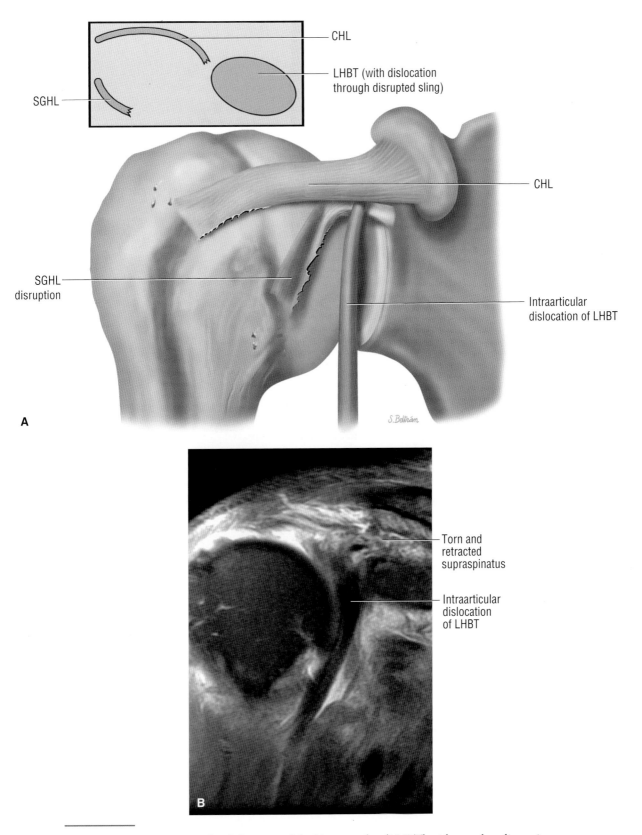

FIGURE 6.171 Intraarticular dislocation of the biceps tendon (LHBT) with complete disruption of the SGHL on a coronal color illustration (**A**) and on coronal (**B**) FS PD FSE images. Both the insertion of the subscapularis tendon and the SGHL component of the CHL–SGHL complex are disrupted.

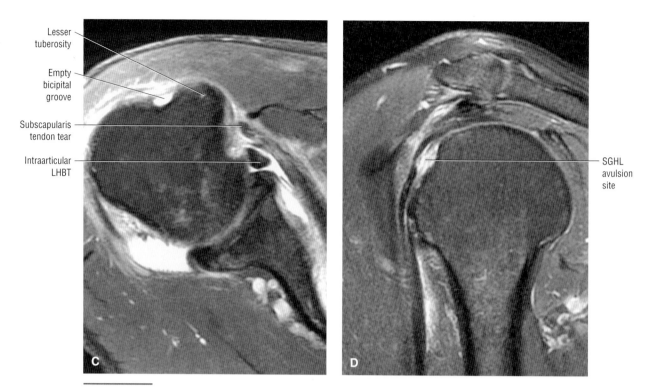

Lesser tuberosity

Empty bicipital groove

Subscapularis tendon tear

Intraarticular LHBT

SGHL avulsion site

FIGURE 6.171 (*Continued*) Intraarticular dislocation of the biceps tendon (LHBT) with complete disruption of the SGHL (**C**) FS PD FSE image. Both the insertion of the subscapularis tendon and the SGHL component of the CHL–SGHL complex are disrupted. (**D**) Sagittal FS PD FSE image in a separate case demonstrates avulsion of the SGHL attachment associated with an intraarticular biceps tendon dislocation.

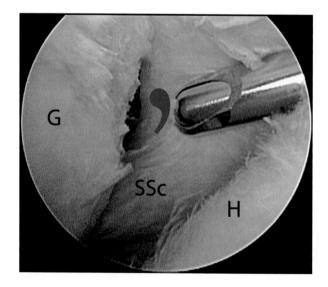

FIGURE 6.172 Right shoulder, posterior viewing portal. In the setting of a retracted subscapularis tear, the medial sling tears away from the bone with the subscapularis tendon. The medial sling forms a distinctive comma-shaped arc of soft tissue (*blue comma shape*) at the superolateral corner of the subscapularis. As demonstrated in this photo, the comma sign serves as a landmark for locating a retracted subscapularis tendon. G, glenoid; H, humeral head, SSc, subscapularis tendon. (Reprinted from Burkhart S, Lo IK, Brady PC, Denard PJ. *The Cowboy's Companion: A Trail Guide for the Arthroscopic Shoulder Surgeon.* Philadelphia, PA: Lippincott Williams & Wilkins; 2012, with permission.)

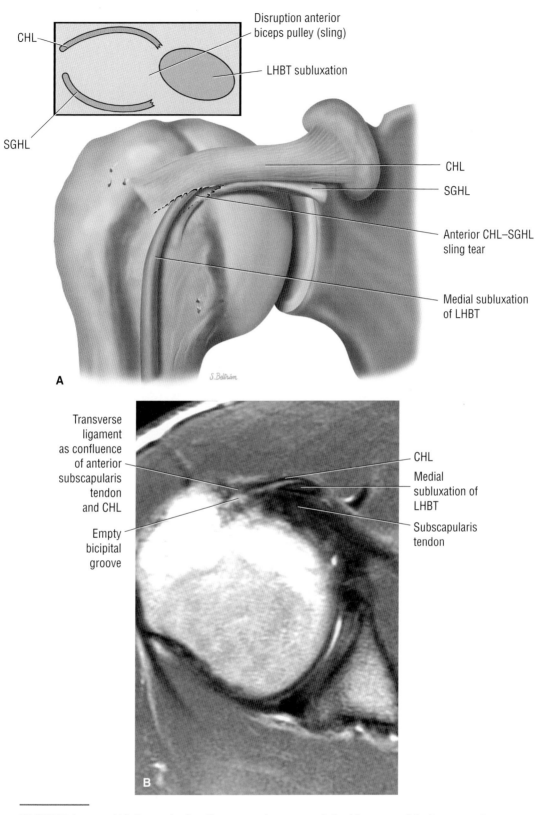

FIGURE 6.173 (**A**) Coronal color illustration showing medial subluxation of the biceps tendon anterior to the subscapularis tendon and deep to the CHL. This pathology is made possible by disruption of the anterior sling with intact lateral fibers of the CHL. The medial fibers of the CHL that directly contribute to the CHL–SGHL complex are torn in conjunction with the SGHL. (**B**) Axial PD FSE image showing medial subluxation of the biceps anterior to the subscapularis tendon and deep to the CHL.

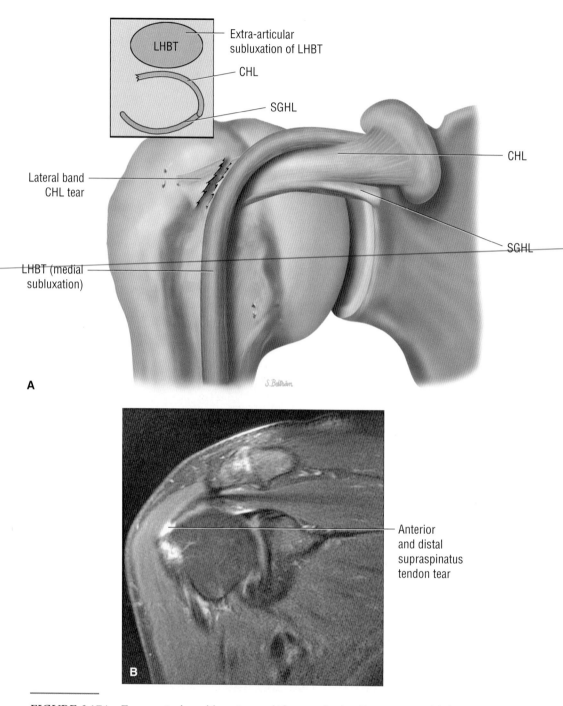

FIGURE 6.174   Extra-articular subluxation on (**A**) coronal color illustration and (**B**) coronal FS PD FSE image. The extra-articular subluxation is seen with the biceps perched anterior to the lesser tuberosity and anterior to both the coracohumeral ligament and the subscapularis tendon. The lateral band of the coracohumeral ligament is torn as a result of the anterior extension from an anterior leading edge supraspinatus tear. Since the medial fibers of the coracohumeral ligament and subscapularis tendon are intact, the biceps dislocates anterior to the intact subscapularis tendon.

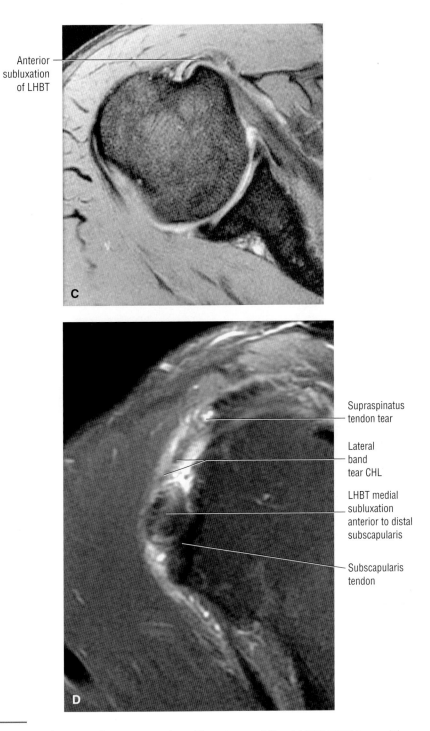

FIGURE 6.174 (*Continued*) Extra-articular subluxation on (**C**) axial T2* GRE image. The extra-articular subluxation is seen with the biceps perched anterior to the lesser tuberosity and anterior to both the coracohumeral ligament and the subscapularis tendon. The lateral band of the coracohumeral is torn as a result of the anterior extension from an anterior supraspinatus tear. (**D**) Sagittal FS PD FSE image demonstrates disruption of the lateral fibers of the coracohumeral ligament in a separate case.

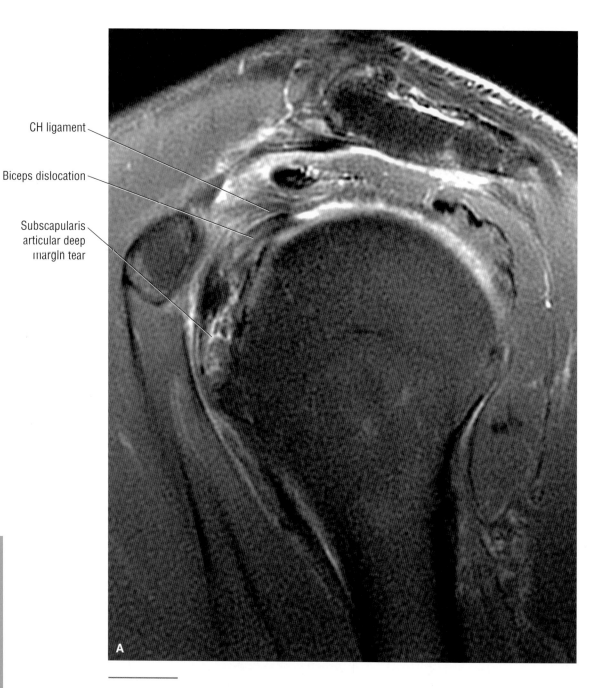

CH ligament

Biceps dislocation

Subscapularis
articular deep
margin tear

FIGURE 6.175 Ruptured biceps pulley with torn SGHL and thickened CH ligament. In the sagittal plane, the biceps will be displaced inferiorly, while in the axial plane, it will be dislocated medially in the presence of a torn pulley. The dislocated biceps tendon is flattened and deformed with tendinosis. (**A**) Sagittal FS PD image.

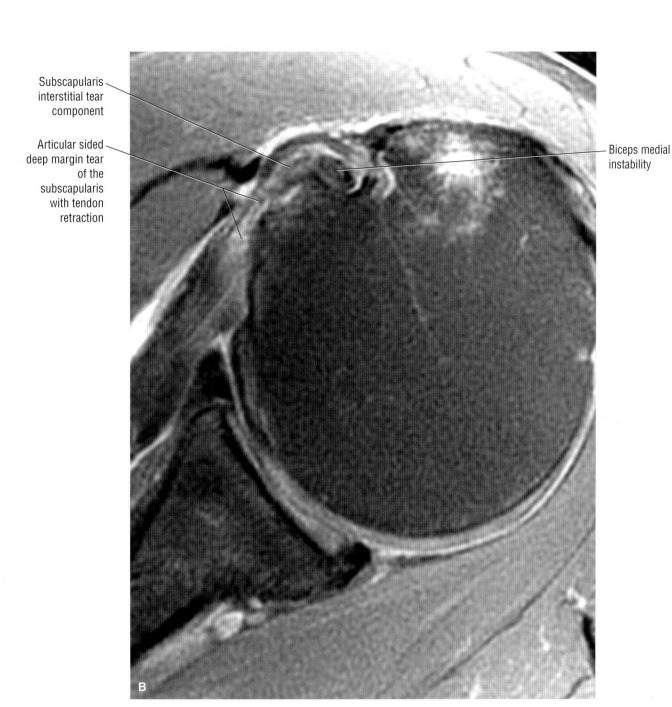

FIGURE 6.175   (*Continued*) (**B**) Axial FS PD. There is interstitial and articular-sided tear of the subscapularis tendon from its footprint.

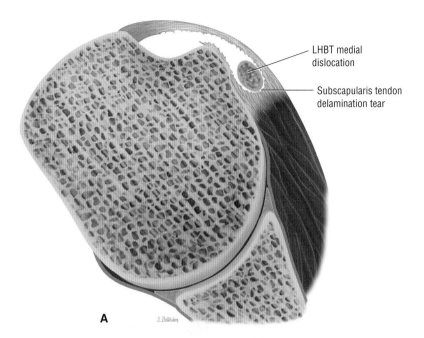

LHBT medial
dislocation

Subscapularis tendon
delamination tear

A

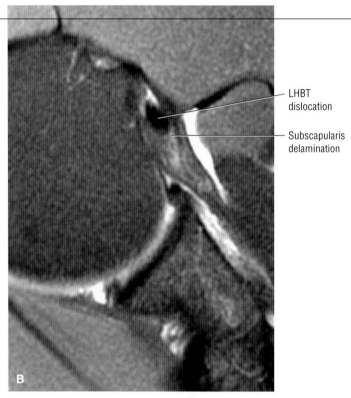

LHBT
dislocation

Subscapularis
delamination

B

FIGURE 6.176   Dislocation of the biceps tendon (LHBT) directly
into a delamination of the subscapularis tendon on (**A**) axial color
illustration and (**B**) axial FS PD FSE image. The pulley is in direct
contact with the insertion of the subscapularis tendon. The superior
glenohumeral ligament forms a semicircular anterior support for the
lateral part of the intraarticular biceps tendon. The pulley must be
torn if the biceps tendon is medial to the groove.

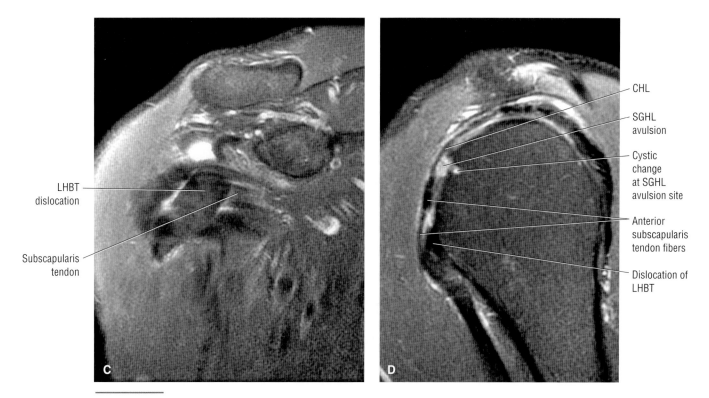

FIGURE 6.176 (*Continued*) Dislocation of the biceps tendon (LHBT) directly into a delamination of the subscapularis tendon on (**C**) coronal FS PD FSE image and (**D**) sagittal FS PD FSE image. The subscapularis tendon is visualized imbedded within the substance of the subscapularis tendon. An associated SGHL tear with reactive osseous erosion is shown in the sagittal plane (**D**).

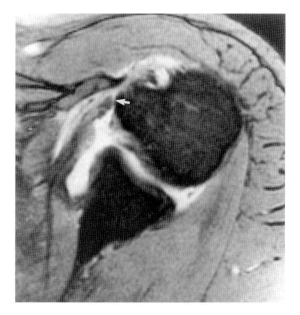

FIGURE 6.177 A T2*-weighted axial image illustrates a subscapularis tendon tear with proximal retraction (*arrow*) to the level of the lesser tuberosity. There is free communication of fluid between the glenohumeral joint subscapularis bursa and the subcoracoid bursa anterior to the subscapularis tendon. The normal subscapularis tendon inserts onto the lesser tuberosity anterior to the superior glenohumeral ligament. Even if the biceps is located within the groove, the pulley will appear abnormal (thickened) on sagittal images in the presence of subscapularis tendon pathology.

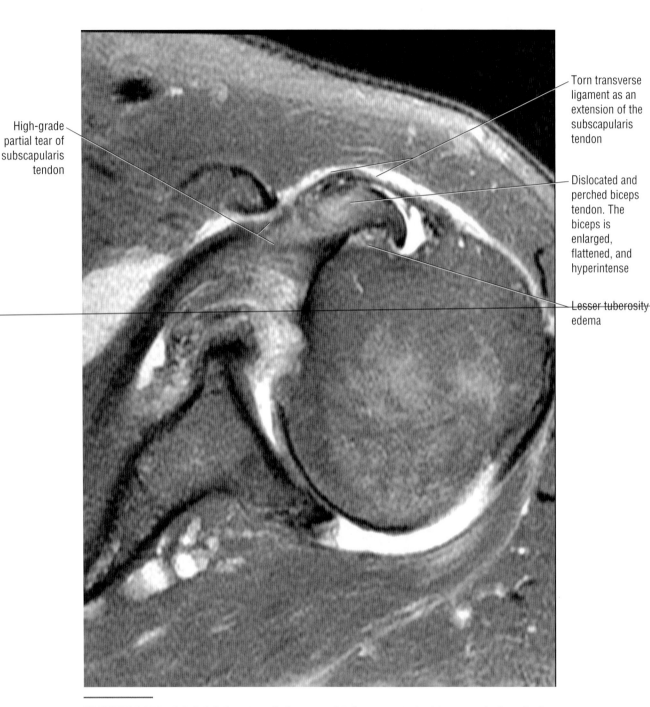

High-grade
partial tear of
subscapularis
tendon

Torn transverse
ligament as an
extension of the
subscapularis
tendon

Dislocated and
perched biceps
tendon. The
biceps is
enlarged,
flattened, and
hyperintense

Lesser tuberosity
edema

FIGURE 6.178   Medial dislocation of a hypertrophied extra-articular biceps perched on the lesser tuberosity. There is a partial tear of the subscapularis tendon involving interstitial and deep articular fibers. The normally wider proximal subscapularis footprint has lost at least 50% of its tendon insertion as a result of retracted fibers.

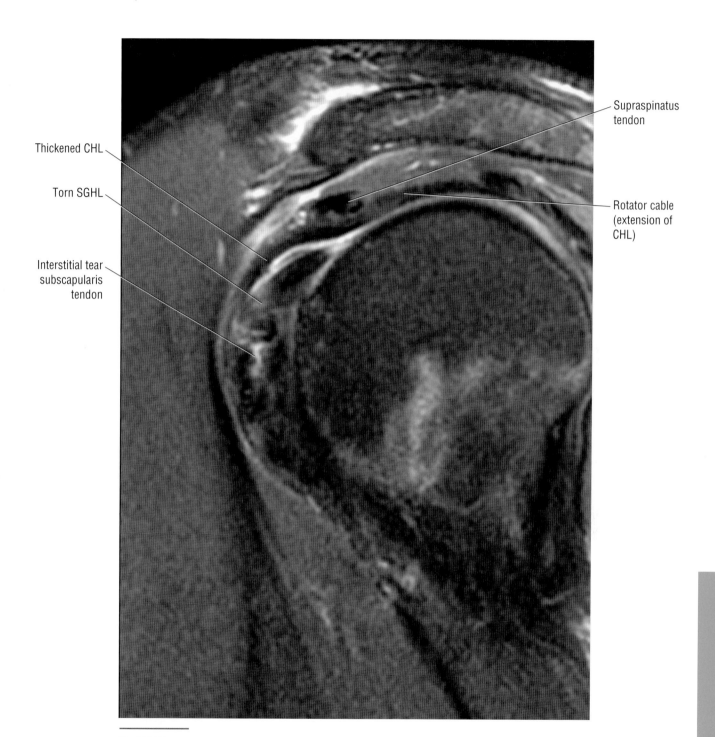

FIGURE 6.179   Interstitial longitudinal tears of the subscapularis tendon are associated with a torn biceps pulley. The coracohumeral ligament is thickened as the roof of the pulley. The superior glenohumeral ligament is torn and the biceps tendon is displaced inferiorly. The normal anterior convexity of the SGHL is absent.

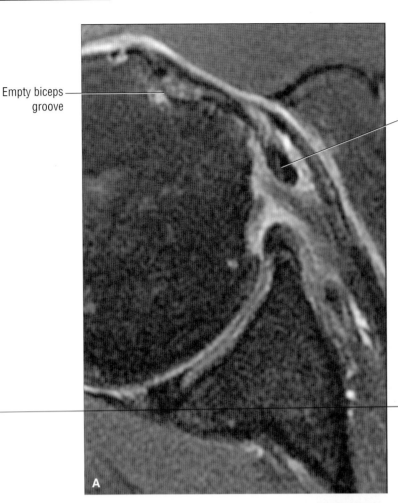

Empty biceps groove

Medial dislocation of biceps tendon into interstitial tear of the subscapularis

A

FIGURE 6.180   (**A**) Empty biceps groove as a result of medial dislocation of the biceps into an interstitial tear of the subscapularis.

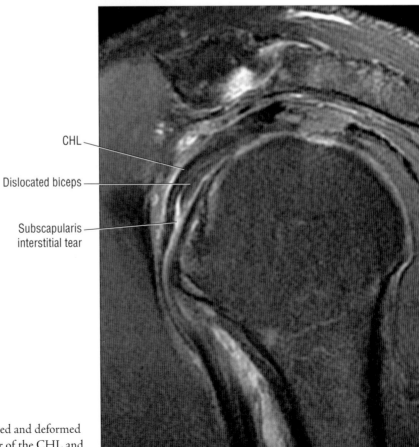

CHL

Dislocated biceps

Subscapularis interstitial tear

B

FIGURE 6.180   (*Continued*) (**B**) Flattened and deformed dislocated biceps tendon between the layer of the CHL and the torn subscapularis.

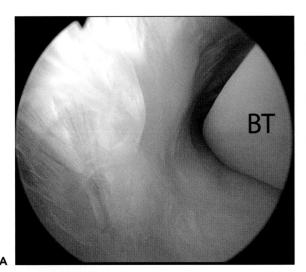

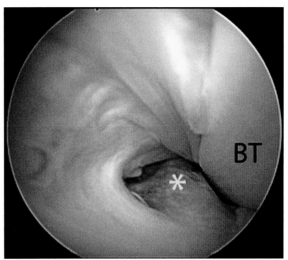

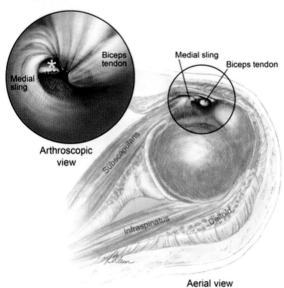

Arthroscopic view

Aerial view

FIGURE 6.181 (**A**) Right shoulder, posterior viewing portal with a 70° arthroscope, shows approximately 2.5cm of the floor and sidewalls of the bicipital groove in this normal right shoulder. (**B**) In a different right shoulder, there is disruption in the medial sidewall with a bare lesser tuberosity footprint distally. (**C**) Depiction of a disrupted medial sidewall, indicating a mid to distal tendon tear of the subscapularis. asterisk, disrupted medial sidewall; BT, biceps tendon. The insertion of subscapularis tendon is directly medial to the insertion of the SGHL-CHL complex. The superior glenohumeral and coracohumeral ligaments and the subscapularis tendon all insert by means of interdigitating fibers. (Reprinted from Burkhart S, Lo IK, Brady PC, Denard PJ. *The Cowboy's Companion: A Trail Guide for the Arthroscopic Shoulder Surgeon*. Philadelphia, PA: Lippincott Williams & Wilkins; 2012, with permission.)

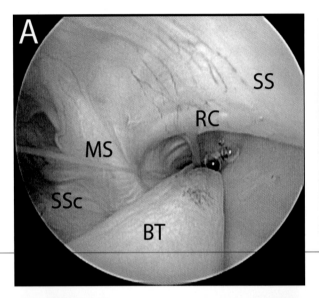

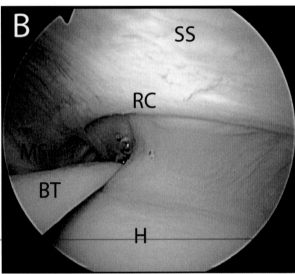

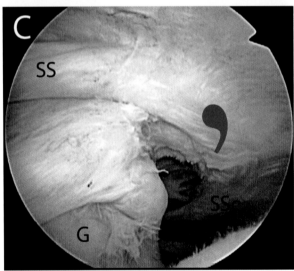

FIGURE 6.182 Right shoulder, posterior viewing portal, demonstrating the connection between the subscapularis (SSc) and the supraspinatus (SS) via the medial sling (MS). (**A**) The rotator cable (RC) of the rotator cuff merges with the medial sling anteriorly. As such, when the medial sling detaches during a subscapularis tear, the comma sign may be followed to locate the anterolateral corner of the supraspinatus tendon. (**B**) A profile view of the rotator cable further shows this constant relationship. (**C**) In the case of a massive contracted rotator cuff tear, the relationship between the subscapularis and the supraspinatus is maintained and the comma sign (*blue comma symbol*) can be used to identify the anterolateral supraspinatus tendon. BT, biceps tendon; G, glenoid; H, humerus. (Reprinted from Burkhart S, Lo IK, Brady PC, Denard PJ. *The Cowboy's Companion: A Trail Guide for the Arthroscopic Shoulder Surgeon*. Philadelphia, PA: Lippincott Williams & Wilkins; 2012, with permission.)

Management of Biceps Pulley Lesions

- Type 1 lesions may require a suture repair of the lax pulley.

- Treatment of type 2 lesions involves débridement of the supraspinatus with a transtendon repair.

- Subscapularis and biceps tendon stabilizations are performed in a type 3 pulley lesion.

- Type 4 biceps pulley lesions are managed by both the subscapularis and supraspinatus tendons plus a biceps tenodesis/tenotomy.

Classification of Biceps Tendon Instability

- Biceps tendon instability can be classified as either intraarticular dislocation (between the coracohumeral ligament and the subscapularis tendon) or extra-articular dislocations.[380]
  - Intraarticular dislocation of the LHBT with the biceps displaced medially and anterior to the glenohumeral joint space occurs in association with disruption of both the insertion of the subscapularis tendon and the SGHL–medial CHL complex.
    - Disruption of the SGHL–medial CHL complex with an intact lateral band of the coracohumeral ligament is associated with biceps subluxation anterior to the subscapularis but deep to the lateral band.
  - Extra-articular subluxation exists when there is an anterolateral supraspinatus tendon tear with extension into the lateral coracohumeral ligament. This permits the biceps tendon to subluxate in a medial direction (anterior to the lesser tuberosity), superficial to both the coracohumeral ligament and subscapularis tendon.
    - Delamination of the deep surface of the subscapularis produces injury to the SGHL–medial CHL complex. The biceps tendon is subluxated directly into the substance of the subscapularis tendon at the location of the delamination tear.

- An isolated subscapularis tendon tear without disruption of the biceps pulley may demonstrate a normal position of the biceps tendon in the groove without subluxation or dislocation.

- The pulley ligaments may become thickened and scarred with plastic deformation of the medial portion of the ligamentous biceps sling (SGHL–medial CHL complex).

Anterosuperior Impingement

Key Concepts

- Anterosuperior impingement is associated with both a tear of the biceps pulley and involvement of the deep subscapularis tendon.
  - A partial articular-side supraspinatus tendon tear may coexist.

- Anterosuperior labral tearing exists with decentralization of the humeral head occurring with adduction and internal rotation.

- Anterosuperior impingement (ASI) represents an internal impingement developing as a result of pulley lesions, including partial tears of the subscapularis and supraspinatus tendons.[199]

- The progressive lesions of the biceps pulley lead to instability of the biceps, which in turn results in an increased passive anterior translation and superior ascent of the humeral head, leading to the development of ASI.

- A partial articular-side subscapularis and supraspinatus tendon tear further contributes to the condition of ASI.

- Impingement of the biceps pulley occurs at the undersurface of the reflection formed by the confluence of the CHL and SGHL.

- In horizontal adduction and internal rotation of the arm, both the pulley and subscapularis tendon impinge against the anterosuperior aspect of the glenoid rim.

- The probability of ASI increases with subscapularis tendon involvement and secondarily with supraspinatus tearing.

- The addition of a partial articular-side tear or a lesion of the deep subscapularis to an existing pulley lesion is required for the development of ASI.

- The frequency of an anterosuperior labral lesion as part of ASI is greater with the involvement of the biceps pulley, subscapularis, and supraspinatus.

- Normally, the LHBT is an anterior stabilizer of the glenohumeral joint during rotation of the arm.
  - This anterior stabilizing effect on the glenohumeral joint is lost as the LHBT undergoes medial subluxation because of the pulley tear.
  - The subluxation of the LHBT and decentralization of the humeral head represent the initial steps of the progressive cascade concluding in ASI.

- The superior fibers of the articular surface of the subscapularis are most frequently affected, and the tearing of deep fibers of the subscapularis is caused by the medial subluxation of the LHBT.

- Deep surface tears of the subscapularis tendon allow further anterior superior translation of the humeral head and potentiate ASI.

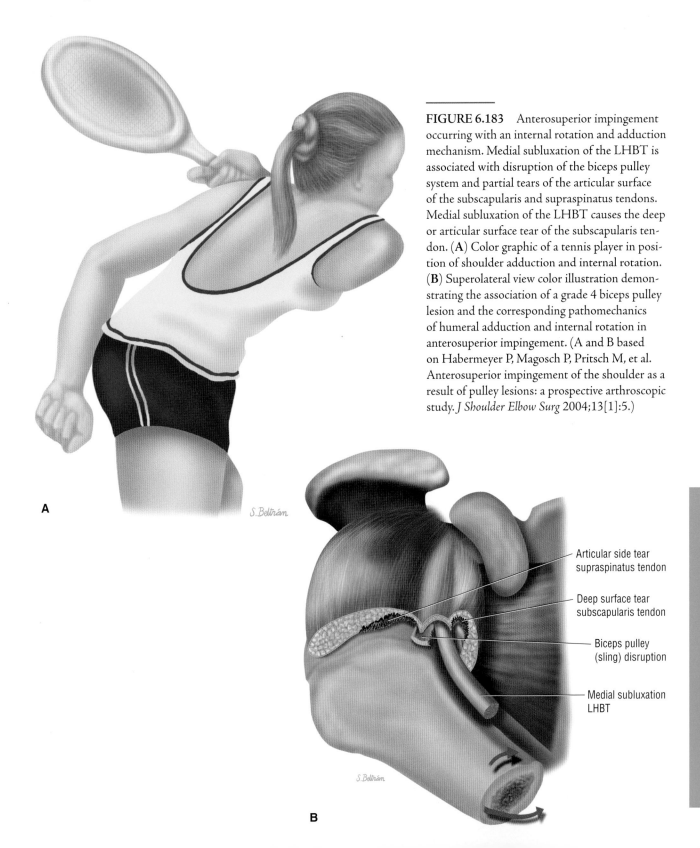

FIGURE 6.183 Anterosuperior impingement occurring with an internal rotation and adduction mechanism. Medial subluxation of the LHBT is associated with disruption of the biceps pulley system and partial tears of the articular surface of the subscapularis and supraspinatus tendons. Medial subluxation of the LHBT causes the deep or articular surface tear of the subscapularis tendon. (**A**) Color graphic of a tennis player in position of shoulder adduction and internal rotation. (**B**) Superolateral view color illustration demonstrating the association of a grade 4 biceps pulley lesion and the corresponding pathomechanics of humeral adduction and internal rotation in anterosuperior impingement. (A and B based on Habermeyer P, Magosch P, Pritsch M, et al. Anterosuperior impingement of the shoulder as a result of pulley lesions: a prospective arthroscopic study. *J Shoulder Elbow Surg* 2004;13[1]:5.)

Articular side tear supraspinatus tendon

Deep surface tear subscapularis tendon

Biceps pulley (sling) disruption

Medial subluxation LHBT

A

B

S. Beltrán

S. Beltrán

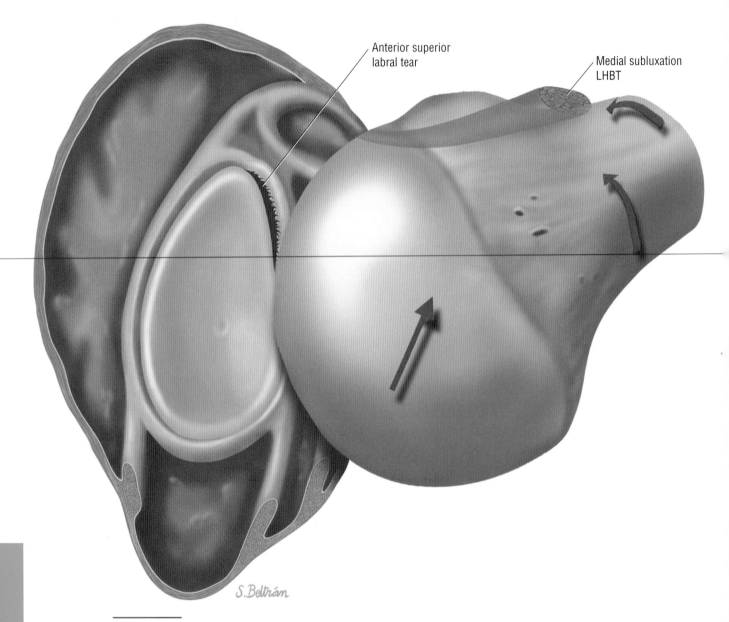

Anterior superior labral tear

Medial subluxation LHBT

S. Beltrán

FIGURE 6.184 Color graphic of the glenohumeral joint as viewed from a superolateral exposure with the humerus adducted and internally rotated. In anterosuperior impingement (ASI), the antero-superior labral tear occurs as the humeral head migrates into the anterosuperior quadrant against the anterior glenoid rim. The normal posterior and compressive joint retraction function of the LHB is lost in ASI secondary to the unstable medially subluxed LHB. Anterosuperior impingement may be related to repetitive trauma of any of the superior complex structures against the anterior superior labrum or coracoid process in flexion and internal rotation. (Based on Habermeyer P, Magosch P, Pritsch M, et al. Anterosuperior impingement of the shoulder as a result of pulley lesions: a prospective arthroscopic study. *J Shoulder Elbow Surg* 2004;13[1]:5.)

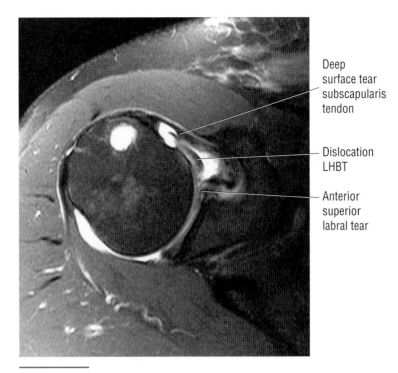

Deep surface tear subscapularis tendon

Dislocation LHBT

Anterior superior labral tear

FIGURE 6.185 Anterosuperior impingement. Medial subluxation of the LHBT is associated with disruption of the biceps pulley system and partial tears of the articular surface of the subscapularis and supraspinatus tendons. Medial subluxation of the LHB causes the deep or articular surface tear of the subscapularis tendon. Axial FS PD FSE image with biceps dislocation tear of distal subscapularis articular fibers and anterosuperior labral tear.

LHBT subluxation

Deep surface tear subscapularis

Lesser tuberosity edema

Empty bicipital groove

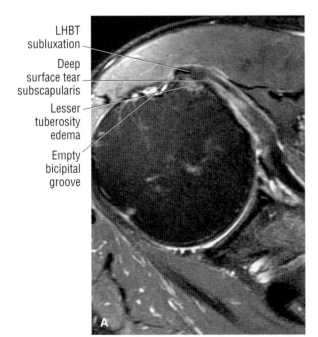
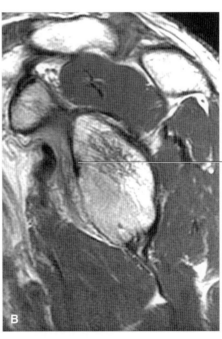

Anterosuperior glenoid rim sclerosis

FIGURE 6.186 (**A**) Axial FS PD FSE image shows ASI with medial subluxation of the biceps tendon, partial distal tearing of the subscapularis tendon, and an associated antero-superior labral tear. (**B**) Corresponding sagittal PD FSE image with sclerosis of the anterior superior glenoid rim. The hypointense signal on all pulse sequences represents an adaptive pattern of sclerosis not usually seen unless there is repetitive adduction and internal rotation.

Throwing Shoulder

Key Concepts

- A SLAP 2 or posterior SLAP 2 lesion causes the dead arm.

- Repetitive tensile loading during follow-through results in a tight posterior band of the IGHL.

- The tight posterior band bowstrings the humeral head in the late cocking phase, resulting in a posterosuperior shift of the glenohumeral contact point.

- Glenohumeral internal rotation deficit (GIRD) is an acquired loss of internal rotation resulting from the tight posterior band of the IGL.

- Peel-back posterior SLAP 2 lesions and posterior articular surface tears of the supraspinatus represent the net effect of the shift of the glenohumeral rotation contact point with a loss of internal rotation and gain of external rotation.

- Pseudolaxity of the anterior IGHL results from a reduced cam effect of the proximal humerus, which allows for an even greater degree of external rotation.

- On sagittal MR images, eccentric posterior glenoid rim sclerosis may precede the development of the peel-back labral lesion.

- The disabled throwing shoulder represents a pathologic cascade that culminates in the "dead arm."[72–74]

- There is a sudden onset of mechanical pain with the development of a posterior type 2 SLAP lesion.[74]

- Prior to the development of the posterior type 2 SLAP tear, there may be a prodromal phase or pre-SLAP stage where the thrower describes posterior shoulder tightness.

  - At this stage, MR studies frequently demonstrate eccentric posterior glenoid rim sclerosis without a SLAP lesion.

  - There may also be associated remodeling (including retroversion) of the posterior glenoid rim.

Dead Arm

- Is a pathologic shoulder condition characterized by the sudden loss of the ability to throw a fastball

    - Sharp pain and discomfort occur as the arm moves forward during the late cocking or early acceleration phase of throwing.

- Is caused by a posterior type 2 SLAP lesion or a combined anteroposterior type 2 SLAP

- Internal shoulder impingement, which occurs in the position of 90° of abduction and 90° of external rotation (the 90°–90° position), was originally thought to describe entrapment of the rotator cuff between the greater tuberosity and the posterosuperior glenoid in abduction and external rotation of the shoulder.

- The pathology in the disabled throwing shoulder involves contraction or tightening of the posterior band of the IGHL and not, except in the older elite thrower, internal impingement.

Glenohumeral Internal Rotation Deficit

- Repetitive tensile loading occurring during the follow-through phase of throwing predisposes to the development of a tight or contracted posterior band of the IGHL.[72]

- Glenohumeral internal rotation deficit (GIRD) is an acquired loss in the degree of glenohumeral internal rotation.

    - Loss of internal rotation in abduction is the most important pathologic process that occurs in throwers and is the result of posteroinferior capsular contracture of the tight posterior band of the IGHL evident in the late cocking phase of throwing.

- The majority of throwers with symptomatic GIRD (>25°) respond to posteroinferior capsular stretching.

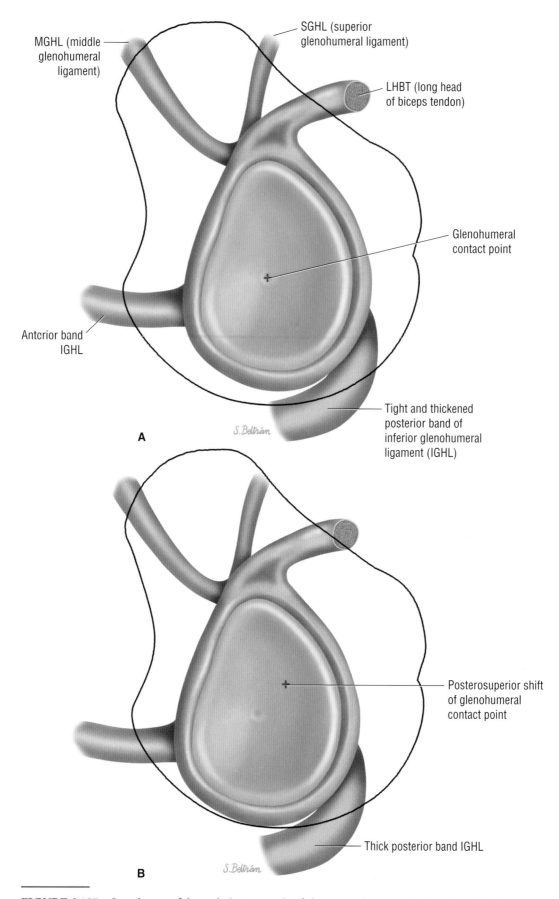

FIGURE 6.187 Initial steps of the pathologic cascade of changes in the throwing shoulder. (**A**) Abduction and external rotation with a tight and thickened posterior band of the inferior glenohumeral ligament. (**B**) Posterosuperior shift of the glenohumeral contact point.

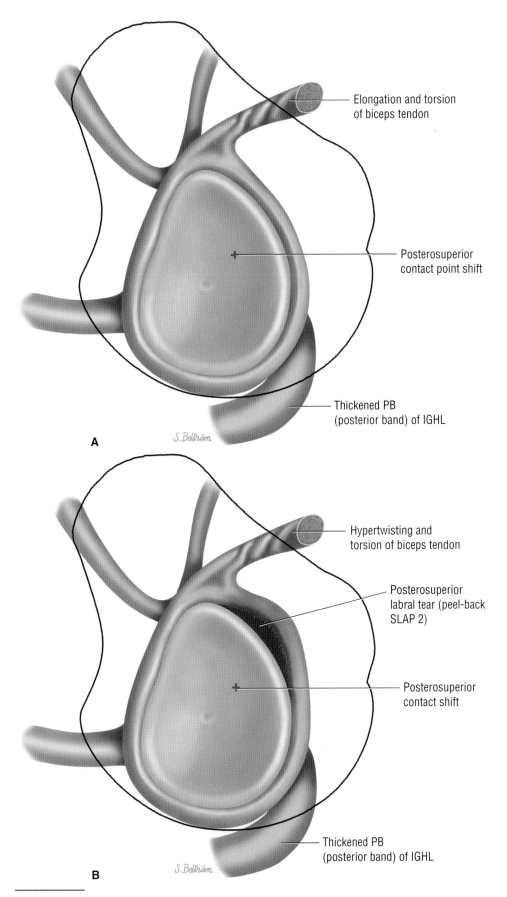

FIGURE 6.188   Dead arm with the development of a posterior SLAP 2 lesion. Color illustrations of glenohumeral joint from a lateral perspective. Hypertwisting and torsion of the intraarticular biceps are shown on (**A**), and a peel-back posterosuperior labral tear is shown on (**B**).

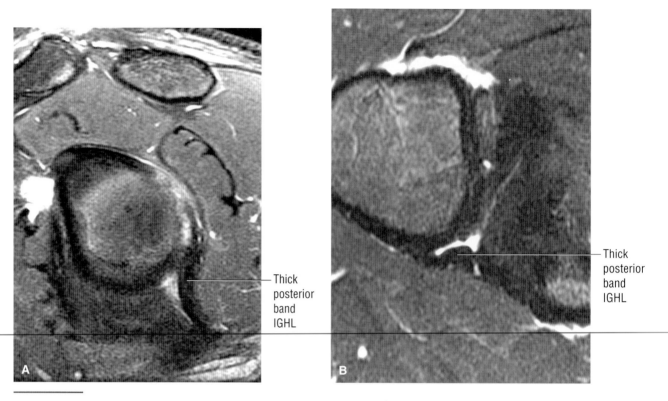

FIGURE 6.189   Initial steps of the pathologic cascade of changes in the throwing shoulder. Thickened cross-section of the posterior band of the inferior glenohumeral ligament on sagittal (**A**) and axial (**B**) FS PD FSE images. It is more common to identify adaptive changes of posterior glenoid rim sclerosis than a thick posterior band.

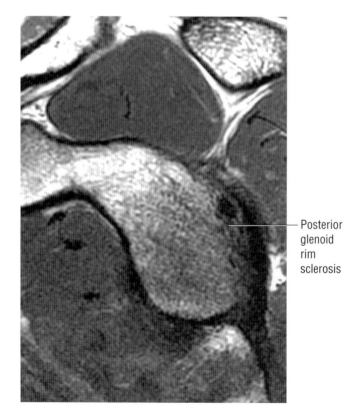

FIGURE 6.190   Dead arm with the development of a posterior SLAP 2 lesion. Sagittal PD FSE image of posterosuperior glenoid rim sclerosis associated with both the posterosuperior cam shift and the posterior SLAP 2 or peel-back lesion. The peel-back may extend to involve the posterior labrum contiguous with the posterosuperior quadrant. Remodeling including retroversion of the posterior glenoid rim may be associated.

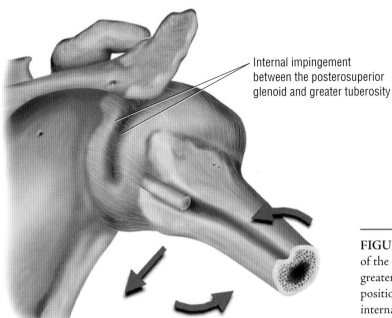

Internal impingement between the posterosuperior glenoid and greater tuberosity

FIGURE 6.191 Internal impingement of the articular surface of the rotator cuff between the posterior superior glenoid and the greater tuberosity is appreciated as a normal mechanism in the position of shoulder abduction and external rotation. Therefore, internal impingement is usually not responsible for the pathologic cascade in the throwing shoulder.

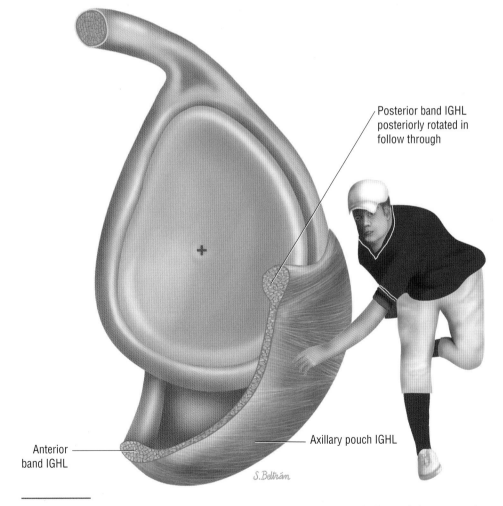

Posterior band IGHL posteriorly rotated in follow through

Anterior band IGHL

Axillary pouch IGHL

FIGURE 6.192 Repetitive tensile loading during the follow-through phase of throwing is the primary mechanism responsible for the development of the tight posteroinferior capsule. Large distraction forces must be resisted by the posteriorly rotated IGL during follow-through. (Based on Burkhart SS, Morgan CD, Kibler WB. The disabled throwing shoulder: spectrum of pathology. Part I: pathoanatomy and biomechanics. *Arthroscopy* 2003;19[4]:404.)

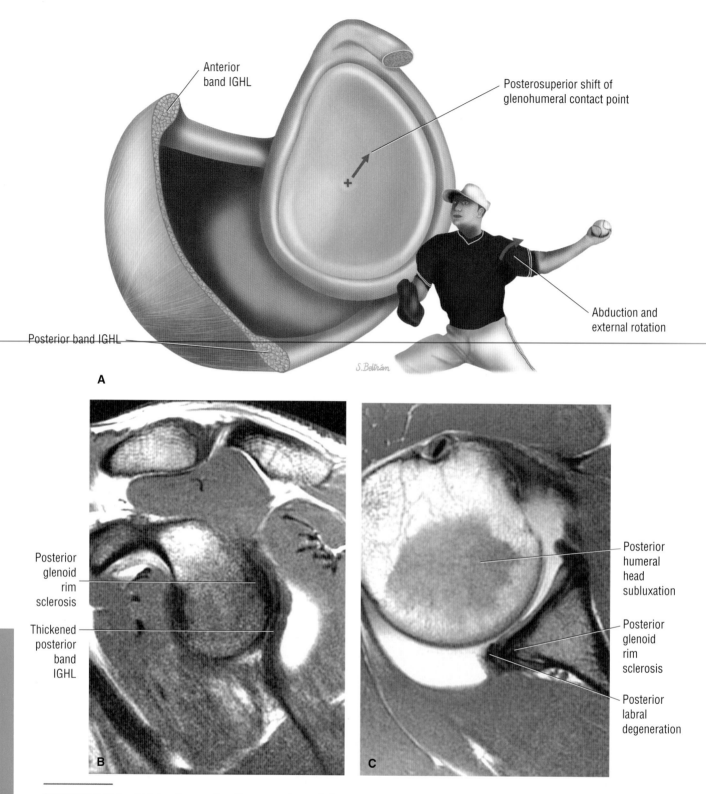

FIGURE 6.193   (**A**) A color graphic illustrating hyperabduction and external rotation in the late cocking phase of throwing. In the late cocking phase of throwing, the posterior band of the IGHL is bowstrung underneath the humeral head, causing a posterosuperior shift in the glenohumeral contact or rotation point. An acquired tight or contracted posterior band of the IGHL thus initiates the pathologic cascade (evident in abduction and external rotation causing GIRD). A posterosuperior shift of the humeral head causes increased shear and peel-back forces to the posterosuperior glenoid labrum, increased greater tuberosity clearance, and scapular protraction. (Based on Burkhart SS, Morgan CD, Kibler WB. The disabled throwing shoulder: spectrum of pathology. Part I: pathoanatomy and biomechanics. *Arthroscopy* 2003;19[4]:404.) (**B**) The thickened posterior band of the IGL with mild posterior glenoid rim sclerosis in a baseball pitcher capable of throwing 100 miles an hour on a sagittal PD FSE MR arthrogram. (**C**) Corresponding posterior subluxation of the humeral head secondary to early changes of posterior glenohumeral wear and a tight posteroinferior capsule on an axial PD MR arthrogram.

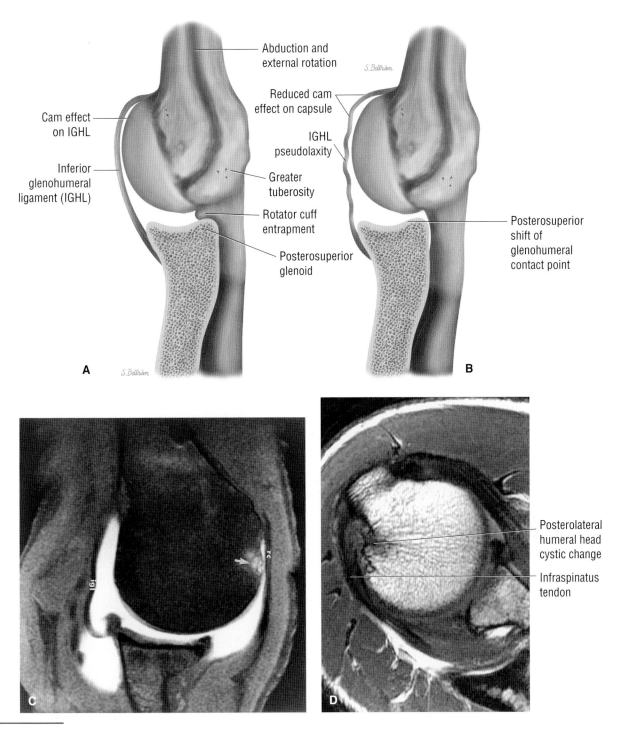

FIGURE 6.194 (**A**) Internal impingement, a normal phenomenon in all shoulders, is demonstrated with abduction and external rotation of the shoulder. The greater tuberosity abuts against the posterosuperior glenoid, which entraps the rotator cuff between these two osseous structures. In throwers, the posterosuperior shift of the glenohumeral contact point produces a reduction of the cam effect as the space-occupying effect of the proximal humerus on the anteroinferior capsule (IGL) is reduced. (**B**) The resultant relative laxity (shown here) or redundancy of the IGL should not be misinterpreted as anteroinferior instability. Hyperexternal rotation of the rotator cuff results in repetitive hypertwisting with torsional overload and shear failure of cuff fibers. A partial thickness articular surface tear then develops in the posterior supraspinatus or anterior infraspinatus tendon. (**A,B:** Based on Burkhart SS, Morgan CD, Kibler WB. The disabled throwing shoulder: spectrum of pathology Part I: pathoanatomy and biomechanics. *Arthroscopy* 2003;19[4]:404.) (**C**) Axial FS PD FSE image in abduction and external rotation confirms the relative laxity of the IGL and posterior shift of the humeral head. Note the proximity of the greater tuberosity to the rotator cuff. The nonarticular humeral erosion has been attributed to posterosuperior glenoid rim contact in internal impingement. (**D**) Axial PD FSE image of posterolateral humeral head cyst changes in a 30-year-old elite baseball player. The subchondral sclerosis and erosions are posterior to the greater tuberosity deep to the distal infraspinatus and involve the bare area of the humeral head. Associated posterosuperior glenoid rim remodeling is characteristic.

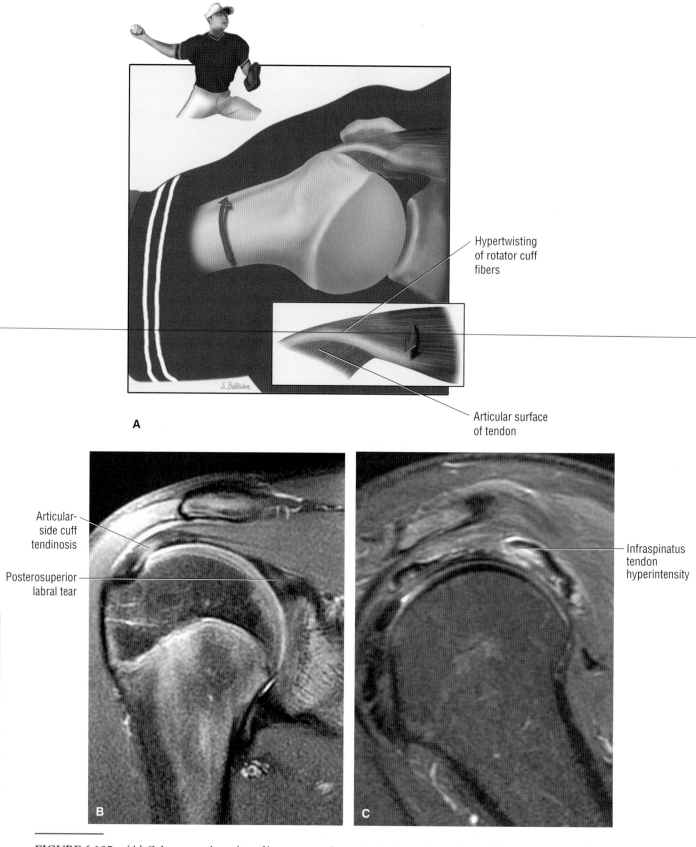

FIGURE 6.195 (A) Color coronal graphic of hyperexternal rotation during cocking phase of throwing, causing hypertwisting of the rotator cuff fibers. (Based on Burkhart SS, Morgan CD, Kibler WB. The disabled throwing shoulder: spectrum of pathology. Part I: pathoanatomy and biomechanics. *Arthroscopy* 2003;19[4]:404.) (**B**) Coronal FS PD FSE image with articular-side cuff hyperintensity and posterosuperior labral tear in a pitcher. (**C**) Sagittal FS PD FSE image in a separate case with posterior articular-side cuff overload. This may occur in the posterior supraspinatus or anterior portion of the infraspinatus. Hyperintensity is demonstrated in the infraspinatus musculotendinous junction tearing.

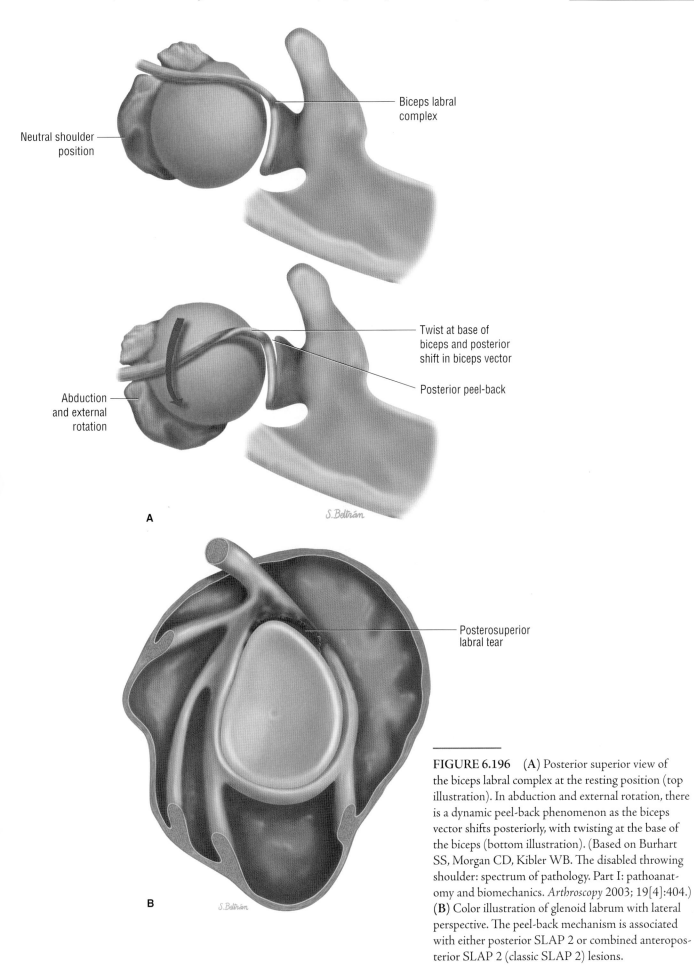

Biceps labral complex

Neutral shoulder position

Twist at base of biceps and posterior shift in biceps vector

Posterior peel-back

Abduction and external rotation

S. Beltrán

A

Posterosuperior labral tear

B S. Beltrán

FIGURE 6.196 **(A)** Posterior superior view of the biceps labral complex at the resting position (top illustration). In abduction and external rotation, there is a dynamic peel-back phenomenon as the biceps vector shifts posteriorly, with twisting at the base of the biceps (bottom illustration). (Based on Burhart SS, Morgan CD, Kibler WB. The disabled throwing shoulder: spectrum of pathology. Part I: pathoanatomy and biomechanics. *Arthroscopy* 2003; 19[4]:404.) **(B)** Color illustration of glenoid labrum with lateral perspective. The peel-back mechanism is associated with either posterior SLAP 2 or combined anteroposterior SLAP 2 (classic SLAP 2) lesions.

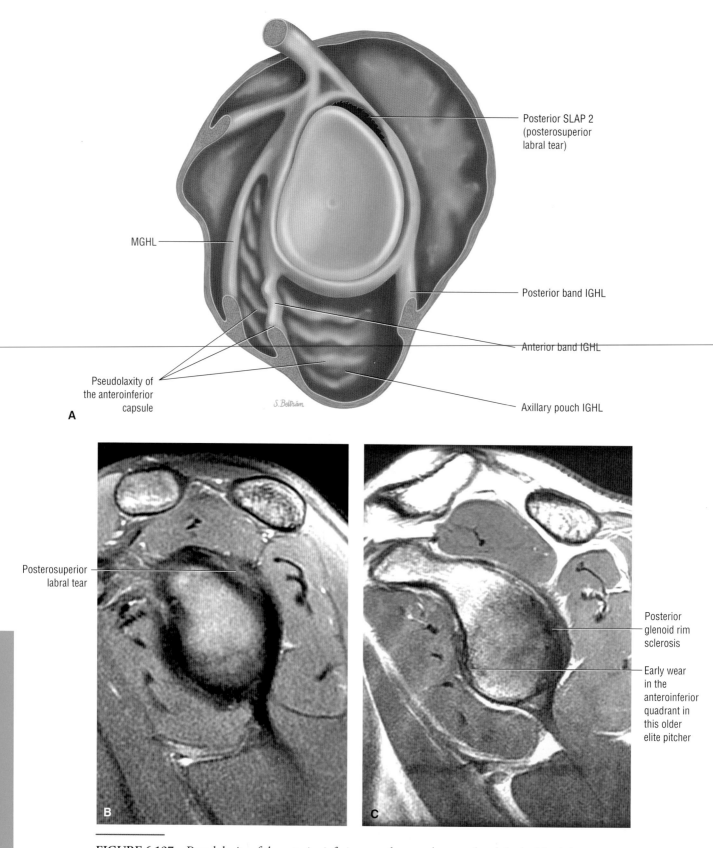

FIGURE 6.197   Pseudolaxity of the anterior inferior capsule secondary to a break in the labral ring associated with a posterior SLAP 2 lesion is shown on a sagittal color graphic (**A**) and a sagittal FS PD FSE image (**B**). (**C**) Moderate posterior glenoid rim sclerosis associated with mild anteroinferior rim sclerosis. The anteroinferior rim changes may be the initial changes of anteroinferior labral injury in the older elite pitcher or may be anterior rim wear secondary to pseudolaxity of the anteroinferior capsule.

Posterior Band of the IGHL

- The tight posterior band of the IGHL acts as a tether and shifts the glenohumeral contact point posterosuperiorly during abduction and external rotation.[72]

- The arc of motion of the greater tuberosity is also shifted posterosuperiorly and, in the position of abduction and external rotation, no longer abuts the expected posterosuperior glenoid contact area described in internal impingement.

- Because of the increased clearance of the greater tuberosity (tuberosity clearance provides additional external rotation of the shoulder), the posterosuperior shift of the glenohumeral contact point preserves hyperexternal rotation and also reduces the cam effect of the humeral head and proximal humeral calcar, creating a relative redundancy of the anterosuperior capsule.

  - This pseudolaxity or redundancy of the anteroinferior capsule produces functional lengthening of the anterior IGHL and also contributes to a secondary increase in external rotation.

- The tight posteroinferior capsule thus facilitates hyperexternal rotation of the humerus by a shift in the glenohumeral contact point posterosuperiorly before internal impingement can occur and by minimizing the cam effect of the proximal humerus on the anterior inferior capsule.

  - Internal impingement is avoided because the posterosuperior shift of the glenohumeral contact point occurs before the greater tuberosity contacts the posterior glenoid.

- Increased retroversion in the dominant or throwing shoulder is associated with increased external rotation (hyperexternal rotation) at 90° of abduction and corresponds with both a decrease in the cam effect and increased tuberosity clearance.

- Hyperexternal rotation may be due to functional lengthening of the IGHL (caused by a tight posterior band and posterosuperior shift of the glenohumeral contact point); chronic hyperexternal rotation associated with a protracted scapula may partially stretch the IGHL directly.

- In the older elite thrower, hyperexternal rotation may lead to chronic failure of the anteroinferior capsule in the Bankart zone.[72]

- IGHL disruption is not typically seen in the younger pitcher presenting with dead arm.

- Hyperexternal rotation in the older pitcher/thrower may contribute to the pseudolaxity associated with combined internal impingement.

  - It is only considered pathologic, however, in the older elite thrower in whom excessive hyperexternal rotation in the late phase of cocking causes abrasion of the undersurface of the cuff against the posterosuperior glenoid. Increased posterolateral humeral cystic changes may also be seen in this group of elite throwers.[184]

  - These older elite throwers achieve maximal external rotation in excess of 130°.

- Cystic lesions of the posterosuperior region of bare area of the humeral head are lined with collagen and connective tissue and are connected to the joint space.[249]

- Since internal impingement is a normal phenomenon, it is not surprising that humeral head cystic changes are seen in asymptomatic patients as a normal variation.

- Bare area cysts are more extensive in older elite throwers, and it appears that internal impingement becomes a pathologic process because excessive hyperexternal glenohumeral rotation produces abrasion of the cuff and bare area against the posterosuperior glenoid.[77]

- In the younger throwing athlete, the greater tuberosity usually has clearance over the posterosuperior glenoid rim through a greater arc of external rotation before internal impingement occurs.[444]

- Hyperexternal rotation also results in repetitive hypertwisting of the rotator cuff fibers, causing torsional overload and shear failure of articular-side cuff fibers.

- The external rotation proprioceptive set point of high-level pitchers is referred to as "the slot," and it allows for high-velocity throws of a baseball at speeds above 90 mph.

- The shift of the glenohumeral contact point with a tight posterior band of the IGHL allows the pitcher to more effectively externally rotate back to the set point.

Peel-Back Lesion

■ Occurs with the shoulder in abduction and external rotation[72]

■ Pitchers with a tight posteroinferior capsule and GIRD throw with deranged mechanics and are at risk for increased peel-back and shear forces on the superior labrum.

■ There is a posterior shift of the biceps vector and twist at the base of the biceps in the late cocking phase of throwing.

■ Increased torsional force is transmitted to the posterior aspect of the BLC and results in a posterior type 2 SLAP or peel-back lesion.

■ Sometimes called "thrower's" SLAP, this lesion is treated with a suture anchor to resist torsional forces generated in the peel-back mechanism.

■ In abduction and external rotation, acceleration of the arm occurs in the late cocking phase and produces a type 2 or posterior type 2 SLAP lesion as the biceps and superior labral complex are peeled (medial rotation of the superior labrum onto the posterosuperior scapular neck and medial shift of the biceps root relative to the supraglenoid tubercle).

■ A protracted scapula will potentiate the pathologic cascade initiated by the acquired capsular contracture (tight posterior band of the IGHL); with the development of the SLAP or posterior peel-back lesion, the posterosuperior shift and hyperexternal rotation components of the cascade are further emphasized, and thus the pathologic cascade continues.

■ The associated partial thickness articular surface rotator cuff tears occur in the posterior portion of the rotator crescent posterior to the supraspinatus contribution to the cuff.

■ The posterior type 2 SLAP lesions produce a break in the labral ring contributing to posterosuperior subluxation of the humerus, which in turn produces high tensile forces in the posterosuperior cuff.

SICK Scapula

- The SICK scapula[74] = Scapular malposition, Inferior medial border prominence, Coracoid pain and malposition, and dysKinesis of scapular movement

  - Is an overuse muscular fatigue syndrome seen in the throwing athlete who presents with dead arm

  - It represents an extreme form of scapular dyskinesis.

- The type I (inferior medial scapular border prominence) and type II (medial scapular border prominence) patterns are associated with posterosuperior labral lesions.

- The type III pattern (prominence of the superomedial border of the scapula) is associated with impingement and rotator cuff lesions.

- Clinical presentation in the SICK scapula syndrome is of an apparent "dropped" scapula in the dominant shoulder of a thrower, subsequent to initial scapular protraction (tilting).

- There is associated coracoid tenderness on the medial aspect of the coracoid tip, corresponding to the insertion of the pectoralis minor tendon.

- In the scapular retraction test, the scapula is manually repositioned in retraction and posterior tilt by the examiner.

- Full forward flexion without coracoid pain is diagnostic of the SICK scapula syndrome. As the scapula tilts anteriorly, it protracts and abducts and displaces up and over the top of the thorax.

- Impingement-like symptoms are associated with anteroinferior angulation of the acromion secondary to scapular protraction.

- Traction and pain related to the levator scapulae muscle result from the tilt and lateral rotation of the scapula.

- The combination of a SICK scapula and GIRD may result in injury to the posterosuperior labrum, the articular surface of the posterior supraspinatus, and the anterior inferior capsular structures.

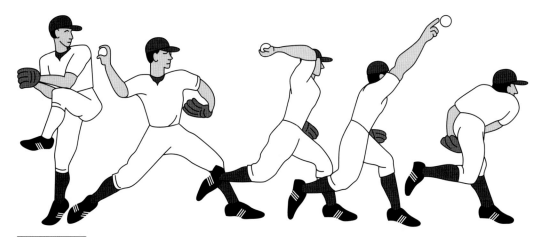

FIGURE 6.198 The kinetic chain. The five phases of pitching a baseball (from left to right): windup, early cocking, late cocking, acceleration, and follow-through. Windup or preparation: Preliminary activity dominated by flexion of the upper extremity, with both hands holding the ball. Early cocking: A period of abduction and external rotation of the shoulder that begins as the ball is released from the nondominant hand. Late cocking: Contact of the forward foot with the ground divides this stage from early cocking. Late cocking continues until maximum external rotation at the shoulder is attained. Acceleration: Starts with the posture of maximum abduction and external rotations at the shoulder and continues until release of the ball, as the ball leaves the fingers. Follow-through: The final interval of motion as the arm flexes and internally rotates across the chest and is decelerated. (Reprinted from Craig EV. *Master Techniques in Orthopaedic Surgery: Shoulder.* 3rd. ed. Philadelphia, PA: Lippincott Williams & Wilkins; 2013, with permission.)

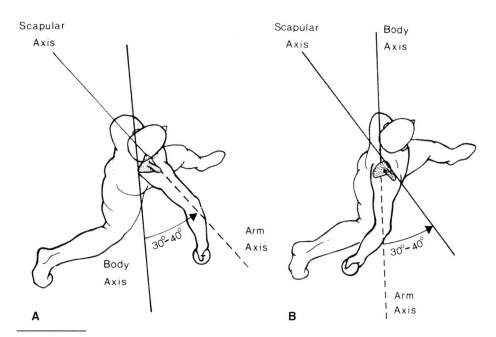

FIGURE 6.199 Hyperangulation during the overhead throwing motion. During the late cocking phase of the overhead throw, as the thrower's humerus excessively abducts horizontally, posterosuperior impingement of the shoulder joint may occur. To prevent this, the thrower must stay in the plane of the scapula. (**A**) Normal angular relationship. (**B**) Hyperangulation. (Reprinted from Craig EV. *Master Techniques in Orthopaedic Surgery: Shoulder.* 3rd ed. Philadelphia, PA: Lippincott Williams & Wilkins; 2013, with permission.)

Summary of the Throwing Athlete and Dead Arm

- The throwing athlete often presents with a sudden onset of mechanical pain caused by a posterior type 2 or type 2 SLAP lesion.[74]

- Prior to the development of the peel-back tear, there may be a prodromal phase or pre-SLAP stage of posterior shoulder tightness.
  - At this stage, MR studies frequently demonstrate eccentric posterior glenoid rim sclerosis and sometimes associated remodeling of the posterior glenoid rim and less commonly a thickened posterior band.

- The shoulder at risk for dead arm symptoms exhibits mild to moderate GIRD and/or a malpositioned SICK scapula.
  - When GIRD exceeds the external rotation gain (ERG), the GIRD/ERG ratio is greater than 1.

- A posterosuperior shift of the glenohumeral rotation point then follows, with abduction and external rotation during the late cocking phase of throwing.

- The SICK scapula syndrome is an extreme form of scapular dyskinesis.

- In a thrower with a dropped elbow, the upper arm hyperangulates posterior to the plane of the scapula.

- Hyperangulation of the humerus on the glenoid and poor throwing mechanics may further contribute to increased humeral external rotation and the peel-back effect.

- The dead arm is characterized by the following pathologic changes:
  - A tight posterior band of the IGHL (a response to the follow-through phase of throwing)
  - GIRD
  - A posterosuperior shift in glenohumeral rotation point
  - Increased clearance of the greater tuberosity over the glenoid
  - Reduced humeral head cam effect on the anterior inferior capsule
  - Hyperexternal rotation of the humerus relative to the scapula
  - Peel-back forces in late cocking phase, which cause a posterior type 2 SLAP lesion
  - Scapular protraction

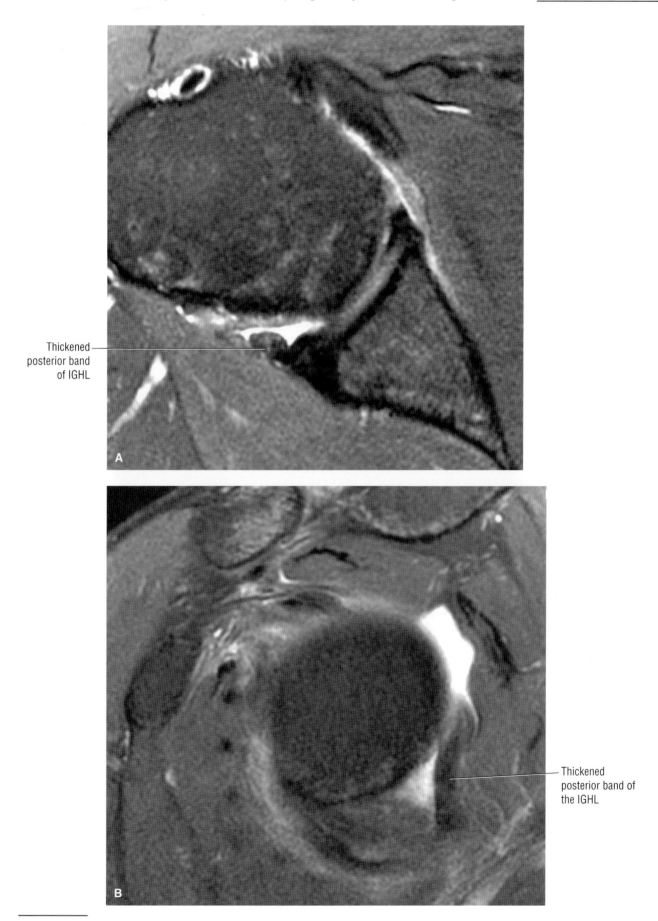

Thickened
posterior band
of IGHL

Thickened
posterior band of
the IGHL

FIGURE 6.200   Thickened posterior band of the inferior glenohumeral ligament (**A**) Axial FS PD. (**B**) Sagittal FS PD. The thickened posterior band that is responsible for the CAM shifting of the humeral head is not the most common MR finding in the throwing athlete as the posterior band may become stiff or contracted without appearing enlarged in cross-sectional diameter on MR.

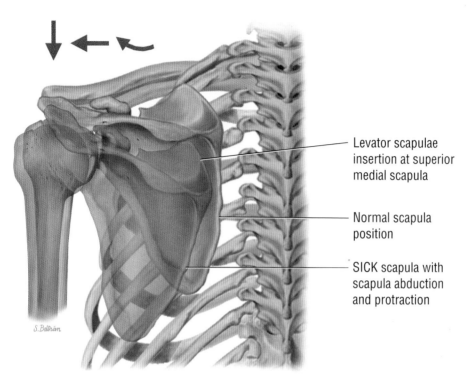

S.Beltrán

- Levator scapulae insertion at superior medial scapula
- Normal scapula position
- SICK scapula with scapula abduction and protraction

FIGURE 6.201 SICK scapula associated with scapular abduction and protraction. Tension on the superomedial scapular insertion of the levator scapulae produces a painful tendinopathy between the medial angle and root of the scapular spine. (Based on Burkhart SS, Morgan DC, Kibler WB. The disabled throwing shoulder: spectrum of pathology. Part III: the SICK scapula, scapular dyskinesis, the kinetic chain, and rehabilitation. *Arthroscopy* 2003;19[6]: 641.)

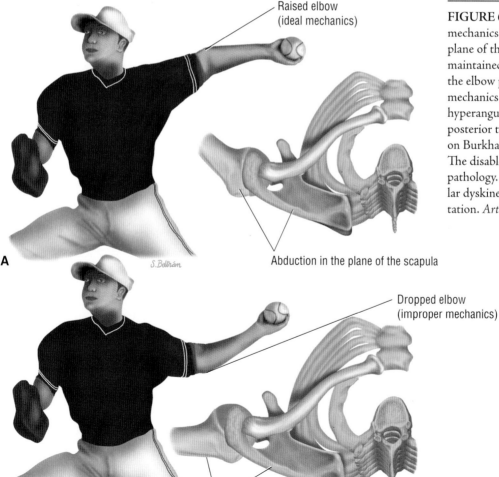

Raised elbow (ideal mechanics)

Abduction in the plane of the scapula

S.Beltrán

A

Dropped elbow (improper mechanics)

Hyperangulation of upper arm posterior to the plane of the scapula

B

FIGURE 6.202 (**A**) Proper throwing mechanics with abduction of the arm in the plane of the scapula. Note the upper arm is maintained above the horizontal plane with the elbow positioned high. (**B**) Improper mechanics with a dropped elbow position and hyperangulation of the upper arm (humerus) posterior to the plane of the scapula. (Based on Burkhart SS, Morgan DC, Kibler WB. The disabled throwing shoulder: spectrum of pathology. Part III: the SICK scapula, scapular dyskinesis, the kinetic chain, and rehabilitation. *Arthroscopy* 2003;19[6]: 641.)

7

Glenohumeral Joint Instability

Glenohumeral Joint Instability

Anterior Instability

Key Concepts

- The IGHL (IGL) can fail at its attachment to the inferior pole of the glenoid (Bankart), midligament, or at the attachment to the anatomic neck of the humerus (HAGL).
- Bankart, Perthes, ALPSA, and HAGL lesions may all produce anterior instability.
- The Bankart lesion may be osseous or primarily soft tissue.
- Atraumatic anterior instability is a component of multidirectional instability (MDI).

- Anterior instability, particularly that produced by lesions of the IGHL-labral complex, is most common of all glenohumeral joint instabilities.

- The anterior band of the IGHL, which forms the anterior labrum, is the primary restraint to anterior translation of the humeral head at 90° of abduction.[605]

  - The anterior band is best demonstrated on sagittal oblique MR images.

- Avulsion of the IGLLC from the glenoid rim, known as a Bankart lesion, involves the detachment of the anterior labrum and the IGLC from the anterior glenoid rim.[502]

- Bankart lesions are described based on the detachment of the labrum and capsule from the anterior glenoid.

  - A Bankart lesion can involve labral avulsion without a bony inferior glenoid rim fracture.
  - The IGL complex can also tear at its midportion or be avulsed from its humeral insertion.
  - An HAGL lesion can be demonstrated arthroscopically and may be responsible for shoulder instability.[641]

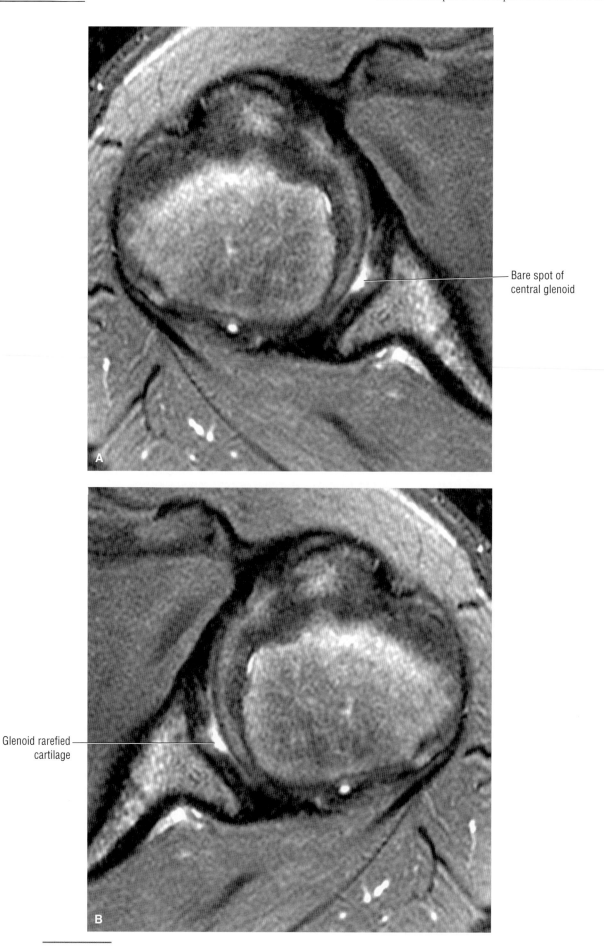

FIGURE 7.1　Bare spot of articular cartilage thinning of the central glenoid in the rarefied cartilage area of contact. (**A**) Axial FS PD. (**B**) Axial FS PD.

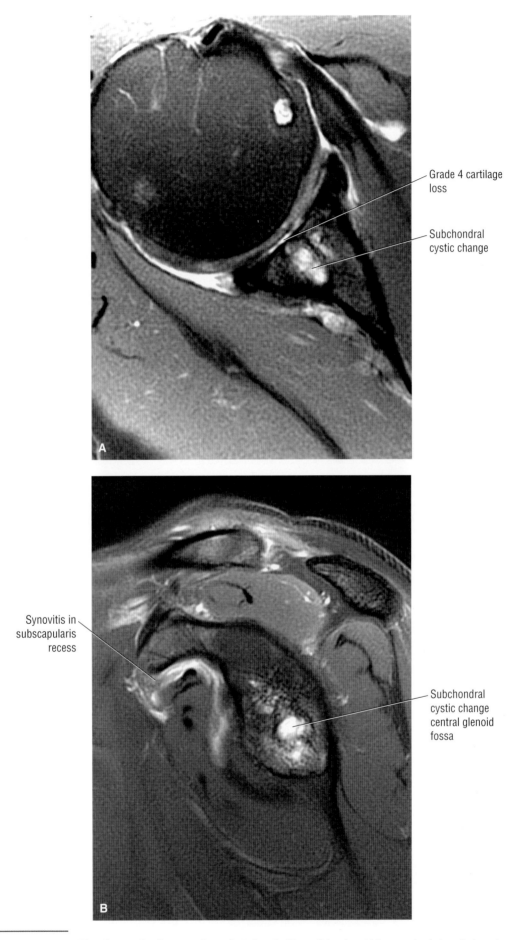

FIGURE 7.2 Glenohumeral arthrosis with grade 4 chondral loss of the glenoid fossa and subchondral cystic change. The articular cartilage loss is associated with synovitis in the subscapularis recess. (**A**) Axial. (**B**) Sagittal.

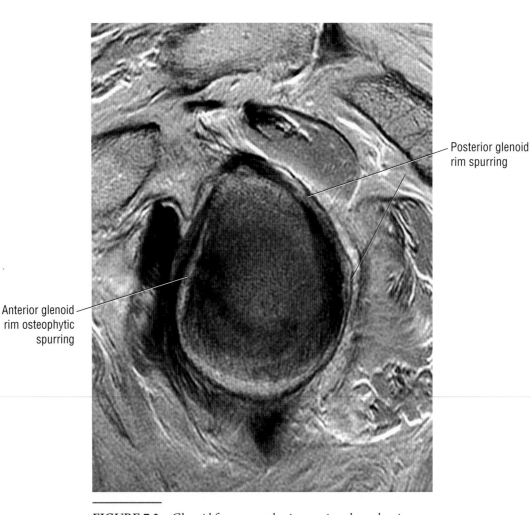

Posterior glenoid
rim spurring

Anterior glenoid
rim osteophytic
spurring

FIGURE 7.3 Glenoid fossa osteophytic spurring along the circumference of the glenoid rim.

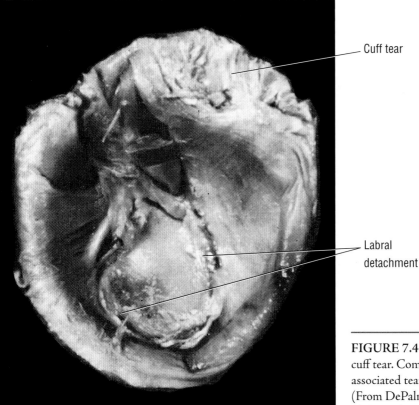

Cuff tear

Labral
detachment

FIGURE 7.4 Glenoid fossa arthrosis associated with cuff tear. Complete detachment of the labrum with associated tear of the supraspinatus and infraspinatus. (From DePalma AF. *Surgery of the Shoulder*. 3rd ed. Philadelphia, PA: JB Lippincott; 1983.)

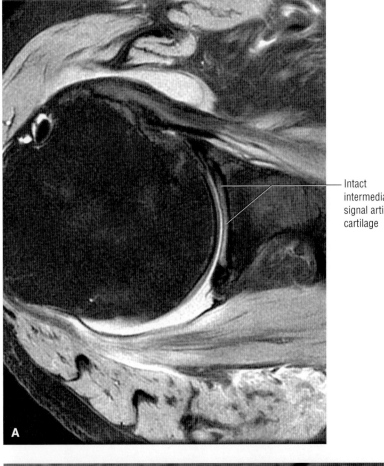

Intact intermediate signal articular cartilage

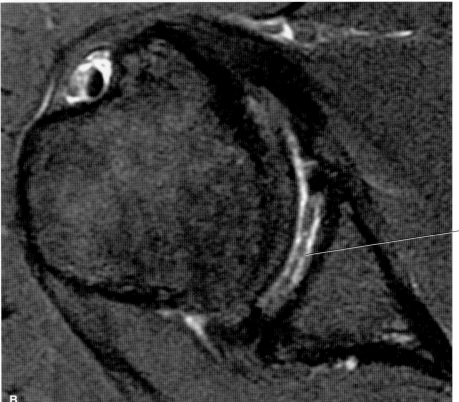

Glenoid chondral delamination

FIGURE 7.5 (**A**) Intact glenoid articular cartilage. (**B**) Delamination with unstable glenoid fossa chondral surface. Hyperintense fluid signal undermines the articular cartilage surface.

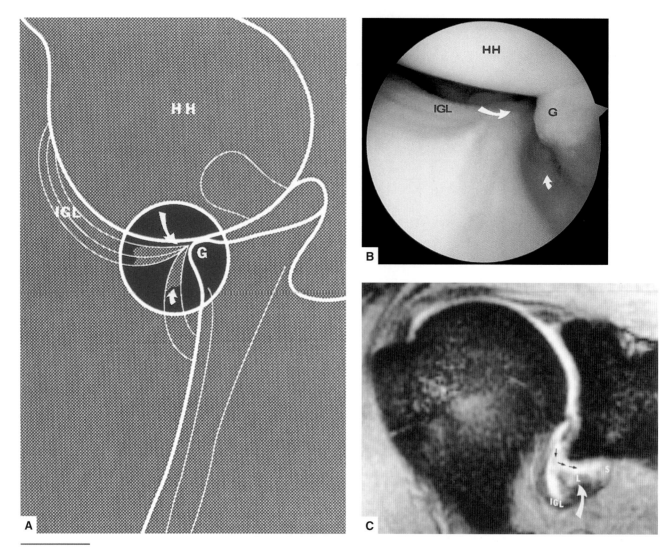

FIGURE 7.6   Bankart lesion. (**A**) A tear (*large curved arrow*) of the inferior glenoid and labral attachment of the inferior glenohumeral ligament (IGL) is present. Scarred muscle of the subscapularis
is shown along the inferior glenoid neck (*small curved arrow*). The humeral head (HH) is subluxed
inferiorly. G, glenoid. (**B**) The arthroscopic view from inferior to anterior is seen with the scope in
the axillary pouch, oriented toward the anterior inferior pole of the glenoid. Note the avulsed labrum
from the glenoid rim (G) and torn inferior pole attachment (*large curved arrow*) of the IGL. HH,
humeral head. Scarred tearing of subscapularis muscle from the scapular neck is also identified (*small
curved arrow*). (**C**) Avulsed anterior glenoid labrum (L; *curved arrow*) and IGL attachment are shown
on a T2*-weighted coronal oblique image. Fluid extension (*straight arrows*) is identified between the
inferior glenoid neck, detached labrum, and subscapularis muscle (S). The IGL consists of anterior
and posterior bands and intervening axillary pouch. The anterior band of the IGL attaches to the
glenoid through its anterior labral connection in the 2–4 o'clock position in the right shoulder or
the 8-10 o'clock position for the left shoulder. The IGL courses diagonally downwards towards the
humerus. In a Bankart lesion the tension on the anterior band will result in both anteroinferior labral
tearing and capsular stretching or avulsion.

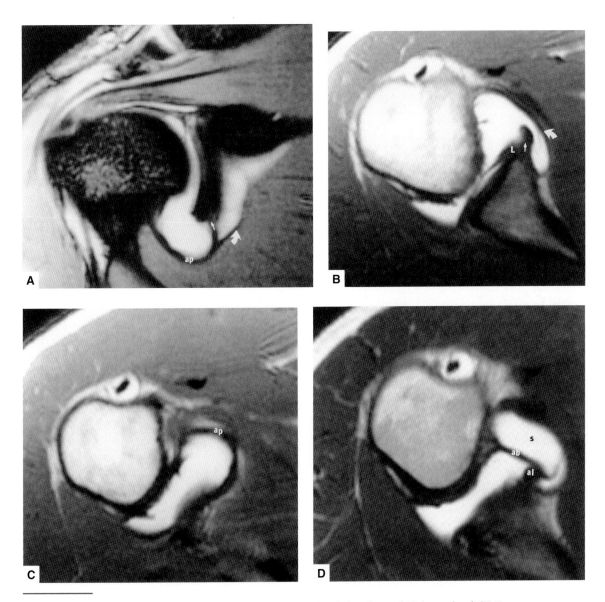

FIGURE 7.7 Inferior glenohumeral ligament labral complex. (**A**) Enhanced T2*-weighted GRE coronal oblique images demonstrate the normal inferior glenoid pole attachment of the axillary pouch (ap) of the inferior glenohumeral ligament (*straight arrow*). Note gadolinium contrast in normal inferior extension of subscapularis bursa (*curved arrow*). (**B**) An enhanced T1-weighted axial image displays the subscapularis bursa (*curved arrow*) and glenoid origin (*straight arrow*) of the inferior glenohumeral ligament complex (IGLC). The IGLC may originate from the glenoid, the labrum (L), or the neck of the glenoid immediately adjacent to the labrum. There is no anterior lateral tear on this image. (**C**) An enhanced T1-weighted axial image below the level of the glenoid displays the normal axillary pouch (ap) of the inferior glenohumeral ligament. (**D**) An enhanced T1-weighted axial image in a different patient identifies the anterior band (ab) of the IGLC and its continuation as the anterior labrum (al). Gadolinium contrast is shown in the subscapularis bursa (s) anterior to the anterior band. There is no tear of the anterior inferior labrum. The hammock effect of the IGL complex cradles the humeral head and functions as the primary static restraint against anterior translation in abduction. The axillary pouch is formed by the fasciculus obliquus medially and by the junction of the anterior and posterior bands on the humerus laterally.

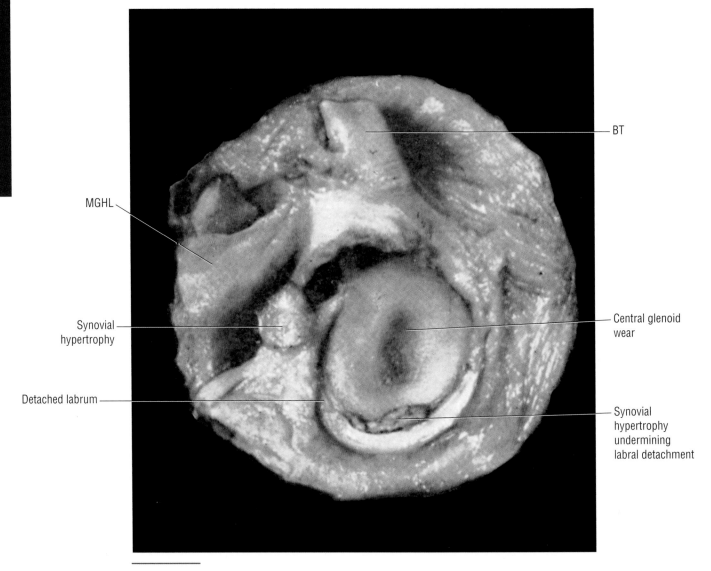

FIGURE 7.8   Extensive tear with synovial hypertrophy involving the BLC and IGLLC. The glenoid chondral degeneration and synovial reaction are associated with the areas of labral detachment. (Modified from DePalma AF. *Surgery of the Shoulder*. 3rd ed. Philadelphia, PA: JB Lippincott; 1983.) The normal labrum is formed by a circular periarticular system of fiber bundles. This system receives fiber bundles from the surrounding ligaments and tendons (e.g., the bicepss labral complex). The glenoid labrum and its related connections can be considered as a single functional unit. The labrum allows for a mechanism to anchor the capsuloligamentous structures to the glenoid rim. The creation of negative pressure allows the labrum to seal the glenohumeral joint.

- It is important to evaluate the IGLLC from its humeral origin throughout its course to its labral insertion.

- The anterior band is the thickest region, followed by the anterior and posterior aspects of the axillary pouch.[459]

- Failure of the IGHL can occur

  - At the glenoid insertion site (40%)

  - In the ligament substance (35%)

  - At the humeral insertion site (25%)

- Avulsions occur more frequently in the anterior band and the anterior aspect of the axillary pouch.

- Ligament substance tears are more common in the posterior aspect of the axillary pouch.

- Bankart avulsions represent failure of the IGHL at the glenoid insertion, and IGHL capsule laxity represents intrasubstance ligament failure.

  - A traumatic anterior dislocation is usually associated with a Bankart lesion (80–85% of cases with detachment of the capsulolabral tissue from the anterior glenoid rim), a Hill-Sachs posterolateral humeral head impaction fracture (>50% of cases), and an anterior inferior labral injury (tear and separation of labrum and capsule as a Bankart lesion or detached/displaced capsulolabral tissue, as an ALPSA lesion).

- The tensile properties of the IGHL allow for significant stretching before failure.

  - Redundancy of the IGHL may be as important as avulsions of the glenoid insertion of the IGHL in producing glenohumeral instabilities.

  - Since the glenohumeral ligaments attach directly to the glenoid labrum, there is always an element of capsular stretching when a labral tear is identified.

    - It is possible to have capsular stretching or laxity without an associated finding of an anterior glenoid labral tear.

Operative Stabilization for Anterior Instability

■ Tightening of the anterior structures to limit external rotation (Magnuson-Stack and Putti-Platt procedure)

■ Coracoid transfer procedures (Bristow operation) to provide a bony block and a tenodesis effect to prevent anterior translation of the humeral head over the anterior glenoid rim

■ Osteotomies of the glenoid or humerus

■ Reconstruction of the avulsed or stretched IGLC structures (Bankart procedure and its modifications)

■ Indications for open surgery include:

    ■ Anterior rim glenoid fracture (>20%)

    ■ Large posterior humeral head defect

    ■ Severe ligament damage (previous capsular shrinkage with failure or HAGL lesion)

■ Arthroscopic stabilization procedures[123] involve a capsular plication combined with reattachment of the IGLLC (arthroscopic Bankart repair).

■ Arthroscopic stabilization can be used in the following circumstances:

    ■ First-time traumatic dislocations

       ■ Hill-Sachs, Bankart, or Perthes lesions, without hyperlaxity

    ■ Recurrent posttraumatic dislocation with or without hyperlaxity

    ■ Injuries not involving compromise of IGHL and MGHL competence

    ■ Injuries without osteochondral lesions

    ■ Symptomatic subluxation

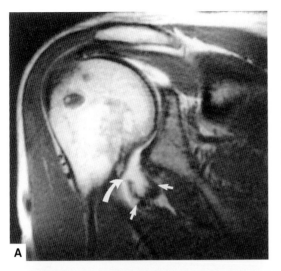
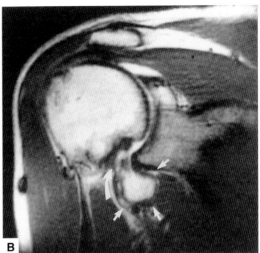

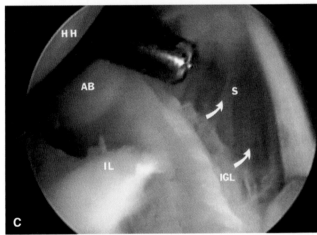

FIGURE 7.9 (**A,B**) Anterior coronal oblique images display an abnormally capacious axillary pouch (*straight arrows*) secondary to avulsion of the IGL humeral insertion (*curved arrows*) as a HAGL lesion. (**C**) An arthroscopic image also shows the avulsed humeral attachment of the IGL (*curved arrows*). AB, anterior band; HH, humeral head; IL, torn inferior labrum; S, subscapularis muscle.

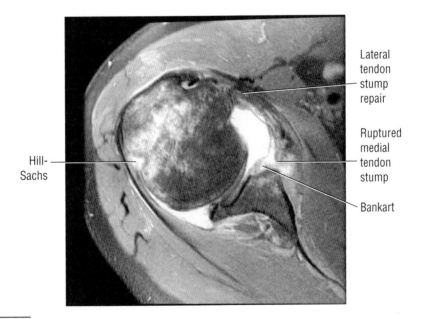

FIGURE 7.10 Axial FS PD FSE image showing a failed Putti-Platt with recurrent anterior instability and deficiency of the anterior inferior glenoid rim. In the Putti-Platt procedure, the subscapularis tendon is divided. The lateral stump of the subscapularis is attached to soft tissue along the anterior rim of the glenoid and the medial stump is lapped over the lateral stump to the greater tuberosity to effect shortening of the capsule and subscapularis muscle.

■ **Arthroscopic stabilization is contraindicated in the following situations:**

  ■ **Osseous or bony Bankart lesions**

  ■ **Labral hypoplasia**

  ■ **Severe injury of the IGHL or MGHL**

  ■ **HAGL lesions**

  ■ **Injuries with concomitant cuff lesions**

  ■ **Voluntary instability and multidirectional instability**

  ■ **Posterior instability**

  ■ **Nondisplaced fracture of the greater tuberosity**

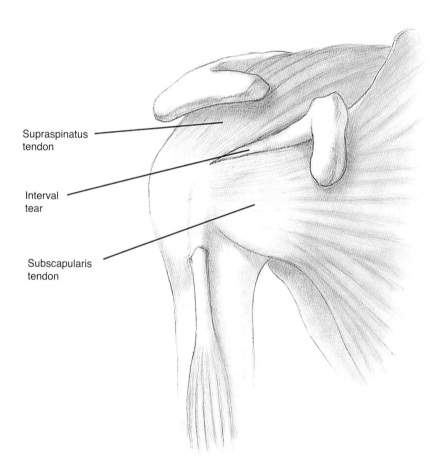

Supraspinatus tendon

Interval tear

Subscapularis tendon

FIGURE 7.11   A common pathologic lesion in shoulders that have recurrent anterior glenohumeral dislocation is an enlargement of the seam separating the supraspinatus and subscapularis tendons. The humeral head can be palpated in this interval. This interval should be closed as part of the repair in cases where the interval is patulous. (Reprinted from Craig EV. *Master Techniques in Orthopaedic Surgery: Shoulder.* 3rd ed. Philadelphia, PA: Lippincott Williams & Wilkins; 2013, with permission.)

Classification of Anterior and Multidirectional Instability

- Eighty-five percent of dislocations are anterior.

  - Subcoracoid dislocations, caused by abduction, extension, and external rotation, are the most common.

- Other types of anterior dislocation include:

  - Subglenoid

  - Subclavicular

  - Intrathoracic

  - Retroperitoneal

- Anterior shoulder instability can be classified as either traumatic or nontraumatic.[338,472]

- Any severe trauma, such as fracture of the greater tuberosity or rotator cuff avulsions, may cause anterior instability.

- Unidirectional (anterior) traumatic dislocation, accounting for 95% of shoulder instability, is referred to as traumatic unidirectional instability treated with Bankart surgery (TUBS).

- Multidirectional atraumatic subluxation is referred to as atraumatic multidirectional and bilateral instability (AMBRI) or multidirectional instability (MDI).

  - This instability is often bilateral and is treated with rehabilitation or reconstruction of the rotator interval capsule–coracohumeral ligament mechanism and an inferior capsular shift.

  - Symptomatic shoulder laxity in one or more directions (anterior, posterior, inferior). The presence of a Bankart lesion or Hill-Sachs fracture does not exclude the diagnosis of MDI. An instability event may occur in a patient with underlying laxity of the glenohumeral joint.

- Patients may have a combination of TUBS and AMBRI (MDI).

  - TUBS patients present in pain with anterior prominence of the humeral head.[405]

    - There is usually a history of an anterior force applied to an abducted, externally rotated arm.

    - This force results in the shoulder "popping out of its socket."

  - AMBRI patients are often difficult to diagnose; many report a sensation of their shoulder sliding forward or their arm going numb.

- In true MDI of the glenohumeral joint, force applied distally in the upper extremity with the patient's arm abducted causes inferior subluxation of the humeral head.

  - This produces a visible sulcus (i.e., the sulcus sign) between the prominence of the acromion and the inferior subluxed humeral head.

  - The positive subacromial sulcus sign indicates laxity of the inferior capsule.

- Positive apprehension and apprehension suppression signs with the arm placed in the ABER position

- Positive anterior-posterior glide (APG) test with the shoulder joint translated anterior and posterior over the edge of the glenohumeral joint

- Positive early warning sign of voluntary muscular instability (with little or no pain) versus positional subluxators

- In classic MDI, the ligament laxity is bilateral and atraumatic.

- No visible ligament labral lesions are seen in patients with true MDI of the glenohumeral joint.

- The capsular ligaments are redundant, and the labrum is often hypoplastic in MDI.

  - Some patients with multidirectional laxity, however, present with unidirectional pathology and experience dislocation predominantly in only one direction.

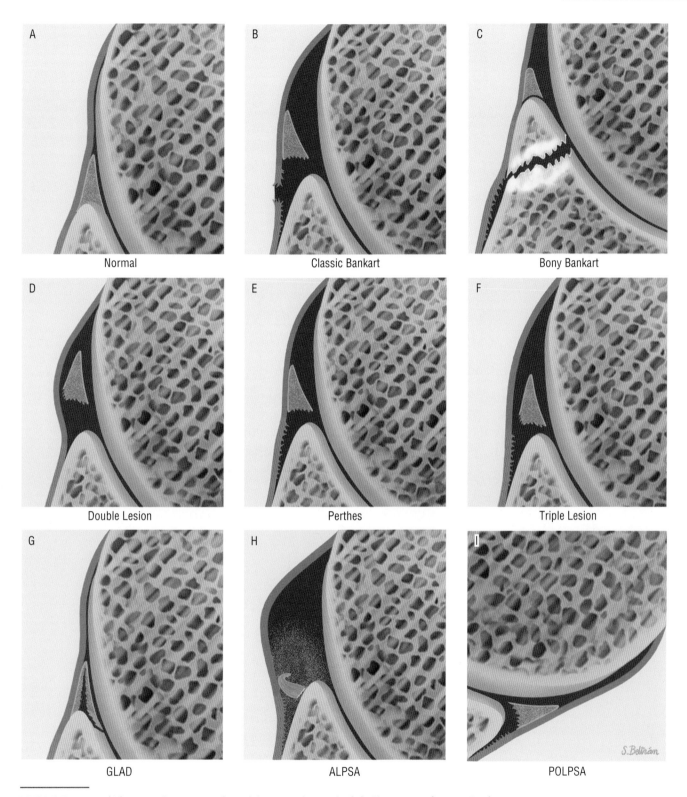

FIGURE 7.12 (**A**) Normal anterior inferior labrum and capsule. (**B**) Classic or soft tissue Bankart with disruption of scapular periosteum. (**C**) Bony or osseous Bankart with a double labral lesion. (**D**) Double labral lesion with labral disruption from both the glenoid rim and adjacent IGHL. (**E**) Perthes avulsion of the labrum and IGHL from the anterior scapular neck without periosteal disruption. (**F**) Triple labral lesion with disruption of the labrum from the glenoid rim and IGHL, with additional tearing of the IGHL from the scapular neck. (**G**) A GLAD lesion (glenoid labrum articular disruption) is also known as a GARD lesion (glenoid articular rim divot). These lesions involve a partial tear of the anterior inferior glenoid labrum with adjacent articular cartilage defect in clinically stable patients. (**H**) The ALPSA lesion is an anterior labroligamentous periosteal sleeve avulsion. (**I**) The POLPSA lesion (posterior labrocapsular periosteal sleeve avulsion).

Related Injuries

- Injuries associated with anterior ligament and capsule dislocations include[338]:

  - Avulsion of the anterior inferior glenohumeral ligament (AIGHL) and capsule from the glenoid (more common in younger individuals)

  - HAGL lesion with or without bone flecks

  - Fractures of the glenoid, humeral head, tuberosities, or coracoid process

  - Cuff tears associated with anterior and inferior glenohumeral dislocation (30% incidence in patients less than 40 years of age and 80% incidence in patients over 60 years of age)

  - Vascular injury, which may occur during dislocation or reduction and is more common in elderly patients

  - The structures at risk include the axillary artery or vein or branches of the axillary artery—the thoracoacromial, subscapular, circumflex, and less commonly the long thoracic nerve.

  - Neurovascular injuries, usually affecting the brachial plexus and axillary nerves

MR Findings in Anterior Instability

Bankart Lesions

- Anterior labral pathology in the anteroinferior quadrant may vary based on the degree of involvement of the anterior inferior labrum, the scapular periosteum, the IGHL, the osseous glenoid rim, and the articular cartilage of the anterior inferior glenoid and displacement of the anterior labrum.[621]

- Subcoracoid dislocation

  - Is the most common form of anterior dislocation

  - Mechanism is usually a combination of shoulder abduction, extension, and external rotation.

- The humeral head is impacted on the anterior inferior glenoid rim, producing a Hill-Sachs posterolateral humeral head fracture.

■ MR studies[96,165,442,591] are used to distinguish between soft tissue (labral only) and osseous (labrum and glenoid rim) Bankart lesions:

   ■ In soft tissue Bankart lesions, the anteroinferior labrum is avulsed without fracture, deformity, or blunting of the anteroinferior glenoid rim.

      ■ There may be only minimal subchondral edema of the anteroinferior glenoid.

   ■ The osseous or bony Bankart lesion presents with a small to large anterior inferior glenoid rim fracture that may extend anterior and superior to the equator.

■ MR is also used to describe associated rotation of the fractured glenoid rim and to quantify associated medial displacements of the IGHL underneath the glenoid.

■ Superior extension of a Bankart lesion into a SLAP tear represents a SLAP 5 (SLAP 2 or 3 plus Bankart) lesion.

■ Sagittal MR images are used to accurately assess the entire area of glenoid fossa involved in the fracture between the equator and the inferior pole of the glenoid.

■ The ABER technique, although not routinely used, is helpful in postoperative assessment of labral repair, properly displaying the labral scar complex in abduction and external rotation.

■ Medial displacement of the avulsed labrum, when it occurs, is secondary to medial and inferior pull from the anterior band of the IGHL.

■ A linear area of hyperintensity is seen in the area of stretching or plastic deformation across the axillary pouch of the IGHL.

■ It is important to differentiate between acute and chronic Bankart lesions.

   ■ A chronic osseous Bankart frequently heals with hypertrophic bone, producing a convex contour anterior to the anterior inferior glenoid rim on sagittal images.

■ Recurrent instability is more likely to occur in patients who are under the age of 20 years at the time of the initial dislocation.[338]

   ■ There is a lower incidence (as low as 10%) of recurrence in patients between 30 and 40 years of age.

- Most recurrences occur within 2 years following the first traumatic dislocation.

- The recurrence rate of instability is lower when a first-time dislocation is associated with a greater tuberosity fracture.

  - An associated greater tuberosity fracture is up to three times more common in patients over 30 years of age.

- Older patients who stretch the IGHL complex or sustain a greater tuberosity fracture are more likely to heal with a static shoulder than younger patients who have nonhealing injuries, including IGHL avulsions and posterolateral humeral head fracture defects (Hill-Sachs defects).

- Recurrence is high in atraumatic instability because there is no traumatic lesion to heal.

- A Hill-Sachs posterolateral compression fracture can be seen in patients with subluxation and single or multiple episodes of dislocation.[644]

  - The compression defect is identified on the posterolateral humeral head.

- There is a normal bare area of bone where the capsule attaches laterally to the anatomic neck of the humerus posteriorly.

  - This bare area shows normal flattening of the posterior aspect of the humeral head in its inferior portion and should not be mistaken for a Hill-Sachs defect.

  - Normal posterolateral cysts or erosions may also occur in the region of the bare area and extend deep to the distal fibers of the infraspinatus tendon posterior to the greater tuberosity.[486]

- Treatment of posttraumatic anterior instability must address:

  - The Bankart lesion

  - Anterior labroligamentous periosteal sleeve avulsion (ALPSA)

  - HAGL

  - Capsular laxity

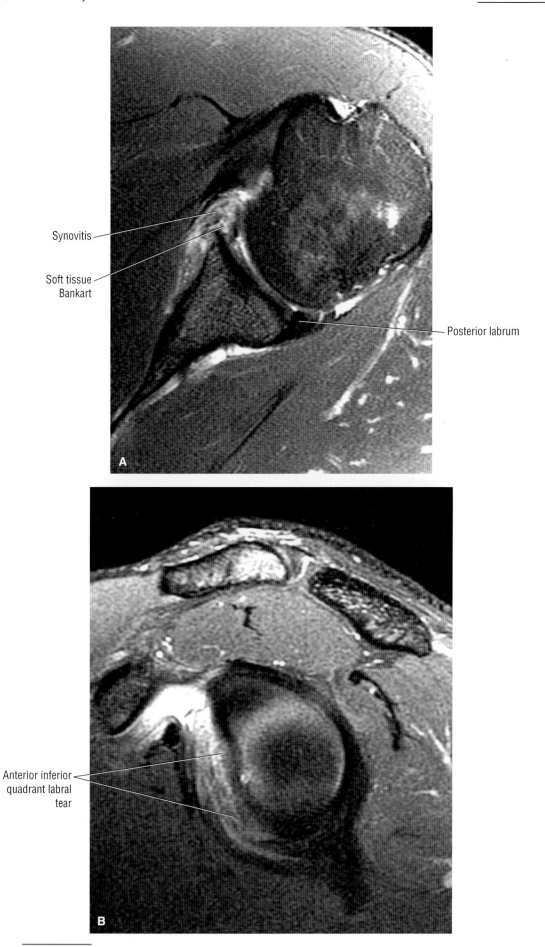

Synovitis

Soft tissue
Bankart

Posterior labrum

Anterior inferior
quadrant labral
tear

FIGURE 7.13 Soft tissue Bankart lesion without fracture or compression of the anterior glenoid rim. FS PD FSE images. (**A**) Axial. (**B**) Sagittal.

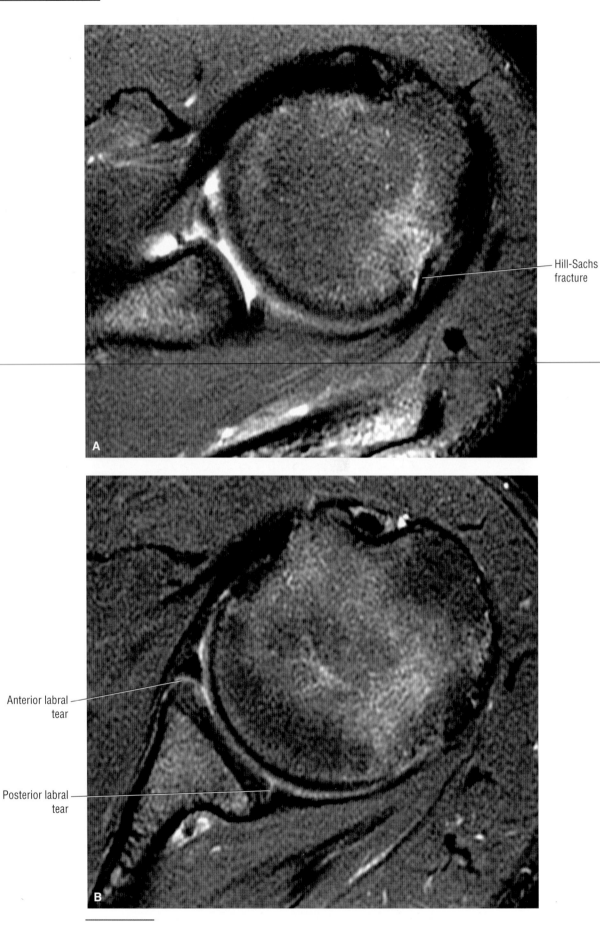

FIGURE 7.14   Posterolateral Hills-Sachs impaction fracture associated with tears of both the anterior and posterior glenoid labrum. (**A**) and (**B**) FS PD FSE.

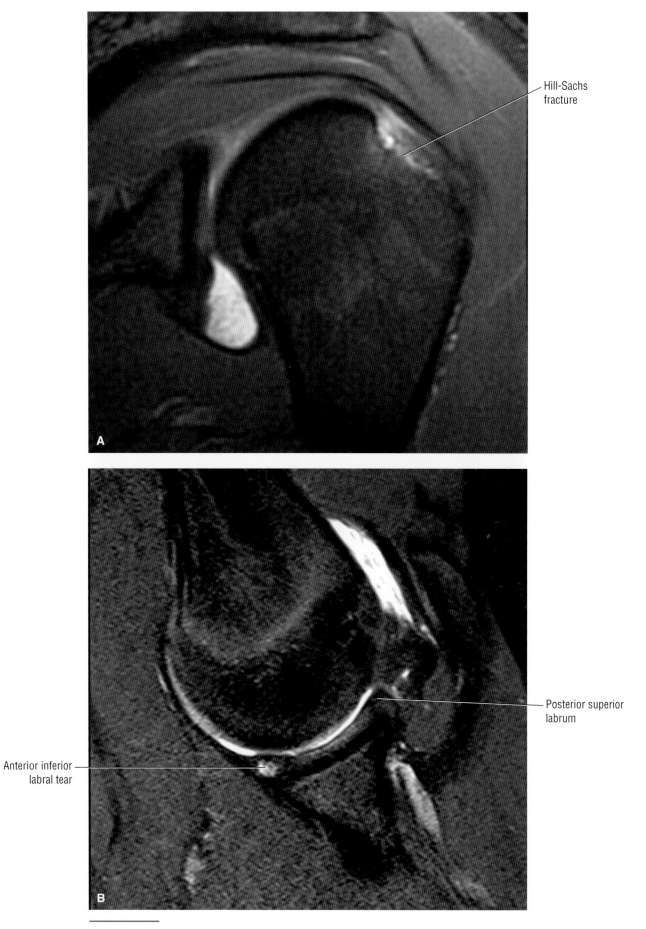

Hill-Sachs
fracture

Posterior superior
labrum

Anterior inferior
labral tear

FIGURE 7.15 Macroinstability with Hills-Sachs fracture and soft tissue Bankart lesion with the addition of ABER sequence. (**A**) Coronal view. (**B**) ABER view.

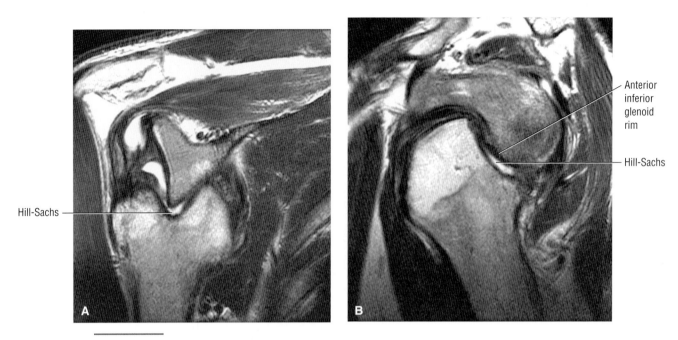

FIGURE 7.16 (**A**) Coronal and (**B**) sagittal T2 FSE images showing fixed anterior subcoracoid dislocation with a large posterolateral humeral head Hill-Sachs fracture.

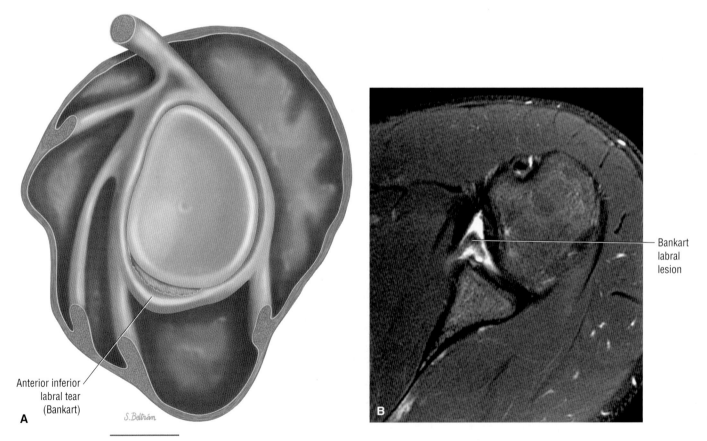

FIGURE 7.17 (**A**) Sagittal color graphic illustrating a soft tissue Bankart lesion. (**B**) Axial FS PD FSE image of anterior displaced anterior inferior labrum (Bankart lesion).

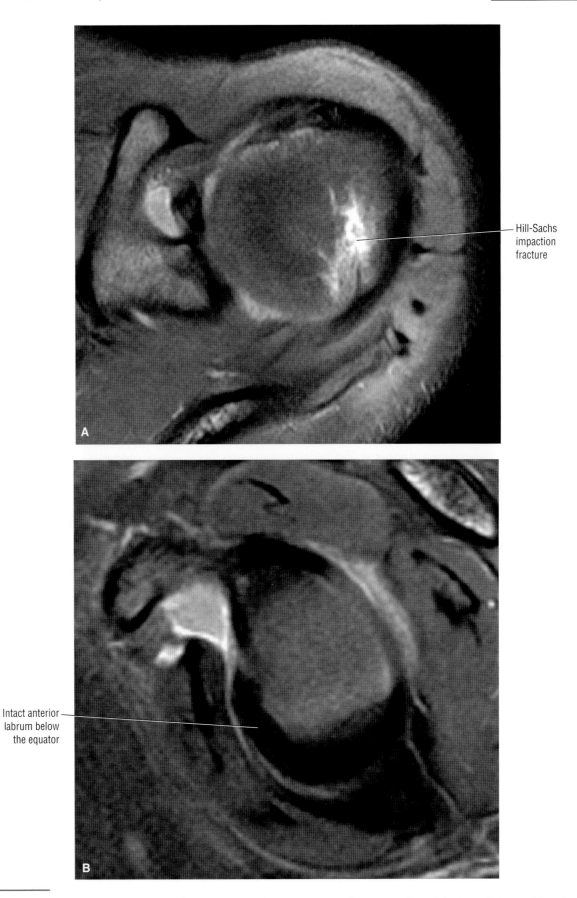

FIGURE 7.18   Posterolateral Hills-Sachs impaction without an associated anterior inferior labral tear. It is possible to have a macroinstability event with capsular stretching without an associated labral tear. Since the capsular ligaments attach directly to the labrum, instability events are associated with both capsular stretching and labral pathology. Subtle degrees of capsular stretching of the IGHL without actual stripping or displacement of the ligament maybe difficult to appreciate on MRI. (**A**) Axial FS PD FSE. (**B**) Sagittal FS PD FSE.

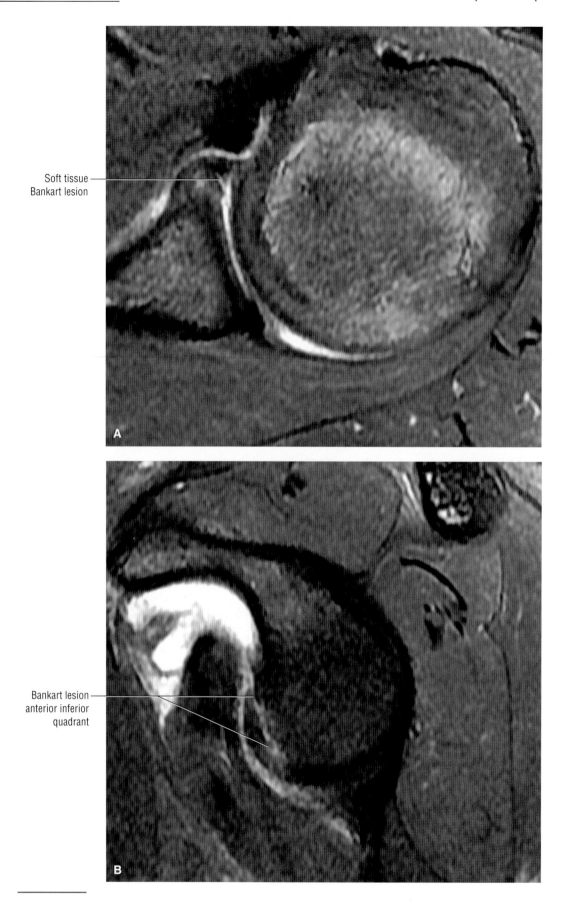

FIGURE 7.19   Soft tissue Bankart lesion involving the entire quadrant of the anterior inferior glenoid labrum below the equator. Close inspection of the contour of the osseous glenoid rim is required to exclude either a compression or fracture of the anterior glenoid fossa which would change the classification to a bony Bankart lesion. On the sagittal image in this case, there is subtle irregularity of the anterior inferior glenoid rim that is more difficult to appreciate in the axial plane. (**A**) Axial FS PD. (**B**) Sagittal FS PD.

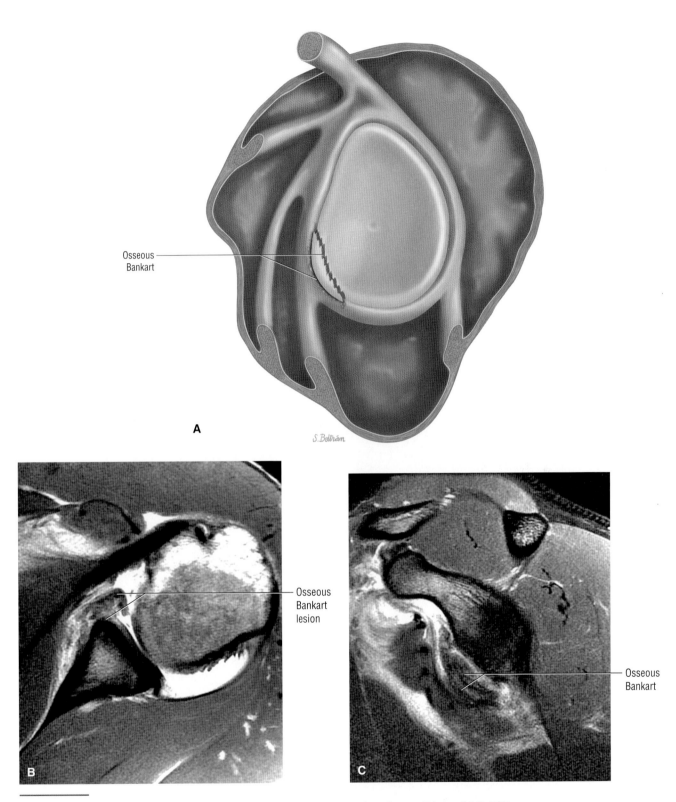

FIGURE 7.20 (**A**) Sagittal color graphic illustrating an osseous Bankart lesion. (**B**) Axial PD FSE MR arthrogram shows an anteroinferior osseous Bankart with avulsion of the labrum and involvement of the anterior glenoid rim. (**C**) Sagittal FS PD FSE MR arthrogram shows the extent of an anteroinferior glenoid rim fracture from the equator to the inferior pole.

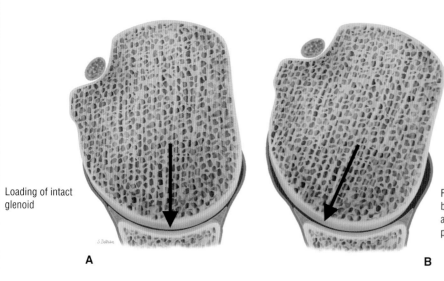

FIGURE 7.21 The normal glenoid arc length resists changes in angles of humeral rotation throughout the glenoid arc length. (**A**) Neutral position. (**B**) External rotation. (Based on Burkhart SS, Lo IKY, Brady PC. *Burkhart's View of the Shoulder: A Cowboy's Guide to Advanced Shoulder Arthroscopy*. Philadelphia, PA: Lippincott Williams & Wilkins; 2006.)

Loading of intact glenoid

Force vector directed beyond the edge of the anterior glenoid may produce a Bankart lesion

A   B

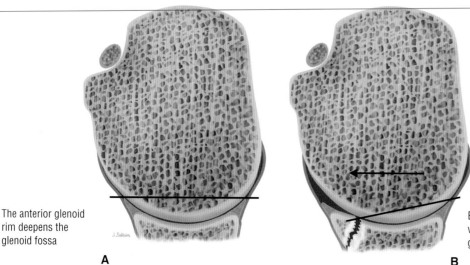

FIGURE 7.22 Osseous Bankart lesion with loss of the full glenoid arc as required to buttress against shear forces as seen in dislocation. (**A**) Normal glenoid fossa. (**B**) Bony Bankart lesion. (Based on Burkhart SS, Lo IKY, Brady PC. *Burkhart's View of the Shoulder: A Cowboy's Guide to Advanced Shoulder Arthroscopy*. Philadelphia, PA: Lippincott Williams & Wilkins; 2006. [See Bankart Lesions pp. 1329 and 1333, in Stoller's 3rd edition.])

The anterior glenoid rim deepens the glenoid fossa

Bony Bankart with decreased glenoid arc

A   B

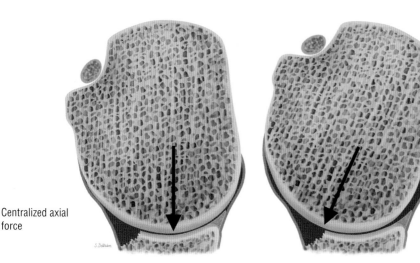

FIGURE 7.23 (**A**) Centrally applied axial force maintains osseous glenohumeral loading in an anterior osseous deficient glenoid. (**B**) The bony Bankart shortens the "safe arc" for the glenoid to overcome axial forces. A Bankart repair may fail if the axial forces are applied beyond the edge of the deficient glenoid. *Based on Burkhart SS, Lo IKY, Brady PC.* (Based on Burkhart SS, Lo IKY, Brady PC. *Burkhart's View of the Shoulder: A Cowboy's Guide to Advanced Shoulder Arthroscopy*. Philadelphia, PA: Lippincott Williams & Wilkins; 2006.)

Centralized axial force

Axial force applied to a point beyond the edge of a deficient glenoid

A   B

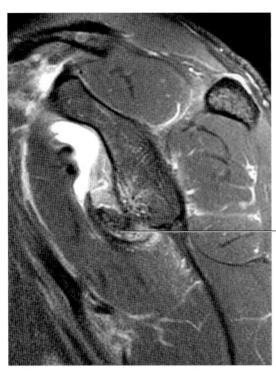

Rotation of osseous Bankart fragment

FIGURE 7.24 Sagittal FS PD FSE image demonstrates rotation of an anteroinferior osseous Bankart fracture.

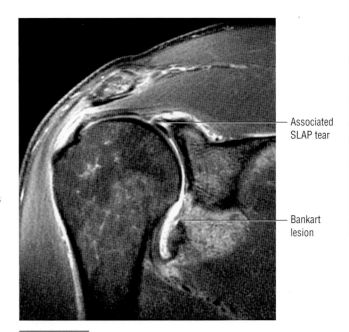

Associated SLAP tear

Bankart lesion

FIGURE 7.25 Coronal FS PD FSE image showing a SLAP 5 lesion. A type 5 SLAP is a combination of a type 2 or 3 SLAP and a Bankart lesion.

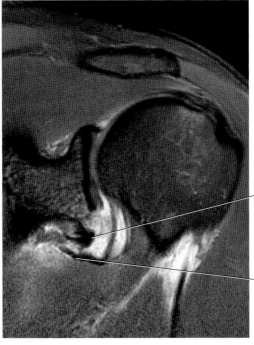

Inferior and medial displacement of anteroinferior labrum (an inferior ALPSA)

Medial displacement of IGHL

FIGURE 7.26 Coronal FS PD FSE image displays medial displacement of the anterior inferior labrum and axillary pouch of the IGHL in a Bankart lesion.

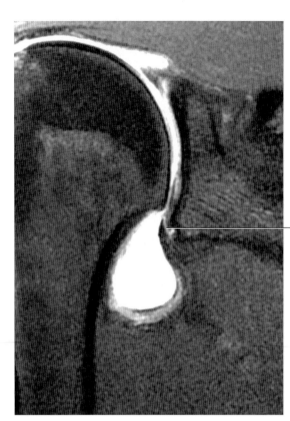

FIGURE 7.27 In the absence of the rare circumferential meniscoid labral variant, no contrast should extend between the inferior labrum and adjacent glenoid articular cartilage. Coronal FS PD FSE image.

Inferior labral tear (6 o'clock)

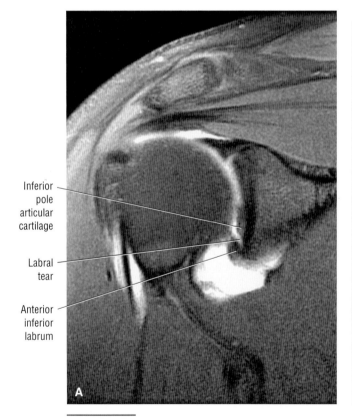

Inferior pole articular cartilage

Labral tear

Anterior inferior labrum

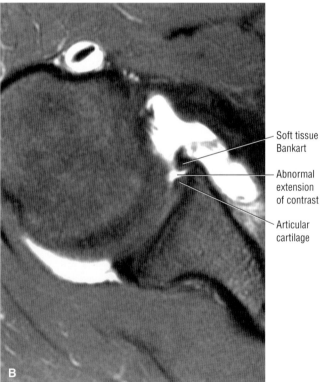

Soft tissue Bankart

Abnormal extension of contrast

Articular cartilage

FIGURE 7.28 Soft tissue Bankart lesion on coronal (**A**) and axial (**B**) FS PD FSE images. Note detection of contrast between the inferior labrum and glenoid inferior pole articular cartilage on the coronal image (**A**). An anteroinferior labral tear can be seen at the inferior glenoid pole using an axial oblique acquisition. This technique matches the anteroinferior glenoid rim with the corresponding posterior inferior glenoid rim and thus minimizes partial volume effects in evaluating anterior inferior labral tears.

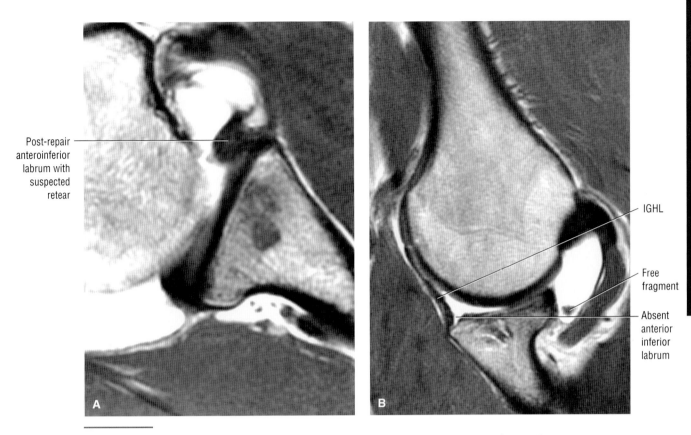

Post-repair anteroinferior labrum with suspected retear

IGHL

Free fragment

Absent anterior inferior labrum

FIGURE 7.29 Retear of the anteroinferior labrum, difficult to appreciate on an axial PD MR arthrogram (**A**), is easily identified on the corresponding abduction external rotation (ABER) sequence (**B**).

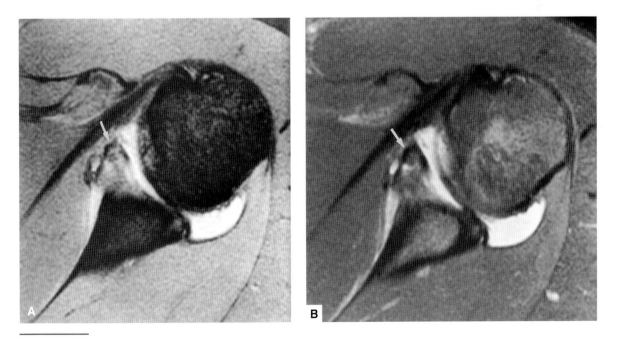

FIGURE 7.30 Chronic Bankart lesion (*arrow*) in an injured football player is seen on T2* (**A**), FS PD FSE (**B**), axial images. On the FS PD FSE, image there is a lack of bone marrow edema at the fracture site or in adjacent glenoid subchondral bone marrow. Sclerotic changes in the anterior inferior glenoid rim would be visible on a T1- or PD-weighted image.

Bankart Repair

- Bankart Labral Detachment
  - Is the primary lesion after initial traumatic dislocation
  - Is associated with coexistent capsular redundancy or laxity at the time of the initial dislocation
    - With chronic recurrent instability, there is even further capsule attenuation.[338]

- A Bankart repair and capsular shifting or plication may be required to restore and maintain stability.
  - Metallic devices such as staples, rivets, or screws are no longer used because of high instability recurrence rates.

- Common Bankart Repair Techniques
  - Bioabsorbable tacks
  - Transglenoid sutures
  - Suture anchors (used for both soft tissue and osseous Bankart repair)[574]

- Bankart Repair Procedures
  - The goal of repair procedures is to fix the detached labrum to the anterior glenoid rim.
    - Capsular shift techniques involve advancing redundant anteroinferior capsular tissue proximally and medially and then attaching the capsule to the glenoid rim.
    - Arthroscopic Bankart repair may be used in acute anterior instability in patients with first-time traumatic dislocation.
      - Particularly in younger patients, who have an 80% to 90% recurrence rate
    - In cases of chronic instability with recurrent dislocation and capsular laxity, a Bankart repair and inferior capsular shift are performed simultaneously.
    - Arthroscopic capsular imbrication is used to reduce capsular volume in patients with small amounts of capsular redundancy.
    - Thermal capsulorrhaphy, using a heat probe with radiofrequency heat energy to reduce capsular laxity, has been associated with high failure rates and tissue necrosis.
    - AMBRI (MDI) patients undergo rehabilitation for at least 3 to 6 months after repair.

Complications in Operative Management of Anterior Instability

- Infection

- Recurrent instability

- Loss of external rotation

- Neurovascular injury

- Hardware migration

Engaging Hill-Sachs Defect and Remplissage

- Located at the posterolateral humeral head, the humeral head may contact the anterior glenoid rim in abduction and external rotation.[71]

- Can be treated by an arthroscopic remplissage for significant bone defects (3 to 7mm) with the addition of a capsular shift
  - To fill the Hill-Sachs lesion with infraspinatus fibers and capsular tissue
  - Since many Hills-Sachs lesions are associated with PASTA lesions of the infraspinatus, the repair of the PASTA and the insetting of the infraspinatus into the Hills-Sachs defect could be done concurrently.

Inverted Pear Glenoid

- Is created by an anterior inferior glenoid rim fracture (an osseous Bankart lesion), which results in an inferior glenoid fossa that is narrower than the superior glenoid

- Less shearing resistance and decreased resistance to humeral axial forces

- Effective glenoid available for humeral rotation is therefore shortened secondary to loss of bone.

■ Treated by lengthening the glenoid and by restoring the glenoid bone stock (e.g., Latarjet reconstruction using a coracoid graft)

   ■ Congruent-arc Latarjet reconstruction used to orient the coracoid graft such that the arc of its inferior surface is a congruent extension of the glenoid articular arc

■ Post arthroscopic Bankart repair, the arc of the humeral head should be centered on the bare spot of the glenoid.

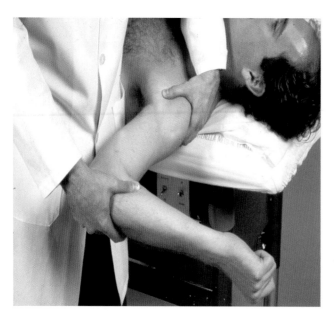

FIGURE 7.31   Apprehension test. Abduction, external rotation, and anterior humeral force recreate the patient's symptoms of anterior instability. (Reprinted from Miniaci A, Iannotti JP, Williams GR, Zuckerman, JD. *Disorders of the Shoulder: Sports Injuries.* 3rd ed. Philadelphia, PA: Lippincott Williams & Wilkins; 2014, with permission.)

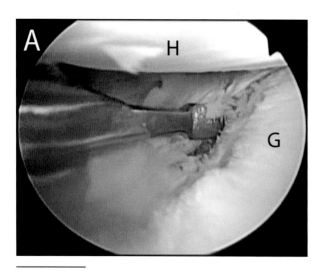
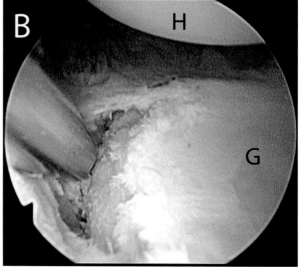

FIGURE 7.32   Right shoulder, anterosuperolateral portal demonstrating mobilization of a Bankart lesion. (**A**) A 15° arthroscopic elevator is introduced through an anterior portal to mobilize the labrum. (**B**) A shaver assists in the mobilization. Mobilization is complete when subscapularis muscle fibers are visualized medially, deep to the capsule. G, glenoid; H, humerus. (Reprinted from Burkhart S, Lo IK, Brady PC, Denard PJ. *The Cowboy's Companion: A Trail Guide for the Arthroscopic Shoulder Surgeon.* Philadelphia, PA: Lippincott Williams & Wilkins; 2012, with permission.)

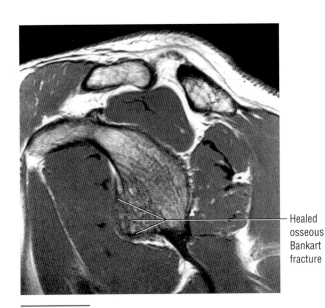

FIGURE 7.33 Sagittal PD FSE image showing a chronic healed osseous Bankart lesion with prominent convex anterior inferior glenoid rim contour (the "beer gut sign").

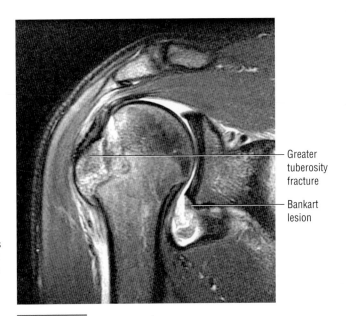

FIGURE 7.34 Coronal FS PD FSE image of a greater tuberosity fracture and a Bankart lesion. The association of a greater tuberosity fracture is more common in patients over 30 years of age.

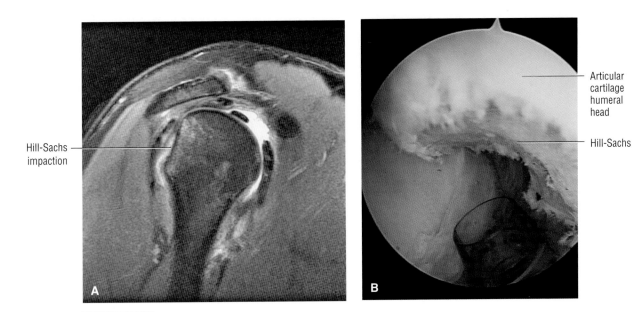

FIGURE 7.35 (**A**) Posterolateral Hill-Sachs deformity with flattening of the posterior humeral head contour on a sagittal FS PD FSE image. (**B**) Arthroscopic view of Hill-Sachs fracture. A deep (>1cm) Hill-Sachs fracture is usually associated with an inverted pear glenoid. Hill-Sachs lesions between 3 to 7mm in depth may be either engaging or nonengaging.

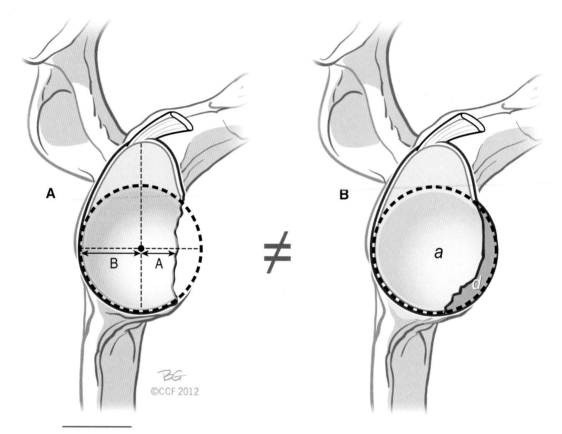

FIGURE 7.36 Methods used to quantify glenoid bone loss. Computer software–assisted calculations of glenoid bone loss using (**A**) linear method and (**B**) surface area method. Although calculated bone loss between the two methods is similar (i.e., absolute value ~20% to 25%), the measurements represent different dimensions and locations of bone loss. Since most biomechanical data regarding glenoid bone loss is based on linear measurements (using an inferior glenoid circle) the linear and surface-area calculations cannot be interchanged. (Adapted from Burkhart SS, De Beer JF, Tehrany AM, et al. Quantifying glenoid bone loss arthroscopically in shoulder instability. *Arthroscopy* 2002;18:488–491; and from Baudi P, Righi P, Bolognesi D, et al. How to identify and calculate glenoid bone deficit. *Chir Organi Mov* 2005;90:145-152. Reprinted from Miniaci A, Iannotti JP, Williams GR, Zuckerman, JD. *Disorders of the Shoulder: Sports Injuries.* 3rd ed. Philadelphia, PA: Lippincott Williams & Wilkins; 2014, with permission.)

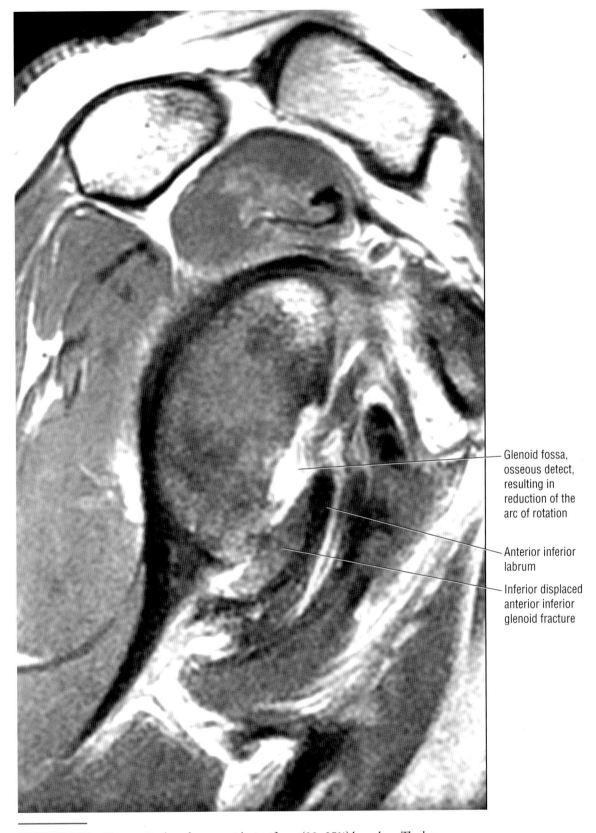

Glenoid fossa,
osseous detect,
resulting in
reduction of the
arc of rotation

Anterior inferior
labrum

Inferior displaced
anterior inferior
glenoid fracture

FIGURE 7.37 Osseous Bankart fracture with significant (20–25%) bone loss. The hypointense glenoid labrum is still adherent to the displaced osseous Bankart fragment. The decrease in inferior glenoid diameter results in an inverted-pear glenoid. A glenoid fossa with bone loss has a decreased congruent arc. There is a decreased resistance to applied shear forces and to obliquely applied off-axis loads.

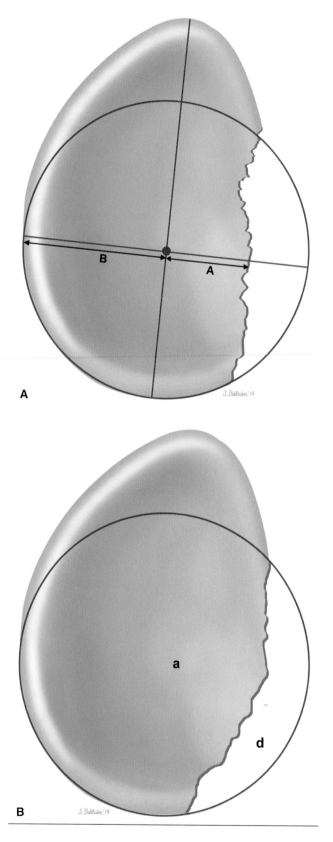

FIGURE 7.38 (**A,B**) Surface area method of calculating bone loss in an osseous Bankart. Comparison of linear method versus surface area method for calculation of glenoid bone loss. In addition, the osseous Bankart fragment should be reported in long and short axis measurement. At arthroscopy glenoid bone loss can be assessed by use of a calibrated probe marking the distance from the glenoid bare spot to the posterior rim and then from the remaining anterior rim to the glenoid bare spot.

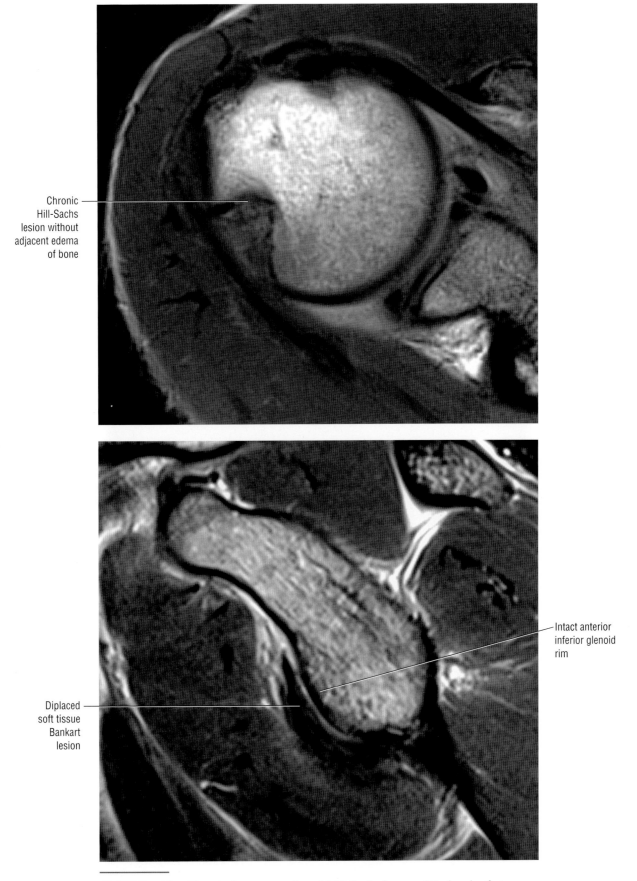

Chronic
Hill-Sachs
lesion without
adjacent edema
of bone

Intact anterior
inferior glenoid
rim

Diplaced
soft tissue
Bankart
lesion

FIGURE 7.39 Chronic deep posterolateral Hill-Sachs fracture. Displaced soft tissue Bankart lesion with medially displaced labrum and capsule. A deep Hill-Sachs lesion can engage in a position of 90° abduction plus 90° external rotation.

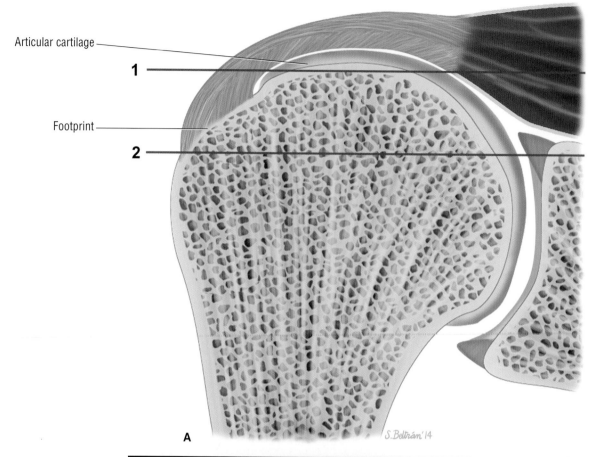

Articular cartilage

1

Footprint

2

A

S.Beltrán'14

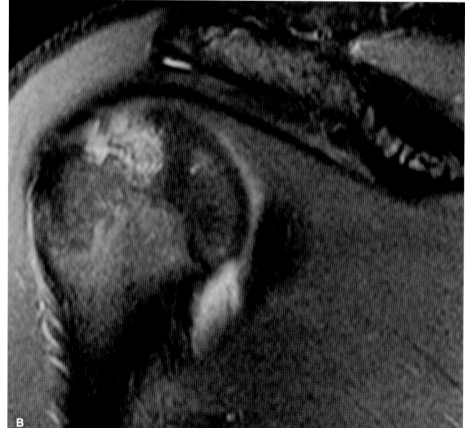

B

FIGURE 7.40   Position number 1 at the level of the humeral head articular cartilage is the region in which a Hills-Sachs lesion must occur. The corresponding axial image must show a posterolateral contour defect at this level. In position number 2, flattening of the humeral head may occur as a variation. Changes of internal impingement may also occur in this area and should not be mistaken for a Hills-Sachs lesion. An extensive Hills-Sachs lesion, however, may extend from position 1 to position 2. Changes of internal impingement, however, may not be seen at the level of the humeral head articular cartilage in position 1. (A) Coronal illustration. (B) Coronal MRI shows the posterior superior location of the Hill-Sachs lesion which involves the articular cartilage surface and is located superior to the footprint of the rotator cuff.

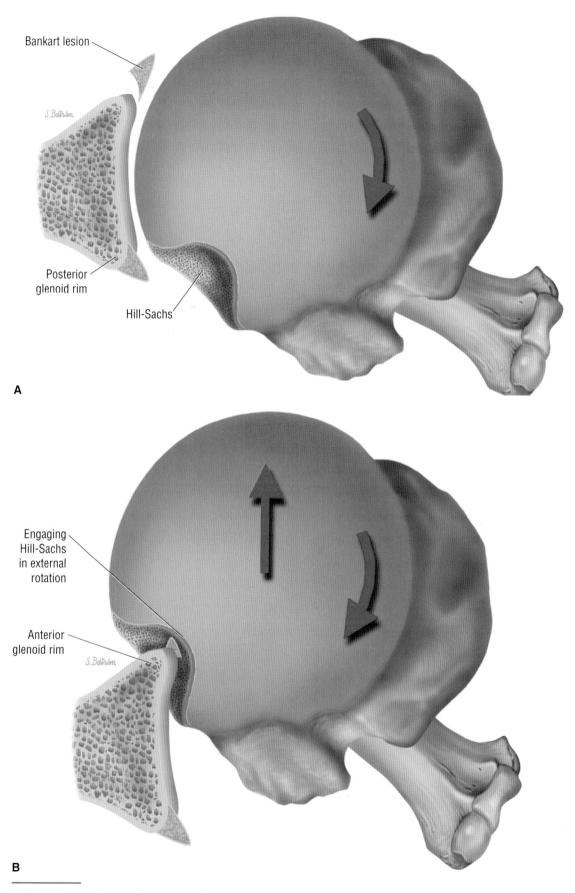

FIGURE 7.41 Stages of engaging Hill-Sachs lesion with posterolateral humeral head defect contacting the posterior glenoid rim (**A**) and subsequently engaging the anterior rim (**B**). The engaging Hill-Sachs reproduces the anterior inferior instability event with humeral head displacement.

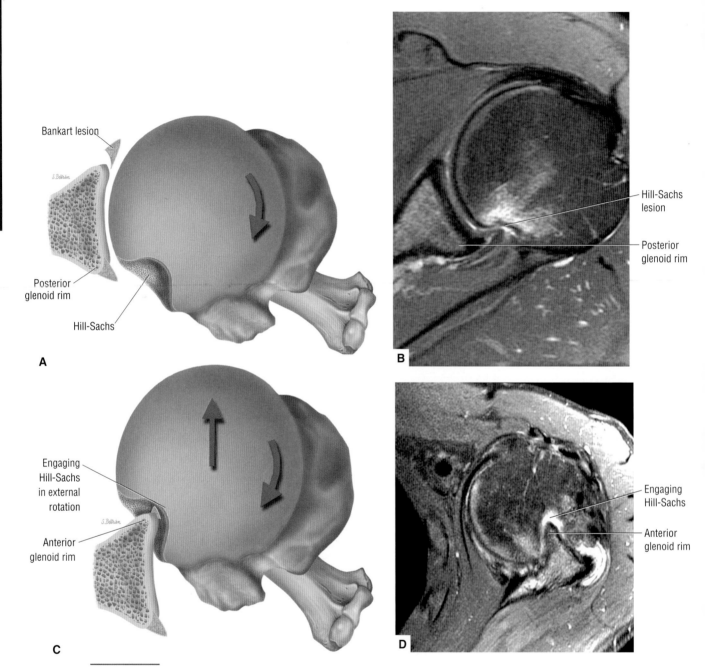

FIGURE 7.42   Stages of engaging Hill-Sachs lesion with posterolateral humeral head defect contacting the posterior glenoid rim (**A,B**) and subsequently engaging the anterior rim (**C,D**). The engaging Hill-Sachs reproduces the anterior inferior instability event with humeral head displacement. (**A,C**) Superior axial views illustrating stages of engagement. (**B,D**) Axial PD FSE images in external rotation. A Remplissage can be performed in patients with a large Hill-Sachs even without associated glenoid bone loss. The remplissage is an infraspinatus transfer that fills the Hill-Sachs defect. This converts the defect to an extra-articular lesion and thereby prevents engagement. A moderate-to-large Hill-Sachs lesion is greater than 4 to 5 mm in depth.

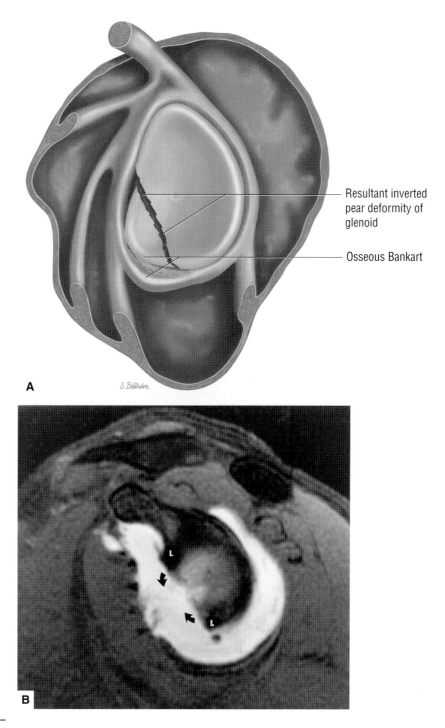

FIGURE 7.43 (**A**) Sagittal color illustration and (**B**) sagittal FS T1-weighted MR arthrogram illustrate an inverted pear deformity with loss of the anterior inferior glenoid rim bone stock in an osseous Bankart lesion. Glenohumeral stability depends on a long congruent articular arc. There is a high recurrence rate of anterior instability in patients with a loss of ≥25% of the inferior glenoid diameter or an engaging Hill-Sachs lesion. L, labrum; curved arrows, deficient anteroinferior glenoid rim.

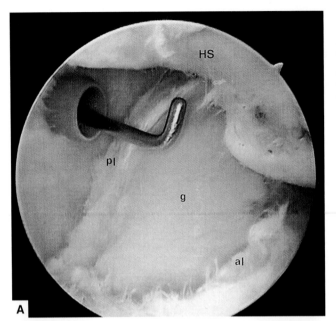

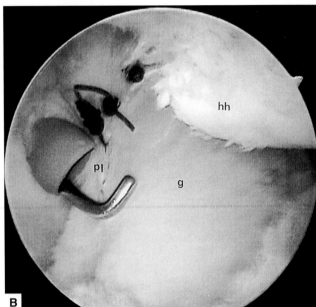

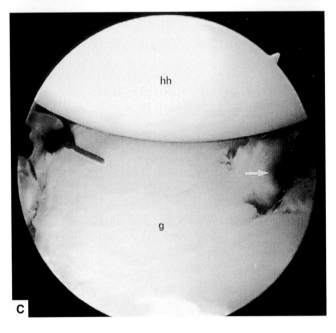

FIGURE 7.44 Arthroscopic repair of the anterior and posterior labrum help centralize an anteriorly dislocated humeral head as viewed from the level of the biceps tendon. (**A**) Frayed posterior labrum (pl) and anterior labrum (al) associated with a Hill-Sachs (HS) fracture of the humeral head are identified. g, glenoid. (**B**) Repair begins with the posterior inferior capsule sutured to the posterior labrum (pl). hh, humeral head; g, glenoid. (**C**) Anteriorly placed sutures (*arrow*) complete the arthroscopic stabilization centralizing the humeral head (hh) on the glenoid (g).

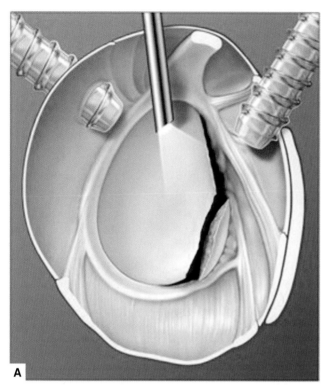

A

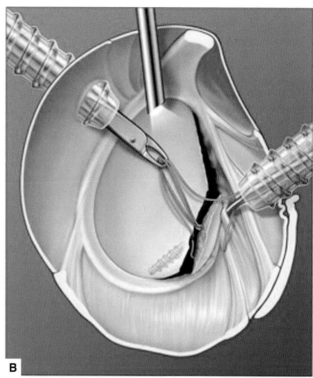

B

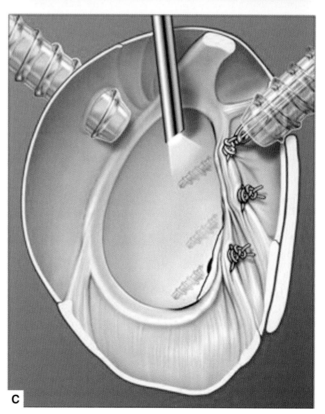

C

FIGURE 7.45   Bony Bankart lesion (**A**). A suture anchor is inserted into the scapular neck and sutures are passed around the bony fragment (**B**). The sutures are then fixed with a knotless anchor at the glenoid rim, and with that, the bony fragment is secured (**C**). (Reprinted from Craig EV. *Master Techniques in Orthopaedic Surgery: Shoulder*. 3rd ed. Philadelphia, PA: Lippincott Williams & Wilkins; 2013, with permission.)

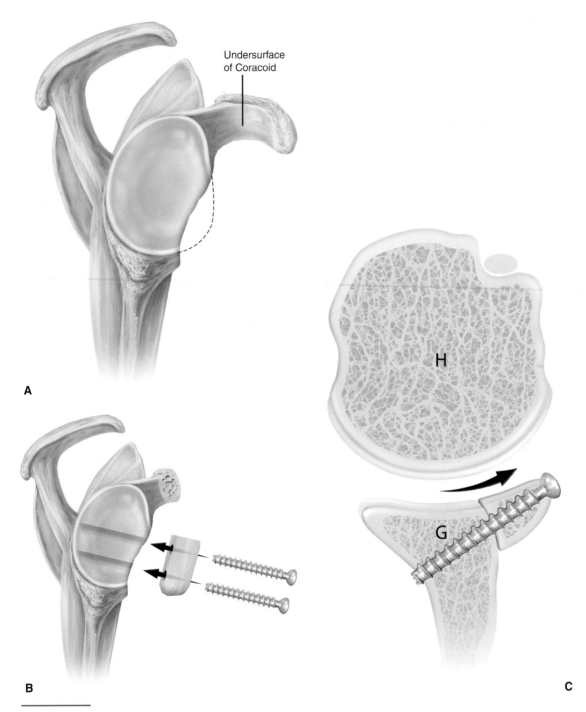

FIGURE 7.46　Schematic of the Burkhart-DeBeer modification of the Latarjet reconstruction. (**A**) Sagittal view demonstrates glenoid bone loss. The undersurface of the coracoid is shaded in blue. (**B**) Following coracoid osteotomy, the graft is rotated 90° on its long axis, so the undersurface of the coracoid is flush with the glenoid and forms a continuation of the concave glenoid articular arc. The graft is secured with two screws. (**C**) Axial view demonstrates how the orientation provides a contour that more closely matches the native glenoid concavity and also provides greater length extension of the articular arc. G, glenoid; H, humerus. (Reprinted from Burkhart S, Lo IK, Brady PC, Denard PJ. *The Cowboy's Companion: A Trail Guide for the Arthroscopic Shoulder Surgeon.* Philadelphia, PA: Lippincott Williams & Wilkins; 2012, with permission.)

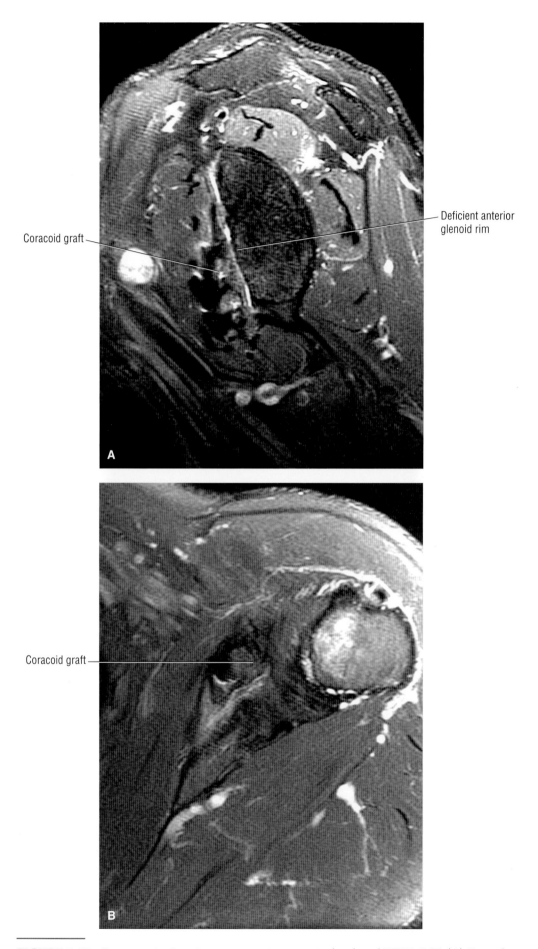

FIGURE 7.47 Postoperative Latarjet reconstruction on sagittal and axial FS PD FSE. (**A**) Sagittal FS PD FSE. (**B**) Axial FS PD FSE. There is incomplete osseous incorporation of the graft.

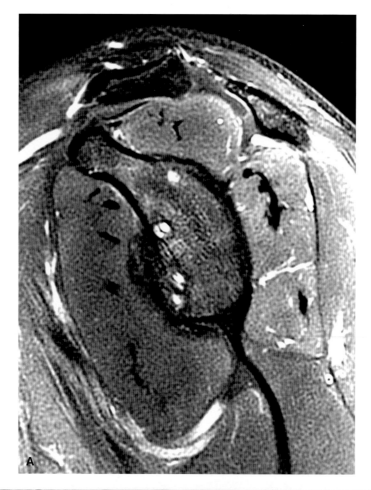

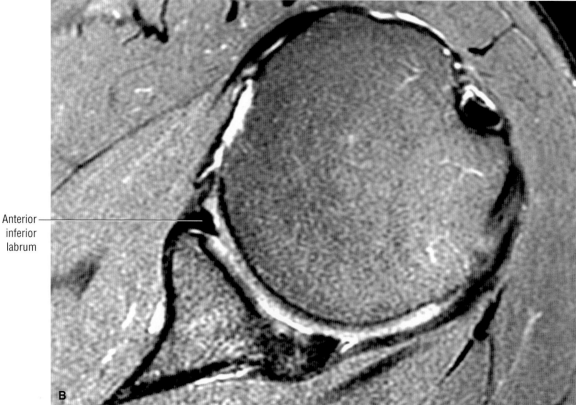

Anterior
inferior
labrum

FIGURE 7.48   Bankart repair using multiple glenoid rim anchors. There is no displacement of the anterior inferior labrum although linear hyperintense fluid undermines the labrum. There is hypertrophic bone on the posterior glenoid rim. **(A)** Sagittal. **(B)** Axial. FS PD FSE images.

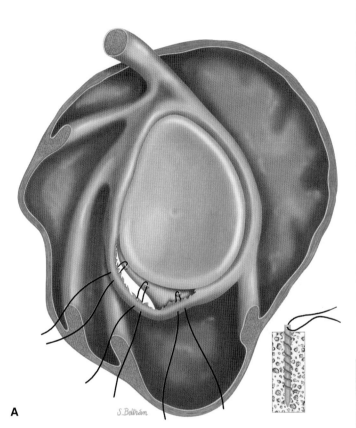

A

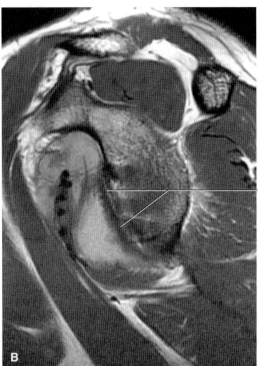

B

Bankart
repair

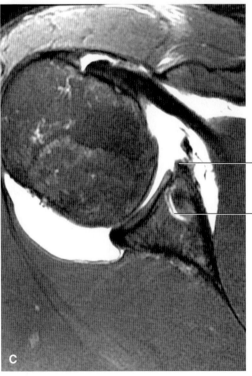

C

Reattached
labrum

Suture
anchor
artifact

FIGURE 7.49 (**A**) Illustration of a Bankart repair with anterior inferior suture anchors shown. Anterior capsule and posterior-inferior capsule plication are further techniques used to improve surgical success for anterior-inferior reconstructions. The goal is to restore anterior and posterior capsular integrity and rebuild the anterior labral wedge. Associated SLAP lesions and middle gleno-humeral ligament detachments are also repaired. The reattached anterior inferior labrum is seen from the equator to the inferior pole of the glenoid on sagittal FS PD FSE image (**B**) and axial FS PD FSE image (**C**). A 2mm strip of articular cartilage is removed along the damaged glenoid rim at arthroscopy to provide for bleeding bone for capsular healing. Remplissage is usually reserved for cases with near normal glenoid fossa width of the inferior glenoid diameter coupled with a deep (>4mm) Hill-Sachs lesion. After a Latarjet reconstruction the shoulder does not engage even with a large-deep Hill-Sachs lesion.

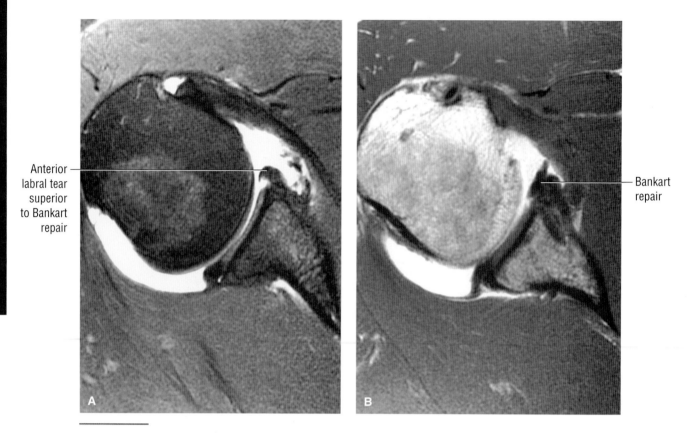

FIGURE 7.50   Axial FS PD FSE MR arthrogram (**A**) shows anterior band superior to the intact Bankart repair (**B**), a PD FSE MR arthrogram.

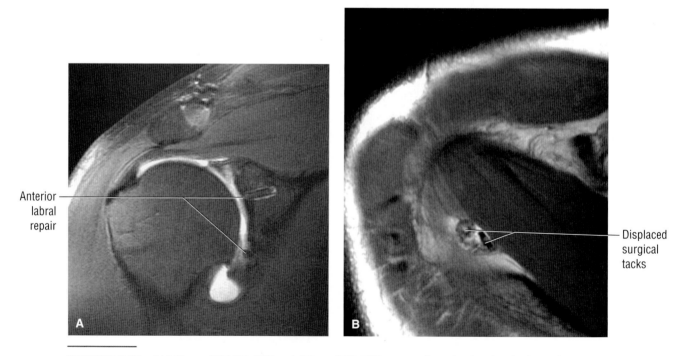

FIGURE 7.51   (**A**) Coronal FS PD FSE and (**B**) axial T2 FSE images show displaced tacks located posterior to the supraspinatus muscle after extensive Bankart repair. These dislodged tacks may lead to degenerative glenohumeral arthrosis and synovitis. The axillary recess, subscapularis, and bursa are common locations.

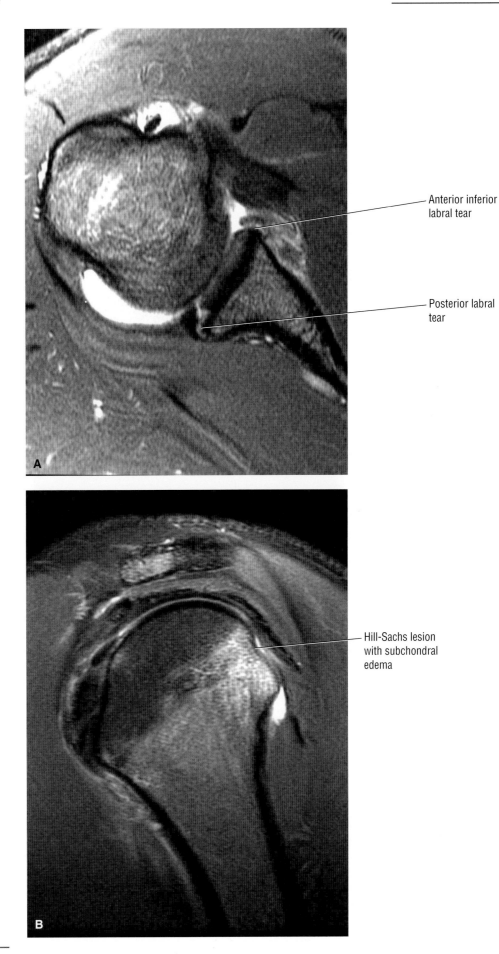

Anterior inferior labral tear

Posterior labral tear

Hill-Sachs lesion with subchondral edema

FIGURE 7.52   Ring concept of glenohumeral instability with both anterior and posterior labral tears after a macroinstability event. (**A**) Axial. (**B**) Sagittal. FS PD FSE images.

Perthes Lesion

■ A labral ligamentous avulsion with an intact scapular periosteum[638]

   ■ Anteroinferior labral tear from its osteochondral attachment to the glenoid. The periosteal sleeve is not torn.

■ The periosteum is stripped medially from the anterior glenoid without medial displacement of the labral periosteal complex.

■ The IGHL and labrum are positioned normally relative to the underlying glenoid. Perthes lesions often occur after the initial dislocation.

■ In chronic cases, there may be fibrosis and resynovialization of the labrum and periosteum.

■ Bankart and Hill-Sachs fractures may be associated findings.

■ May be difficult to identify at arthroscopy or MR because of both minimal labral displacement and granulation tissue at its base. The ABER position which places traction on the anterior band may improve the visualization of Perthes lesions as the labrum partially displaces from the glenoid rim.

ALPSA Lesions (Anterior Labroligamentous Periosteal Sleeve Avulsion)

■ An avulsion of the IGHL through its anterior band attachment to the anterior labrum, similar to the Bankart lesion[409]

   ■ The ALPSA lesion is associated with chronic instability in contrast to the Bankart or Perthes lesion.

■ Differs from a Bankart lesion in that an ALPSA lesion has an intact anterior scapular periosteum that allows the labroligamentous structures to displace medially and rotate inferiorly on the scapular neck

   ■ In a Bankart lesion, the anterior scapular periosteum ruptures, resulting in displacement of the labrum and attached ligaments anterior to the glenoid rim.

   ■ The anteroinferior labroligamentous complex scars anteriorly onto the scapular neck and undergoes a synovialized process with its attached periosteum.

■ After the ALPSA lesion heals, there may be recurrent anterior dislocations secondary to IGHL incompetence.

■ Arthroscopically, an ALPSA lesion is converted to a Bankart lesion to allow reconstruction of the anterior inferior structures of the capsule (capsulorrhaphy).

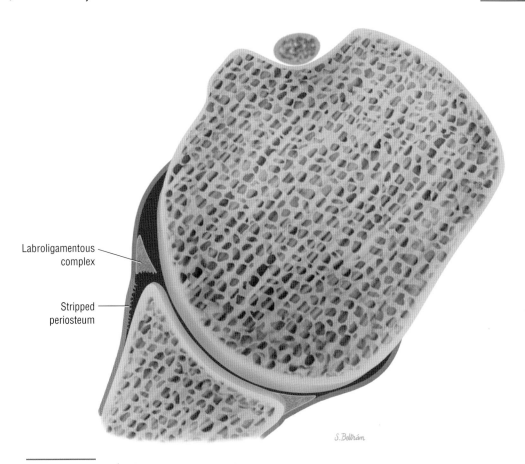

Labroligamentous complex

Stripped periosteum

FIGURE 7.53 Axial color graphic of Perthes lesion, a labral ligamentous avulsion with intact but medially stripped periosteum along the anterior glenoid neck.

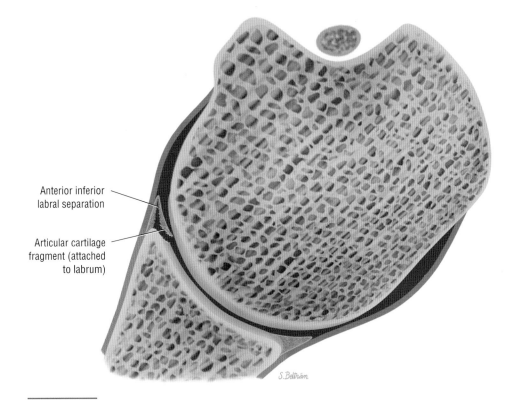

Anterior inferior labral separation

Articular cartilage fragment (attached to labrum)

FIGURE 7.54 Axial color section of GLAD (glenolabral articular disruption) or GARD (glenoid articular rim divot) lesion with flap tear of the anterior inferior labrum and chondral defect of the adjacent articular cartilage. The labrum is connected to the glenoid rim in the GLAD lesion.

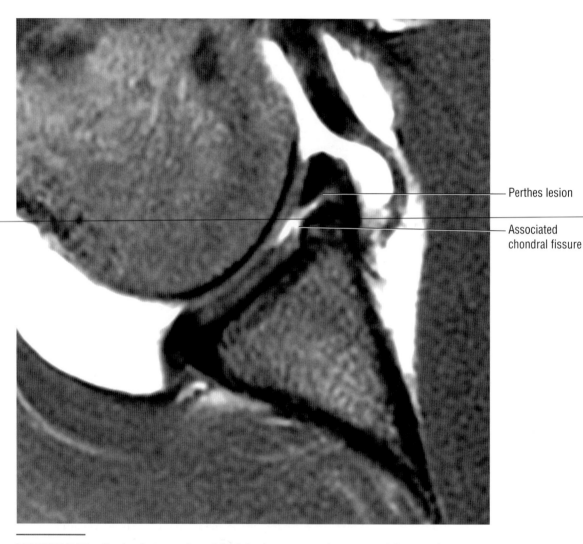

FIGURE 7.55   Perthes lesion without labral displacement or disruption of the scapular periosteum. The lesion occurs from its osteochondral attachment as demonstrated by the hyperintense linear fluid collection between the labrum and the articular cartilage. The periosteal sleeve is intact. MR identifies the closely apposed anterior inferior labrum to the glenoid rim which would not be the case in a Bankart lesion. Associated scarring may make the detection of fluid undermining the labrum more difficult.

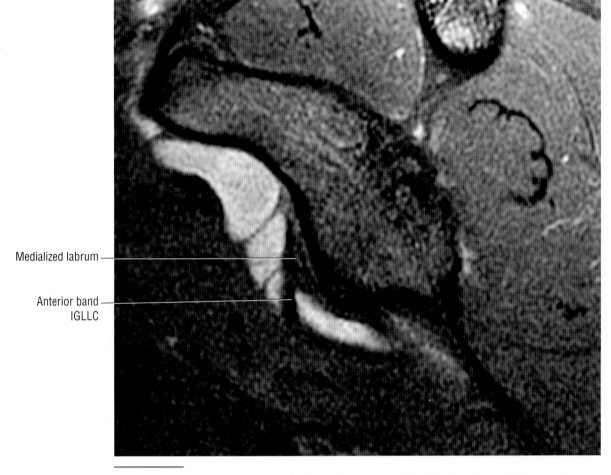

Medialized labrum

Anterior band
IGLLC

FIGURE 7.56 ALPSA lesion with the medialization of a displaced and rotated inferior gleno-humeral ligament labral complex. Note that the labrum and anterior band are located medial to the glenohumeral joint line. Sagittal FS PD. The ALPSA lesion is associated with chronic instability and is usually associated with a history of multiple instability events. The anterior band connects to the medialized anterior inferior labrum and abnormal periosteal sleeve. The association of ALPSA with instability is greater compared with Perthes lesions.

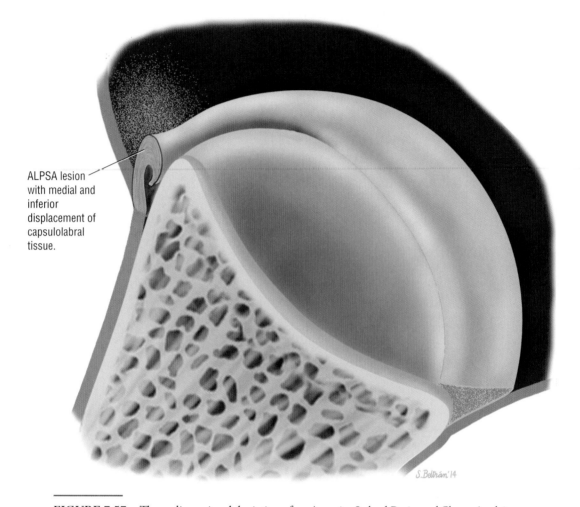

ALPSA lesion
with medial and
inferior
displacement of
capsulolabral
tissue.

S.Beltrán'14

FIGURE 7.57   Three-dimensional depiction of an Anterior Labral Periosteal Sleeve Avulsion or ALPSA lesion retracted along the anterior glenoid neck medial to the glenoid articular surface. In the ALPSA lesion the capsulolabral tissue is detached and healed medially on the glenoid neck. ALPSA lesions are associated with an increase number of presurgical dislocations. There is a higher failure rate with arthroscopic repair compared with Bankart lesions related to the progressive damage to the capsulolabral tissues with multiple episodes of instability.

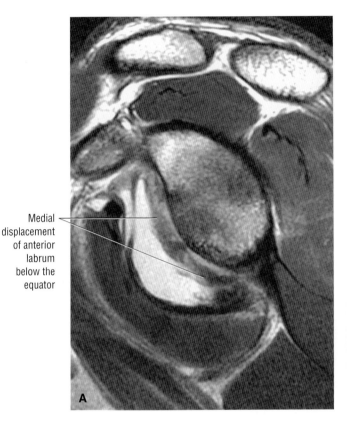

Medial displacement of anterior labrum below the equator

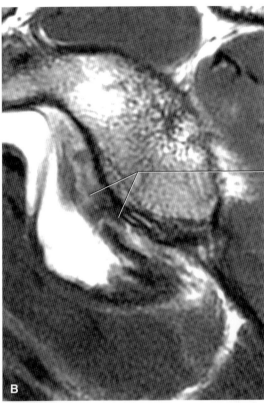

Medialization of anterior inferior labrum

FIGURE 7.58   (**A,B**) Sagittal PD FSE MR arthrograms demonstrate progressive (B is medial to A) medialization of the displaced and rotated inferior glenohumeral ligament labral complex. The medially displaced labral tissue always connects with the anterior band of the IGHL which actually pulls the entire capsulolabral complex in the direction of anterior band (medial and inferior). The key to the MR diagnosis on sagittal images relates to the visualization of labral tissue on medial images of the anterior glenoid rim (several images medial to the glenohumeral joint). (**C**) Corresponding arthroscopic view of a displaced ALPSA lesion. The labrum and fibrous tissue may resynovialize anterior to the neck of the glenoid.

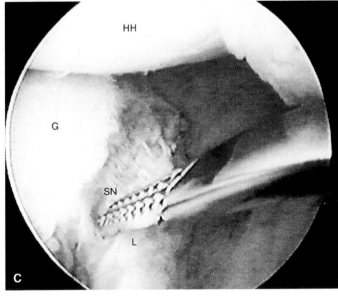

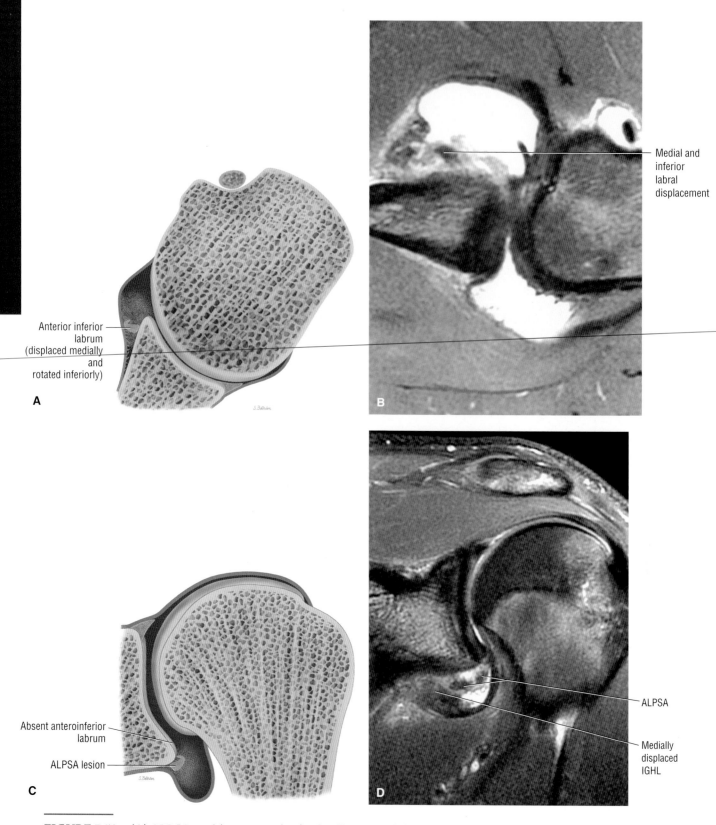

FIGURE 7.59   (**A**) ALPSA axial (transverse plane) color illustration, (**B**) axial FS PD FSE image, (**C**) coronal color illustration, and (**D**) coronal FS PD FSE image of an ALPSA lesion (anterior labroligamentous periosteal sleeve avulsion) with medial and inferior rotation of the anteroinferior labroligamentous complex. The ALPSA is also referred to as a medialized Bankart lesion.

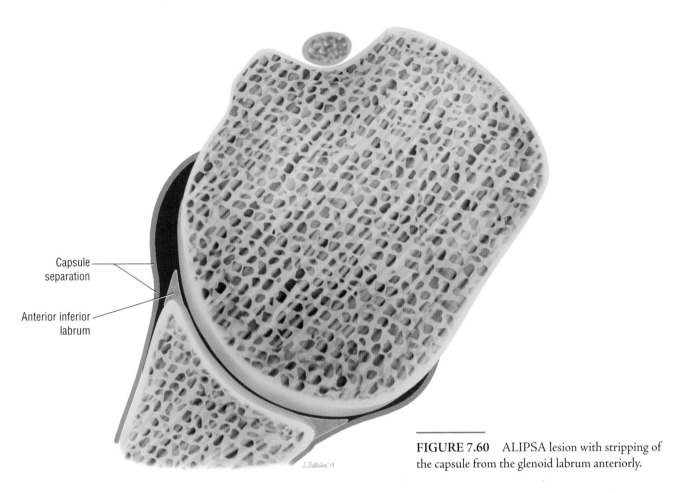

Capsule separation

Anterior inferior labrum

FIGURE 7.60   ALIPSA lesion with stripping of the capsule from the glenoid labrum anteriorly.

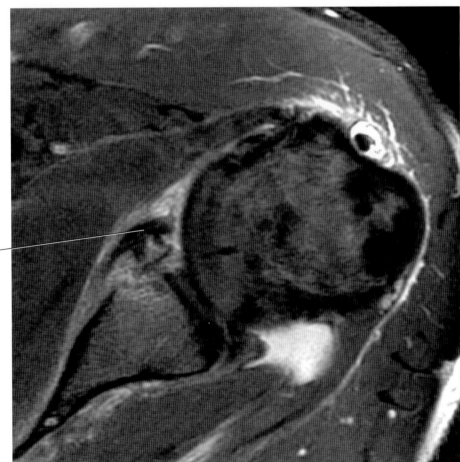

Anterior capsular stripping from Bankart component

FIGURE 7.61   Bankart lesion with ALIPSA component showing capsular stripping.

GLAD Lesions (Glenolabral Articular Disruption)

■ Result from a forced adduction injury occurring from the position of abduction and external rotation of the shoulder[410]

■ There is a superficial anterior inferior labral tear associated with an anterior inferior glenoid articular cartilage injury.

■ There are no signs of clinical or surgical anterior instability.

■ Identification of anterior inferior labral tears may require imaging of the shoulder with the arm positioned in external rotation and abduction.

Capsular-Related Lesions

■ In addition to anterior dislocation associated with failure of the IGHL at the inferior glenoid attachment, the IGHL may fail at other locations, causing the following lesions:[369]

  ■ Failure at the anatomic neck of the humerus causes HAGL and bony HAGL lesions.

      ■ Anterior failure-HAGL

      ■ Posterior failure-HAGL

  ■ Failure at both the humerus and glenoid causes AIGHL lesions.

  ■ Posterior capsular detachment and failure of the posterior band attachment to the humerus causes reverse HAGL lesions.

      ■ RHAGL also includes both ligament and bony RHAGL.

  ■ Failure of the IGHL glenoid attachment without labral avulsion causes glenoid avulsion of the glenohumeral ligament (GAGL) lesions.

  ■ Medial displacement of the IGHL associated with a Bankart causes an inferior ALPSA lesion.

  ■ Midaxillary pouch tears

  ■ Axillary pouch sprain and scarring of the IGHL at the glenoid attachment (partial or healed GAGL)

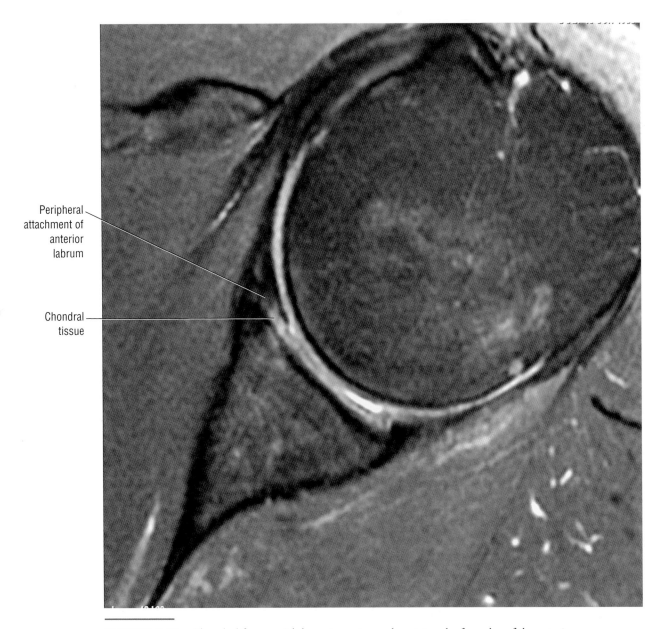

Peripheral
attachment of
anterior
labrum

Chondral
tissue

FIGURE 7.62 Chondral fissure with hyperintensity undermining the free edge of the anterior inferior labrum with stable labral peripheral attachment. GLAD lesions are the result of a forced adduction injury. There is a free edge or superficial anterior inferior labral tear associated with an adjacent anterior inferior chondral injury (tissue or defect). The anterior inferior labrum maintains its peripheral/connection to bone.

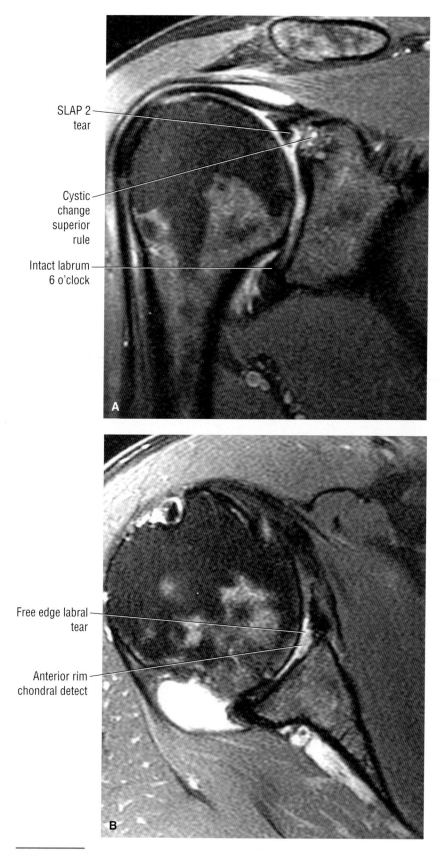

FIGURE 7.63   GLAD lesion with chondral defect and free edge labral tear without labral avulsion. Thus this is considered a clinically stable event. There is an associated tear along the glenoid side of the superior labrum at the level of the biceps labral complex. The cystic change of the superior pole of the glenoid is opposite the superior labral pathology. (**A**) Coronal FS PD. (**B**) Axial FS PD.

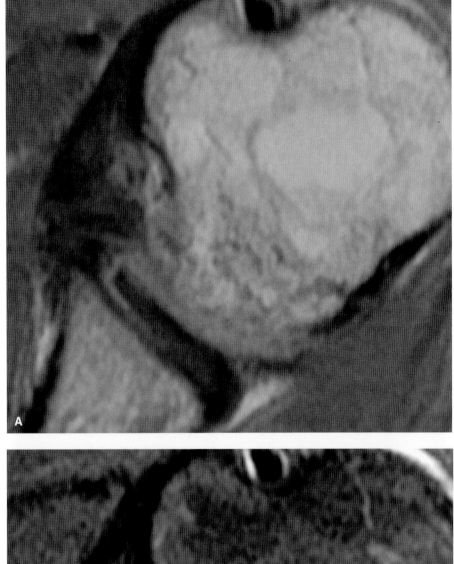

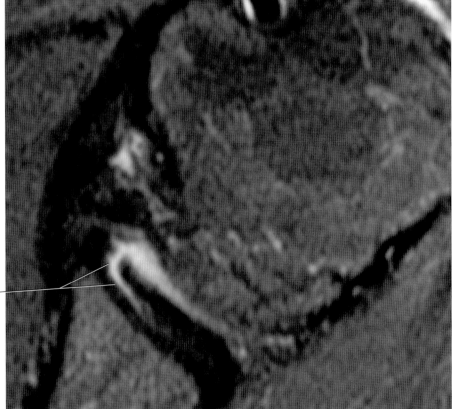

Delaminating chondral injury (unstable chondral surface)

FIGURE 7.64 Unstable articular cartilage of the glenoid fossa with delaminating chondral shear injury which will result in subsequent fragmentation of the articular cartilage surface. (**A**) Axial PD. (**B**) Axial FS PD.

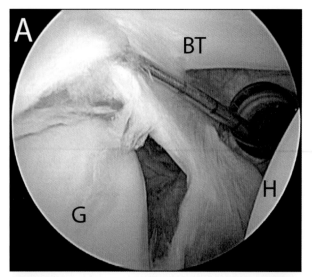

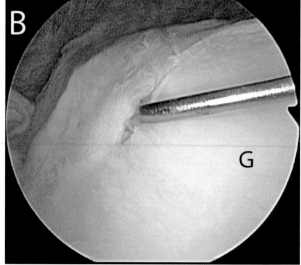

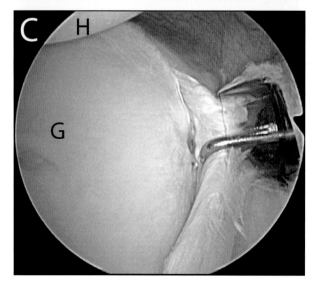

FIGURE 7.65 Triple labral lesion in a right shoulder. A triple labral lesion are combined tears of the anterior, posterior and superior labrum (Bankart, reverse Bankart, and SLAP). Clinical history in patients with triple labral lesions involve anterior instability and recurrent instability episodes, following trauma. There are symptoms of chronic pain and discomfort between instability episodes in contrast to patients with isolated Bankart lesions. (**A**) Posterior viewing portal demonstrates a SLAP lesion Bankart lesion. (**B**) Anterosuperolateral viewing portal demonstrates a Bankart lesion and (**C**) posterior Bankart lesion. BT, biceps tendon; G, glenoid; H, humerus. (Reprinted from Burkhart S, Lo IK, Brady PC, Denard PJ. *The Cowboy's Companion: A Trail Guide for the Arthroscopic Shoulder Surgeon.* Philadelphia, PA: Lippincott Williams & Wilkins; 2012, with permission.)

HAGL Lesion (Humeral Avulsion of the Glenohumeral Ligament)

- Anterior dislocation without a Bankart lesion

- HAGL and Bankart may be concurrent lesions

- Three HAGL Variants
    - Avulsion from the bone humerus (anterior anatomic neck)
    - Capsular split (least common)
    - Combined bone avulsion and capsular split

- Significantly less frequent than the classic Bankart lesion as a cause of anterior shoulder instability

- May exist in patients with anterior instability with or without an associated anterior labral tear[25]

- Is produced by external rotation of the abducted shoulder (compared to the Bankart lesion, which is produced by external rotation of the abducted shoulder with simultaneous compression)

- The axillary pouch is converted from a fluid-distended U-shaped structure to a J-shaped structure as the IGHL drops inferiorly.

- The direct extension of fluid or contrast can be identified between the humerus and the avulsed IGHL.

- Coronal images display HAGL lesions as either partial or complete, with primary involvement of the attachment of the anterior capsule (centered on the anterior band of the IGHL) to the humerus.

- Bony humeral avulsion of the glenohumeral ligament (BHAGL) lesions are also associated with traumatic anterior dislocation but are relatively rare compared to HAGL.[422]
    - In BHAGL lesions, there is a small avulsed osseous fragment attached to the torn end of the humeral attachment of the IGHL.
    - Repair consists of excising the fragment and reattaching the IGHL to the anatomic neck of the humerus.

- In a reverse HAGL lesion,[554] there is detachment of the posterior capsule or reverse humeral avulsion of the glenohumeral ligament.

- At arthroscopy, the HAGL lesion is found in the anterior inferior quadrant of the humeral origin of the IGHL.

- The goal of arthroscopic HAGL repair is to mobilize and suture the avulsed capsular edge.
    - HAGL lesions are treated by surgical reattachment of the glenohumeral ligament to its humeral insertion.

Reverse HAGL (RHAGL) Lesion

- Occurs posteriorly

- Avulsion of posterior capsuloligamentous tissue from humerus (reverse or mirror image of HAGL)

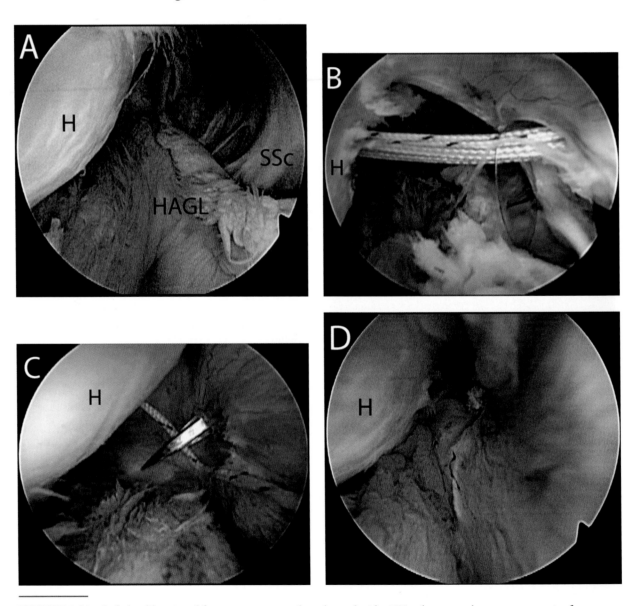

FIGURE 7.66   Left shoulder, viewed from an anterosuperolateral portal with a 70° arthroscope, demonstrates repair of an HAGL lesion. (**A**) View of the HAGL lesion. Note: The muscle of the subscapularis tendon is visible anteriorly (right in the image). (**B**) An anchor has been placed in the humeral head. (**C**) Sutures are passed retrograde through the avulsed ligaments. (**D**) Final repair demonstrates restoration of the glenohumeral ligament insertion. H, humerus; HAGL, humeral avulsion of the glenohumeral ligament; SSc, subscapularis tendon. (Reprinted from Burkhart S, Lo IK, Brady PC, Denard PJ. *The Cowboy's Companion: A Trail Guide for the Arthroscopic Shoulder Surgeon.* Philadelphia, PA: Lippincott Williams & Wilkins; 2012, with permission.)

- Capsular split or avulsion of bone or combination of both

- Neurovascular structures are not at risk in a posterior approach repair of RHAGL

Combined Humeral and Glenoid Lesions

- HAGL + Bankart

- RHAGL + Reverse Bankart

- First, repair the glenoid disruption to stabilize one end and then repair the humeral side.

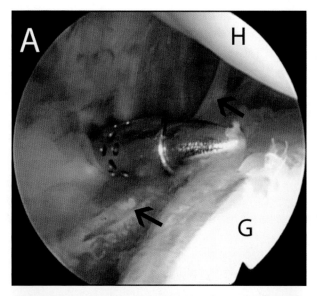

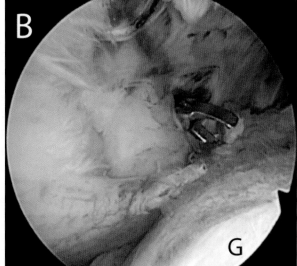

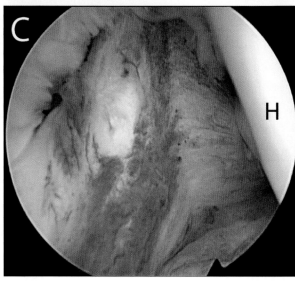

FIGURE 7.67   Left shoulder, anterosuperolateral viewing portal demonstrates (**A**) a reverse humeral avulsion of the glenohumeral ligaments (RHAGL lesion) (*black arrows*). (**B**) A grasper is introduced from a posterior portal to assess capsular mobility. (**C**) View demonstrating sufficient mobility of the RHAGL lesion to reach the posterior humerus. G, glenoid; H, humerus. (Reprinted from Burkhart S, Lo IK, Brady PC, Denard PJ. *The Cowboy's Companion: A Trail Guide for the Arthroscopic Shoulder Surgeon*. Philadelphia, PA: Lippincott Williams & Wilkins; 2012, with permission.)

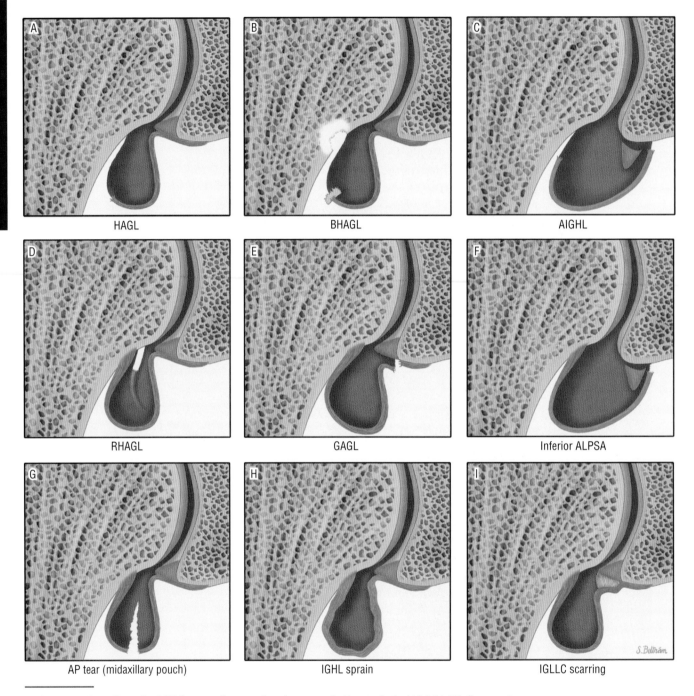

FIGURE 7.68 Capsular IGL lesions illustrated in the coronal plane include (**A**) HAGL (humeral avulsion of the glenohumeral ligament), (**B**) BHAGL (bony humeral avulsion of the glenohumeral ligament), (**C**) AIGHL (anterior inferior glenohumeral ligament), (**D**) RHAGL (reverse HAGL), (**E**) GAGL (glenohumeral avulsion of the glenohumeral ligaments), (**F**) inferior ALPSA (anterior labroligamentous periosteal sleeve avulsion), (**G**) midaxillary pouch (AP) tear, (**H**) IGHL sprain, and (**I**) IGLLC (inferior glenohumeral ligament labral complex) scarring.

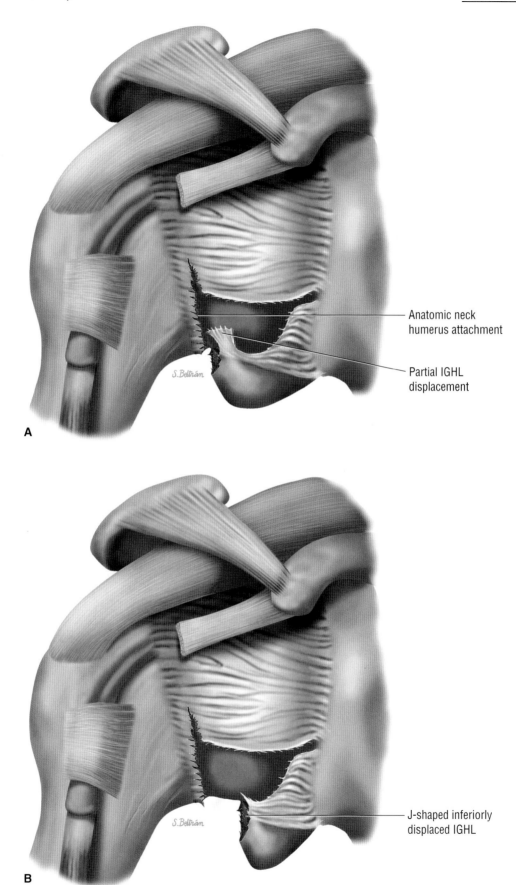

Anatomic neck
humerus attachment

Partial IGHL
displacement

J-shaped inferiorly
displaced IGHL

FIGURE 7.69 Stages of a displaced HAGL tear in the anterior anatomic neck attachment of the IGHL (IGL). (**A**) Coronal illustration with partial IGL inferior displacement. (**B**) Coronal illustration of a J-shaped or inferiorly displaced IGL.

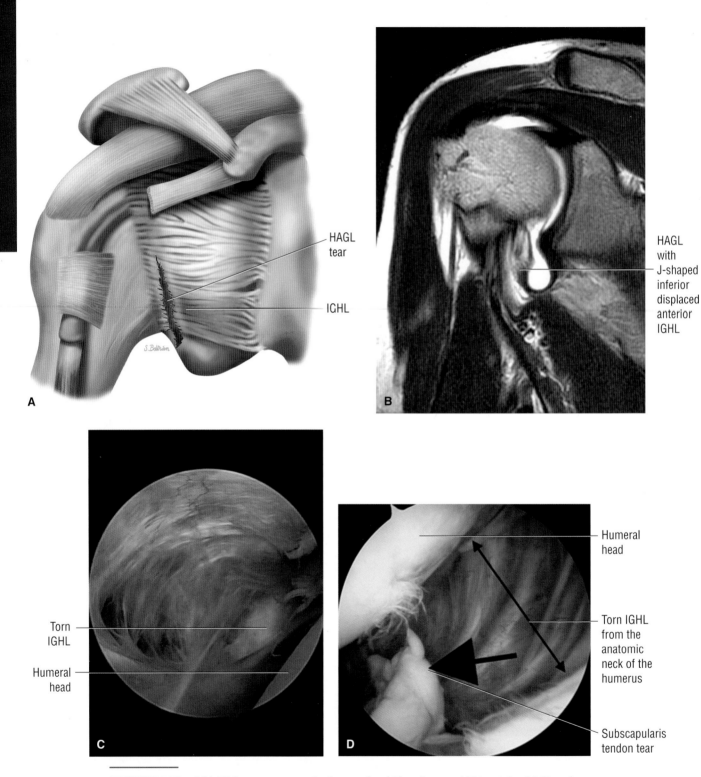

FIGURE 7.70   HAGL lesion on coronal color graphic (**A**) and coronal T1-weighted MR arthrogram (**B**). Arthroscopic view (**C**) demonstrates avulsion of the anterior capsule. (**D**) Arthroscopic view of a torn subscapularis tendon (*short arrow*) and humeral avulsion of the IGL (*double-headed long arrow*) creating the J-shaped axillary pouch.

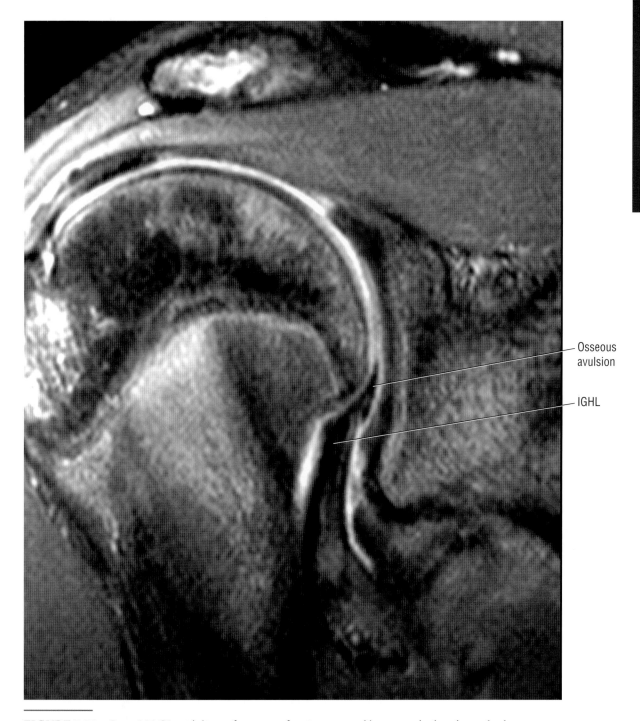

Osseous
avulsion

IGHL

FIGURE 7.71 Bony HAGL with linear fragment of periosteum and bone attached to the avulsed IGL from the anatomic neck of the humerus. Coronal FS PD.

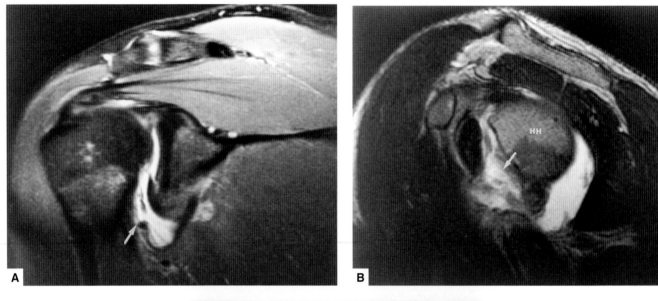

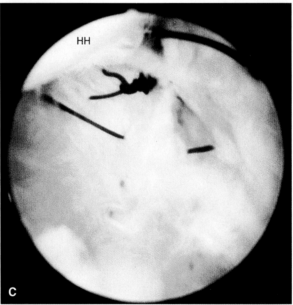

FIGURE 7.72   HAGL lesion wth avulsion of the humeral attachment of the inferior glenohumeral ligament (*arrow*) on FS PD-weighted FSE coronal oblique (**A**) and T2-weighted FSE sagittal oblique (**B**) images. Corresponding arthroscopic photograph (**C**) shows suturing with coaptation of the detached portion of the IGHL. HH, humeral head. HAGL lesions may present as an avulsion from bone, capsular split or combined bone avulsion and capsular split. The presence of a Bankart lesion does not preclude a HAGL lesion.

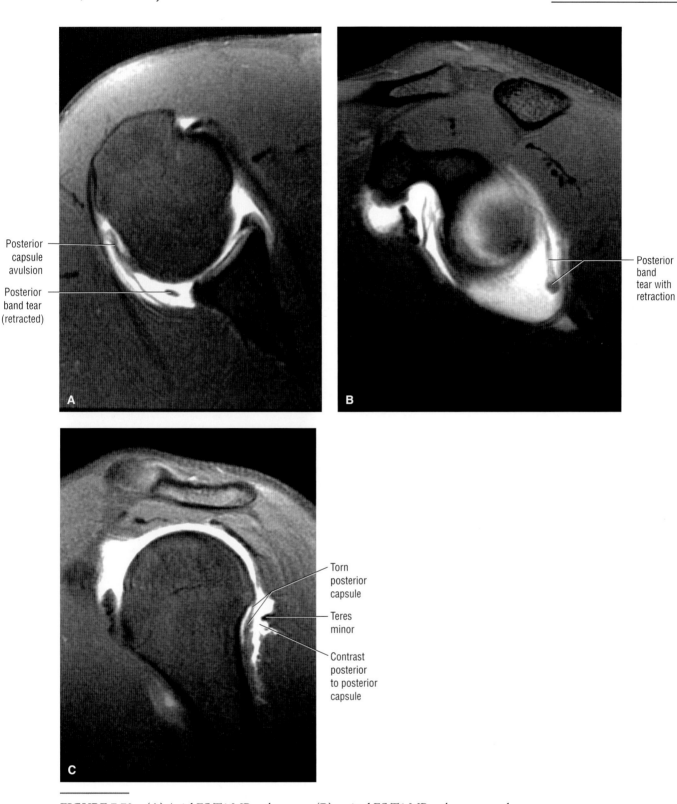

FIGURE 7.73 (**A**) Axial FS T1 MR arthrogram, (**B**) sagittal FS T1 MR arthrogram, and (**C**) sagittal FS T1-weighted image showing reverse humeral avulsion of the glenohumeral ligaments (RHAGL) associated with both posterior capsular avulsion and rupture of the posterior band of the IGL. There is extension of contrast between the torn posterior capsule and teres minor.

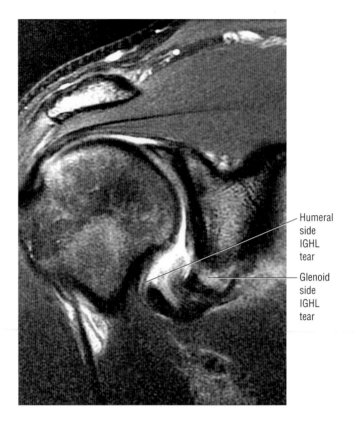

FIGURE 7.74   Coronal FS PD FSE image of floating anterior inferior glenohumeral ligament (AIGL) with unattached glenoid (Bankart) and humeral (HAGL) components.

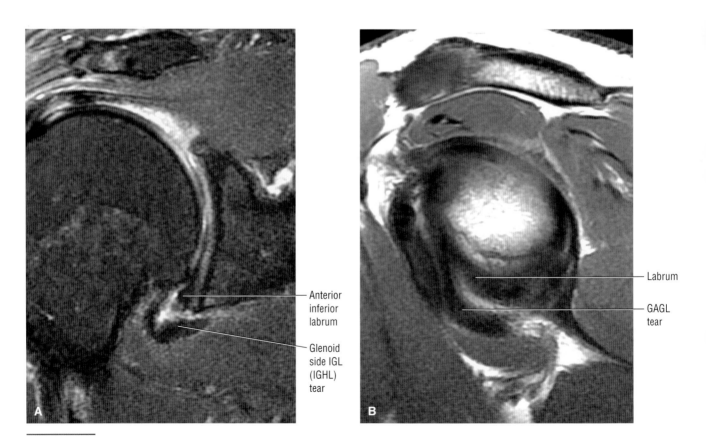

FIGURE 7.75   (**A**) Coronal FS PD FSE and (**B**) sagittal PD FSE images show glenoid avulsion of the glenohumeral (GAGL) with intact anterior inferior labrum.

"Floating" AIGHL Lesions (Anterior Inferior Glenohumeral Ligament)

- Rare injury that involves both disruption of the IGHL attachment at the inferior pole of the glenoid (Bankart component) and tearing of the IGHL from its attachment to the anatomic neck of the humerus (HAGL component)[666]

- Restoration of function requires reattachment of the humeral and glenoid capsular disruptions.

- Although it is unusual to see disruptive forces produce both HAGL and Bankart lesions, we have observed ALPSA lesions with associated tearing of the anterior attachment of the IGHL to the anatomic neck of the humerus.

  - These compound ALPSA lesions also demonstrate a greater degree of medial IGHL displacement associated with the labral or Bankart component.

GAGL Lesions (Glenoid Avulsion of the Glenohumeral Ligament)

- GAGL lesions are uncommon.

- There is avulsion of the IGHL from the inferior pole of the glenoid without associated disruption of the inferior labrum.

- The Bankart lesion is more common at the location of the inferior pole with involvement of both the anteroinferior labrum and medial capsular displacement.

- The GAGL lesion will be associated with a reverse "J" sign configuration on coronal images (compared to the HAGL lesion). GAGL lesions tend to involve younger patients with an instability episode.

Inferior ALPSA Lesions (cul-de-sac-lesions)

- There is medial displacement of both the anterior inferior labrum and the IGHL underneath the inferior neck of the glenoid.

- Involvement of the anterior inferior labrum establishes the existence of a Bankart lesion.

- The additional displacement of the labrum and IGHL represents a variation of the Bankart lesion.

- Coronal MR images characteristically demonstrate greater medial displacement of the capsule relative to the anterior inferior labrum.

- There is complete absence of labral fibrocartilage in the 6 o'clock position of the glenoid at the expected location of the labral glenoid–chondral interface.

Axillary Pouch Midligament Tears, Sprains, and Scarring

- Midligament (midportion of the IGHL) tears are less common than axillary pouch sprains.

- Coronal MR images demonstrate disruption or discontinuity centered in the middle third of the IGHL.

- Posttraumatic IGHL sprains are characterized by partial or diffuse hyperintensity and thickening of the IGHL as an isolated finding or in association with other IGHL-related lesions, including the Bankart lesion.

- Adhesive capsulitis, more common than posttraumatic axillary pouch sprain, may present with identical findings, including IGHL thickening and hyperintensity on FS PD FSE images.

- Scarring of the IGHL attachment to the anterior inferior labrum and/or inferior glenoid may represent a partial or healed GAGL lesion.[369]

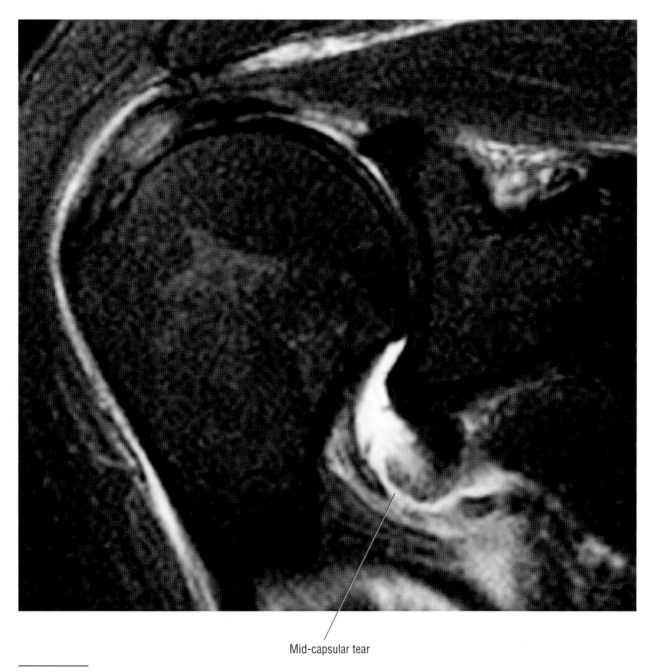

Mid-capsular tear

FIGURE 7.76 Mid-capsular (IGHL ligament) tear with extension of fluid halfway between the capsular attachment to the humeral side and inferior pole of the glenoid. Coronal FS PD. IGHL injuries can occur either at the glenoid side (Bankart), mid-capsular or the humeral side (HAGL). The intermediate signal intensity within the axillary pouch represents synovitis.

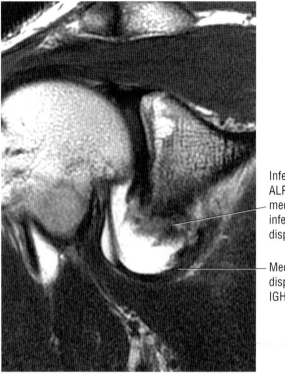

Inferior
ALPSA with
medial and
inferior labral
displacement

Medial
displacement of
IGHL

FIGURE 7.77   Coronal T1-weighted MR arthrogram of inferior ALPSA with medial displacement
of both the anterior inferior labrum and IGHL (IGL) underneath the inferior pole of the glenoid and
along the inferior neck.

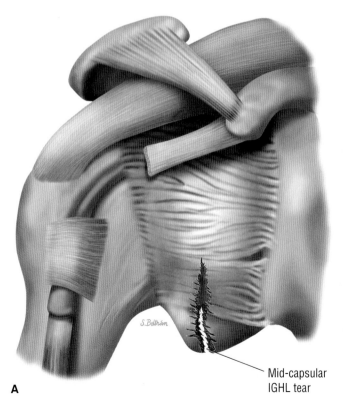

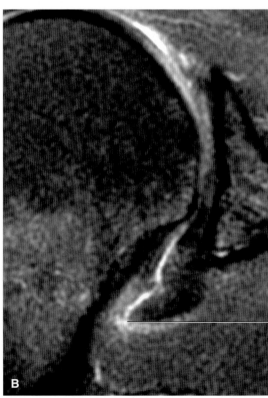

Mid-capsular
IGHL tear

Axillary
pouch
capsular
tear

A

B

FIGURE 7.78   Midaxillary pouch tear of the IGHL (IGL) on a coronal color graphic centered
on the axillary pouch (**A**) and a coronal FS PD FSE image (**B**).

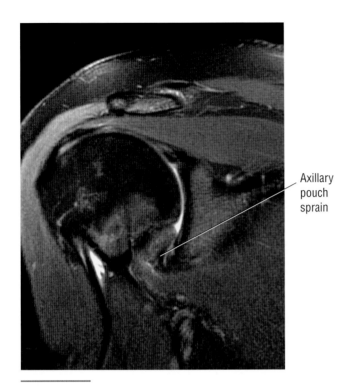

Axillary pouch sprain

FIGURE 7.79 Coronal FS PD FSE image of axillary pouch hyperintensity after traumatic injury with abduction and external rotation component.

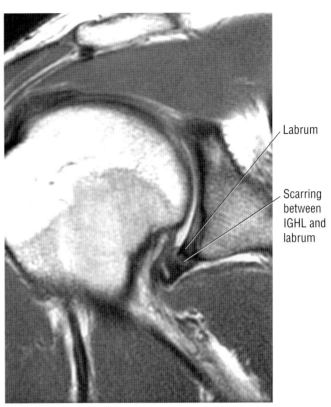

Labrum

Scarring between IGHL and labrum

FIGURE 7.80 Intermediate-signal-intensity scarring of the IGL attachment to the inferior labrum and inferior pole of the glenoid without labral disruption on a coronal PD FSE image.

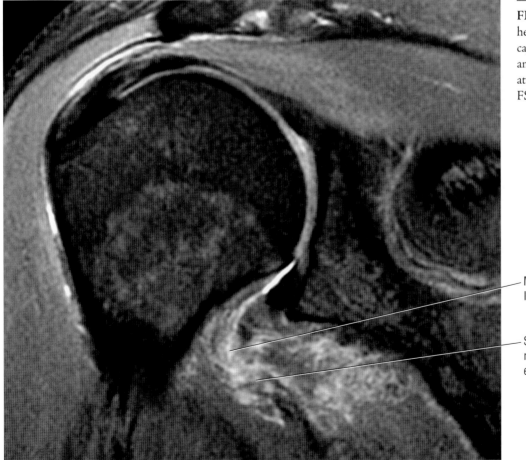

FIGURE 7.81 Extensive hemorrhage associated with mid-capsular tear of the IGHL with anatomic neck and inferior pole attachments still intact. Coronal FS PD.

Mid-capsular tear IGHL

Soft tissue reaction with edema

Posterior Instability

Key Concepts

- The reverse Hill-Sachs and the reverse Bankart lesions are associated with posterior instability.

- The reverse HAGL lesion is characterized by tearing of the posterior capsule at the humeral attachment.

- Posterosuperior labral tears may occur as part of posterior SLAP 2 or posterior peel-back lesions.

- The Bennett lesion occurs in the throwing athlete and is visualized as an extra-articular posterior ossification.

- Kim lesion as an incomplete and concealed posterior inferior labral tear with intact peripheral attachment between the posterior labrum and glenoid

  - Seen in posterior or multidirectional instability.

- POLPSA (posterior labrum periosteal sleeve avulsion) lesions are associated with scapular periosteal stripping along with the posterior labral tear.

- Retroversion of the glenoid

- May occur after trauma and presents with pain and apprehension on examination with forward flexion and adduction of the shoulder[22]

- The jerk test (a jerking motion on posterior shoulder displacement near the midline or as the shoulder reduces anteriorly) is used to demonstrate the instability or apprehension.

- A redundant posterior capsule, posterior labral tearing, and osteochondral defects (including reverse Hills-Sachs and Bankart lesions) may be found.

- Posterior inferior instability occurs as a component of MDI.

  - Additional findings in MDI include abnormal anterior and inferior laxity.

  - Global pathology in MDI thus includes the labrum, the capsule (IGHLC), and the rotator cuff interval.

- The posterior band of the IGLC is primarily responsible for capsuloligamentous restraint to posterior translation in 90° of abduction.[519,563]

- The anterior-superior capsule, or rotator interval capsule, has also been shown to be important in limiting posterior and inferior translation.

- Posterior dislocation occurs only with combined dysfunction of the posterior capsule and anterior superior capsule.[391]

    - The incidence of posterior instability has been reported to be between 2% and 4% of patients with shoulder instability.

- Acute posterior dislocation may occur secondary to indirect forces (such as electric shock procedure) that produce adduction, flexion, and internal rotation.

- A fall on the outstretched hand with the arm abducted is another mechanism of injury in posterior instability.

- A direct posterior force on an anteriorly flexed, abducted, and internally rotated arm (e.g., football pass blocking) may also produce acute posterior shoulder subluxation.

- Posterior instability may also occur as an operative complication in patients with MDI after a misdirected anterior capsular procedure.

    - With arthroscopy, it is possible to assess associated intraarticular lesions, including labral tears, avulsions, and articular surface rotator cuff, SLAP, and biceps lesions.[391]

- Posterior instability should be suspected in the presence of posterior labral disruption or fragmentation.[518]

    - A detailed examination with the patient under anesthesia (EUA) is critical in identifying this type of instability.

MR Findings in Posterior Instability

- A reverse Hill-Sachs lesion (notch sign or trough lesion) in the anteromedial humeral head[603]

- Fractures of the posterior glenoid margin (reverse osseous Bankart lesion) associated with a posterior labral tear

- Deficiency of the posterior glenoid rim[205]

- Fractures of the lesser tuberosity associated with a posterior dislocation secondary to the pull of the subscapularis tendon insertion with or without tears of the subscapularis tendon and teres minor tendon

- Fracture of the acromion/distal clavicle

- A posterior labrocapsular periosteal sleeve avulsion (POLPSA)[603]
    - Normally, the posterior capsule attaches directly to the posterior aspect of the posterior labrum.
    - The posterior labrum is secured to the glenoid by the posterior scapular periosteum.
    - Stripping of the posterior labrum produces the POLPSA lesion.

- A posterior capsular tear with an intact posterior labrum (the opposite or reverse of the GAGL lesion of the anterior inferior glenoid)

- Reverse HAGL with or without associated posterior labral tear

- Posterior superior labral tears as part of a posterior SLAP 2 (posterior peel-back lesion) or posterosuperior to posterior labral tear in association with a paralabral cyst.

- Posterior labral tears in the throwing athlete at the mid-glenohumeral joint level as a posterior continuation of a posterior peel-back lesion

- PLIPSA or posterior ligamentous inferior periosteal sleeve avulsion without posterior labral tear (opposite lesion of ALIPSA)

- Kim lesion
    - Axial images identify the intermediate to increased signal between the free edge of the posterior labrum and the articular cartilage. Probing the labrum will establish detachment of the deep portion of the posteroinferior labrum with intact peripheral margin.
        - Treatment may require converting the concealed incomplete lesion to a complete tear to facilitate repair.

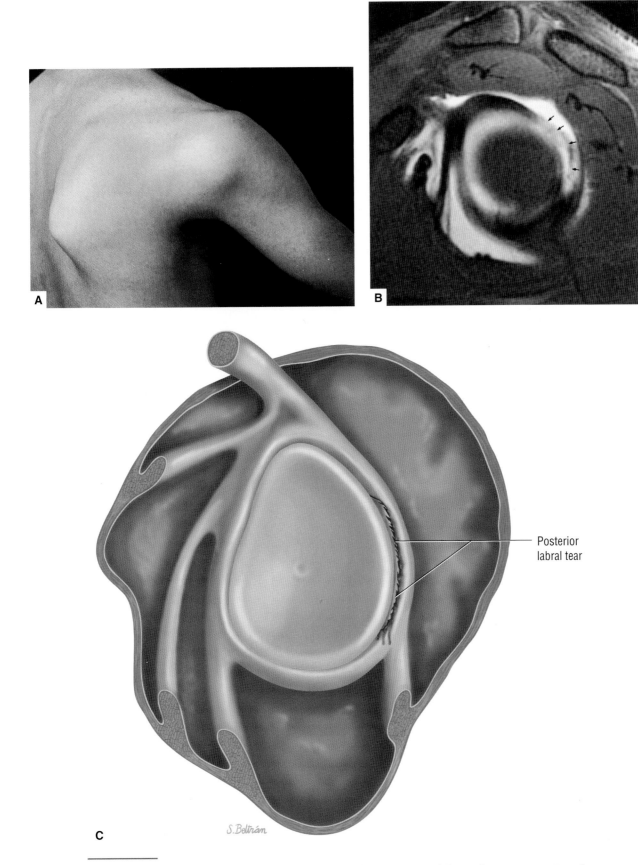

FIGURE 7.82 Posterior instability and labral tear. (**A**) Posterior instability with anterior rotation of the scapula after dislocation. (**B**) FS T1-weighted sagittal oblique MR arthrogram with posterior labral avulsion and discontinuity (*arrows*). (**C**) Posterior labral tear centered on the posterior quadrant of the glenoid fossa.

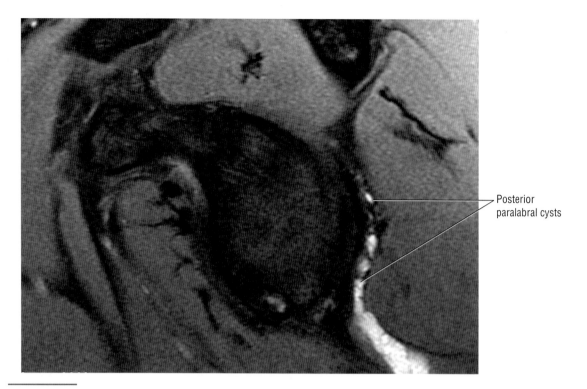

Posterior
paralabral cysts

FIGURE 7.83   Multiple paralabral cysts parallel to the posterior aspect of the glenoid fossa communicating with a posterior labral tear from the posterior superior to the posterior inferior quadrant of the glenoid. In weight lifters, AC joint arthrosis, SLAP tears, and posterolabral tears are common findings. In addition, sclerosis of the posterior glenoid rim and/or sclerosis of the anterior and posterior glenoid rim as well as teres minor muscle atrophy may be seen in weight lifters. The changes on the anterior and posterior glenoid rim usually indicate rocking of the humeral head in the glenoid fossa from heavy weight lifting, creating a secondary component of MDI. Sagittal FS PD.

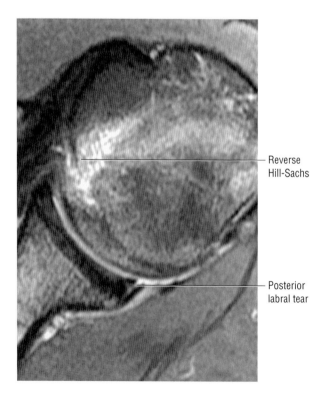

Reverse
Hill-Sachs

Posterior
labral tear

FIGURE 7.84   Reverse Hill-Sachs with hyperintense marrow edema and associated posterior labral tear (reverse Bankart) on an axial FS PD FSE image. Traumatic posterior instability is less common than anterior instability and is more frequently seen with multidirectional instability or as a component of a complex laxity pattern associated with anterior dislocation.

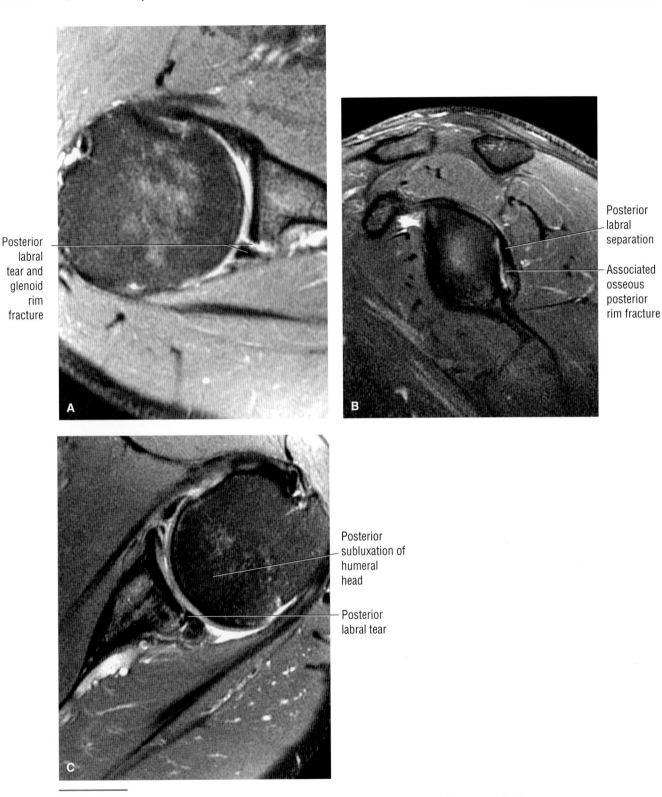

Posterior labral tear and glenoid rim fracture

Posterior labral separation

Associated osseous posterior rim fracture

Posterior subluxation of humeral head

Posterior labral tear

FIGURE 7.85　(**A**) Axial FS PD FSE and (**B**) sagittal FSE PD FSE images of posterior labral tear with associated glenoid rim fracture. This represents a reverse bony Bankart lesion. (**C**) Axial FS PD FSE image shows increased glenoid version associated with a posterior labral tear and mild posterior subluxation. Patients with posterior instability frequently have pain exacerbated by activities that posteriorly load the glenohumeral joint in shoulder adduction.

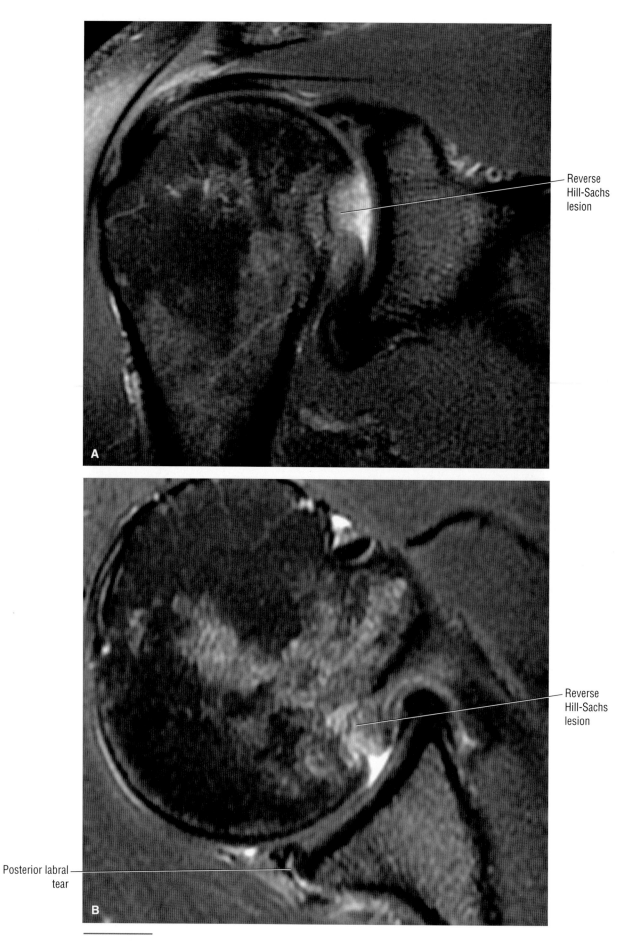

FIGURE 7.86   Reverse Hills-Sachs and reverse Bankart with posterior labral in a case of posterior instability. (**A**) Coronal FS PD. (**B**) Axial FS PD.

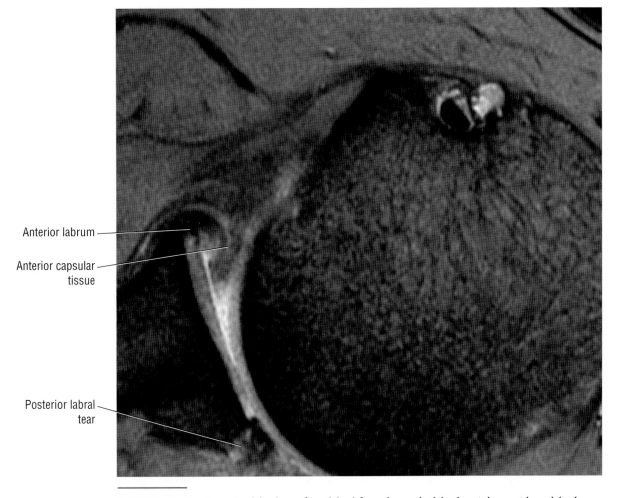

Anterior labrum

Anterior capsular tissue

Posterior labral tear

FIGURE 7.87 Posterior labral tear from labral free edge to the labral periphery without labral displacement. The infolding of anterior capsular tissue should not be mistaken for entrapped labral tissue. There is posterior subluxation of the humeral head relative to the glenoid. Acute posterior dislocations are the result of high energy trauma or seizures. Recurrent posterior instability in athletes is associated with injuries related to shear stresses applied to the posterior labrum (FOOSH or direct impact to the anterior shoulder while blocking in football). Repetitive trauma as occurs in bench-pressing heavy weights or capsular stretching in swimming may result in posterior instability.

FIGURE 7.88 Kim lesion with concealed undersurface tear of the posterior glenoid labrum that does not extend through the capsular periphery. Thus the Kim lesion is an incomplete avulsion of the posterior labrum. (**A**) Axial color illustration. (**B**) Axial FS PD.

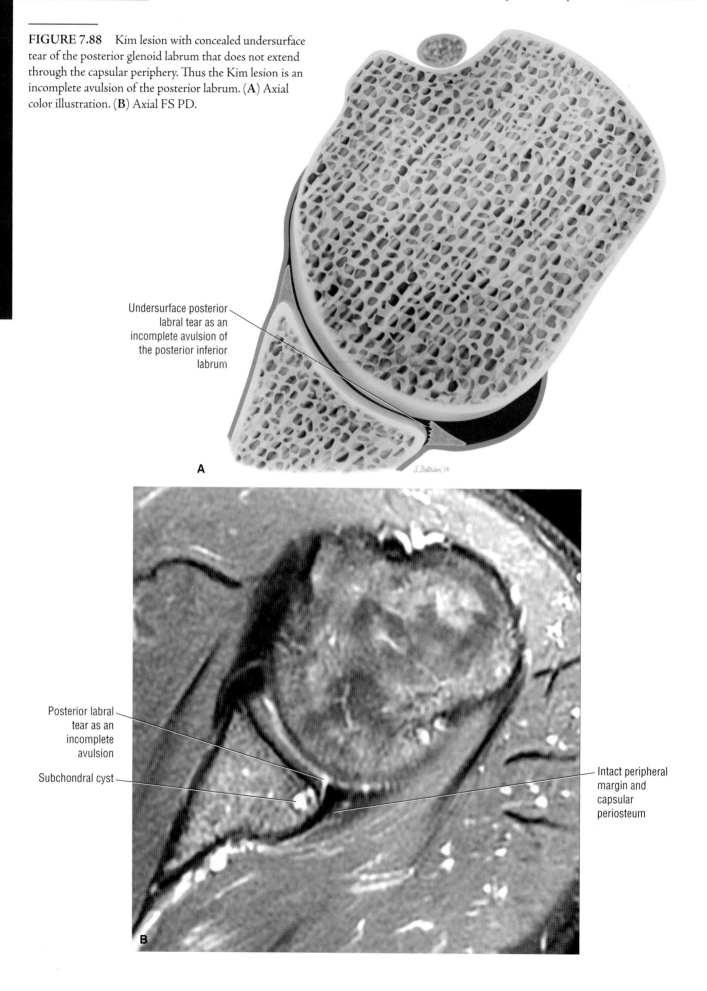

Undersurface posterior labral tear as an incomplete avulsion of the posterior inferior labrum

A

S. Beltran '14

Posterior labral tear as an incomplete avulsion

Subchondral cyst

Intact peripheral margin and capsular periosteum

B

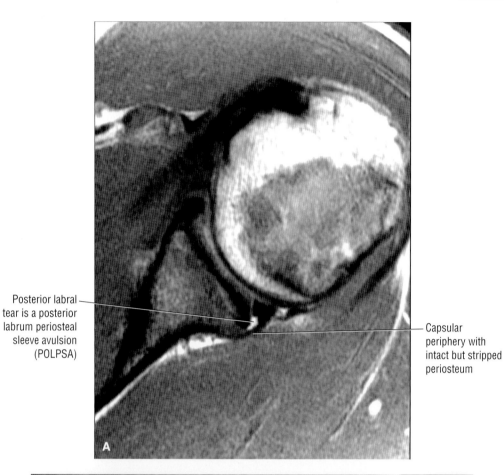

Posterior labral tear is a posterior labrum periosteal sleeve avulsion (POLPSA)

Capsular periphery with intact but stripped periosteum

A

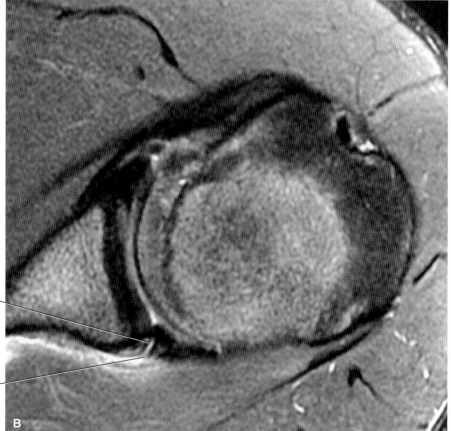

Complete posterior labral tear from central free edge to capsular margin

Disruption of posterior periosteal sleeve

B

FIGURE 7.89 (**A**) Posterior labral tear that extends to the scapular periosteum (**B**) Posterior labral tear that extends through the scapular periosteum. In both cases, the humeral head remains centered on the glenoid fossa. (**A**) Axial PD. (**B**) Axial FS PD.

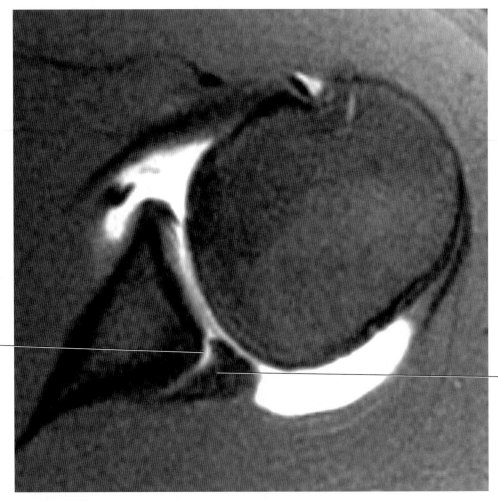

Posterior labral avulsion

Osseous posterior glenoid rim fracture

FIGURE 7.90   Posterior labral tear associated with posterior glenoid rim fracture that extends to the chondral surface of the glenoid. Axial FS PD MR arthrogram. The glenoid rim fracture is a finding often associated with a direct impact injury and not repetitive trauma. Patients with posterior instability may present with shoulder pain and weakness instead of instability.

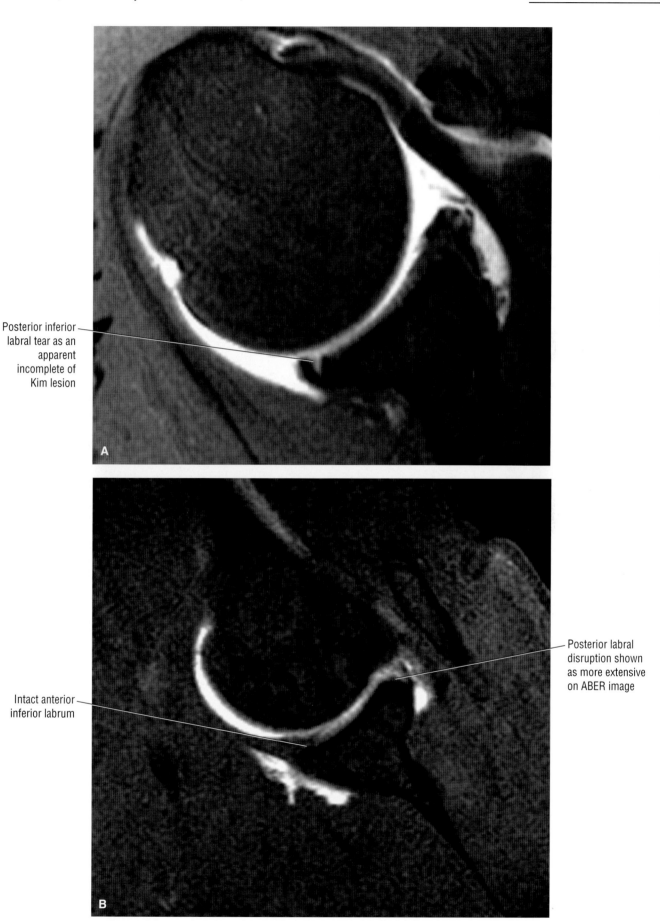

Posterior inferior labral tear as an apparent incomplete of Kim lesion

A

Posterior labral disruption shown as more extensive on ABER image

Intact anterior inferior labrum

B

FIGURE 7.91 Posterior labral tear defined on axial and ABER images. On ABER images, the posterior labrum is located opposite the IGHL anterior labral complex. (**A**) Axial FS PD (**B**) ABER.

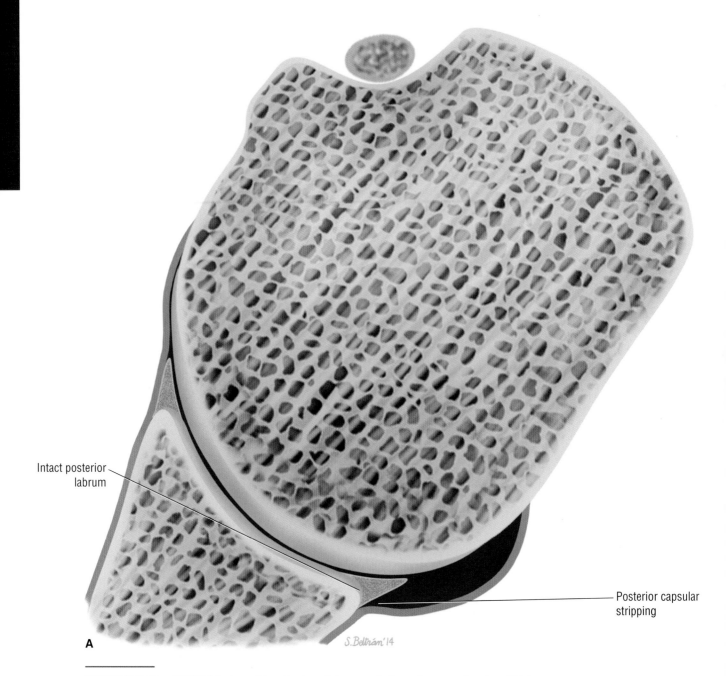

Intact posterior
labrum

Posterior capsular
stripping

A

S. Beltrán '14

FIGURE 7.92 PLIPSA lesion with stripping of the capsule from the posterior glenoid labrum without labral avulsion. (**A**) 2D axial illustration.

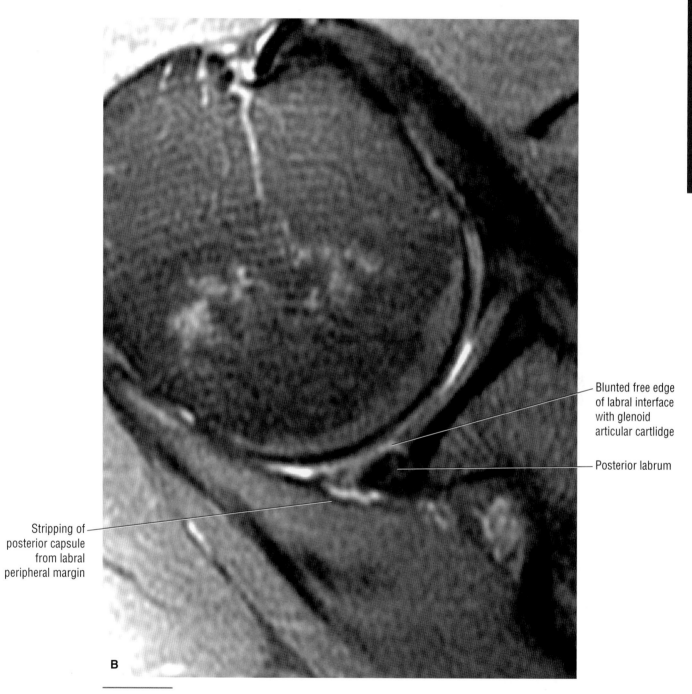

Blunted free edge of labral interface with glenoid articular cartlidge

Posterior labrum

Stripping of posterior capsule from labral peripheral margin

B

FIGURE 7.92 *(Continued)* (**B**) Axial FS PD.

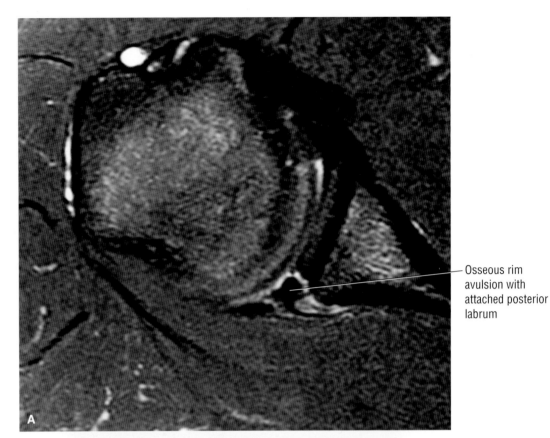

Osseous rim avulsion with attached posterior labrum

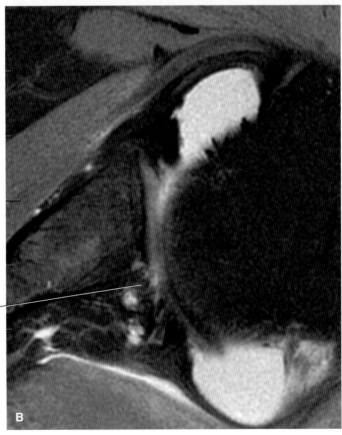

Chronic posterior rim remodeling with chondral loss and subchondral cystic degeneration

FIGURE 7.93   (**A,B**) Posterior labral osseous avulsion both from contact sports. (**A**) Osseous labral avulsion with capsular stripping secondary to football impact. (**B**) Chronic changes of remodeling from previous history of direct contact injury resulting in labral tear and rim fracture. Eccentric loss of articular cartilage is present in the posterior glenoid rim which will predispose to posterior subluxation. (**A,B**) Axial FS PD.

Reverse HAGL

- Posterior instability is sometimes associated with a complete avulsion of the posterior attachment of the shoulder capsule from the posterior humeral neck (reverse HAGL or RHAGL lesion).[554]

- Both the posterior band and the posterior capsule of the IGHL may be disrupted, and there may also be an associated posterior labral tear.

- Humeral avulsion of the posterior band of the IGHL (RHAGL or PHAGL lesion) has discontinuous avulsed posterior capsule that can be identified on axial images.[110]

  - At arthroscopy, the posterior capsule appears absent and the muscle of the posterior cuff is visualized.

- Sagittal images display fluid or contrast forming an irregular outline of the anterior surface of the teres minor muscle or infraspinatus muscle.

- Frequently, there is extension of fluid through a capsular defect anterior to the junction between the infraspinatus and teres minor muscles.

- The laxity of the medial retracted posterior capsule is evident on axial images.

- The reverse HAGL lesion is repaired with anchors and side-to-side sutures to close the remaining capsular flap.

- The reverse HAGL lesion if associated with an osseous avulsion from the humerus can be referred to as an osseous reverse HAGL lesion.

  - The osseous fragment from the humerus is usually a thin fragment which if not looked for can easily be missed. The fragment of bone is usually hypointense on PD and fluid sensitive images.

- In addition to sagittal images, the axial plane is used to identify the posterior capsular tear.

  - Similar to findings in the sagittal plane, there is usually fluid and or contrast extending posterior to the site of capsular tear on axial images.

- The reverse HAGL when occurring in combination with a posterior labral tear can produce a posterior floating ligament (PIGL) analogous to an HAGL lesion that occurs in combination with a Bankart lesion anteriorly as a floating anterior ligament (AIGL).

Bennett Lesion

- An extra-articular posterior ossification associated with posterior labral injury and posterior articular surface rotator cuff damage

- Believed to be the result of a posterior capsular avulsion secondary to traction of the posterior band of the IGHL (during the deceleration phase of pitching, for example) or to the posterior subluxation that occurs during cocking of the arm[166]

- Frequently asymptomatic, but a fracture of the spur or a fibrous union at its base may interfere with the throwing motion.

  - The calcification can contribute to posterior inferior capsular contracture.

- The crescentic extra-articular ossification, which extends from the posterior inferior medial glenoid posterior to the posterior labrum, can be demonstrated on CT or MR scans.

  - There may be associated reactive posterior inferior glenoid rim sclerosis.

- MR findings include low-signal-intensity calcification, posterior humeral subluxation, and a posterior labral tear.[166]

  - The ossification cannot be identified arthroscopically because of its extra-articular location.

- Posterior labral tears are most frequent in the posterior superior quadrant of the glenoid labrum.

- May represent a further progression on the spectrum of concentric glenoid wear or posterior glenoid fossa sclerosis associated with a posterosuperior cam shift of the humeral head in the throwing athlete

- A Bennett lesion that may occur in the throwing athlete is usually associated with sclerosis of the posterior glenoid fossa; however, the more common situation is to see posterior glenoid rim sclerosis without a Bennett lesion.

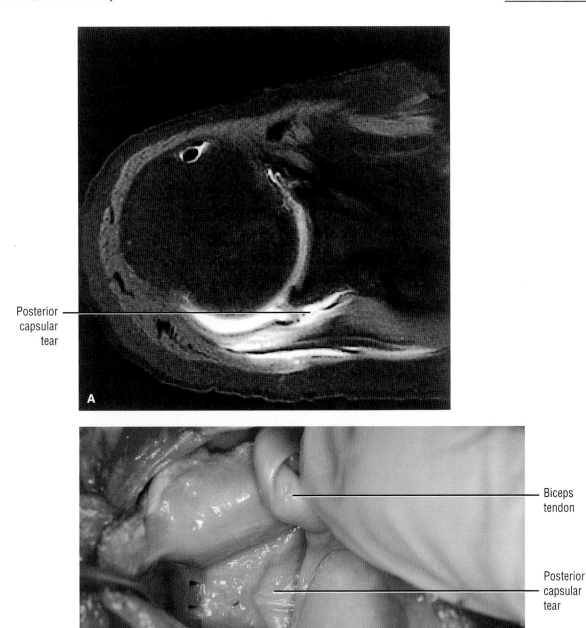

Posterior capsular tear

Biceps tendon

Posterior capsular tear

Glenoid

FIGURE 7.94 (**A**) Posterior capsular tear with firmly attached posterior labrum shown on an axial FS T1-weighted MR arthrogram. (**B**) Corresponding surgical exposure of torn posterior capsule. The location of this injury is a mirror image of the GAGL injury. The RHAGL more commonly will involve the distal or humeral attachment of the posterior capsule.

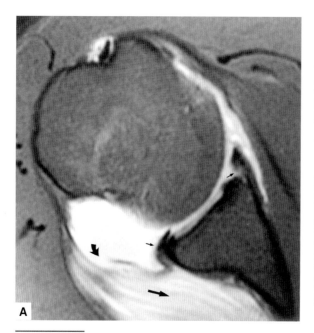

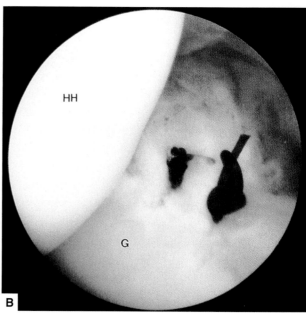

FIGURE 7.95   (**A**) FS T1-weighted MR arthrogram of reverse humeral head avulsion of the glenohumeral ligaments (RHAGL). There is discontinuity of the humeral attachment of the posterior capsule (*curved arrow*) with extravasation (*large straight arrow*) of contrast and associated tears of the anterior (Perthes) and posterior labrum (*small arrows*). Repair of both the posterior labrum and RHAGL is required. (**B**) Arthroscopic view of posterior labral repair. The RHAGL repair uses two or three anchors and several side-to-side sutures for closure of the capsular flap and reattachment of the capsule to the humeral head.

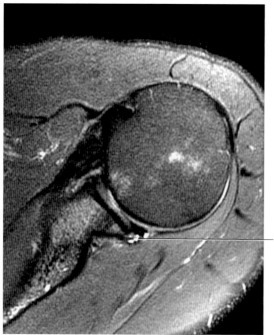

Posterior paralabral cyst and labral tear

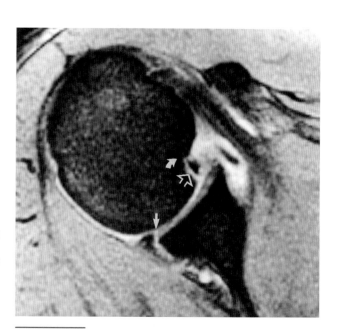

FIGURE 7.96   Axial FS PD FSE image showing association of a posterior labral tear with a paralabral cyst. These posterior paralabral cysts should also be evaluated on sagittal images since they may be extensive and reach from the BLC to the inferior glenohumeral ligament labral complex.

FIGURE 7.97   A reverse Bankart lesion with anteromedial humeral head impaction (*curved arrow*), anterior labral avulsion, and posterior labral tear. Note fluid undermining the posterior labrum (*straight arrow*) and anterior fracture fragment (*open arrow*). The anteromedial defect creates the notch sign or trough lesion.

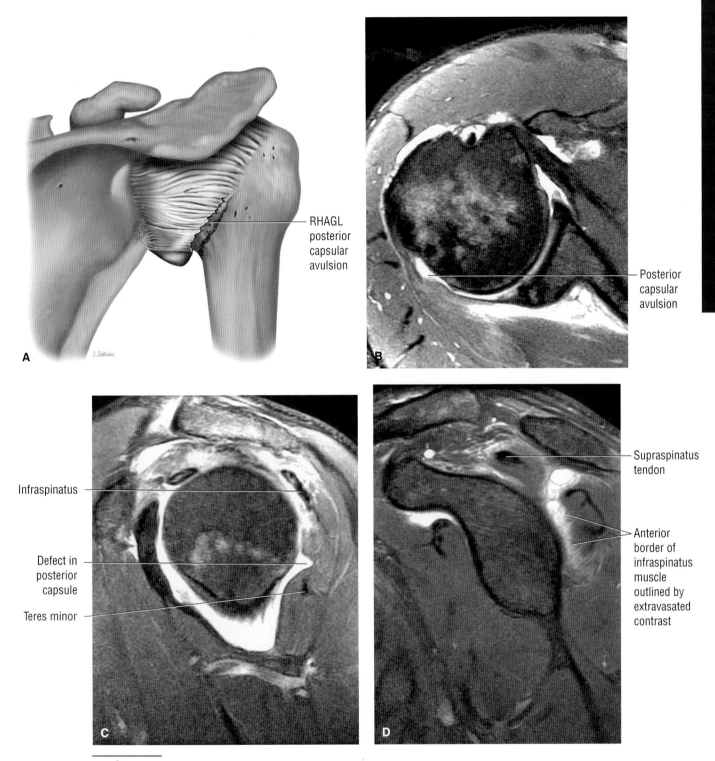

RHAGL posterior capsular avulsion

Posterior capsular avulsion

Infraspinatus

Defect in posterior capsule

Teres minor

Supraspinatus tendon

Anterior border of infraspinatus muscle outlined by extravasated contrast

FIGURE 7.98 (**A**) Posterior coronal color view of RHAGL with avulsion of the posterior humeral attachment of the shoulder capsule. (**B**) Axial FS PD FSE image shows posterior humeral detachment of the posterior capsule associated with capsular laxity or a wavy contour. (**C**) A characteristic dimple or defect in the posterior capsule between the infraspinatus and teres minor on a sagittal FS PD FSE image. (**D**) Direct extension of fluid outlining the anterior muscle of the infraspinatus secondary to posterior capsular rupture can be seen on this sagittal FS PD FSE image.

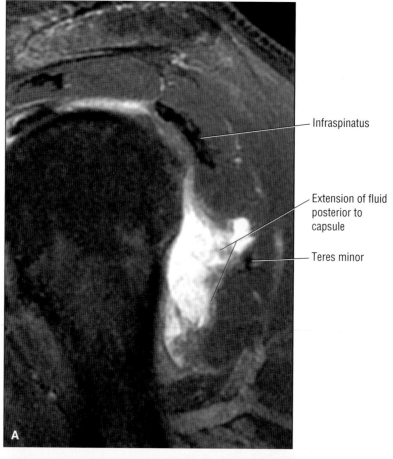

Infraspinatus

Extension of fluid
posterior to
capsule

Teres minor

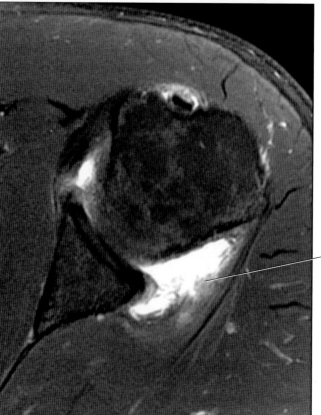

Posterior capsular
disruption

FIGURE 7.99 Reverse HAGL lesion
with disruption of the posterior capsule
with fluid directly outlining the anterior
surface of the infraspinatus and teres
minor secondary to capsular discontinuity
and extravasation. (**A**) Sagittal FS PD.
(**B**) Axial FS PD.

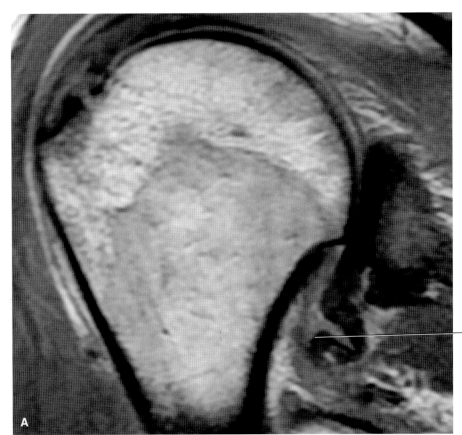

Reverse HAGL on posterior coronal image

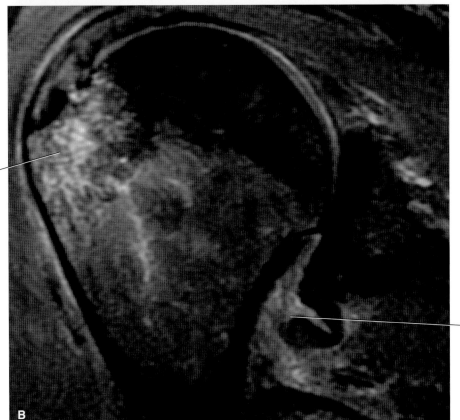

Greater tuberosity trabecular fracture

Posterior capsular avulsion with J-sign

FIGURE 7.100 Reverse HAGL with J-sign from inferior displacement of the anatomic neck attachment of the IGHL. The HAGL lesion involves the anterior component of the IGHL on the humeral side while the RHAGL involves the posterior component of the IGHL on the humeral side. (**A**) Coronal T2. (**B**) Coronal FS PD.

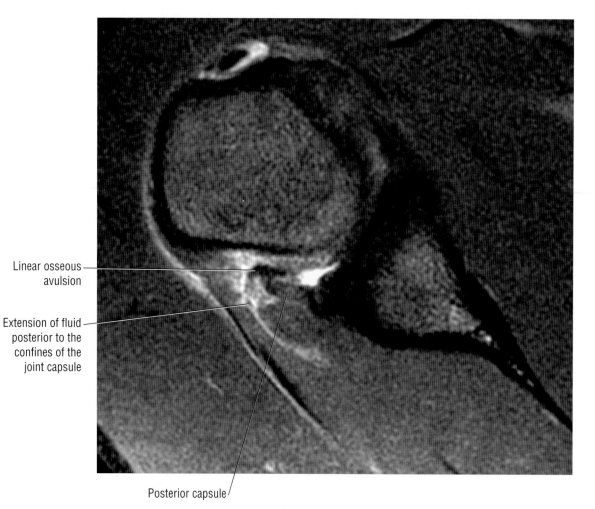

Linear osseous
avulsion

Extension of fluid
posterior to the
confines of the
joint capsule

Posterior capsule

FIGURE 7.101   RHAGL with osseous component (bony RHAGL). The osseous component of an RHAGL usually presents as a thin shell or fragment of bone with linear morphology. Axial FS PD. The RHAGL is a mirror image of the HAGL lesion. There is an avulsion of the posterior capsuloligamentous tissue from the humerus. Similar to the HAGL lesion there may be a capsular split, avulsion from bone or a combination lesion.

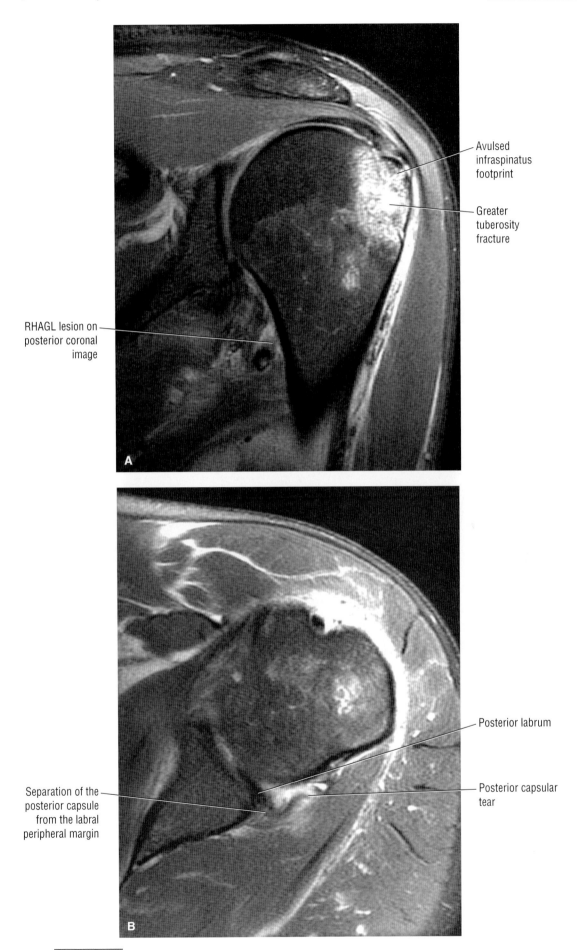

Avulsed infraspinatus footprint

Greater tuberosity fracture

RHAGL lesion on posterior coronal image

Posterior labrum

Posterior capsular tear

Separation of the posterior capsule from the labral peripheral margin

FIGURE 7.102 RHAGL associated with a greater tuberosity fracture. (**A**) Coronal. (**B**) Axial.

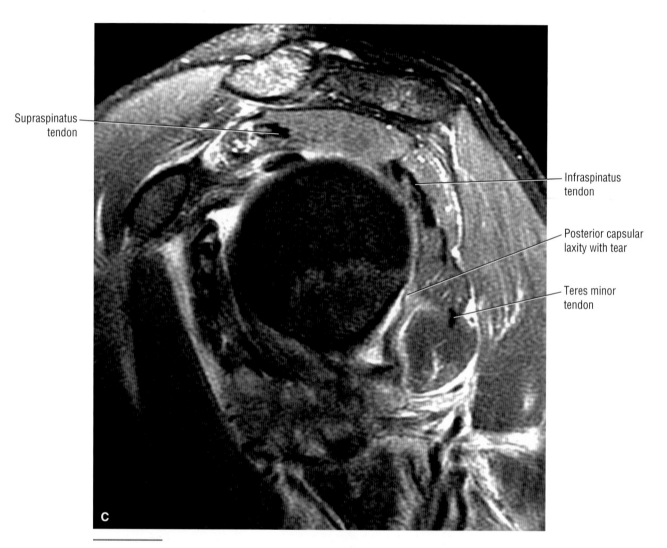

Supraspinatus tendon

Infraspinatus tendon

Posterior capsular laxity with tear

Teres minor tendon

C

FIGURE 7.102 (*Continued*) (**C**) Sagittal. The torn posterior capsule is thickened and lax. The extension of fluid through the posterior capsule results in the loss of the sharp anterior contour of the anterior inferior infraspinatus and teres minor muscles.

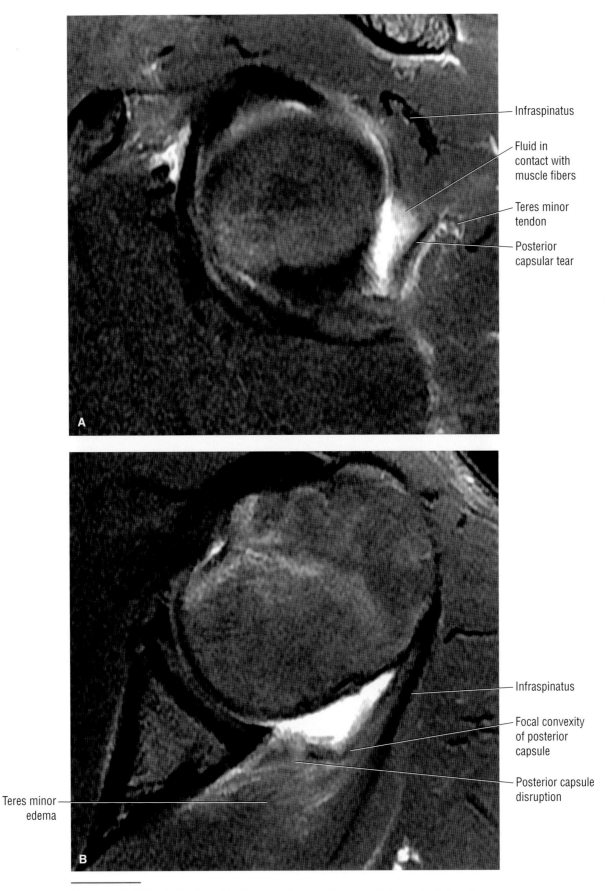

FIGURE 7.103 RHAGL with the posterior capsule torn inferior to the infraspinatus muscle. This permits contrast to coat the anterior muscle fibers of the teres minor and inferior infraspinatus. (**A**) Sagittal FS PD. (**B**) Axial FS PD.

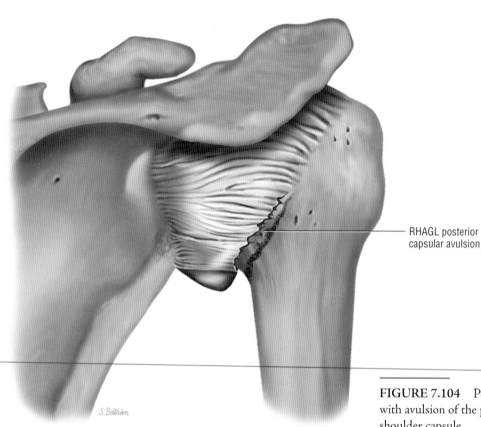

RHAGL posterior
capsular avulsion

FIGURE 7.104   Posterior coronal color view of RHAGL
with avulsion of the posterior humeral attachment of the
shoulder capsule.

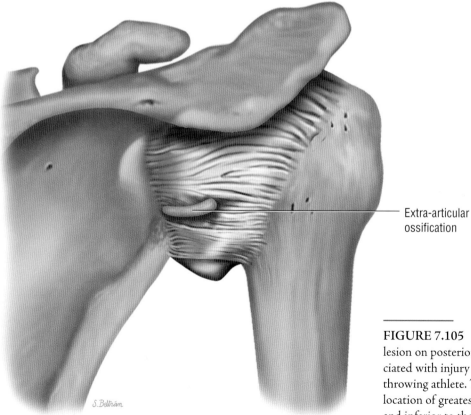

Extra-articular
ossification

FIGURE 7.105   Extra-articular ossification of a Bennett
lesion on posterior coronal view. The Bennett lesion is associated with injury to the posterior superior labrum in the
throwing athlete. The Bennett lesion usually occurs in the
location of greatest posterior glenoid rim wear or sclerosis
and inferior to the posterosuperior peel-back lesion.

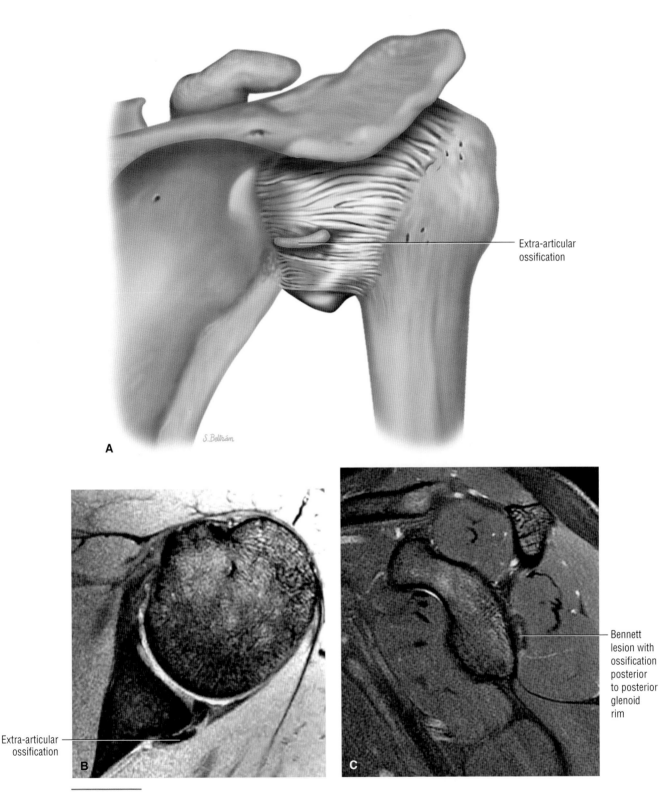

Extra-articular
ossification

Bennett
lesion with
ossification
posterior
to posterior
glenoid
rim

Extra-articular
ossification

FIGURE 7.106 (**A**) Extra-articular ossification of a Bennett lesion on posterior coronal view (color illustration). The Bennett lesion is associated with injury to the posterior superior labrum in the throwing athlete. (**B**) Axial T2*-weighted GRE image with linear crescentic ossification corresponding to the course of the posterior capsule. This ossification is usually in contact with the posterior glenoid neck. (**C**) Corresponding sagittal FS PD FSE image with hypertrophic buildup or ossification along the posterior rim. The Bennett lesion usually occurs in the location of greatest posterior glenoid rim wear or sclerosis and inferior to the posterosuperior peel-back lesion.

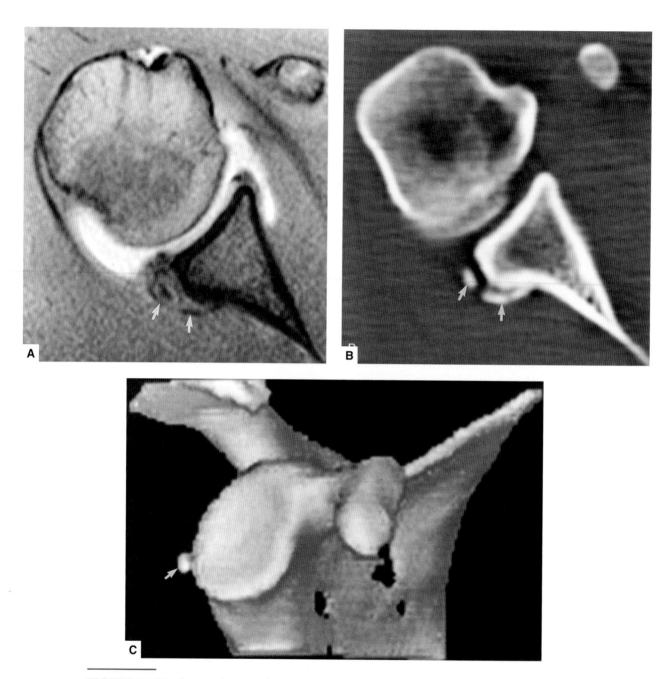

FIGURE 7.107   Bennett lesion with posterior extra-articular ossification (*straight arrows*) on FS T1-weighted axial arthrographic image (**A**), axial CT (**B**), and 3D CT rendering (**C**). The Bennett lesion is seen in the throwing athlete although not as common as posterior glenoid fossa sclerosis. The heterotopic ossification is near the insertion of the posterior band on the glenoid. A traction injury of the IGHL occurs in the cocking or follow-through stages of pitching.

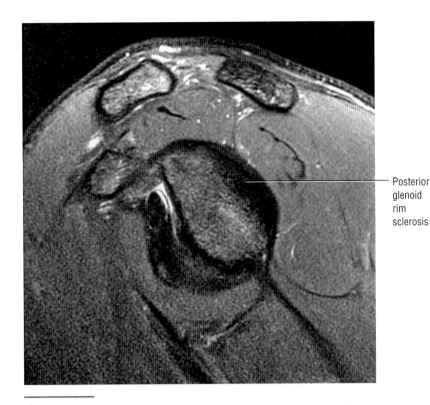

Posterior
glenoid
rim
sclerosis

FIGURE 7.108 Posterior glenoid rim sclerosis can be seen on this sagittal FS PD FSE image prior to the development of a posterior peel-back labral tear or Bennett's ossification. This pitcher has a fastball velocity of over 100 mph.

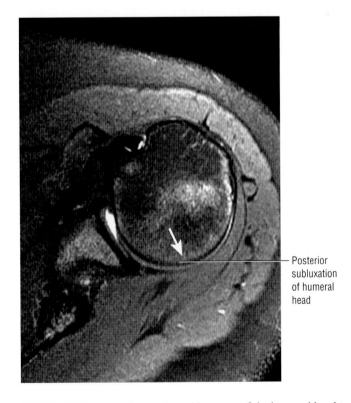

Posterior
subluxation
of humeral
head

FIGURE 7.109 Axial FS PD FSE image of posterior subluxation of the humeral head in a 20-year-old swimmer with a clinical "loose" shoulder. An episode of trauma may aggravate a shoulder with a preexisting or mild underlying laxity.

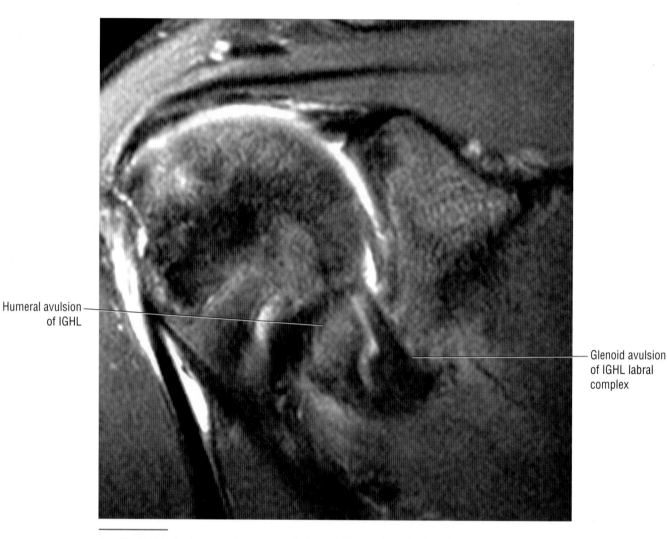

Humeral avulsion of IGHL

Glenoid avulsion of IGHL labral complex

FIGURE 7.110   Floating ligament with the IGHL torn from both its humeral and glenoid attachments as in an AIGL lesion. The anterior floating ligament represents a combination of a Bankart and HAGL lesion. A Hill-Sachs lesion is usually present. The glenoid disruption is repaired first to stabilize one end of the unstable capsular sheet. The humeral component is then addressed. Coronal FS PD.

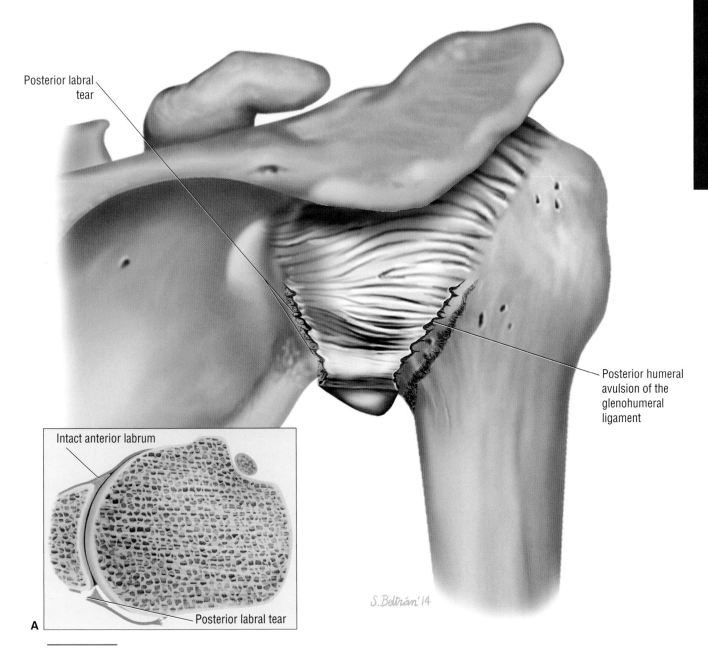

Posterior labral tear

Posterior humeral avulsion of the glenohumeral ligament

Intact anterior labrum

Posterior labral tear

A

S.Beltrán '14

FIGURE 7.111 Floating posterior IGHL with disruption both on the glenoid and posterior humeral neck side. This is the reverse of an anterior floating ligament. There are four subtypes of posterior inferior glenohumeral ligament lesions. (**A**) Soft tissue posterior floating ligament referred to as type 1.

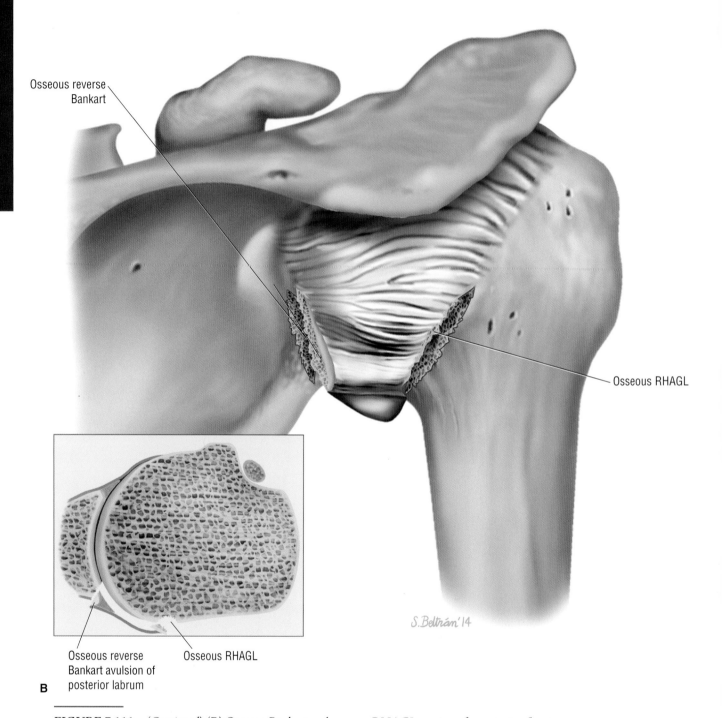

Osseous reverse
Bankart

Osseous RHAGL

Osseous reverse
Bankart avulsion of
posterior labrum

Osseous RHAGL

S. Beltrán '14

B

FIGURE 7.111 (*Continued*) (**B**) Osseous Bankart and osseous RHAGL version of a posterior floating ligament referred to as a type 4.

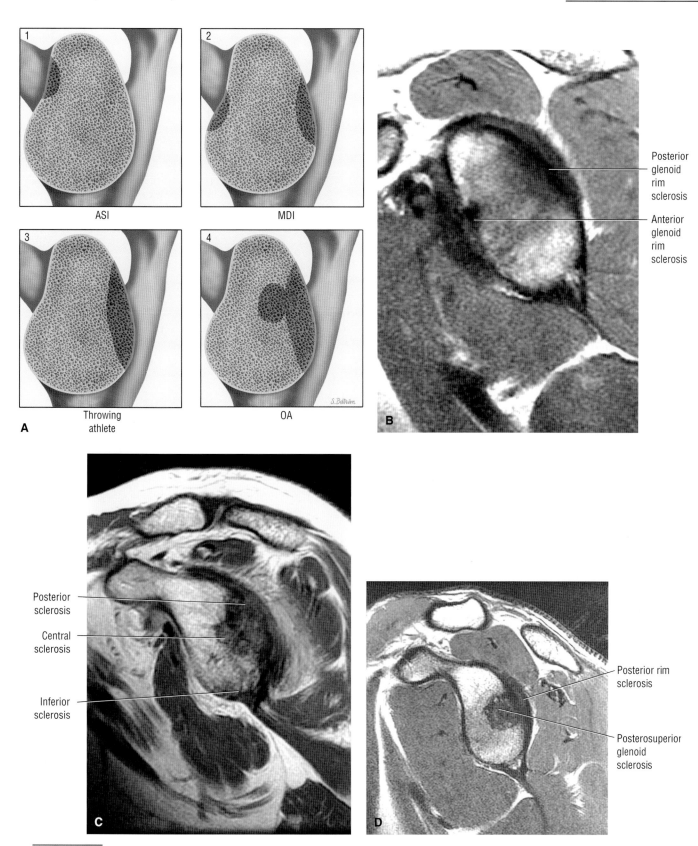

FIGURE 7.112 Four types of glenoid fossa sclerosis. (A1, upper left) Anterosuperior impingement (ASI) pattern. (A2, upper right) Multidirectional instability (MDI). (A3, lower left) Posterior glenoid rim wear in the throwing athlete. (A4, lower right) Osteoarthritis pattern with central glenoid fossa and posterior glenoid wear. (**B**) Sagittal FS PD FSE image showing MDI wear with anterior and posterior glenoid rim sclerosis. (**C**) Osteoarthritis in a 70-year-old patient with posterior wear and central glenoid sclerosis. The initial change of inferior rim sclerosis can also be seen. (**D**) Similar osteoarthritis pattern in the older elite pitcher with central and posterior rim sclerosis without the degenerative changes of the inferior pole. Central or posterosuperior glenohumeral fossa sclerosis is an unusual finding in the younger throwing athlete; instead, wear is initially limited to the posterior rim.

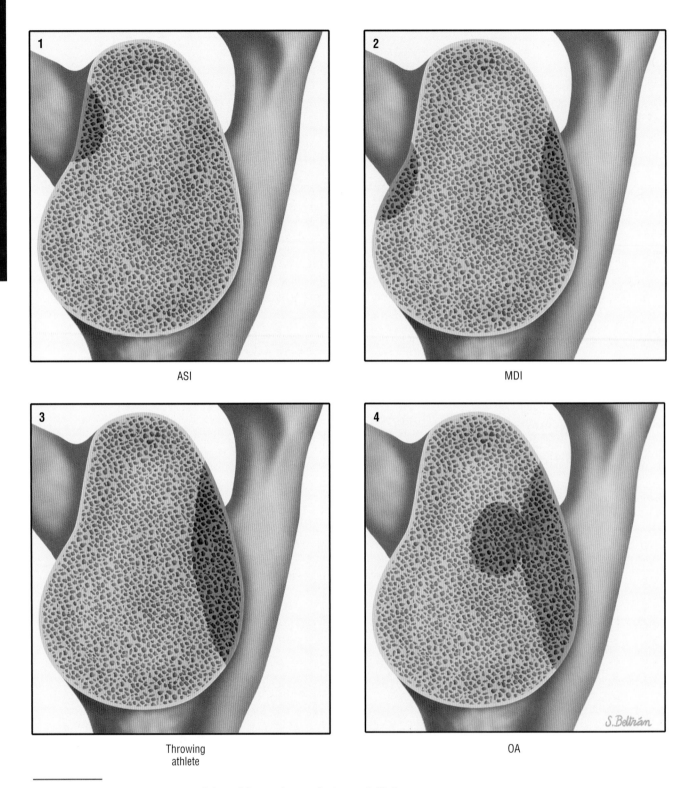

FIGURE 7.113 Four patterns of glenoid fossa sclerosis. (1. Upper left) Anterosuperior impingement (ASI). (2. Upper right) Multidirectional instability (MDI). (3. Lower left) Posterior glenoid rim wear in the throwing athlete. (4. Lower right) Osteoarthritis pattern with central glenoid fossa and posterior glenoid wear. The hypointense signal of adaptive sclerosis demonstrates the location of overhead repetitive use, microinstability and MDI. The involvement of the central glenoid fossa wear is no longer adaptive and instead indicates the development of osteoarthritis.

Multidirectional Instability

Key Concepts

- Referred to as either MDI (multidirectional instability) or AMBRI (atraumatic multidirectional instability, bilateral treated with rehabilitation or inferior capsular shift)

- MDI must include a component of inferior instability (anteroinferior or posteroinferior).

- MR findings in MDI may include subtle anterior and posterior glenoid rim sclerosis or static humeral head subluxation in the axial plane.

- A pancapsular plication is used to selectively tighten lax ligaments.

- Shoulder instability can be grouped into the Bankart lesions (patients with TUBS) and atraumatic MDI.

  - MDI is also referred to as atraumatic multidirectional instability, bilateral, treated with rehabilitation or inferior capsular shift (AMBRI).

- MDI/AMBRI may be seen in both athletic and nonathletic individuals with excessive capsular laxity, and the incidence is higher in females than in males.

- Etiologies range from anatomic defects to neuromuscular or biochemical abnormalities.[494]

- Although a structural lesion is not usually found, the IGHLC is suspect, since all MDI patients have a component of inferior instability, whether anteroinferior or posteroinferior.[26]

- The glenoid labrum and rotator cuff interval are also potential anatomic sites of pathology.

- In athletic patients, MDI may result from overuse and present as instability after minor trauma.

- Symptoms may also appear after minimal trauma in patients with preexistent laxity. Rarely, MDI presents in patients with genetic or inheritable hypermobility syndromes (e.g., Ehlers-Danlos syndrome or Marfan syndrome).

- The primary direction of instability can usually be determined.

- An MR arthrogram may demonstrate an increased capsular volume and capsular or ligamentous injury.

- In the case of posteroinferior MDI, increased chondrolabral and osseous retroversion and variable capsular stretching may be identified.[281]

- Loss of chondrolabral containment of the glenoid and an associated decrease in posterior labral height is a consistent finding in shoulders with atraumatic posteroinferior MDI.

- Retroversion of the chondrolabral portion of the glenoid is seen to be greater than the osseous glenoid at the level of the inferior glenohumeral joint.

  - Eccentric glenoid fossa (rim) sclerosis is directly visualized on sagittal images, even in the absence of an overlying chondral or labral lesion.

  - Patterns of sclerosis or wear may correlate with the direction of underlying laxity.

Surgical Treatment of Multidirectional Instability

- Surgical treatment is indicated if an extended course of rehabilitation for involuntary MDI fails.

- Earlier intervention may be justified in cases of MR-documented IGHLC injury in association with a physical examination for instability.

- A triad repair for MDI addresses the posterior-inferior capsule, anterior repair or shift of IGHLC, and superior capsular closure.[26]

- Snyder[547] recommends arthroscopic pancapsular plication for:

  - Selective tightening of lax ligaments

  - Widening of the surface area of the labrum and thus the weight-bearing capacity of the glenoid

  - Augmentation of the "chock block" effect of the labrum by deepening the relative concavity of the glenoid fossa

  - Closing of the rotator interval, providing a temporary internal splint (the SGHL and MGHL do not heal together) by reducing forces on the inferior capsule and limiting external rotation and inferior subluxation in the early postoperative period

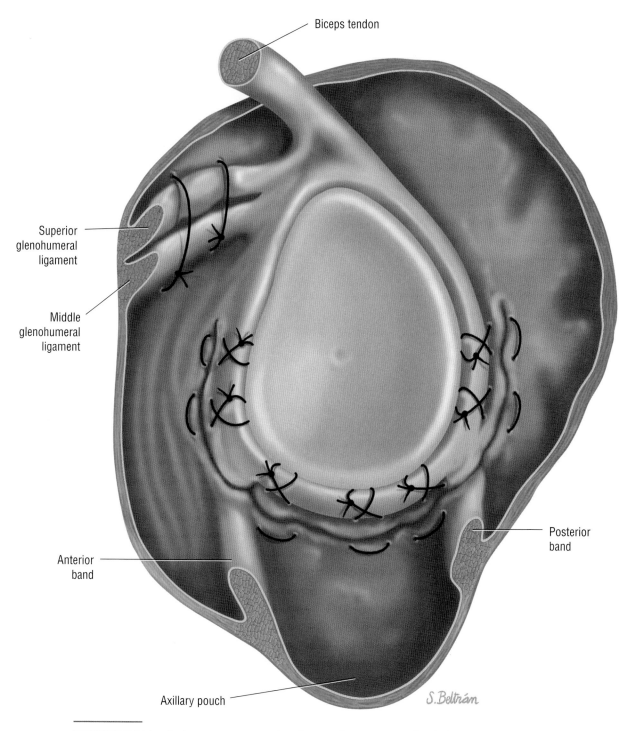

FIGURE 7.114 Arthroscopic pancapsular plication for treatment of multidirectional instability with the IGL and capsule folded to the labrum from the posteroinferior quadrant to the anteroinferior quadrant. The rotator interval is closed, and the final result is to have the humeral head centralized within the glenoid fossa. Arthroscopic assessment of MDI includes: Treating associated pathology of the biceps, labrum or cuff, reducing capsular laxity, augmentation of a hypoplastic labrum with a "chock bock" effect of folded capsule against the glenoid rim, and a suture technique through both the labrum and capsule keeping knots away from the articular cartilage surface.

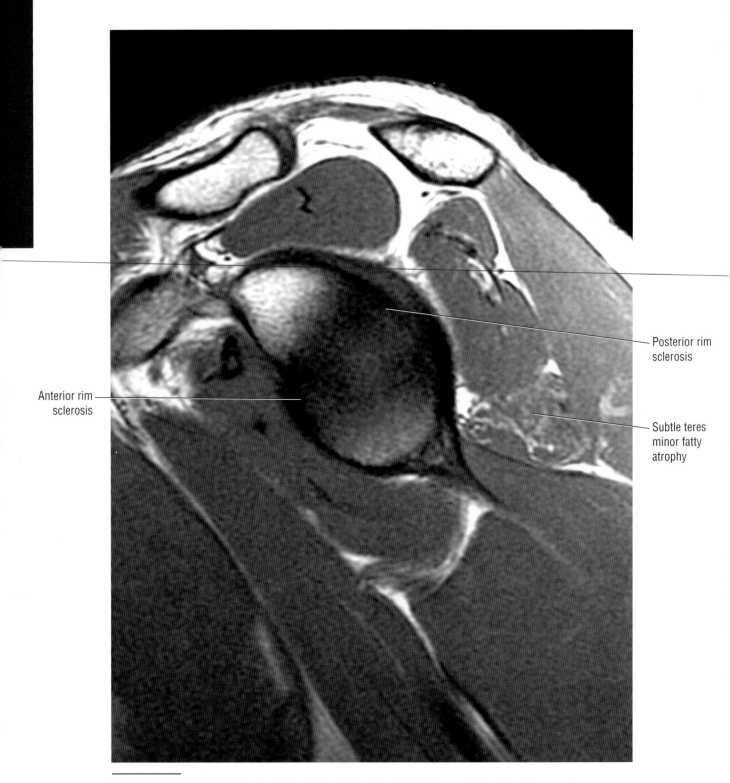

Anterior rim
sclerosis

Posterior rim
sclerosis

Subtle teres
minor fatty
atrophy

FIGURE 7.115   Multidirectional instability inferred by MR findings of sclerosis of the anterior
and posterior glenoid rim. There is mild fatty atrophy of teres minor muscle. Sagittal T2 FSE.

Instability Repair Overview

Bone Loss Criteria

- Significant bone loss
    - Loss of >25% of the inferior glenoid diameter
    - A deep Hill-Sachs lesion that engages the anterior glenoid rim in 90° abduction and 90° external rotation
    - Latarjet reconstruction performed in patients with significant bone loss
        - Extends the articular side of the glenoid so that the Hill-Sachs lesion cannot engage

Instability Associated with Bone Loss

- Evaluation for bone loss
    - Glenoid fossa bone loss
    - Hill-Sachs lesion
    - Percentage of bone loss
        - Width of glenoid on affected side relative to normal shoulder width
        - Bone loss less than or greater than 25% of glenoid width

Bony Bankart Lesions

- Small acute bony Bankart lesions
    - Repair of glenoid bone fragment with suture anchors
- Large acute bony Bankart lesions
    - Arthroscopic reduction and internal fixation using cannulated screws

Gray Zone

- Normal inferior glenoid diameter (<25% bone loss) with a deep posterolateral Hill-Sachs lesion (≥4mm deep)
    - High rate of failure after a Bankart repair
    - Treatment of choice is to augment the arthroscopic Bankart repair with an arthroscopic remplissage.
    - The infraspinatus tendon is inserted into the humeral head defect using suture anchors.
        - Arthroscopic remplissage as an infraspinatus transfer to fill the Hills-Sachs lesion

Soft Tissue Preparation

- Optimal tension at the bone-soft tissue interface

- Capsulolabral sleeve repair so as not too tight or loose

- Plication used to address excessive laxity as in multidirectional instability (MDI)

- Traumatic Instability
    - Recreate bumper of tissue at glenoid rim by achieving physiologic tensioning of the capsule and centering the humeral head on the bare spot of the glenoid.

Bone Bed Preparation

- Bone bed preparation to a base of bleeding bone is critical for a successful instability repair.

- A 2-mm stripe of articular cartilage is removed along the damaged glenoid.
    - Additional bleeding for capsular healing

Ancillary Fixation

- Plication sutures

- Rotator interval closure
    - Nonroutine except for use in the presence of a patulous interval

- Remplissage

Significant Bone Defects

- Latarjet Reconstruction

    - Coracoid bone graft

    - ≥25% loss inferior glenoid diameter

    - ≥4mm deep Hill-Sachs lesion that engages in a 90°-90° position

Anterior Instability without Significant Bone Loss

- Ninety percent of patients with traumatic anterior instability have some degree of glenoid bone loss.

    - Glenoid bone loss or abnormal anterior glenoid rim contour

    - The anterior glenoid rim deepens the glenoid and functions as a buttress to resist dislocation. Glenoid bone loss decreases the congruent arc of the glenoid.

- Majority of cases of bony Bankart lesions involve 25% of the inferior diameter of the glenoid, and suture anchor repair can be used to incorporate the bony fragments.

- Common for residual ossesous Bankart fragment to be smaller than the amount of glenoid bone loss

    - The small bony fragment can still be incorporated into the repair and will improve the surgical outcome.

Bankart Repair

- Most inferior and superior anchors are used to repair the labrum.

    - Middle anchors used to capture the bony Bankart fragment

- Bony Bankart screw fixation

    - If bony Bankart fragment is >20% to 25% of the diameter of the inferior glenoid

Bankart Repair Indications

- Glenoid fragment greater than 25%

- Associated injuries (rotator cuff or proximal humerus fracture)

- Irreducible dislocation

- Nonconcentric reduction
    - Interposed tissue

Coracoid Bone Graft

- Triple Effect
    - Lengthening of the articular arc by the bone graft
    - The sling effect of the conjoined tendon
    - Tensioning of the lower subscapularis by the conjoined tendon in its new position

- Congruent-Arc-Latarjet Reconstruction
    - Coracoid graft orientation with arc of its inferior surface as a congruent extension of the glenoid articular arc

Arthroscopic Remplissage

- To fill the Hill-Sachs defect with the infraspinatus

- Many Hill-Sachs lesions are associated with PASTA lesions of the infraspinatus.
    - The PASTA lesion can be addressed by inserting the infraspinatus into the Hill-Sachs defect.

- Remplissage converts the Hill-Sachs from an intraarticular to an extra-articular defect that will no longer engage on the corner of the glenoid.

- Large and deep (>1cm) Hill-Sachs lesion is commonly associated with inverted pear glenoids.
    - Combined deep Hill-Sachs lesions and glenoid lesions are treated with open Latarjet procedures.

Posterior Instability Repair

- Posterior pain

- Posterior instability

- Acute traumatic injury
    - Posterior translational load
    - Defensive lineman

- Posterior joint line pain
    - Bench press
    - Overhead press
    - Dips

- Positive relocation sign
    - Posterolateral SLAP

- Pain with posterior load and shift
    - Posterolabral tear

- True posterior instability
    - Pain
    - Instability
    - Ligamentous laxity
    - Positive sulcus sign
    - Positive jerk test
    - Instability voluntary but positional

- MR identifies posterior bony Bankart or degenerative lesions.
    - Posterior bony Bankart associated with an acute instability episode
    - Associated paralabral cyst(s)

- Combined posterior labral tear and SLAP lesion
    - Seen in patients with posterior pain following a traumatic injury

- Posterior labral repair with reverse remplissage

8
Inferior Glenohumeral Ligament Capsular Variations, High Attachment Anterior Band, and SLAP Lesions

Inferior Glenohumeral Ligament Capsular Variations, High Attachment Anterior Band, and SLAP Lesions

Labral Pathology

Key Concepts

- The sublabral foramen
    - Is created by the high attachment of the anterior band
    - Is located in the anterosuperior quadrant of the glenoid fossa
- The biceps labral sulcus is identified at the level of the superior pole of the glenoid in the 12 o'clock position.
- The MGL may be cord-like, thin, or absent.
    - An attenuated MGHL(MGL) may be either very thin or fibrous in appearance with no ligamentous thickening. This variation, as well as the absent MGHL, is frequently associated with a high attachment of the anterior band.
- When cord-like, the MGL presents as an isolated variation or in conjunction with a high attachment anterior band of the IGL or as part of the Buford complex.
- Since there is an absent anterosuperior labrum in the Buford complex, a sublabral foramen cannot exist.
    - Although the existence of a sublabral foramen is related to the presence of a high attachment of the anterior band
- In the presence of a high attachment of the anterior band of the IGHL and a Buford complex, the anterior band may form an apparent or pseudo-sublabral foramen above the equator. Because both the Buford complex and the high attachment of the anterior

band have an association with an absent anterior superior labrum, the combination of both these variations will always be seen with an absent labrum in the anterior superior quadrant.

> ■ High attachment of the anterior band without a Buford complex will present most commonly with an absent anterior superior labrum but may also be seen with an attenuated or diminutive anterior superior labrum above the equator.

Normal Variations

Sublabral Foramen

- ■ There is considerable variation in the attachment and morphology of the glenoid labrum.

  - ■ Most significant variation is the relative attachment, or lack thereof, to the glenoid rim in the anterior superior quadrant above the epiphyseal line.

- ■ Frequently between the labrum and the glenoid rim, which is often the cause for misinterpretation of anterior superior labral disruptions or tears

  - ■ Although the glenoid labrum in the superior one third of the glenoid above the epiphyseal line can be firmly fixed in its periphery[137]

- ■ A normal anterosuperior sublabral foramen or hole has been reported in up to 11% to 17% of individuals.[120,552,623]

- ■ Sublabral foramen may in fact be the result of a high attachment of the anterior band of the IGL.

  - ■ This anatomy can be confirmed by correlated axial images with sagittal images to follow the course of the anterior band extending superiorly toward the biceps labral complex with the normal absence of an anterior superior labrum. Thus the anterior band is functioning as if it were the anterior labrum above the equator and thus has been considered a sublabral foramen.

  - ■ The anterior band of the IGL is closely applied to the anterior surface of the anterior inferior labrum below the equator. Above the equator, the anterior band is conspicuous as it moves further anterior relative to the anterior glenoid rim in its course toward the BLC superiorly.

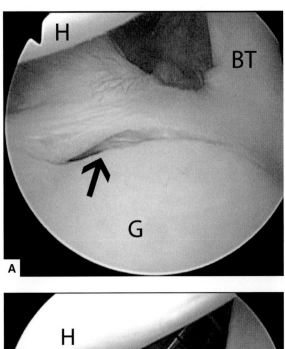

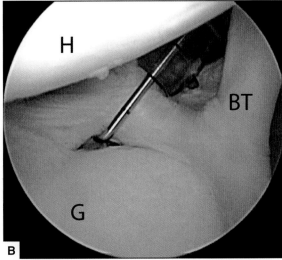

FIGURE 8.1 (**A**) Left shoulder, posterior glenohumeral viewing portal, demonstrates a sublabral foramen (*black arrow*). (**B**) Same shoulder. A probe is used to further show this normal anatomic variant. The anterior edge of the glenoid fossa has an indentation or dimple at arthroscopy corresponding to the equator. The equator demarcates the superior two-fifths from the inferior three-fifths of the glenoid. The high attachment of the anterior band is located anterior to the glenoid rim above the equator (where it is no longer in direct contact with the underlying anterior inferior labrum) and is thus perceived as a sublabral foramen. BT, biceps tendon; G, glenoid; H, humerus. (Reprinted from Burkhart S, Lo IK, Brady PC, Denard PJ. *The Cowboy's Companion: A Trail Guide for the Arthroscopic Shoulder Surgeon*. Philadelphia, PA: Lippincott Williams & Wilkins; 2012, with permission.)

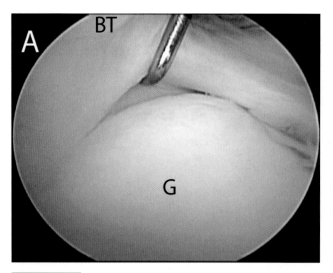
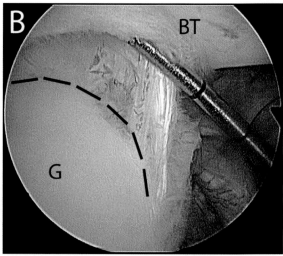

FIGURE 8.2　Right shoulder, posterior viewing portal, demonstrating (**A**) normal superior sublabral sulcus. (**B**) An abnormal sublabral recess >5mm with exposed bone (glenoid rim outlined by *dashed lines*). BT, biceps tendon; G, glenoid. The biceps labral sulcus or sublabral sulcus should be identified in the 12 o'clock location. (Reprinted from Burkhart S, Lo IK, Brady PC, Denard PJ. *The Cowboy's Companion: A Trail Guide for the Arthroscopic Shoulder Surgeon*. Philadelphia, PA: Lippincott Williams & Wilkins; 2012, with permission.)

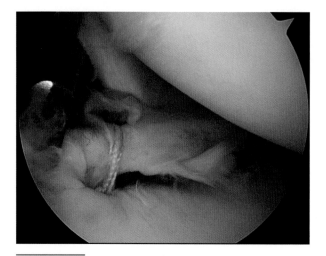

FIGURE 8.3　Inappropriate repair performed of the normal sublabral foramen. The patient complained of significant postoperative pain and stiffness requiring revision surgery. Whether the sublabral foramen is appreciated as a true foramen or the result of a high attachment of the anterior band of the IGL the sublabral foramen should not be repaired. Tacking down the anterior band would convert an unconstrained functional unit to becoming a stiff or constrained or restricted complex which will fail. (Reprinted from Miniaci A, Iannotti JP, Williams GR, Zuckerman, JD. *Disorders of the Shoulder: Sports Injuries*. 3rd ed. Philadelphia, PA: Lippincott Williams & Wilkins; 2014, with permission.)

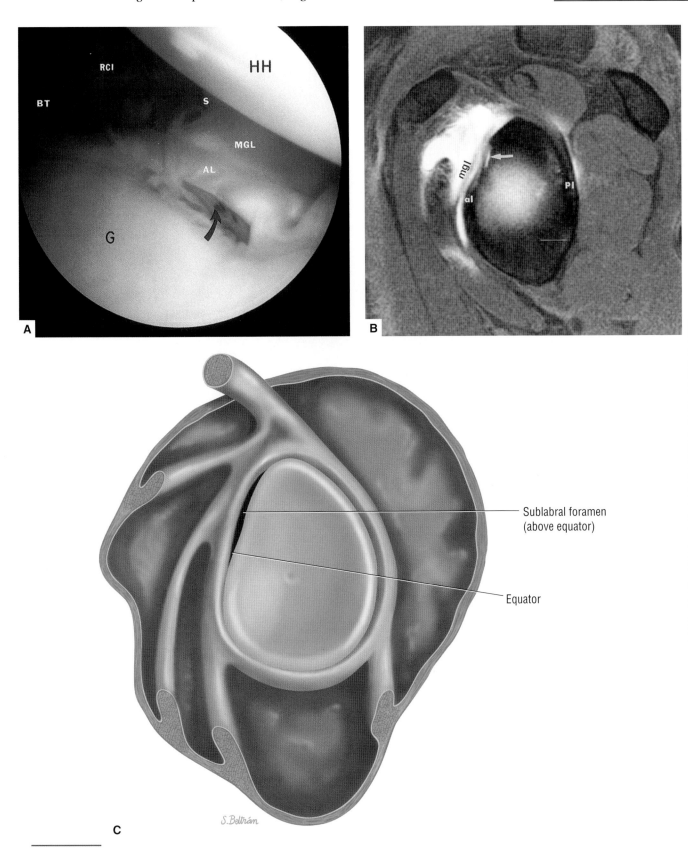

FIGURE 8.4 (**A**) An arthroscopic photograph of a normal anatomic variant of the sublabral foramen with a missing anterior labrum attachment above the epiphyseal line of the glenoid (*curved arrow*). AL, anterior labrum; BT, biceps tendon; G, glenoid; HH, humeral head; MGL, middle glenohumeral ligament; RCI, rotator cuff interval or Weitbrecht's foramen; S, subscapularis tendon. (**B**) Sublabral foramen (*arrow*) shown above the equator (above the anterior glenoid notch) on an FS T1-weighted sagittal oblique MR arthrogram. Contrast extends between the anterosuperior labrum and the glenoid rim as a normal variant. MGL, middle glenohumeral ligament; al, anterior labrum; pl, posterior labrum. (**C**) Lateral view color graphic of a sublabral foramen beneath the anterior superior labrum. The anterior band would have to merge with the anterior labrum near the equator in order to appreciate substantial tissue that would form a firmly attached anterior superior labrum above the equator.

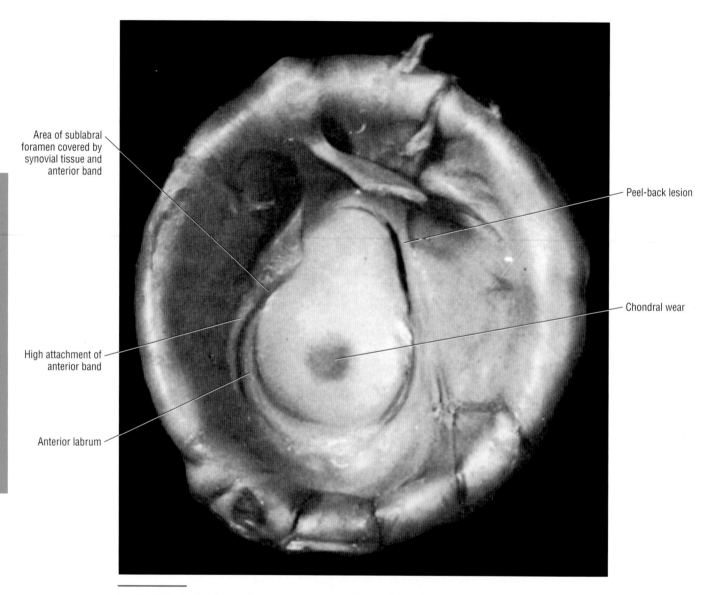

Area of sublabral foramen covered by synovial tissue and anterior band

Peel-back lesion

High attachment of anterior band

Chondral wear

Anterior labrum

FIGURE 8.5   High attachment of the anterior band of the IGHL creating this sublabral foramen in the anterior superior quadrant. The formation of the sublabral foramen by the anterior band of the IGHL is consistent with attributing the anterosuperior labrum as a fold or continuation of capsular tissue. It is the anterior band instead of the labrum that forms a bridge over the glenoid notch. (From DePalma AF. *Surgery of the Shoulder*. 3rd ed. Philadelphia, PA: JB Lippincott; 1983.)

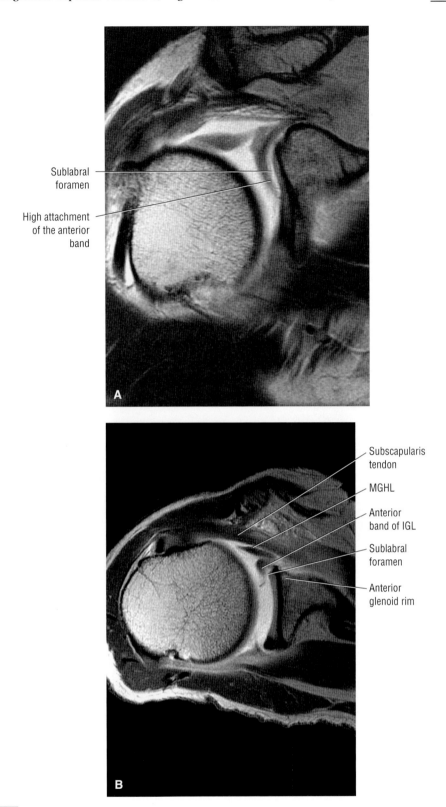

Sublabral foramen

High attachment of the anterior band

Subscapularis tendon

MGHL

Anterior band of IGL

Sublabral foramen

Anterior glenoid rim

FIGURE 8.6   The sublabral foramen is present in 14% of shoulders and can range in size from a few millimeters to the entire anterosuperior quadrant between the superior pole and the equator. The sublabral foramen should not be mistaken for a Bankart labral detachment or a SLAP lesion of the biceps labral complex. The sublabral foramen is often associated with a cord-like middle glenohumeral ligament. This assumes that the cord-like MGL is not associated with a Buford complex since a sublabral foramen cannot exist in this variation (because the anterosuperior labrum is absent). (**A**) Coronal T1 MR arthrogram with a large anterosuperior sublabral foramen. (**B**) Corresponding axial T1 MR arthrogram demonstrating the subscapularis, the middle glenohumeral ligament (MGHL), the anterior labrum, the sublabral foramen, and the anterior glenoid as visualized from anterior to posterior. The sublabral foramen in fact represents a high attachment of the anterior band associated with an absent anterosuperior labrum. The anterior band is perceived of as an unattached anterosuperior labrum above the equator.

Middle Glenohumeral Ligament Variations

- MGHL is identified as a folded thickening of the anterior capsule between the anterior labrum and subscapularis tendon, inserting on the labrum or near the glenoid rim.[382,623]

- In 19% of cases, the MGHL has a cord-like morphology, compared with the more normal sheet-like appearance of ligamentous tissue.

- Complete absence of the MGHL may be associated with a congenitally lax anterior capsule.

- The cord-like MGHL is best demonstrated on axial and sagittal MR images.

  - The thick and low-signal-intensity cord-like MGHL may be mistaken for a detached anterior labrum above the epiphyseal line (Bankart lesion).

  - The high attachment MGHL on multiple axial images, distinct from the normal anterior inferior glenoid labrum below the level of the subscapularis tendon, excludes the presence of a Bankart lesion.

- MGHL arises from the upper periphery of the glenoid fossa and from the glenoid labrum.

  - Courses diagonally and inferiorly to the humerus to join the inferior aspect of the subscapularis tendon and fasciculus obliquus before inserting together on the lesser tuberosity[182]

- The glenoid origin of the MGHL can be as high as the supraglenoid tubercle and scapular neck at the level of the base of the coracoid process.

  - The MGHL may fuse to the SGHL in its proximal course.

- MGHL variations include:

  - Origin only from the glenoid labrum

  - No attachment to the labrum

  - Complete osseous origin without labral attachment

  - Origin is conjoined with the SGHL

  - Less common double MGHL without connection to labrum, scapula, or SGHL[182]

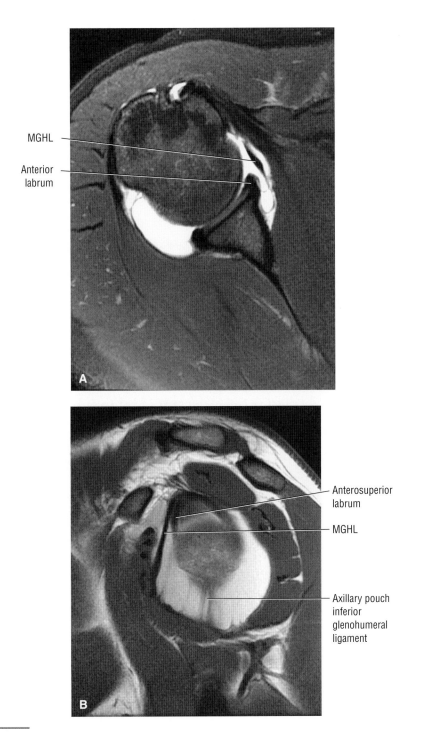

FIGURE 8.7   Normal middle glenohumeral ligament (MGHL or MGL) on axial FS PD FSE (**A**) and sagittal FSE (**B**) images. The MGL is the most variable in morphology of all the anterior glenohumeral capsular ligaments. In the most common appearance (70% of cases), the MGL represents a folded anterior capsular thickening that crosses the subscapularis tendon at a 45° angle. The MGL inserts onto the anterosuperior glenoid neck at the level of or just medial to the labrum. The MGL, superior glenohumeral ligament, and anterosuperior labrum thus converge at the anterior superior pole of the glenoid. This ligament configuration creates one opening into the subscapularis recess anterior to the leading edge of the MGL.

Buford Complex

- In the normal labrum, a thin MGHL is identified anterior to the anterior labrum.

- The normal anterior labrum is found above and below the equator.

- In contrast, the Buford complex consists of three defining elements:
  - A cord-like MGHL
  - An MGHL that attaches directly to the superior labrum anterior to the biceps (at the base of the biceps anchor)
  - An absent anterosuperior labrum[635,636]

- Of 200 shoulder arthroscopies reviewed by Williams and Snyder et al.,[635,636] the Buford complex was found in 1.5%; a sublabral foramen, located between the anterosuperior glenoid quadrant and the articular surface of the anterior glenoid, was found in 12%.

- In 75% of patients who demonstrated a sublabral foramen, a cord-like MGHL was also present.
  - This cord-like MGHL attaches directly to the superior labrum.
  - The additional finding of an absent anterosuperior labrum places patients into the subgroup of the Buford complex.
  - The sublabral foramen is in fact created by a high attachment of the anterior band.

- Several key MR findings help to avoid misinterpretation of the absence of anterosuperior labral tissue in the anterosuperior quadrant of the glenoid fossa.
  - An absent anterior labrum exists above the level of the subscapularis tendon as assessed on axial images. A sublabral foramen can only exist in the presence of an anterior superior labrum (which is functionally represented by a high attachment of the anterior band).
  - The anterior inferior glenoid labrum below the level of the subscapularis tendon is firmly attached to the glenoid with normal morphology.
  - A cord-like MGHL if present is identified anterior to the glenoid rim and anterior to the course of the anterior band.

- There may be remnant or hypoplastic anterosuperior labral tissue identified on axial images at the level of the subscapularis tendon.

  - If the anterior superior labrum is small above the equator, then there should be an associated high attachment of the anterior band (an absent anterior superior labrum, however, is the more common variant in the presence of a high attachment of the anterior band).

- It is easy to distinguish a Bankart lesion from the Buford complex because in a Bankart lesion, the anterior inferior labrum is torn or avulsed and does not appear firmly attached to the anteroinferior glenoid rim.

- The sagittal oblique plane demonstrates the course of the cord-like MGHL attaching directly to the superior labrum at the anterior base of the biceps tendon.

- The anterosuperior labrum is absent both in the Buford complex and in the high attachment of the anterior band.

  - The anterosuperior labrum is also absent if there coexists a Buford complex and the high attachment of the anterior band.

- Intraarticular MR arthrography can be used to improve visualization of the cord-like MGHL distinct from the bare anterior glenoid rim.

  - This complex can be recognized without the routine use of an MR contrast agent.

- If the Buford complex is associated with a SLAP lesion, the cord-like MGHL may be incompetent since it is attached to a lax or loose superior labrum (the superior labrum pulls away from the glenoid under traction).[558]

- Failure to recognize the Buford complex may result in the inappropriate surgical attachment of the cord-like MGHL directly to the anterior glenoid.

  - This fixation leads to limitation of shoulder elevation and external rotation.

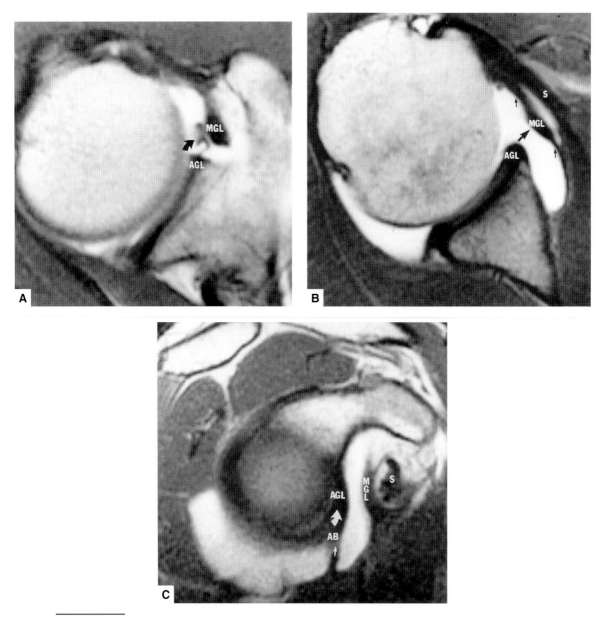

FIGURE 8.8 Cord-like middle glenohumeral ligament (MGHL or MGL) on T1-weighted enhanced axial images at the level of the coracoid (**A**) and inferior to the coracoid at the level of the subscapularis tendon (**B**). Curved arrow, filamentous attachment to cord-like MGL; large straight arrow, cord-like portion of MGL; small straight arrows, thin portion of MGL; AGL, anterior glenoid labrum. (**C**) Corresponding T1-weighted enhanced sagittal oblique image showing the relationship of the MGL to the anterior band of the IGL (AB; straight arrow), the anterior glenoid labrum (AGL; curved arrow), the middle glenohumeral ligament (MGL), and the subscapularis tendon (S). The MGL is located in the plane between the subscapularis tendon and the anterior band of the IGL or anterior glenoid labrum. There is a normal anatomic variation in which the cord-like MGHL attaches to the anterior band in the anterosuperior quadrant. At arthroscopy the sublabral foramen would appear to have a cord-like MGHL attached. The MGHL may exist as a cord-like, thin or absent structure. The cord-like appearance exists in up to 20 percent of normal shoulders. The cord-like MGHL may attach to the neck of the anterior superior glenoid (normal position) or to the anterior superior labrum.

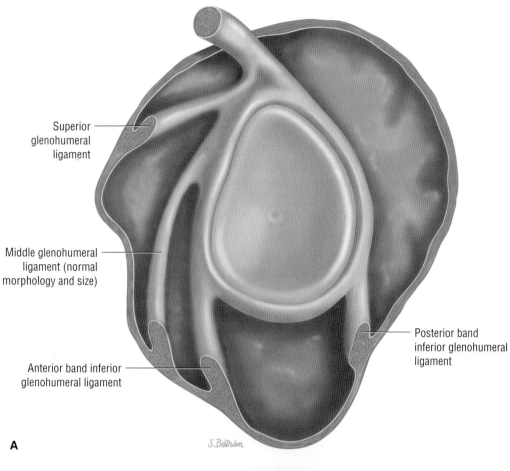

Superior
glenohumeral
ligament

Middle glenohumeral
ligament (normal
morphology and size)

Posterior band
inferior glenohumeral
ligament

Anterior band inferior
glenohumeral ligament

A

S.Beltrán

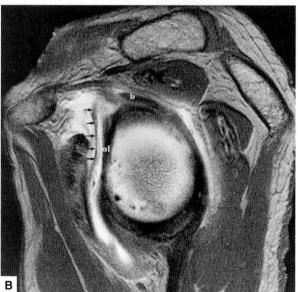

B

FIGURE 8.9 (**A**) Normal MGL morphology on lateral glenoid exposure. In 10% of shoulders, the MGL is a thin attenuated structure or completely absent. The anterior band of the IGL may be inversely prominent in association with an attenuated or fibrous MGL variation. (**B**) Sagittal T1-weighted MR arthrogram demonstrating a thin (with no area of thickening) linear MGL (*arrows*) anterior to the anterior labrum (al). b, biceps. A thin MGHL may appear as a translucent fibrous sheet or a few filmy fibrous bands at arthroscopy. There may be a high attachment of the anterior band in these cases.

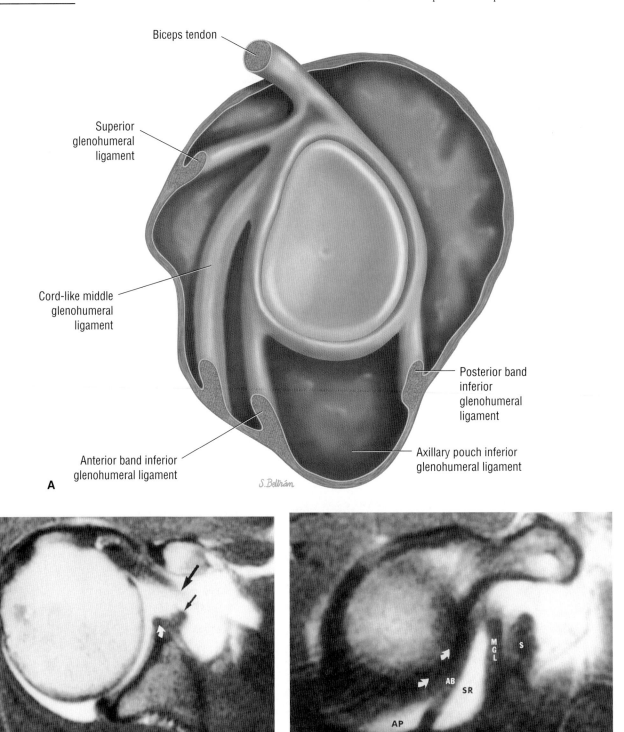

FIGURE 8.10   The cord-like middle glenohumeral ligament (MGL) represents the most common variation of MGL anatomy and is seen in up to 20% of normal shoulders. The cord-like MGL has a smooth rope-like or round cross-section instead of the more linear sheet-like morphology. The cord-like MGL attaches either to the neck of the glenoid superiorly or directly to the anterosuperior labrum. The cord-like MGL may be associated with a sublabral pole in cases where it attaches directly to the anterosuperior labrum. This variation does not represent a labral detachment or Buford complex. (**A**) Lateral color illustration of the cord-like MGL. (**B**) Enhanced T1-weighted axial images showing a cord-like or hypertrophied MGL (*small black arrow*) that simulates an avulsion of the anterior labrum (*curved arrow*). Subscapularis tendon (*large black arrow*) is anterior to cord-like MGL. (**C**) A corresponding enhanced T1-weighted sagittal image displays a normal anterior labrum (*curved arrows*) and anterior band of the IGL (AB). A thick, cord-like MGL and subscapularis tendon (S) can also be identified. Intraarticular gadolinium contrast is shown in the axillary pouch (AP) of the inferior glenohumeral ligament and in a synovial recess (SR) below the MGL.

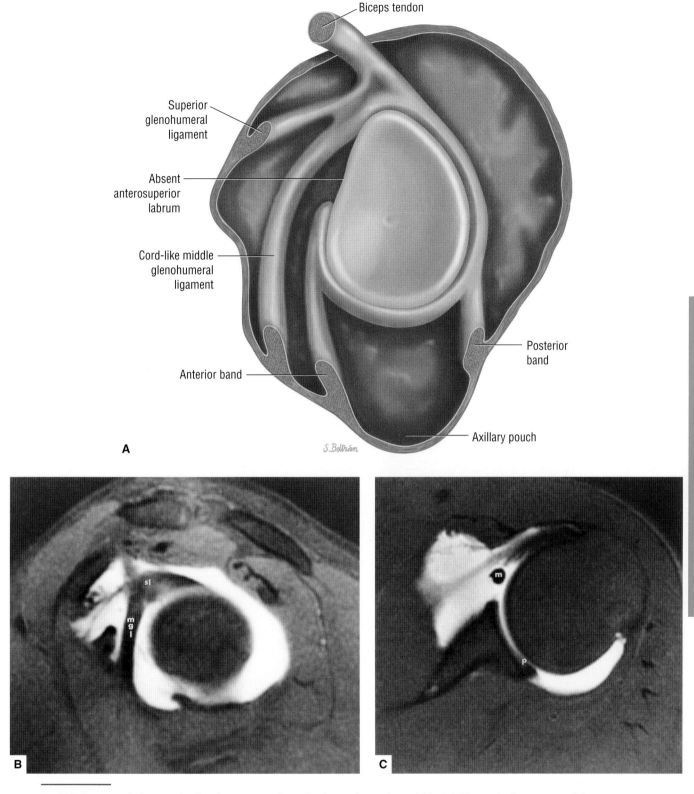

FIGURE 8.11 (**A**) Lateral color illustration of a Buford complex with cord-like MGL attached to superior labrum just anterior to the base of the biceps anchor and absent anterosuperior labrum above the equator. (**B**) Thick cord-like middle glenohumeral ligament (mgl) attaching directly to the superior labrum (sl) on an FS T1-weighted sagittal oblique arthrogram. (**C**) Corresponding FS T1 axial image displays the cord-like middle glenohumeral ligament (m) with an absent anterior superior labrum as a normal variant. Note that the posterior labrum (p) is present.

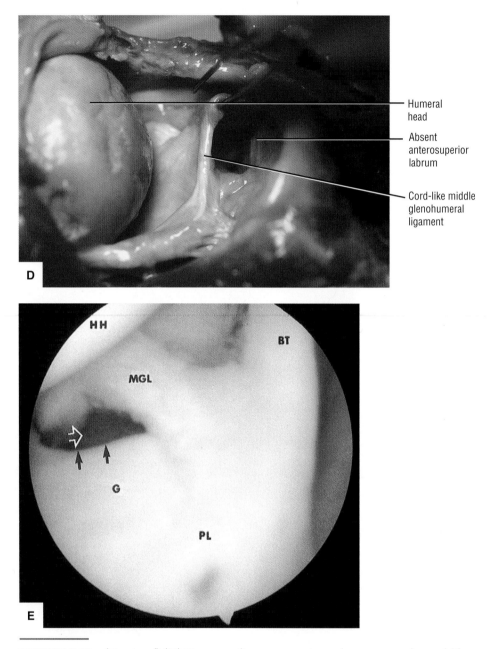

FIGURE 8.11   (*Continued*) (**D**) Corresponding gross specimen demonstrates the cord-like MGL, which attaches directly to the superior labrum. (**E**) An arthroscopic view of cord-like MGL in a Buford complex. The anterior superior glenoid edge (*black arrows*) shows an absence of the labrum as a normal variant in association with prominent MGL. The MGL originates from the anteromedial humeral neck and attaches medially on the glenoid (G) and the neck of the scapula. Open arrow, subscapularis recess; BT, biceps tendon; HH, humeral head; PL, posterior labrum. The Buford complex should not be confused with a pathologic detachment of the anterior superior labrum. At arthroscopy, there is no evidence of fraying or signs of trauma to the labrum or capsular tissues. The edge of the cord-like MGL (MGHL) is smooth consistent with a congenital variation. It is possible to have both a cord-like MGHL and a high attachment of the anterior band in the same shoulder. The anterosuperior labrum would be absent in this variation as well.

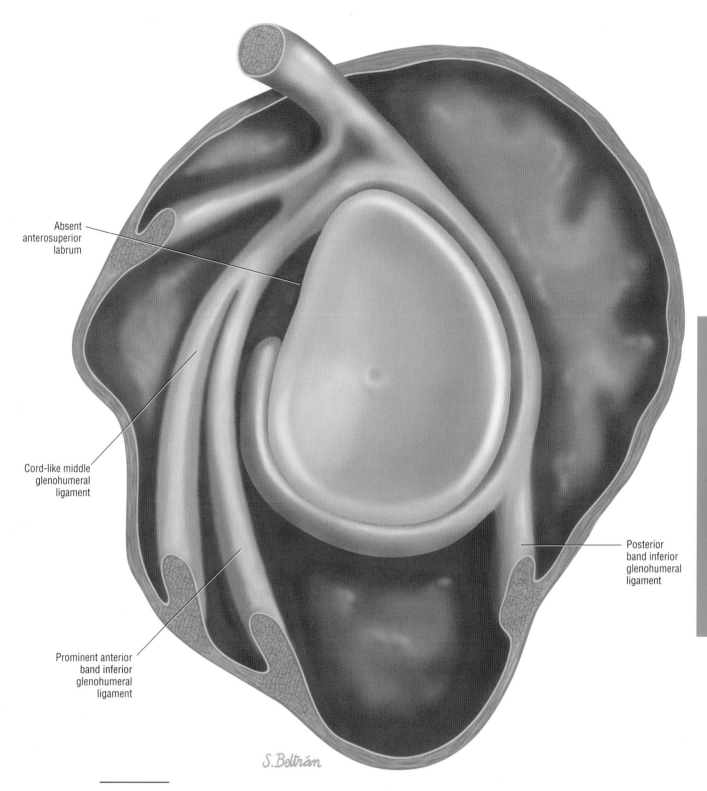

Absent anterosuperior labrum

Cord-like middle glenohumeral ligament

Prominent anterior band inferior glenohumeral ligament

Posterior band inferior glenohumeral ligament

S. Beltrán

FIGURE 8.12   A high attachment of the anterior band associated with a cord-like MGL and absent anterosuperior labrum on a lateral view color illustration. Because the MGL is cord-like, this could be considered a Buford variant. The original description of the Buford complex did not include the variant of a prominent anterior band. Since either a cord-like MGL or a high attachment of the anterior band is associated with an absent anterosuperior labrum, it is consistent that the anterosuperior labrum is also absent when both these anatomic variations coexist.

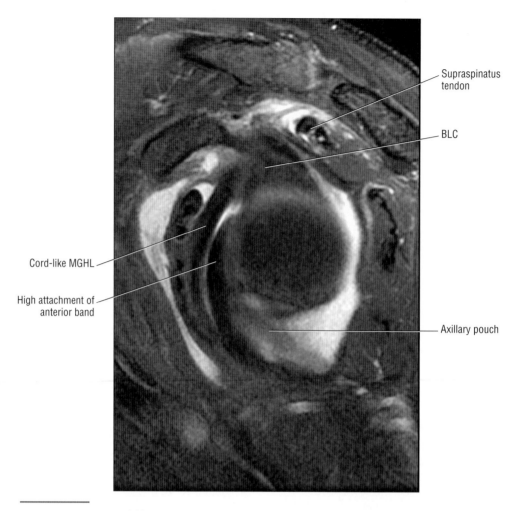

FIGURE 8-13   Cord-like MGHL plus high attachment of the anterior band. There is an absent anterior superior labrum in both the Bufford complex and the case of the Bufford and high attachment of the anterior band. A high attachment of the anterior band without the Bufford complex may be associated with an absent anterior superior labrum or an attenuated anterior superior labrum. Sag FS PD.

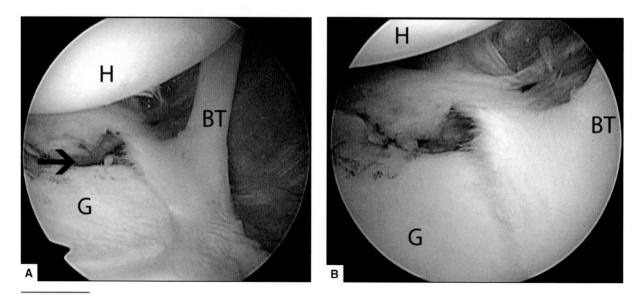

FIGURE 8.14   Left shoulder, posterior glenohumeral viewing portal, demonstrates (**A**) panoramic and (**B**) up-close views of a Buford complex that is characterized by a cord-like middle glenohumeral ligament with absence of the labrum between the biceps root and the midglenoid notch (*black arrow*). BT, biceps tendon; G, glenoid; H, humerus. (Reprinted from Burkhart S, Lo IK, Brady PC, Denard PJ. *The Cowboy's Companion: A Trail Guide for the Arthroscopic Shoulder Surgeon.* Philadelphia, PA: Lippincott Williams & Wilkins; 2012, with permission.)

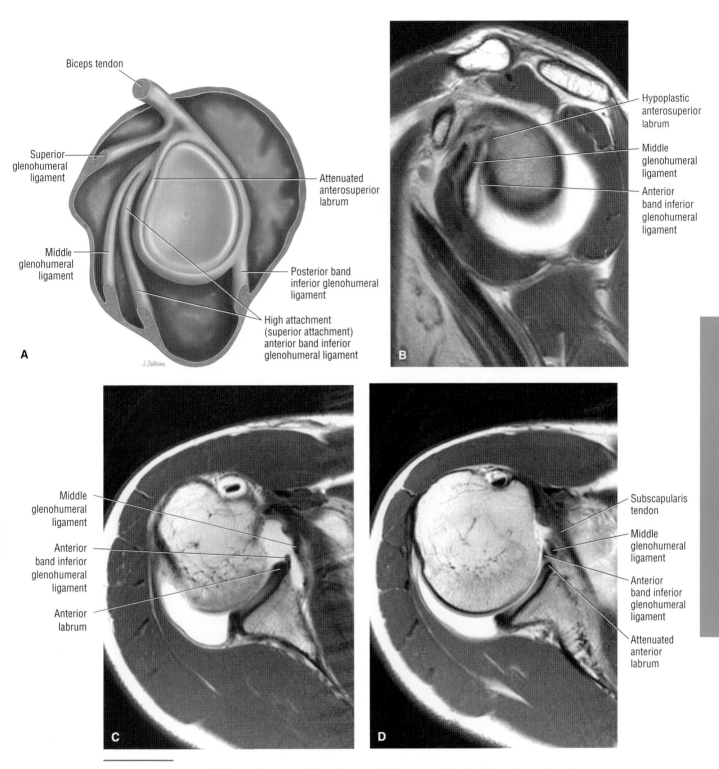

FIGURE 8.15   High (above the equator) attachment of the anterior band of the inferior glenohumeral ligament coursing anterior to a small anterosuperior labrum and attaching at the level of the superior labrum. (**A**) Lateral color illustration. (**B**) Sagittal PD-weighted MR arthrogram. (**C**) Inferior axial PD-weighted MR arthrogram at the inferior edge of subscapularis tendon. (**D**) Axial PD-weighted MR arthrogram at the level of superior edge of subscapularis tendon above the equator.

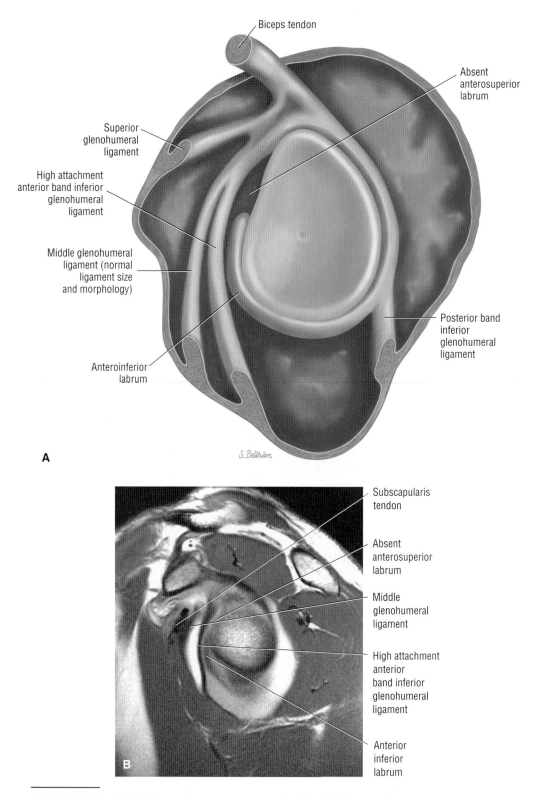

FIGURE 8.16 (**A**) High attachment anterior band of the IGHL with absent anterosuperior labrum. This is not a Buford complex since the MGL is not cord-like. If the anterosuperior labrum is absent, as in the case of a prominent anterior band, Buford complex, or Buford variant (cord-like MGL plus a prominent anterior band), there may be a normal sulcus between the superior labrum and superior pole of the glenoid. This biceps labral sulcus may be seen one image posterior to the biceps labral junction in association with the Buford complex or prominent anterior band of the IGL. (**B**) Sagittal T1-weighted MR arthrogram.

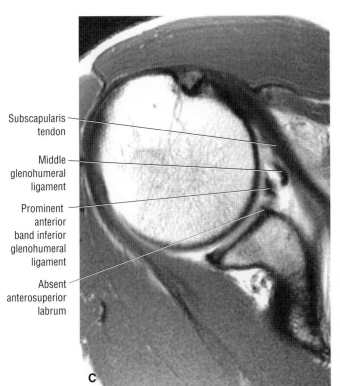

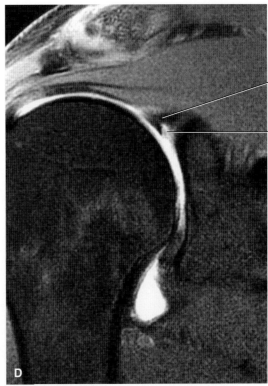

Subscapularis tendon

Middle glenohumeral ligament

Prominent anterior band inferior glenohumeral ligament

Absent anterosuperior labrum

Posterior aspect of biceps labral complex

Biceps labral sulcus maintained on up to one image posterior to intraarticular biceps tendon

FIGURE 8.16 (*Continued*) (**C**) Axial T1-weighted MR arthrogram. (**D**) Coronal FS PD FSE MR arthrogram. Thus the anterosuperior labrum is absent in the presence of either a cord-like MGHL, high attachment of the anterior band, or a combination of both. Also the presence of signal intensity posterior to the biceps anchor as a continuation of the biceps labral sulcus is not necessarily pathologic as shown in this case.

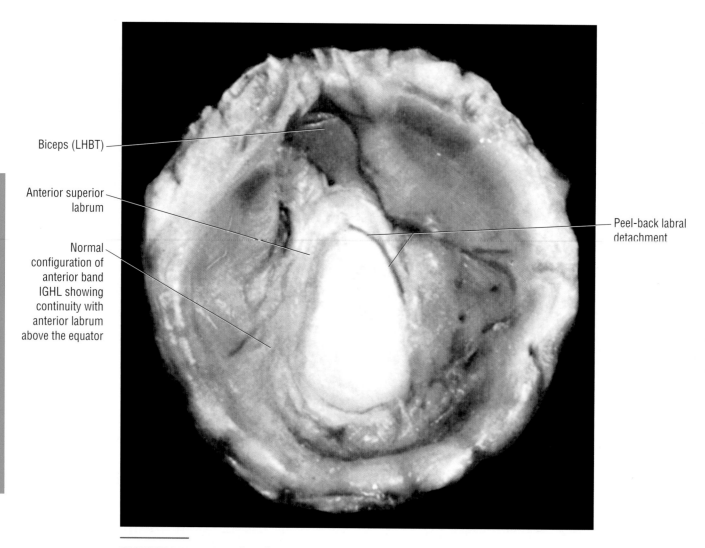

Biceps (LHBT)

Anterior superior labrum

Normal configuration of anterior band IGHL showing continuity with anterior labrum above the equator

Peel-back labral detachment

FIGURE 8.17   Normal configuration of the anterior band showing continuity with the anterior inferior labrum with a well-formed anterior superior labrum. There is no high attachment of the anterior band to the biceps labral complex. There are degenerative changes with peel-back labral detachment posterior to the 12 o'clock position as a separate finding. (Modified from DePalma AF. *Surgery of the Shoulder*. 3rd ed. Philadelphia, PA: JB Lippincott; 1983.) The anterior band contributes and joins the anterior labrum near the equator. This allows for a distinct anterior superior labrum to be appreciated above the equator. In the presence of a high attachment of the anterior band, however the anterosuperior labrum is either attenuated or absent.

High Attachment of the Anterior Band of the IGHL

- A high attachment of the anterior band of the IGHL may be found anterior to the anterior labrum on axial images above the equator.

- Below the equator, the anterior band may appear to be adherent to the anteroinferior labrum and is thus indistinguishable.

- In the presence of a high attachment anterior band, the anterosuperior labrum is either attenuated (hypoplastic) or absent.

- Demonstration of the course of the anterior band deep to the MGHL on corresponding axial images prevents the misdiagnosis of a labral tear.

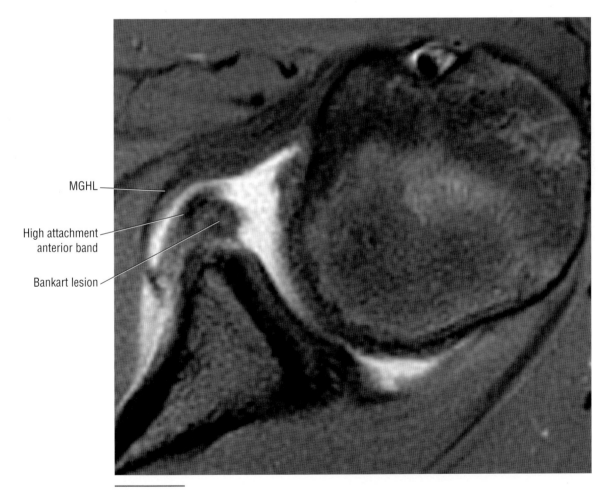

MGHL

High attachment anterior band

Bankart lesion

FIGURE 8.18   High attachment of the anterior band associated with a Bankart lesion. Note the characteristics close relationship of the anterior band applied to the outer surface (periphery) of the anteroinferior labrum. Above the equator, however, a high attachment anterior band will be located more anteriorly so that fluid can be seen along the anterior and posterior surface of the AB.

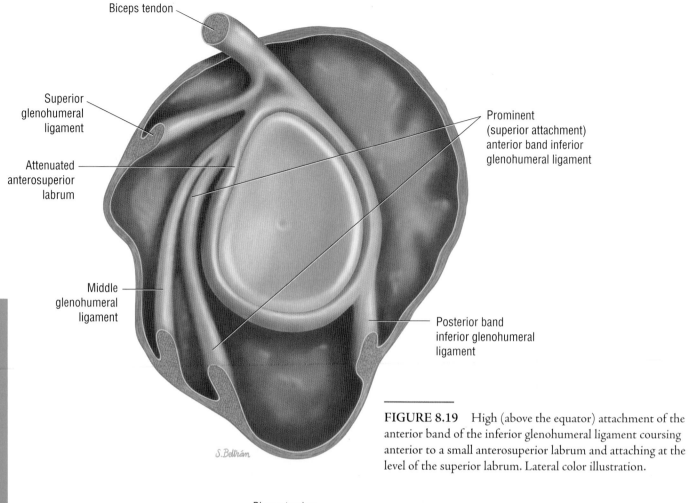

Biceps tendon

Superior glenohumeral ligament

Attenuated anterosuperior labrum

Middle glenohumeral ligament

Prominent (superior attachment) anterior band inferior glenohumeral ligament

Posterior band inferior glenohumeral ligament

S. Beltrán

FIGURE 8.19   High (above the equator) attachment of the anterior band of the inferior glenohumeral ligament coursing anterior to a small anterosuperior labrum and attaching at the level of the superior labrum. Lateral color illustration.

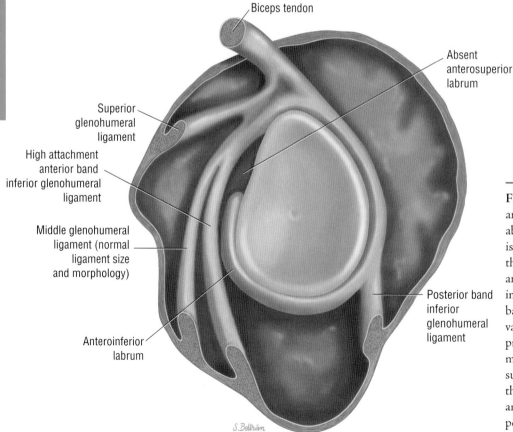

Biceps tendon

Superior glenohumeral ligament

High attachment anterior band inferior glenohumeral ligament

Middle glenohumeral ligament (normal ligament size and morphology)

Anteroinferior labrum

Absent anterosuperior labrum

Posterior band inferior glenohumeral ligament

S. Beltrán

FIGURE 8.20   High attachment anterior band of the IGHL with absent anterosuperior labrum. This is not a Buford complex because the MGL is not cord-like. If the anterosuperior labrum is absent, as in the case of a prominent anterior band, Buford complex, or Buford variant (cord-like MGL plus a prominent anterior band), there may be a normal sulcus between the superior labrum and superior pole of the glenoid. The high insertion of the anterior band and absent anterosuperior labrum effectively creates a sublabral foramen.

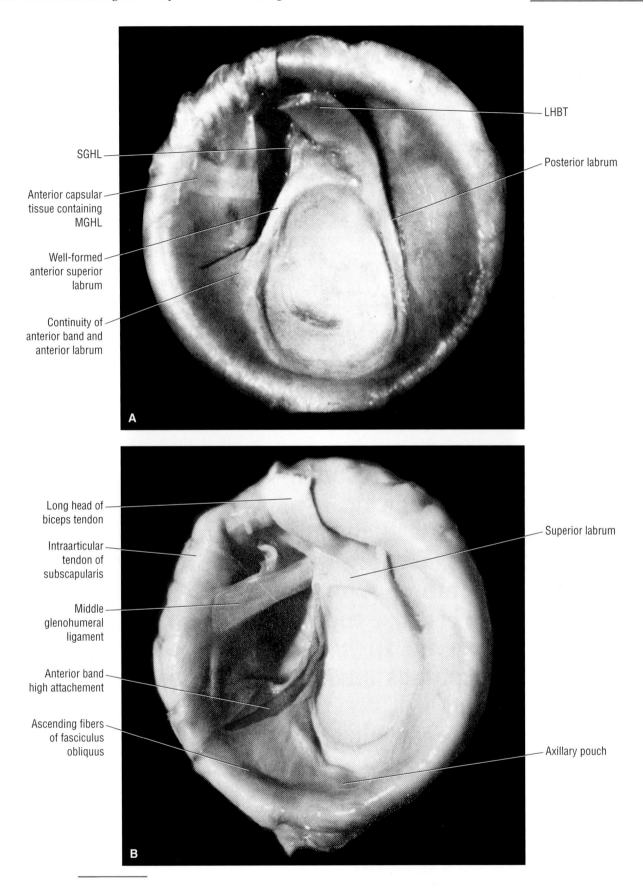

FIGURE 8.21 (**A**) Anterior band contributing to the formation of the anterior superior labrum. Anterior band shows continuity with the labrum at the equator and there is no high attachment of the anterior band to the superior labrum. This explains the normal formation of an anterior labrum in the anterior superior quadrant. (**B**) High attachment of the anterior band with absent anterior superior labrum. Biceps tendon in blue. MGHL in yellow. Anterior band in red. (Modified from DePalma AF. *Surgery of the Shoulder*. 3rd ed. Philadelphia, PA: JB Lippincott; 1983.)

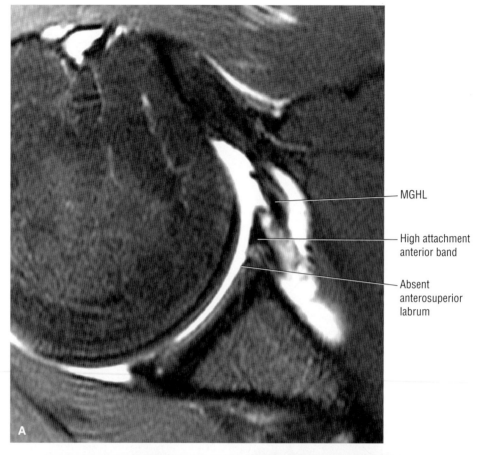

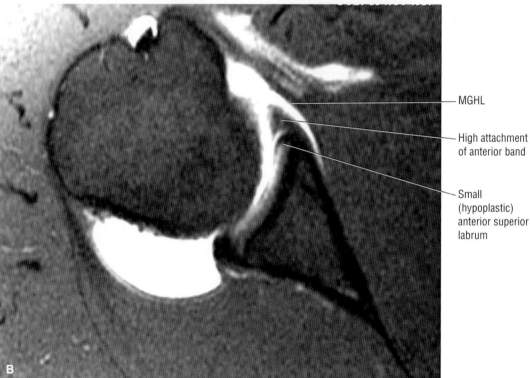

FIGURE 8.22 (**A**) High attachment of the anterior band of the IGL associated with an absent anterior superior labrum as one of two possible associated findings with this variation of the high attachment. The anterior band should not be mistaken for an avulsed labrum since the anterior superior labrum is absent as a normal finding. Axial FS PD. (**B**) In a separate case, high attachment of the anterior band associated with a small or attenuated anterior superior labrum as the second type of associated finding in the presence of a high attachment of the anterior band. It is more common, however, to see an absent anterior superior labrum in the presence of a high attachment anterior band than a small or attenuated anterior superior labrum.

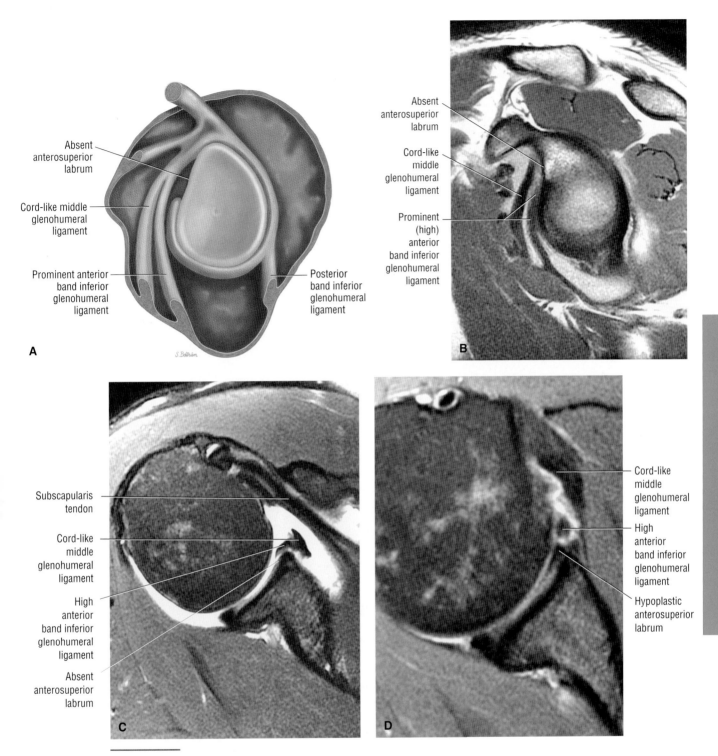

FIGURE 8.23   A high attachment of the anterior band associated with a cord-like MGL and absent anterosuperior labrum on a lateral view color illustration (**A**), a sagittal PD MR arthrogram (**B**), and an axial FS PD FSE MR arthrogram (**C**). Because the MGL is cord-like, this could be considered a Buford variant. The original description of the Buford complex did not include the variant of a high attachment of the anterior band. (**D**) Axial FS PD FSE image in a separate case demonstrating a combination of a cord-like MGL, a prominent anterior band, and hypoplastic anterior labrum.

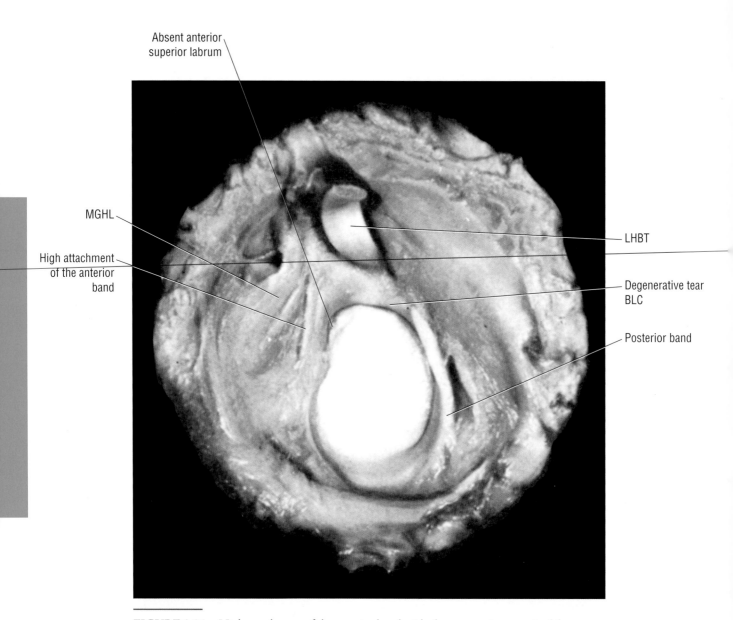

FIGURE 8.24   High attachment of the anterior band with absent anterior superior labrum. (Modified from DePalma AF. *Surgery of the Shoulder*. 3rd ed. Philadelphia, PA: JB Lippincott; 1983.) The absence of the anterosuperior labrum is an anatomical variation which is not associated with instability. The anterior band functions as if it were the anterior labrum in the anterosuperior quadrant. In contrast the inferior labrum is more fibrous and is securely attached to the glenoid rim.

- In the case of a high attachment of the anterior band, the IGHL effectively functions as an anterior labrum and attaches superiorly at the BLC.

- The following variations can exist with a high attachment of the anterior band of the IGHL:

    - High attachment of the anterior band plus a small anterosuperior labrum

    - High attachment of the anterior band plus an absent anterosuperior labrum

    - High attachment of the anterior band plus a cord-like MGHL (associated with an absent or small anterosuperior labrum)

- At arthroscopy, the high attachment of the anterior band is usually interpreted as a sublabral foramen when in fact the anterosuperior labrum is absent.

- The coexistence of a high attachment of the anterior band and a cord-like MGHL could be included as an additional Buford variation if the original description were expanded to include a high attachment of the anterior band associated with an absent anterosuperior labrum and cord-like MGHL.

    - However, referring to the relationship of the anterior band to the anterosuperior glenoid rim as forming a sublabral foramen could lead to confusion since, by definition, there is no sublabral foramen in the Buford complex because the anterior superior labrum is absent.

- A biceps labral sulcus may be seen on one image posterior (in the coronal oblique plane) through the junction of the biceps and labrum in association with either a Buford complex or a prominent (high) anterior band of the IGHL.

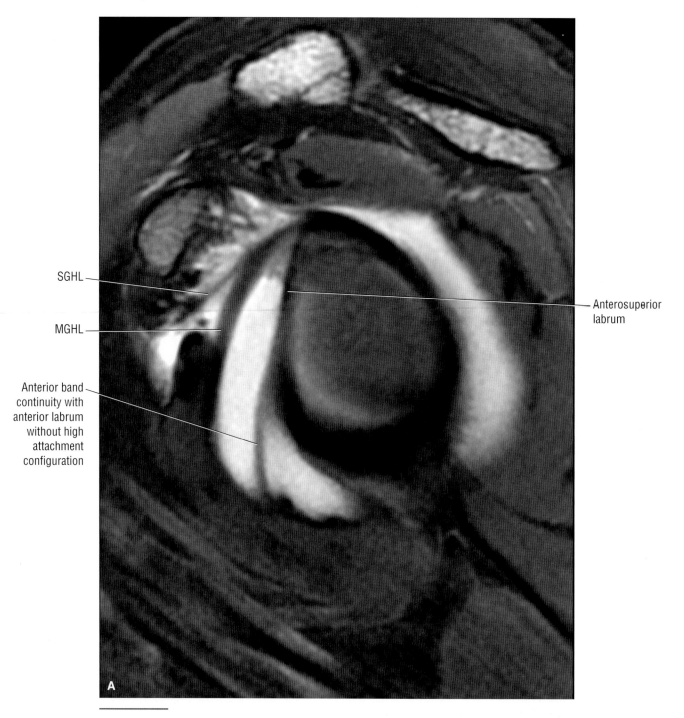

SGHL

MGHL

Anterior band
continuity with
anterior labrum
without high
attachment
configuration

Anterosuperior
labrum

FIGURE 8.25   (**A**) Normal configuration of anterior band and well-formed anterior superior labrum. Sagittal FS PD. The normal anterior band of the inferior glenohumeral ligament attaches to the glenoid at 2 to 4 o'clock in a right shoulder or 8 to 10 o'clock in a left shoulder. The posterior band of the inferior glenohumeral ligament is more difficult to discern than the anterior band. Slight abduction and external rotation of the humerus improves visualization of the posterior band.

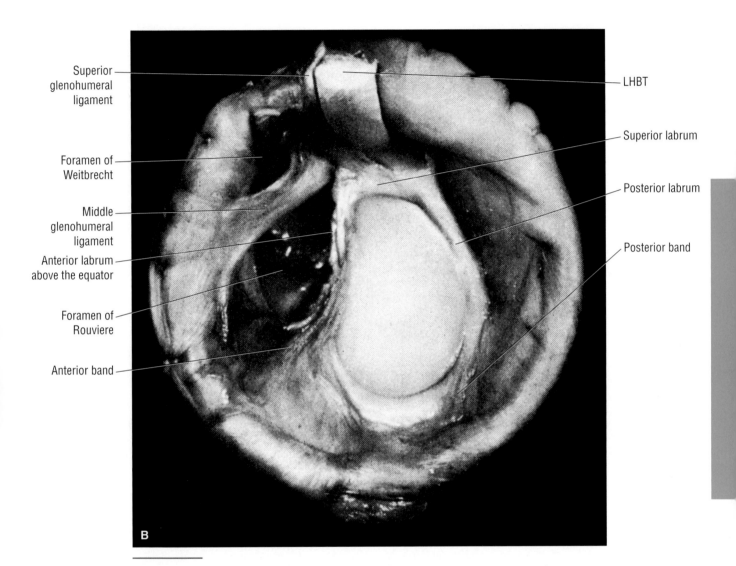

FIGURE 8.25 (*Continued*) (**B**) Normal configuration of the anterior band joining the anterior inferior labrum without a high attachment variation. Thus, the anterior superior labrum is well-formed above the equator. The anterosuperior labrum is designated in yellow. The MGHL also in yellow forms a superior (Foramen of Weitbrecht) and inferior capsular recess (Foramen of Rouviere). The anterior band attaches at the level of equator and does not continue superiorly to the BLC. Without a high attachment of the anterior band, there is no sublabral foramen. (Modified from DePalma AF. *Surgery of the Shoulder*. 3rd ed. Philadelphia, PA: JB Lippincott; 1983.)

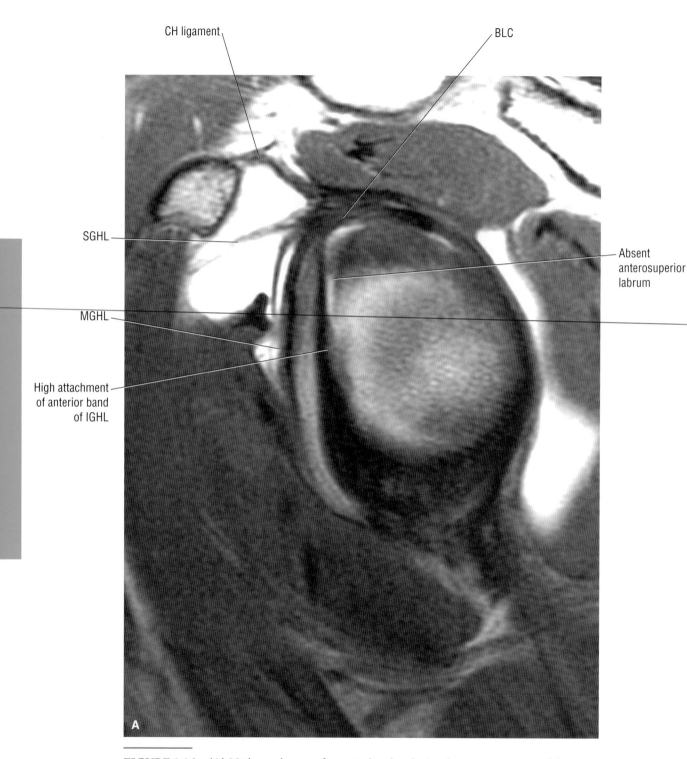

FIGURE 8.26 **(A)** High attachment of anterior band replacing the anterior superior labrum above the equator. The MGHL is parallel and anterior to the high attaching anterior band. Sagittal MR arthrogram.

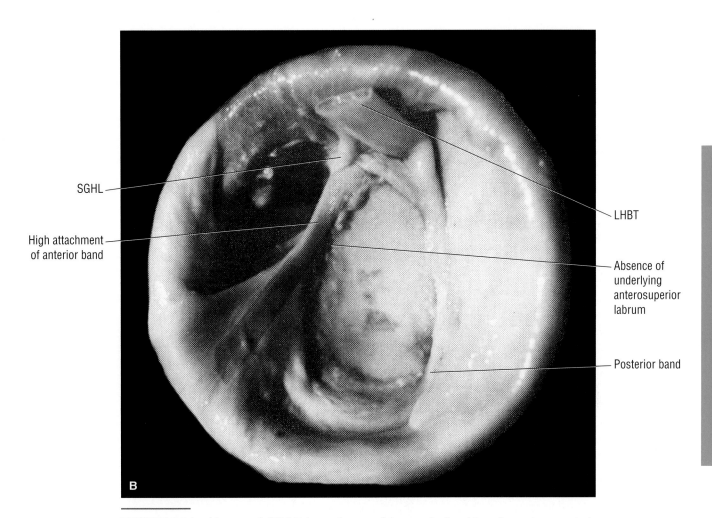

SGHL

High attachment of anterior band

LHBT

Absence of underlying anterosuperior labrum

Posterior band

B

FIGURE 8.26 *(Continued)* (**B**) High attachment of the anterior band in red coursing superiorly to the biceps labral complex with absence of underlying anterior superior labrum. This configuration would appear as a sublabral foramen at arthroscopy. The anterior band (in red) extends superiorly toward the BLC. It is a more common associated finding to have an absent anterosuperior labrum than a hypoplastic or attenuated anterosuperior labrum. (Modified from DePalma AF. *Surgery of the Shoulder*. 3rd ed. Philadelphia, PA: JB Lippincott; 1983.)

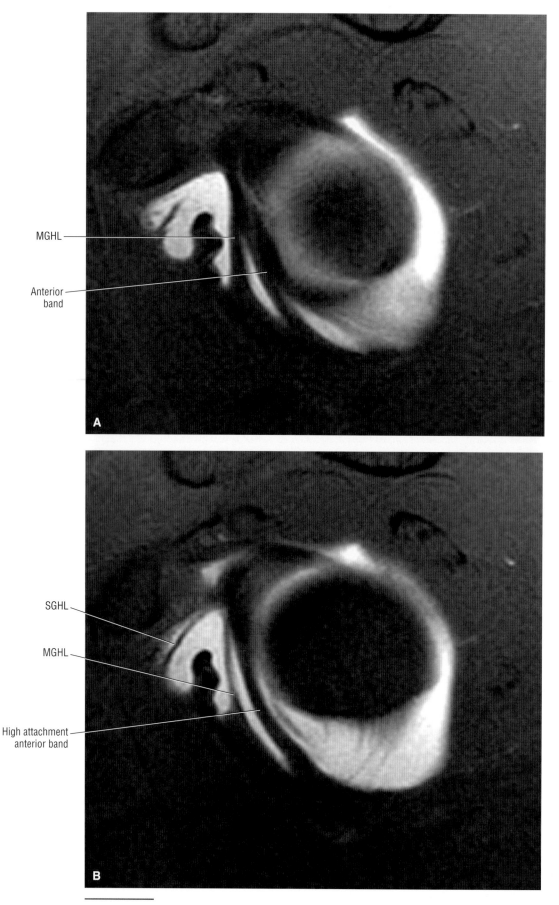

FIGURE 8.27   High attachment of the anterior band on sequential sagittal and axial images. (**A,B**) Sagittal, fat suppressed.

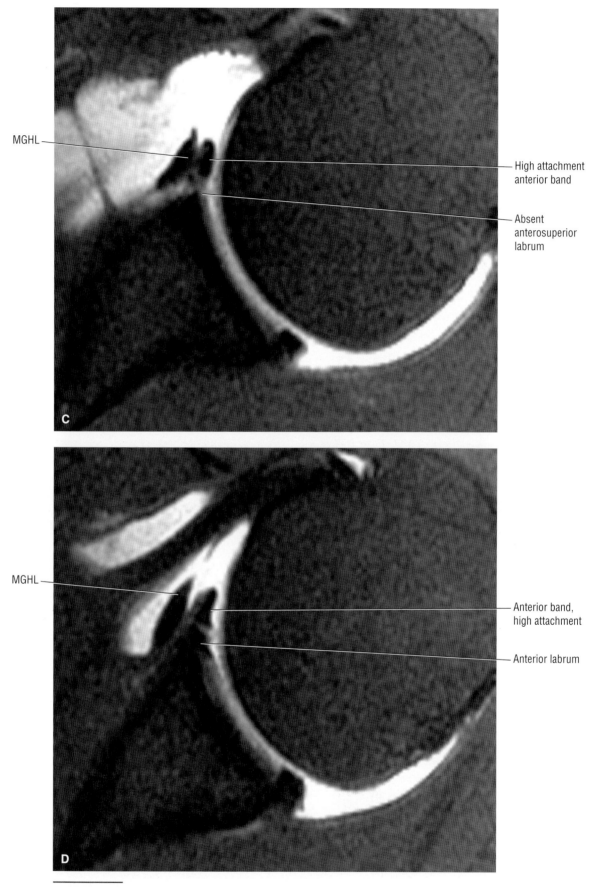

MGHL

High attachment anterior band

Absent anterosuperior labrum

MGHL

Anterior band, high attachment

Anterior labrum

FIGURE 8.27   (*Continued*) (**C,D**) Axial, fat suppressed. The anterior labrum in (**D**) is just below the equator before the AB takes over the role as the functioning anterior labral equivalent above the equator.

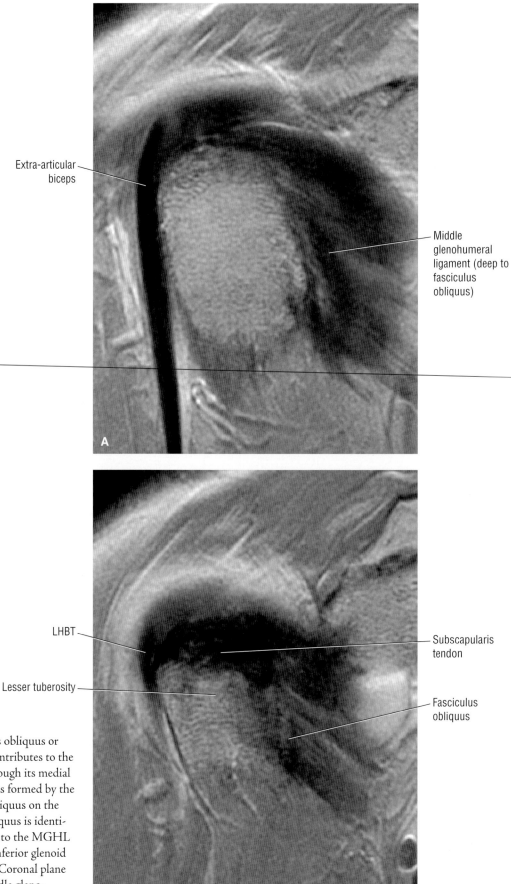

Extra-articular biceps

Middle glenohumeral ligament (deep to fasciculus obliquus)

A

LHBT

Subscapularis tendon

Lesser tuberosity

Fasciculus obliquus

B

FIGURE 8.28 (**A**) Fasciculus obliquus or spiral glenohumeral ligament contributes to the axillary pouch of the IGHL through its medial fibers. Thus, the axillary pouch is formed by the medial part of the fasciculus obliquus on the glenoid side. The fasciculus obliquus is identified on a coronal image anterior to the MGHL and extends from the anterior inferior glenoid rim to the lesser tuberosity. (**B**) Coronal plane identifying the plane of the middle glenohumeral ligament posterior to the fasciculus obliquus.

Superior Labral Tears as a Subtype of Labral Pathology

- The labrum can be arbitrarily divided into six areas:[635]

    - The superior labrum

    - The anterosuperior (superior to the mid-glenoid notch) labrum

    - The anteroinferior labrum

    - The inferior labrum

    - The posteroinferior labrum

    - The posterosuperior labrum

- Labral tear patterns may be:[635]

    - Degenerative lesions

    - Flap tears

    - Vertical split nondetached tears

    - Bucket-handle tears

    - SLAP lesions

Degenerative Labrum

- Degenerative lesions show fraying of the labrum, probably as part of the spectrum of degenerative glenohumeral joint disease.[136,137]

- The degenerative roughened labrum may contribute to the process of joint degeneration by creating an abrasive articular interface in addition to humeral head chondromalacia.

- Osseous findings of the glenoid fossa

    - Glenoid sclerosis (hypointense signal)

    - Glenoid rim spurring

    - Subchondral cystic change glenoid fossa central to posterior

Flap Tears

- Flap tears represent a frequent labral tear pattern in acute or subacute injuries.[635]

- Occur in any location but are frequently identified in the posterosuperior segment of the labrum

- Occur secondary to chronic shear stress,[512] as seen in repetitive subluxation in throwing or overhead athletes

- An unstable flap tear may cause mechanical symptoms of joint clicking, catching, and popping and mimic instability.

Vertical Split and Bucket-Handle Labral Tears

- Vertical split labral tears are the least frequent labral tear pattern.[635] A complete vertical split labrum may be associated with a displaceable fragment and presents as a bucket-handle tear.

- A vertical split labrum is seen in the meniscoid-type labrum, which is most commonly observed in the superior quadrant.

- A type 3 SLAP lesion is a bucket-handle tear of the superior labrum (see SLAP Tears in the following discussion).

- Although a vertical split may occur in the anterior and posterior labrum, this tear pattern is unusual in the inferior labrum.

- The mechanism of injury is thought to be intraarticular compression from a fall on the outstretched arm or extensive humeral rotation associated with anterior or posterior labral compression.

- Symptoms include pseudosubluxation with locking, catching, and popping. Associated clinical instability, however, is uncommon in this lesion.

- Treatment is directed at producing a stable labral rim by excision or repair of the tear.

Superior Labral Tears

- Anterosuperior labral tears with avulsion and fraying of the labrum have been described in throwing athletes.[13]

- There may be involvement of the biceps and associated partial rotator cuff tears.

- Traction by the LHBT on the anterosuperior labrum occurs during the deceleration phase of throwing.

- Treatment is arthroscopic débridement of the frayed labrum, cuff, and biceps tendon.

- The biceps root should be perceived as stable to palpitation with a hook probe at arthroscopy.

- The tactile feedback is that the biceps fibers are anchored to the glenoid medial to the superior labrum.

Triple Labral Lesions

- Triple labral lesions refer to the association of an anterior and posterior labral tear with an associated superior tear at the biceps labral complex.

  - Anterior labral tear

    - 2 o'clock to 6 o'clock (10 o'clock to 6 o'clock for left shoulder)

  - Posterior labral tear

    - 6 o'clock to 10 o'clock (6 o'clock to 2 o'clock for left shoulder)

  - Superior labral tear (SLAP lesions)

    - 10 o'clock to 2 o'clock

  - Triple labral lesion represents a complex tear as there is circumferential labral damage.

  - Triple labral lesions have recurrent instability history with multiple instability events following trauma.

    - In contrast to isolated Bankart lesions, patients with triple labral lesions have chronic pain and discomfort between instability events.

Superior Labral Lesions Relative to the Biceps Labral Sulcus and Biceps Root

- MR evaluation of SLAP lesions should be performed only in the coronal plane.
  - Always establish normal morphology of the superior labrum in the 12 o'clock position and then the peel-back area before evaluating anterosuperior labral extension.
  - The biceps labral sulcus can be mistaken for a SLAP 2 lesion in the axial plane.
- The biceps root and anchor are terms used to describe the relationship between the BLC and the attachment of the intraarticular biceps to the superior labrum and supraglenoid tubercle.
  - At arthroscopy, it is important to evaluate the solidity of the root of the biceps tendon at its anchor point at the supraglenoid tubercle.
    - The anchor to the supraglenoid tubercle is usually located 5mm medial to the edge of the glenoid.[559]
- High-performance baseball players have one or more of the following three surgical lesions:
  - SLAP requiring suture anchor repair
  - Glenohumeral internal rotation defect (GIRD) of >40° requiring posterior capsular release
  - Hyperexternal rotation >130°
    - Throwers internal impingement contact point
- Dead arm syndrome inability to throw hard
  - O'Driscoll's sign
  - O'Brien's sign
- SLAP Arthroscopic Diagnosis (require three of these five)
  - Drive-through sign
  - Superior biceps labral sulcus >5mm
  - Bare sulcus footprint
  - Displaceable biceps root
  - Positive peel-back sign
- Drive-through sign
  - Posterior portal

- ▦ Arthroscopic driven from superior glenohumeral joint to axillary recess with minimal resistance
- ▦ Indicative of the pseudolaxity that may occur with SLAP lesions

- ■ If biceps labral sulcus is >5mm, there is increased exposed bone or a bore sulcus footprint associated with detachment of the superior labrum from superior pole.

- ■ A normal sulcus is associated with articular cartilage covering the superior pole of the glenoid.

  - ▦ Superior labral tears that involve the glenoid side of the superior labrum especially in the 12 o'clock position may be associated with chondral degeneration of the superior pole of the glenoid.

  - ▦ In a SLAP repair (SLAP 2 for example), the articular cartilage of the superior pole of the glenoid is sacrificed in order to develop a bleeding bone surface to facilitate labral fixation. This is one of the reasons why débridement and not labral fixation is becoming more popular when appropriate when treating SLAP lesions.

- ■ A bare footprint with exposed bone indicates attachment of the superior labrum.

- ■ Positive peel-back sign in overhead athletes from disruption of the biceps root detachment into the bone

  - ▦ Arm placed into external rotation creates torsional force from the biceps leading to peel-back.

- ■ Superior labral detachment may affect the stability of the root resulting in a displaceable biceps root that is easily translated medially with a probe.

- ■ Dynamic stability of the superior labrum and biceps root

  - ▦ Evaluated with arm in functional throwing position of 90° of abduction and full external rotation

- ■ When the superior labrum is torn, there is further increased torsional force as created by the twisting motion of abduction and external rotation of the biceps tendon transmitted to the biceps root attachment to the superior pole of the glenoid. This mechanism contributes to the medial displacement of the biceps root and the posterosuperior labrum in SLAP lesions.

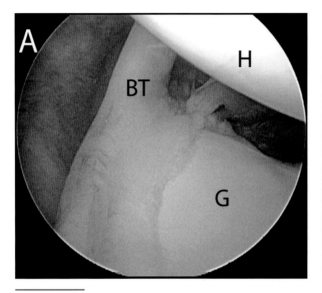
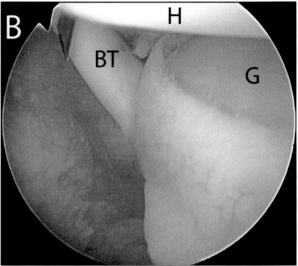

FIGURE 8.29   Right shoulder, posterior viewing portal, demonstrates a positive peel-back sign (**A**) prior to peel-back maneuver. (**B**) Peel-back maneuver results in medial displacement of the superior labrum and biceps root. BT, biceps tendon; G, glenoid; H, humerus. (Reprinted from Burkhart S, Lo IK, Brady PC, Denard PJ. *The Cowboy's Companion: A Trail Guide for the Arthroscopic Shoulder Surgeon*. Philadelphia, PA: Lippincott Williams & Wilkins; 2012, with permission.)

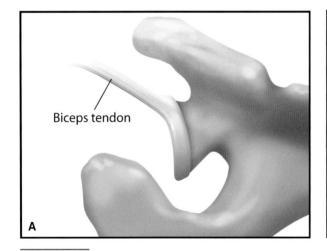
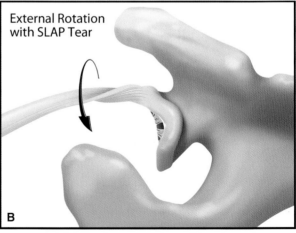

FIGURE 8.30   Schematic of the peel-back maneuver for demonstration of a superior labrum anterior and posterior (SLAP) tear. (**A**) Appearance of the biceps root with the arm at the side. (**B**) Placing the arm in 90° of abduction and maximal external rotation creates a torsional force on the biceps root. In the setting of a SLAP tear, the biceps root and the labrum just posterior to the biceps root displace medially during this maneuver. (Reprinted from Burkhart S, Lo IK, Brady PC, Denard PJ. *The Cowboy's Companion: A Trail Guide for the Arthroscopic Shoulder Surgeon*. Philadelphia, PA: Lippincott Williams & Wilkins; 2012, with permission.)

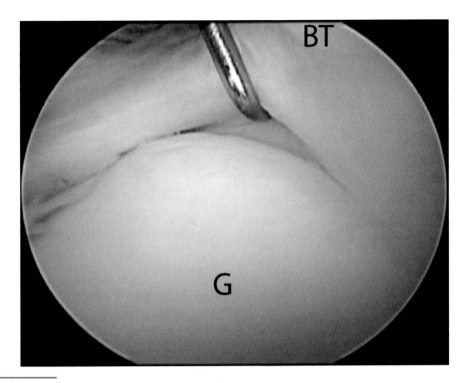

FIGURE 8.31 Left shoulder, posterior viewing portal, demonstrates a normal superior labral recess. The articular cartilage normally extends 2 to 3 mm medial to the superior glenoid. BT, biceps tendon; G, glenoid. (Reprinted from Burkhart S, Lo IK, Brady PC, Denard PJ. *The Cowboy's Companion: A Trail Guide for the Arthroscopic Shoulder Surgeon*. Philadelphia, PA: Lippincott Williams & Wilkins; 2012, with permission.)

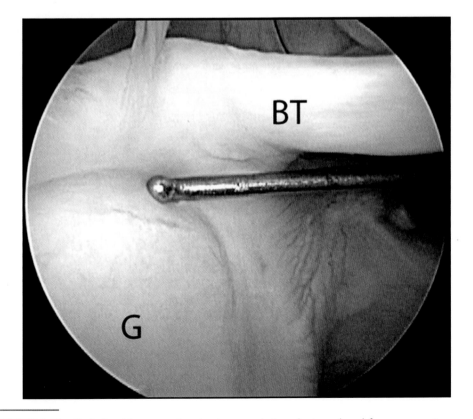

FIGURE 8.32 Left shoulder, posterior viewing portal. A probe introduced from an anterior working portal demonstrates a stable biceps root. BT, biceps tendon; G, glenoid. (Reprinted from Burkhart S, Lo IK, Brady PC, Denard PJ. *The Cowboy's Companion: A Trail Guide for the Arthroscopic Shoulder Surgeon*. Philadelphia, PA: Lippincott Williams & Wilkins; 2012, with permission.)

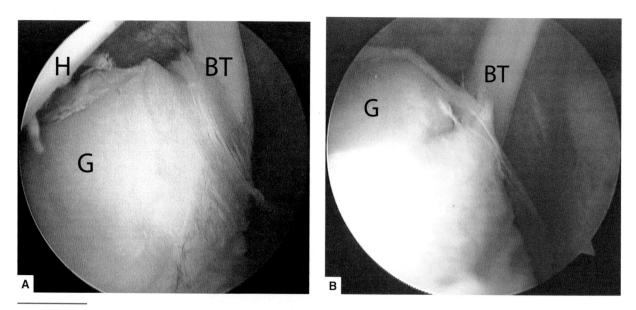

FIGURE 8.33   Peel-back maneuver (**A**) Left shoulder, posterior viewing portal, demonstrates appearance of the biceps root with the arm at the side. (**B**) Same shoulder demonstrates a positive peel-back whereby the biceps root displaces medial to the glenoid rim when the arm is placed in 90° of abduction and maximal external rotation. BT, biceps tendon; G, glenoid; I I, humerus. (Reprinted from Burkhart S, Lo IK, Brady PC, Denard PJ. *The Cowboy's Companion: A Trail Guide for the Arthroscopic Shoulder Surgeon.* Philadelphia, PA: Lippincott Williams & Wilkins; 2012, with permission.)

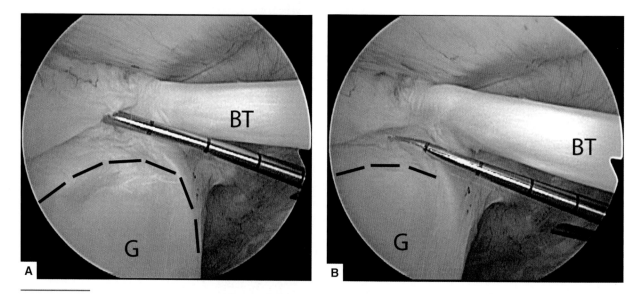

FIGURE 8.34   (**A,B**) Right shoulder, posterior glenohumeral viewing portal, demonstrates a displaceable biceps root. The *dashed black lines* outline the glenoid rim. BT, biceps tendon; G, glenoid. (Reprinted from Burkhart S, Lo IK, Brady PC, Denard PJ. *The Cowboy's Companion: A Trail Guide for the Arthroscopic Shoulder Surgeon.* Philadelphia, PA: Lippincott Williams & Wilkins; 2012, with permission.)

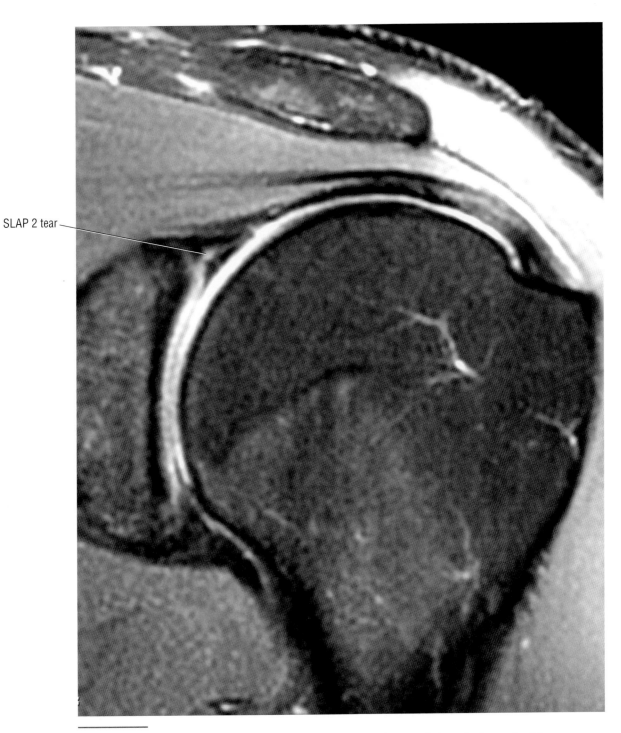

SLAP 2 tear

FIGURE 8.35   SLAP 2 lesion with linear hyperintense signal oriented along the long axis of the superior labrum in the 12 o'clock position. A SLAP lesion may be present, however, without intralabral signal if the labrum is fragmented or displaced from the biceps tendon or has a missing side. Coronal FS PD FSE. If the superior labrum were displaced inferiorly a SLAP 3 pattern would be formed.

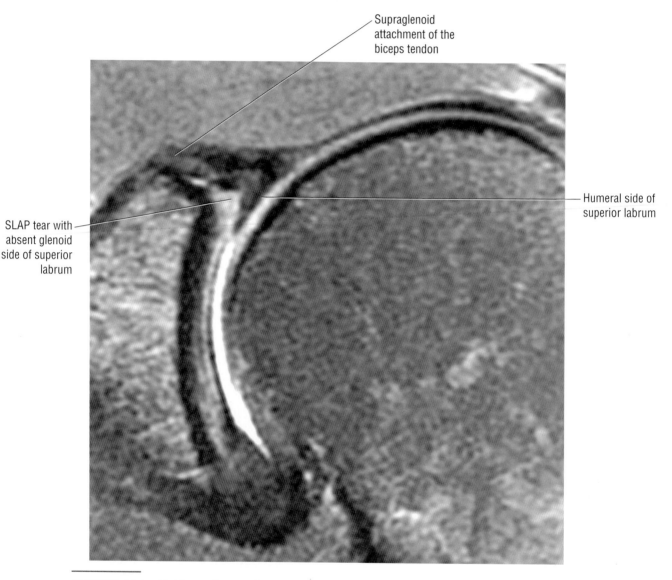

Supraglenoid
attachment of the
biceps tendon

Humeral side of
superior labrum

SLAP tear with
absent glenoid
side of superior
labrum

FIGURE 8.36   SLAP tear (SLAP 2) superior labrum in the 12 o'clock position of the BLC with absent superior labral tissue on the glenoid side of the superior labrum. Thus, it is possible to have a SLAP lesion with abnormal morphology of the superior labrum without the presence of discrete linear or hyperintense signal. Coronal FS PD FSE. In the 12 o'clock position, the superior labrum should have an isosceles triangle morphology. Posterior to the 12 o'clock location (in the peel-back area of the BLC). The posterosuperior labrum is permitted to have a more asymmetric scalene morphology.

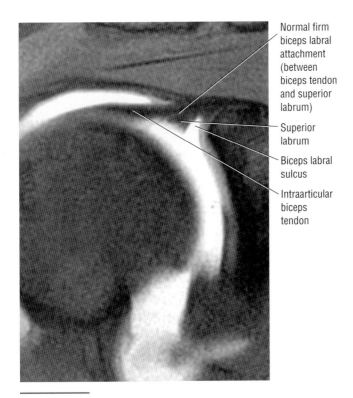

Normal firm biceps labral attachment (between biceps tendon and superior labrum)

Superior labrum

Biceps labral sulcus

Intraarticular biceps tendon

FIGURE 8.37 Coronal FS PD FSE image showing a normal biceps labral sulcus. The medial to lateral measurement is 2.5mm with the shoulder positioned in neutral to external rotation.

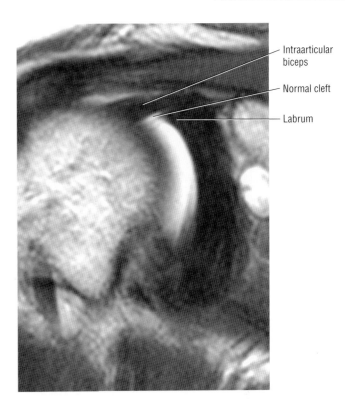

Intraarticular biceps

Normal cleft

Labrum

FIGURE 8.38 Coronal PD FSE MR arthrogram displays the normal cleft between the intraarticular biceps and the superior labrum anterior to the 12 o'clock position of the biceps labral complex.

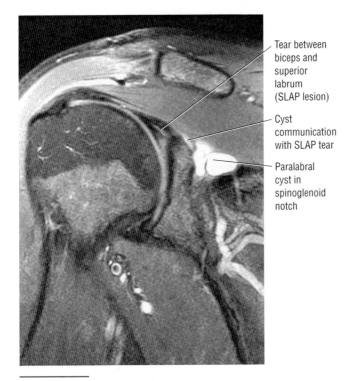

Tear between biceps and superior labrum (SLAP lesion)

Cyst communication with SLAP tear

Paralabral cyst in spinoglenoid notch

FIGURE 8.39 Linear signal between the intra-articular biceps and superior labrum is abnormal if visualized on a coronal oblique image posterior to an established firm attachment between the superior labrum and biceps tendon. Linear hyperintensity can be seen between the biceps tendon and superior labrum, representing posterior extension of the SLAP tear.

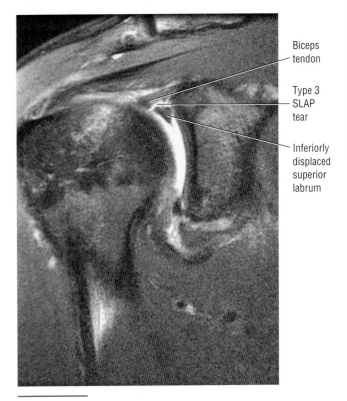

Biceps tendon

Type 3 SLAP tear

Inferiorly displaced superior labrum

FIGURE 8.40 Coronal FS PD FSE image showing inferior displacement (relative to the biceps anchor) of the superior labrum in a type 3 SLAP lesion with bucket-handle morphology.

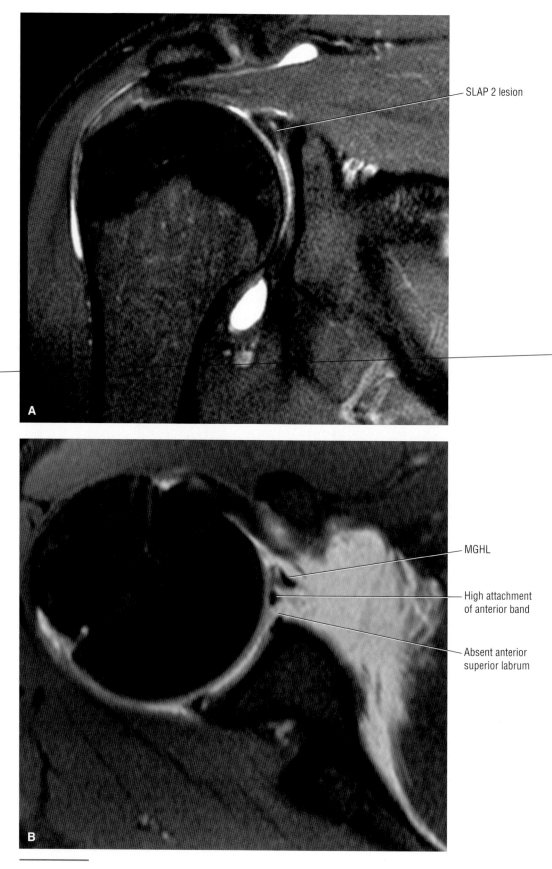

FIGURE 8.41   SLAP 2 tear superior labrum just posterior to the 12 o'clock position in association with a high attachment of the anterior band of the inferior glenohumeral ligament. The diagnosis of a SLAP lesion should only be made off coronal images and not from axial images. In this case, the absence of the anterior superior labrum in the axial plane is a normal finding. (**A**) Coronal FS PD FSE. (**B**) Axial FS PD FSE.

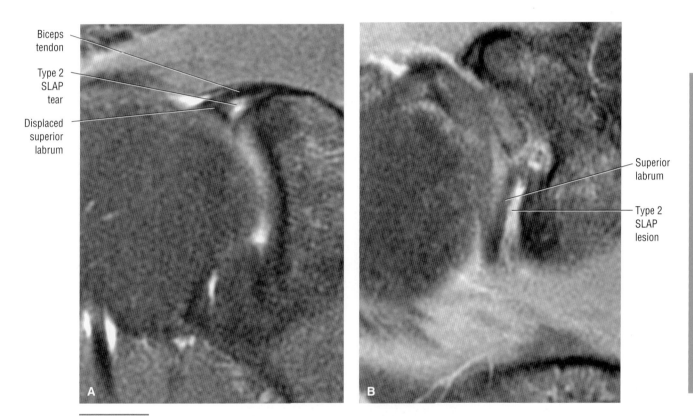

FIGURE 8.42   (**A**) Coronal FS PD FSE and (**B**) axial FS PD FSE images show an avulsed superior labrum from the superior pole of the glenoid. The chemical shift artifact of the superior pole articular cartilage may be mistaken for a small labral fragment. Even though the SLAP tear is evident in both coronal and axial planes, greater specificity is obtained if diagnostic interpretation is restricted to coronal images to avoid mistaking a BLC sulcus for a SLAP lesion.

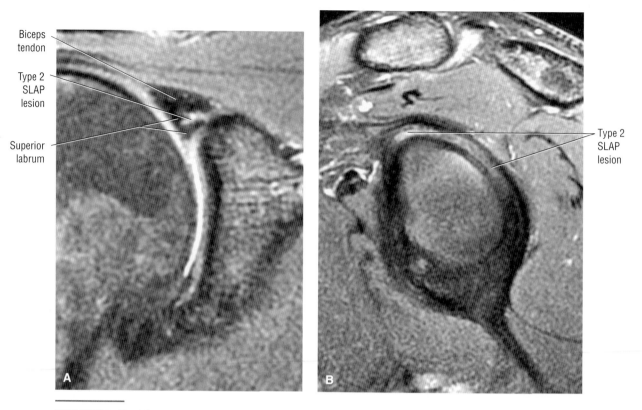

FIGURE 8.43   Eccentric superior labral tear with type 2 SLAP lesion occurring adjacent to the glenoid on (**A**) a coronal FS PD FSE image and (**B**) a sagittal FS PD FSE image.

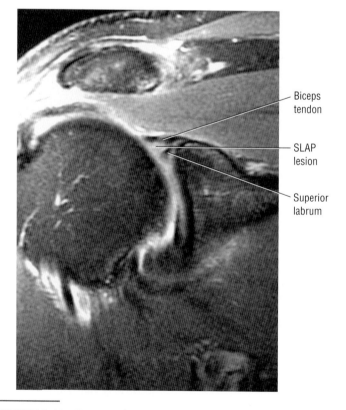

FIGURE 8.44   Eccentric humeral side SLAP tear. If a fragment of the superior labrum is absent or displaced, a type 3 SLAP lesion should be considered. Coronal FS PD FSE image.

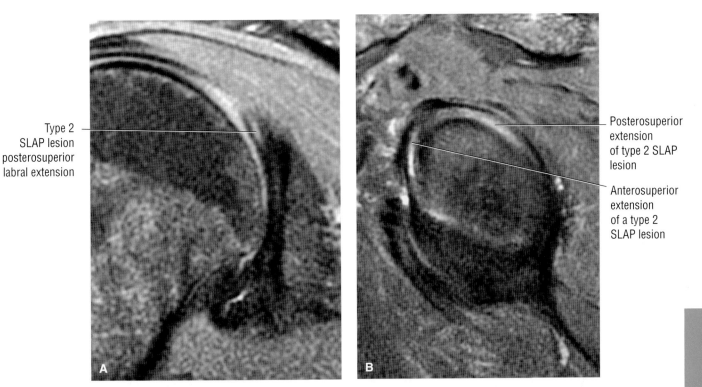

FIGURE 8.45 (**A**) Coronal FS PD FSE image shows characteristic SLAP 2 linear oblique signal intensity of the posterior superior labrum posterior to the biceps anchor attachment to the superior labrum. (**B**) Corresponding sagittal FS PD FSE image.

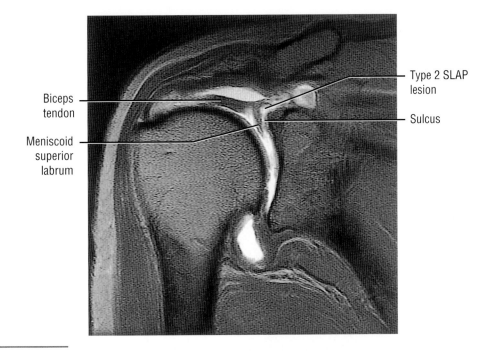

FIGURE 8.46 Coronal T1-weighted MR arthrogram of superior displacement of the biceps anchor and superior labrum (a type 2 SLAP lesion). This may be a difficult MR pattern to distinguish from a normal biceps labral sulcus. Correlation with sagittal images confirms superior displacement of the labrum.

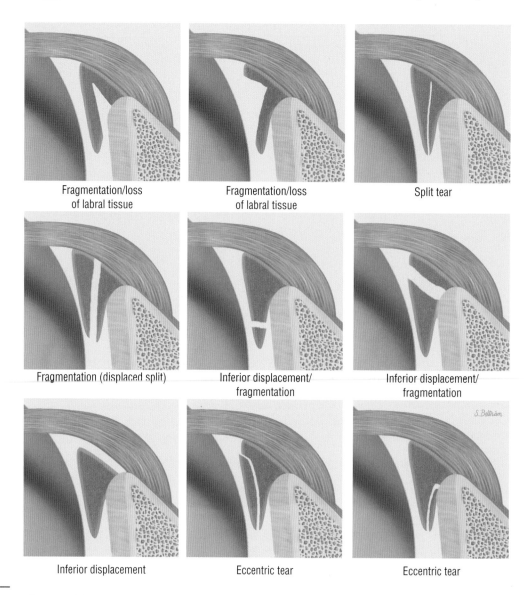

Fragmentation/loss of labral tissue

Fragmentation/loss of labral tissue

Split tear

Fragmentation (displaced split)

Inferior displacement/ fragmentation

Inferior displacement/ fragmentation

Inferior displacement

Eccentric tear

Eccentric tear

FIGURE 8.47   Common SLAP tear variants include labral fragmentation, vertical split, inferior displacement, and eccentric tears (humeral or glenoid side). A fragmented labrum with gross displacement or absence of labral tissue is associated with bucket-handle morphology. A split of the labrum into separated triangles (double triangle sign) is associated also with a bucket-handle tear pattern. Inferior displacement of the entire superior labrum or a portion of the labrum indicates displacement of a bucket-handle tear. Linear signal without loss of labral tissue or labral displacement/fragmentation is associated with SLAP 2 lesions. There also may be complete superior labral separation from the superior pole with a widened biceps labral sulcus.

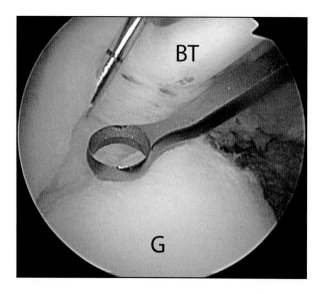

FIGURE 8.48   Right shoulder posterior viewing portal. Preparation of bone bed for SLAP repair is accomplished with a ring curette and subsequent use of a shaver to expose an adequate bone bed for healing. BT, biceps tendon; G, glenoid. (Reprinted from Burkhart S, Lo IK, Brady PC, Denard PJ. *The Cowboy's Companion: A Trail Guide for the Arthroscopic Shoulder Surgeon.* Philadelphia, PA: Lippincott Williams & Wilkins; 2012, with permission.)

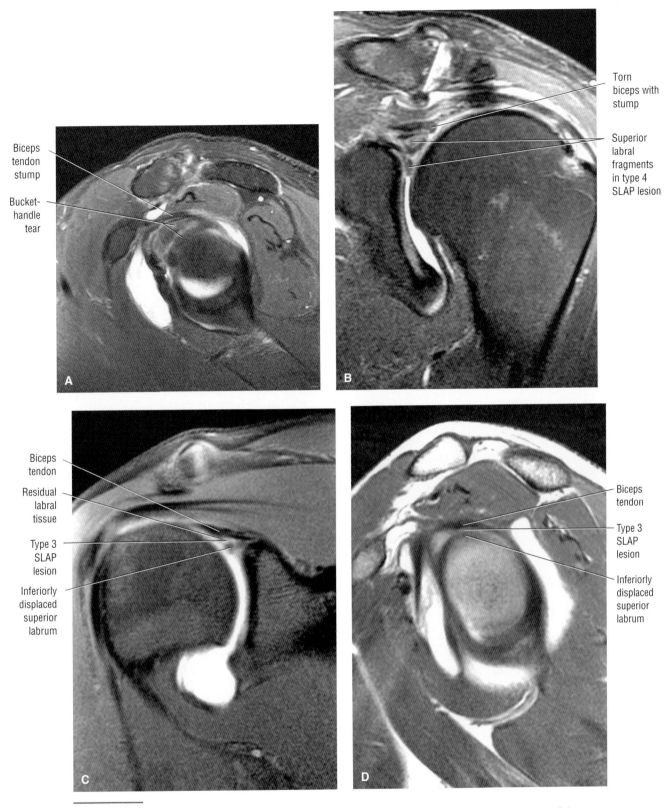

FIGURE 8.49 Type 4 SLAP lesion with the torn biceps stump superior to the two components of the fragmented labrum on (**A**) a sagittal FS PD FSE image and (**B**) a coronal FS PD FSE image. In a separate case, a type 3 SLAP bucket-handle tear with an intact biceps tendon and a separate inferiorly displaced labral fragment is visualized on a coronal FS T1-weighted MR arthrogram (**C**) and a sagittal T1-weighted MR arthrogram (**D**).

SLAP Tears

Key Concepts

- A biceps labral sulcus greater than 5mm is abnormal.

- Superior paralabral cysts that often extend into the spinoglenoid notch communicate with SLAP 2 or posterior SLAP 2 (peel-back) lesions.

- Inferior displacement of the superior labrum (relative to the biceps labral junction) is associated with bucket-handle SLAP morphology.

- SLAP tears are grouped into 10 subtypes. Four primary types were initially described and six further types were subsequently characterized.

- The SLAP 2 or classic SLAP lesion is further subdivided into anterior SLAP 2 in the SLAC lesion and posterior SLAP 2 in the posterior peel-back lesion.

- SLAP fracture is a posterosuperior medial humeral head chondral fracture in association with a SLAP lesion.

- Snyder et al.[548] have described SLAP (superior labrum from anterior to posterior, relative to the biceps tendon anchor) lesions, which vary from simple fraying and fragmentation of the BLC, to a bucket-handle tear, to a tricorn bucket-handle tear in which one rim of the tear actually extends up into the biceps tendon, splitting it as the tear goes up toward the bicipital groove.

- One mechanism of injury is a fall on the outstretched abducted arm with associated superior joint compression and a proximal subluxation force.[284,635]

- Another mechanism is sudden contraction of the biceps tendon that avulses the superior labrum.

- Repetitive stress acting through the biceps tendon may also produce SLAP lesions, as may instability of the glenohumeral joint.

- The normal biceps labral sulcus should not be mistaken for a SLAP lesion.

  - This sulcus may become more prominent in external rotation of the arm.

Guidelines for SLAP Tear Detection

- A biceps labral sulcus measurement of less than 5mm is within a normal range, although the biceps labral sulcus is most commonly less than 3mm on coronal MR images.

    - Inappropriate repair of a normal sulcus may severely restrict motion at the BLC and superior labrum

    - A sulcus of greater than 5mm is abnormal.[558]

    - Since the free edge of the superior labrum is variable in its attachment to the articular cartilage, the BLC should be assessed as either a type 1, 2, or 3.

        - A biceps labral sulcus should not be interpreted as a labral detachment even if present in a younger patient. Signs of labral damage or superior pole chondral pathology should be identified if there is associated pathology of the superior labrum.

        - The biceps labral sulcus may become more prominent or deeper with respect to the superior labrum in the older patient as the BLC becomes more mobile and the superior labrum separates from the underlying articular cartilage of the superior pole of the glenoid.[559]

- On review of coronal oblique images, there should not be hyperintense signal intensity located between the intraarticular biceps tendon and the superior labrum.

- There is frequently a normal lateral oblique cleft of fluid signal intensity between the biceps tendon and the superior labrum anterior to the biceps labral junction.

    - A firmly attached connection between the intraarticular biceps and the superior labrum prevents increased signal intensity between the biceps tendon and the superior labrum.

- A paralabral cyst adjacent to the superior labrum usually communicates with a classic SLAP 2 or the posterior component of a SLAP 2 lesion.

- Inferior displacement of the superior labrum separated from its biceps connection is always associated with bucket-handle SLAP morphology.

- Fragmentation or splitting of the superior labrum into separate fragments is associated with bucket-handle SLAP tear patterns.
    - This SLAP tear pattern should not be mistaken for the normal biceps labral sulcus.
    - Avulsion of the superior labrum from the superior pole of the glenoid will result in an enlarged biceps labral sulcus.
        - Identify frayed, torn, and irregular tissue below the superior labrum. A blood clot or reactive granulation tissue is often associated with an avulsion injury.

- SLAP tears occur either centrally or eccentrically with the superior labrum at the biceps labral junction. Eccentric tears are located adjacent to either the glenoid or humerus.

- SLAP tears are usually parallel to the long axis of the posterosuperior labrum posterior to the biceps tendon.[599]

- Superior displacement of the biceps labral complex relative to the superior pole of the glenoid on sagittal images is associated with SLAP 2 lesions.

- Common patterns of SLAP tears demonstrate a spectrum of lesions from detachment at the biceps labral junction to splitting and fragmentation of the labrum.

- A SLAP tear occurs commonly in one of three locations:
    - Between the biceps tendon and the superior labrum
    - Within the superior labrum
    - Between the superior labrum and the superior pole of the glenoid

- Visualization of three distinct hypointense structures (the biceps tendon and the split superior labrum) on sagittal images through the BLC correlates with bucket-handle morphology.

- Complex or extended SLAP lesions (SLAP 5 through SLAP 10) may be associated with SLAP 2 or SLAP 3 lesions.

- A biceps labral sulcus may be seen one image posterior to the biceps labral junction in association with the Buford complex or prominent (high) anterior band of the IGHL.

- In throwers, SLAP lesions characteristically demonstrate a positive peel-back sign.

- The biceps root shifts medially in the combined motion of abduction and external rotation (90° of abduction and maximal external rotation).

- In contrast, in nonthrowers, SLAP lesions usually do not display a positive peel-back sign, but the biceps root is displaceable.

- With an intact superior labrum:

  - The biceps root and superior labrum remain centered on the superior pole of the glenoid.

  - The intraarticular biceps will only change its angular position (at arthroscopy) relative to the superior labrum with superior labral tears especially those that extend to the posterior superior labrum.

    - The torsional force from the biceps tendon lifts the superior labrum off the glenoid, displacing the labrum medially off the glenoid rim (peel-back sign).

    - In the overhead athlete with a positive peel-back sign, there is posterosuperior labral disruption and some degree of disruption of the biceps root attachment to the superior pole of the glenoid.[75,559]

Classification of SLAP Tears

- Type 1 SLAP lesions[622]

  - Characterized by a frayed and degenerative superior labrum with a normal (stable) biceps tendon anchor

- Type 2 SLAP lesions

  - Have similar labral fraying but also have detachment of the superior labrum and biceps anchor, making them unstable

  - May appear similar to the normal free edge of the meniscoid-like superior labrum

    - However, the articular cartilage of the superior glenoid extends to the attachment of the labrum.

  - There is usually a space or gap between the glenoid articular cartilage and the attachment of the superior labrum and biceps anchor.

  - Displacement of the labrum from the superior glenoid of more than 3 to 4mm is usually associated with an abnormal superior labrum and biceps anchor attachment.

  - May also be associated with anterior glenohumeral joint dislocation

- Tearing of the superior labrum biceps anchor may contribute to anteroinferior instability.
- Subdivided into anterior and posterior SLAP 2 lesions:
  - The anterior SLAP 2 lesion (anterior component of a SLAP 2 lesion) is associated with an anterior supraspinatus articular-side partial cuff tear in the SLAC (superior labrum anterior cuff) lesion.
  - The posterior SLAP 2 lesion (posterosuperior labral tear) is the posterior peel-back lesion in the throwing athlete.
- In SLAP tear assessment, identify an irregular or indistinct border to the superior labrum on either the humeral or glenoid side in the 12 o'clock location.
- The lateral signal direction sign may only be of help in diagnosing SLAP tears if intralabral signal is present.
  - Superior labral tears may exist with abnormal morphology without any increase in intralabral signal. This is possible because of inferior displacement of the labrum or absence of a portion or segment of labral tissue.[75,559]

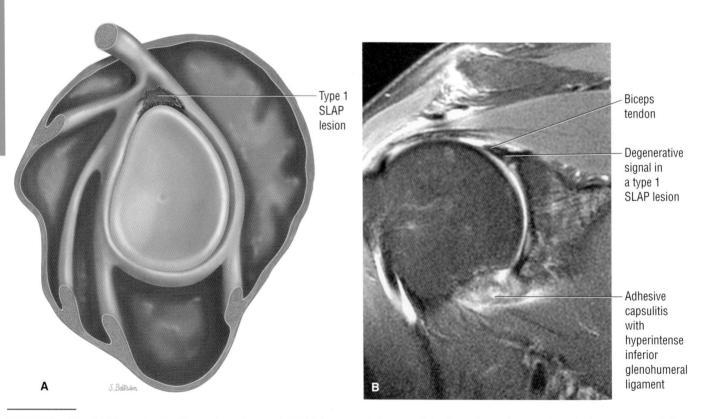

FIGURE 8.50 (A) Lateral color illustration of a type 1 SLAP lesion with fraying of the free edge and intrasubstance degeneration of the superior labrum. This is considered a normal finding in the aging labrum, similar to grade 1 or 2 signal intensity within the degenerative meniscus. This is not considered a symptomatic lesion. (B) Corresponding coronal FS PD FSE image with diffuse intralabral signal intensity without a defined tear, split, fragmentation, or displacement.

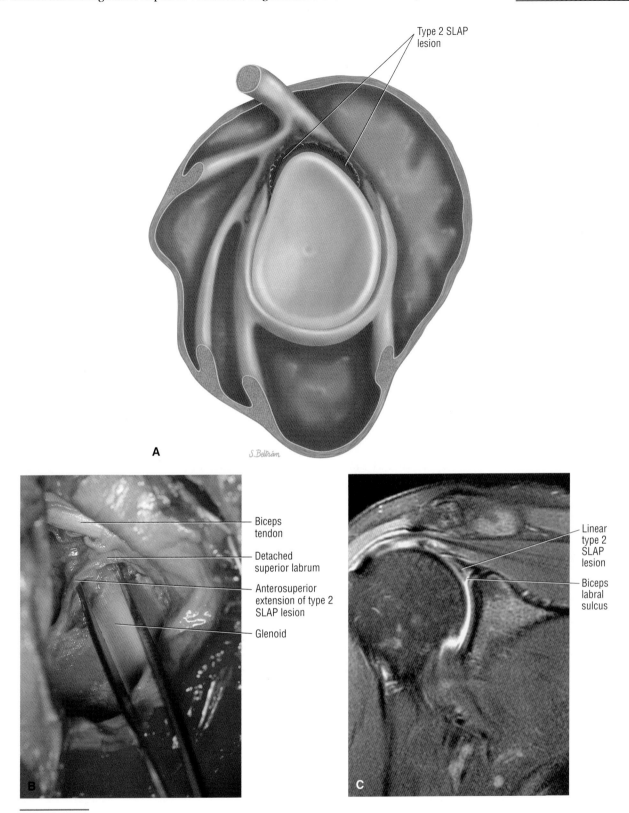

FIGURE 8.51 Type 2 SLAP tear with detached superior labrum and biceps anchor. The labral tear extends from anterior to posterior and may occur within the substance of the labrum or with complete detachment of the biceps and labrum from the superior pole of the glenoid. (**B**) Type 2 SLAP lesion on a corresponding gross dissection identifying superior labral and biceps tendon detachment. The term "biceps expansion" is more accurate and should be used instead of "torn biceps anchor", since the origin of the biceps tendon from the supraglenoid tubercle is not involved. The biceps tendon has a separate expansion or attachment directly to the anterior and posterior glenoid labrum. Except for the frayed appearance of the superior labrum, this SLAP lesion could be mistaken for a prominent biceps labral sulcus on coronal oblique MR images. (**C**) Coronal FS PD FSE image of a type 2 SLAP lesion defined by linear hyperintensity extending across the superior labrum. The associated biceps labrum sulcus is a normal finding. With an intact coapted triangular outline of the superior labrum, the tear represents a type 2 SLAP and not a bucket-handle tear.

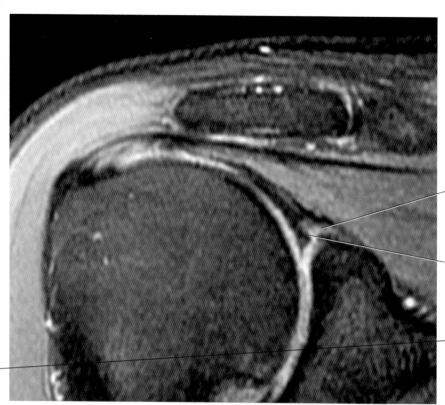

FIGURE 8.52 SLAP 2 lesion demonstrating partial displacement of the biceps root with partial tearing of the origin (anchor) of the bicep tendon from the supraglenoid tubercle and separation of the superior labrum from the intraarticular biceps. This MR would be the equivalent to an arthroscopic examination that revealed a displaceable root. Coronal FS PD.

Partial tear of biceps attachment to supraglenoid tubercle

Separation of superior fibers of biceps

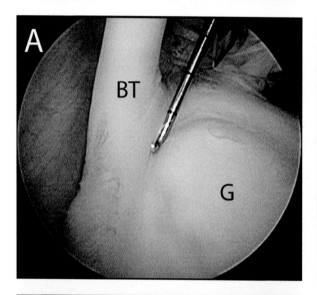

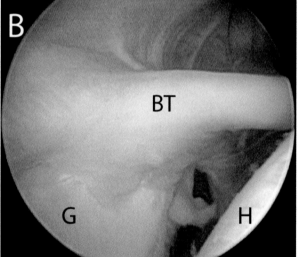

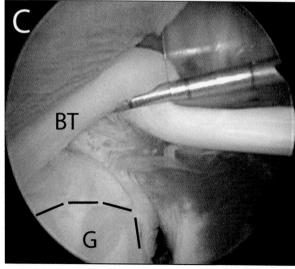

FIGURE 8.53 Probing the biceps root in right shoulder, posterior viewing portal. (**A**) A probe reveals a stable biceps root. (**B**) Right shoulder, posterior viewing portal. The biceps root appears normal initially (**C**), but a probe reveals a displaceable biceps root. The glenoid rim is outlined by *dashed lines*. BT, biceps tendon; G, glenoid; H, humerus. (Reprinted from Burkhart S, Lo IK, Brady PC, Denard PJ. *The Cowboy's Companion: A Trail Guide for the Arthroscopic Shoulder Surgeon.* Philadelphia, PA: Lippincott Williams & Wilkins; 2012, with permission.)

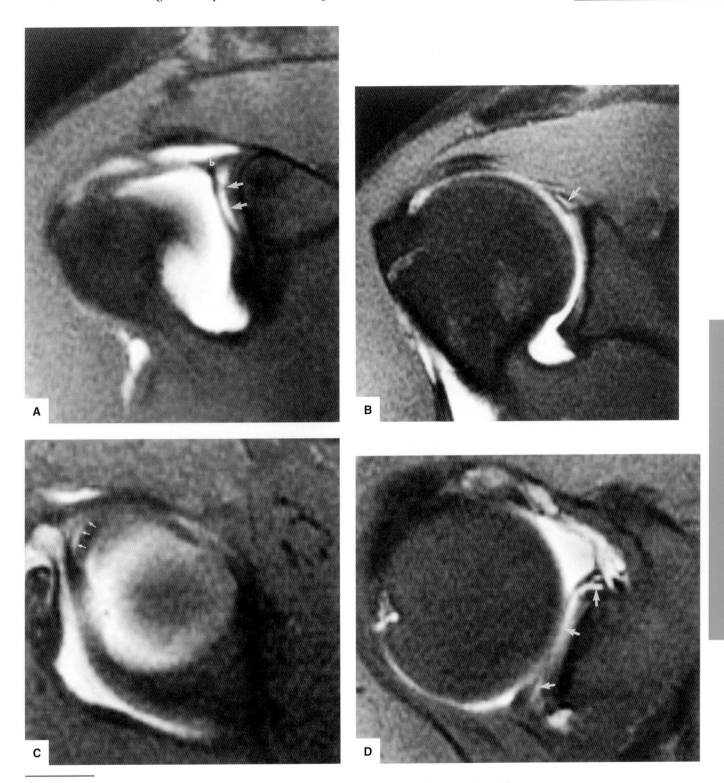

FIGURE 8.54 Type 2 SLAP lesion. (**A**) Separation of the superior labrum and biceps anchor (b) from the underlying anterior glenoid rim. Hyperintense fluid (*arrows*) fills the detachment on this FS T1-weighted coronal oblique MR arthrogram. (**B**) Posterior extension of the tear is shown as a linear hyperintensity through the posterior superior labrum (*arrow*) on this FS T1-weighted coronal oblique MR arthrogram. Corresponding FS T1-weighted sagittal oblique (**C**) and axial (**D**) images display the avulsion (*arrows*) of the BLC (**C**) and anterior-to-posterior extension (*arrows*) of the superior labral tear (**D**).

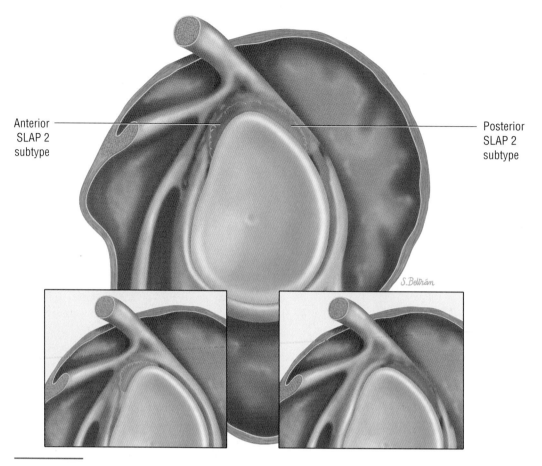

Anterior
SLAP 2
subtype

Posterior
SLAP 2
subtype

S. Beltrán

FIGURE 8.55   Location of anterior SLAP 2 (blue) and posterior SLAP 2 (green) subtypes. Hemorrhage is highlighted in red. A classic type 2 SLAP lesion would involve anterior and posterior components.

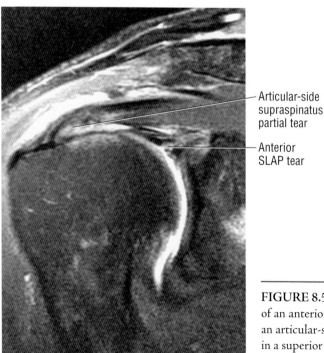

Articular-side
supraspinatus
partial tear

Anterior
SLAP tear

FIGURE 8.56   Coronal FS PD FSE image of an anterior SLAP lesion combined with an articular-side supraspinatus partial tear in a superior labrum anterior cuff (SLAC) lesion.

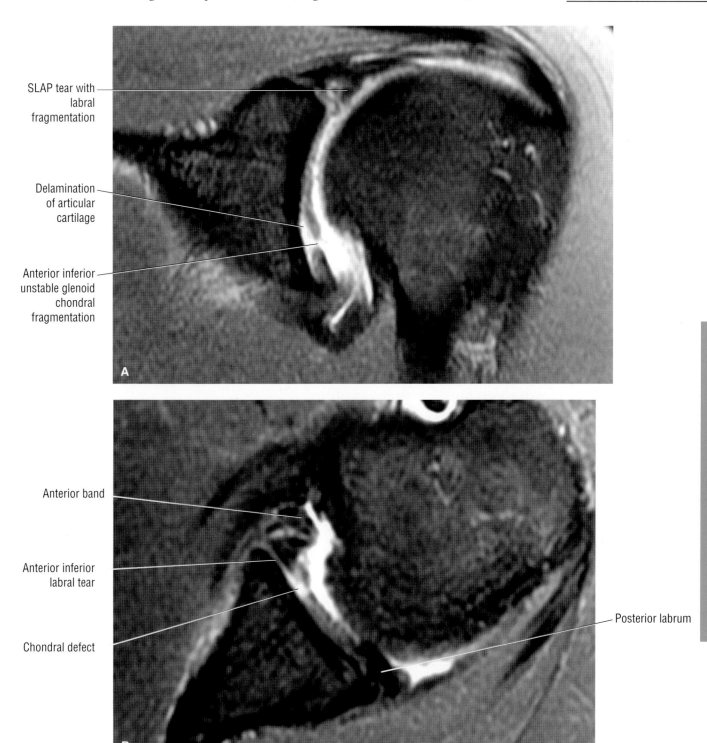

SLAP tear with labral fragmentation

Delamination of articular cartilage

Anterior inferior unstable glenoid chondral fragmentation

Anterior band

Anterior inferior labral tear

Chondral defect

Posterior labrum

FIGURE 8.57   Complex injury from sparring resulting in SLAP 3 lesion of the superior labrum and a GLAD lesion. The superior labrum is fragmented into two components. The fragmentation and/or inferior displacement of superior labral tissue correlates with bucket-handle morphology. The GLAD lesion is associated with delamination or articular cartilage of the anterior inferior glenoid rim. The anterior inferior labrum is stable because there remains an intact attachment to bone peripherally. (**A**) Coronal FS PD. (**B**) Axial FS PD.

- Type 3 SLAP lesions

  - Involve a bucket-handle tear of the superior labrum without extension into the biceps tendon

  - Biceps anchor is stable and the remaining labrum is intact.

  - Multiple hypointense structures on sagittal images represent the biceps tendon and split superior labrum and are associated with a bucket-handle SLAP tear.

  - Commonly associated with anterior labral tears, creating a type 5 SLAP lesion

  - The inferiorly displaced superior labrum may become trapped within the superior glenohumeral joint.

- Type 4 SLAP lesions

  - Involve a bucket-handle tear of the superior labrum, but with extension into the biceps tendon

  - A ruptured biceps tendon represents completion of the biceps tendon tear extension, resulting in a proximal biceps stump.

  - A partially torn biceps tendon may displace the superior labral flap into the joint.

- Type 5 SLAP lesions[372]

  - SLAP 2 or 3 lesion plus superior extension of a Bankart lesion

  - A Hill-Sachs posterolateral humeral head fracture and inferiorly displaced superior labrum may be seen on superior axial images through the glenohumeral joint.

- Type 6 SLAP lesions

  - Usually identified as a type 3 SLAP on coronal images and a SLAP 6 on sagittal images

  - Flap tear morphology of the superior labrum is evident on sagittal images as a flap of labral tissue displaces inferior and rotates.

  - It is more common to classify SLAP 6 lesions as type 3 SLAP tears on MRI unless the displaced flap is visualized directly extending across the superior surface of the glenoid fossa on sagittal images.[75,559]

- Type 7 SLAP lesions
    - SLAP 2 or SLAP 3 lesions with extension into the middle glenohumeral ligament
    - Extension into the MGHL is difficult to assess on MR because of the presence of common variants and normal laxity of the MGHL.

- Type 8 SLAP lesions
    - SLAP 2 or SLAP 3 lesions plus a posterior labral tear

- Type 9 SLAP lesions
    - Circumferential labral tears with anterior and posterior labral involvement
    - Best represented on axial images with superior and inferior labral involvement shown on coronal images
    - The entire circumference of the torn labrum is often displayed on a single sagittal image with associated degenerative changes of the adjacent glenoid rim.

- Type 10 SLAP lesions
    - SLAP 2 or 3 lesions with extension into the rotator cuff interval through the superior glenohumeral ligament

Diagnosis of SLAP Tears

- SLAP 1 lesions are a normal finding.

- SLAP 2 lesions occur in traction injuries with forced extension on a flexed forearm.

- In 31% of cases, SLAP 3, 4, or 5 lesions are associated with a fall on an outstretched hand.

- Anterior dislocation is often associated with SLAP 5 lesion.

- Patients usually present after trauma and approximately one third have symptoms referable to the biceps tendon.[558]

- Rotator cuff pain is common in type 2 or type 2 subtype SLAP lesions.
    - Up to 40% of SLAP lesion may be associated with a full or partial thickness rotator cuff tear.

- Twenty-two percent of SLAP lesions correspond with Bankart instability injuries.

- Twenty-eight percent of SLAP lesions are isolated findings.[559]

- Bicipital groove tenderness is assessed with Speed's test (resisted forward flexion of a supinated arm) or Yergason's test (resisted supination with the elbow in 90° of flexion).

- In a positive crank or clunk test, there is pain and/or popping with compression and rotation.

- O'Brien's active compression test for SLAP lesions elicits pain with resisted elevation with the forearm fully pronated.

- A positive Jobe relocation test indicates a posterior SLAP lesion.

- SLAP tears are associated with microinstability, including rotator cuff interval lesions.

Pathologic Findings in SLAP Tears

- A bare labral footprint

- A sublabral sulcus greater than 5mm (measure between the superior labrum and the superior pole of the glenoid)

- A displaceable biceps (biceps root rolls over the glenoid)

- Associated effects of SLAP lesions include:

  - Biceps root disruption between the intraarticular biceps and the superior labrum with or without associated intralabral tearing (The superior labrum may be directly avulsed from the superior glenoid articular cartilage in a type I BLC.)

  - Increased humeral head translation in microinstability

  - Strain of humeral head restraints

  - Glenohumeral laxity and/or instability

  - Paralabral cysts (commonly associated with type 2 SLAP lesion)

  - SLAP fracture[558] with a superior humeral head chondral fracture and a SLAP lesion

  - SLAP fracture avulsion from the superior pole of the glenoid (rare)

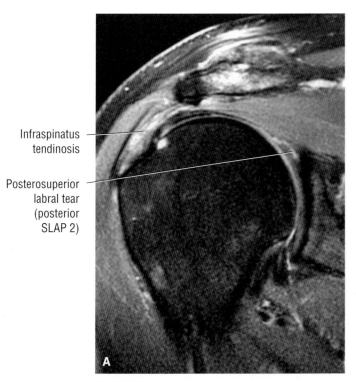
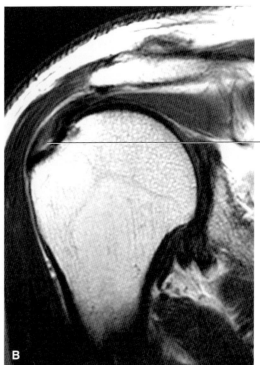

Infraspinatus
tendinosis

Posterosuperior
labral tear
(posterior
SLAP 2)

Articular-sided
infraspinatus
tendon tear

FIGURE 8.58   Coronal FS PD FSE (**A**) and T2 FSE (**B**) images of posterior peel-back lesion with a tear of the posterosuperior labrum associated with an articular-sided posterior cuff partial tear.

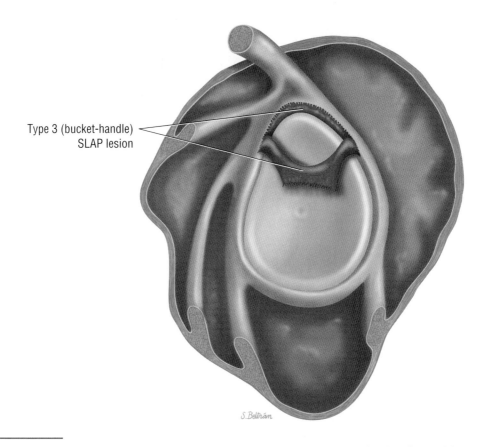

Type 3 (bucket-handle)
SLAP lesion

S. Beltrán

FIGURE 8.59   Sagittal color illustration of a type 3 SLAP lesion with bucket-handle tear. The superior labrum may be meniscoid. The biceps tendon attachment is intact. The bucket fragment may be split into two fragments and displaced inferiorly from the biceps root on MR images.

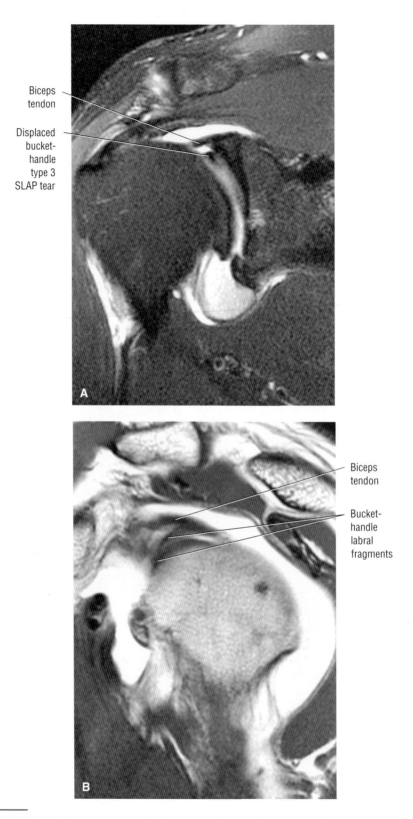

FIGURE 8.60 The "three structure sign" corresponding to the biceps tendon superior to the two bucket-handle components of the superior labrum on (**A**) a coronal FS PD FSE MR arthrogram and (**B**) a sagittal PD FSE MR arthrogram.

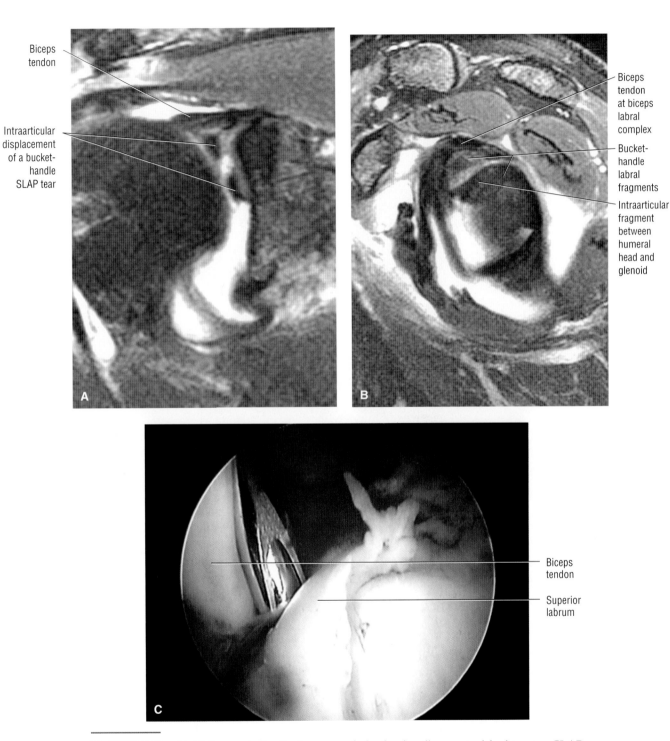

FIGURE 8.61 **(A,B)** Intraarticular displacement of a bucket-handle superior labral tear in a SLAP 3 associated with a Bankart lesion (a SLAP 5 equivalent). **(A)** Coronal FS PD FSE. **(B)** Sagittal FS PD FSE. **(C)** Arthroscopic view of type 3 SLAP tear at the superior pole of the glenoid. There is separation from the biceps anchor at the probe site in this bucket-handle tear. A SLAP 2 or 3 plus a Bankart lesion represents a SLAP 5. The inferior displaced superior labral fragments identified in the coronal plane correlate with bucket-handle SLAP morphology.

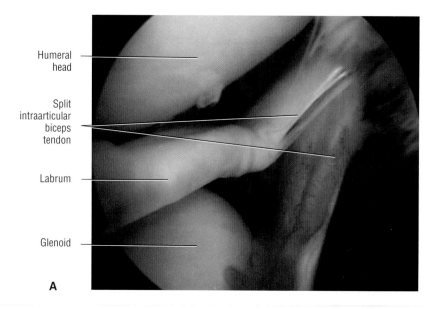

Humeral head

Split intraarticular biceps tendon

Labrum

Glenoid

A

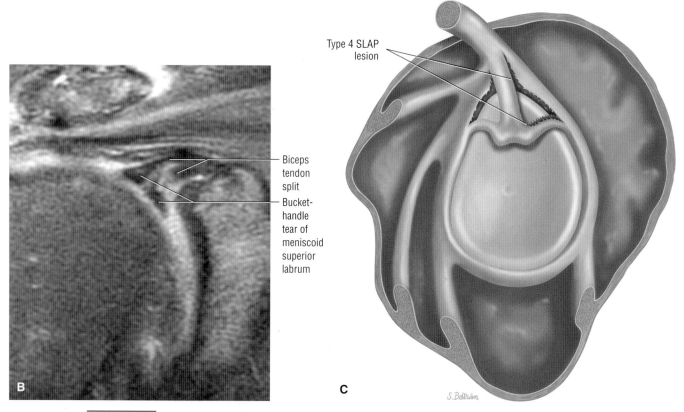

Type 4 SLAP lesion

Biceps tendon split

Bucket-handle tear of meniscoid superior labrum

B

C

S. Beltrán

FIGURE 8.62 (**A**) Arthroscopic view of type 4 SLAP with extension of the superior labral tear into the biceps root. (**B**) Coronal FS PD FSE image with bucket-handle tear and split of the intraarticular biceps. (**C**) Lateral color graphic illustrating a SLAP 4 lesion with a split or bucket-handle tear of the superior labrum that continues into the biceps tendon. A SLAP 4 may be inferred either by tracing a fluid signal intensity extension of the SLAP tear into the intraarticular biceps or by observing a complete tear of the biceps tendon. The orientation of the superior labrum in the 12 o'clock position may be obliquely shifted when there is an biceps tear.

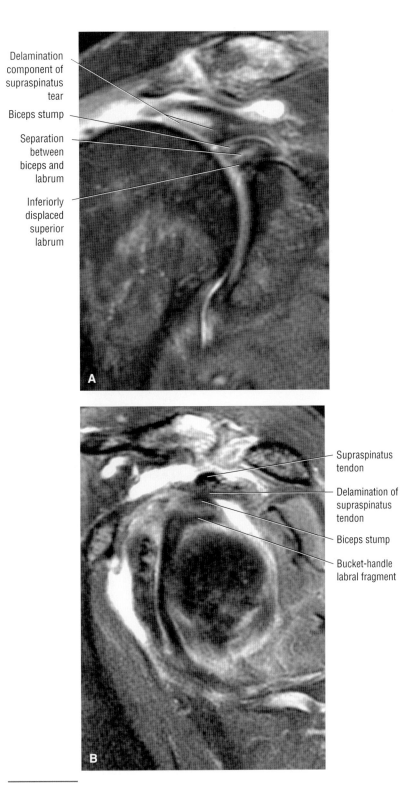

Delamination component of supraspinatus tear

Biceps stump

Separation between biceps and labrum

Inferiorly displaced superior labrum

Supraspinatus tendon

Delamination of supraspinatus tendon

Biceps stump

Bucket-handle labral fragment

FIGURE 8.63 (**A**) Coronal FS PD FSE and (**B**) sagittal FS PD FSE images of a SLAP 4 lesion with associated rupture of the intraarticular biceps. The intraarticular biceps stump is visible superior to the superior labrum. The course of the biceps should always be traced from its intraarticular location to its extraarticular course. The finding of a biceps stump should not be mistakened for an intact LHBT.

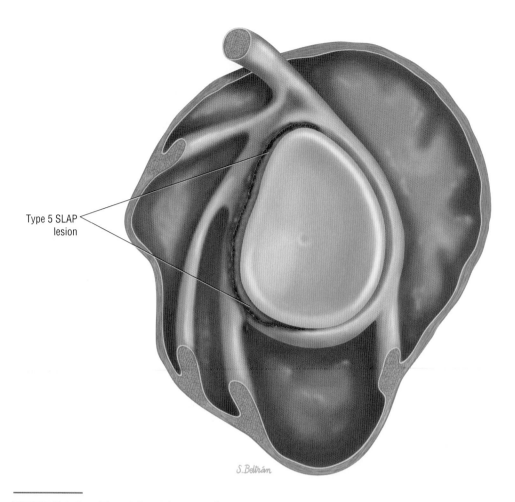

Type 5 SLAP
lesion

S.Beltrán

FIGURE 8.64 Type 5 SLAP lesion with superior extension of a Bankart lesion into a superior SLAP lesion. The superior labral lesion may be type 2 or 3. Lateral color illustration with anterosuperior and anteroinferior SLAP 5 extension.

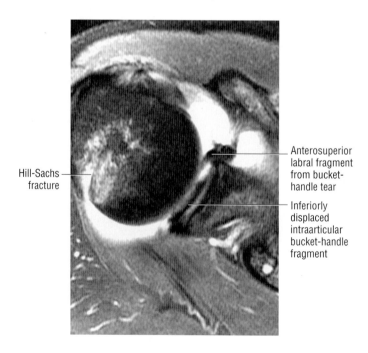

Hill-Sachs
fracture

Anterosuperior
labral fragment
from bucket-
handle tear

Inferiorly
displaced
intraarticular
bucket-handle
fragment

FIGURE 8.65 An axial FS PD FSE image displaying a SLAP 5 lesion with an associated postero-lateral Hill-Sachs humeral head fracture. Superior glenohumeral joint entrapment of bucket-handle labral fragments is visualized in the same axial section.

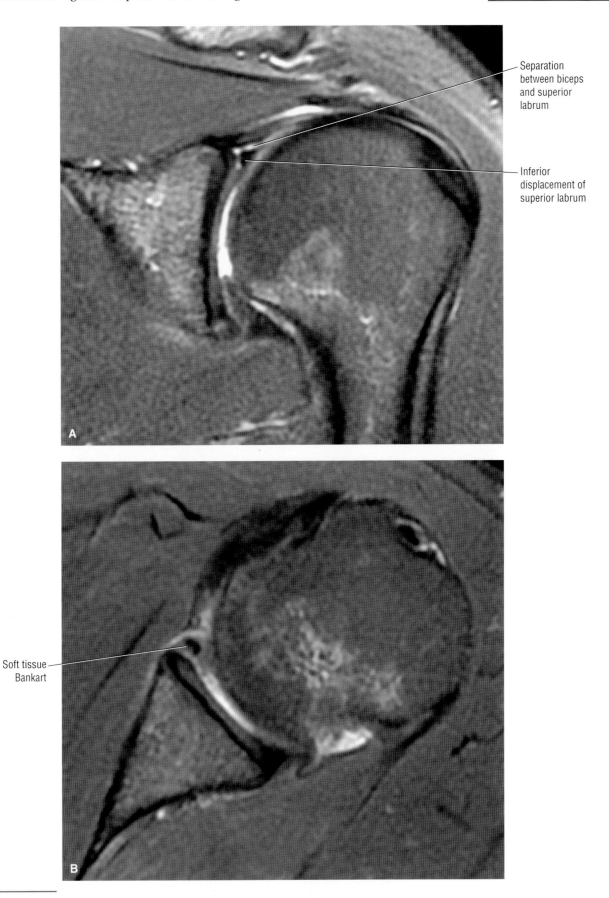

Separation between biceps and superior labrum

Inferior displacement of superior labrum

Soft tissue Bankart

FIGURE 8.66   SLAP 5 lesion with SLAP 3 component of the superior labrum at the level of the BLC and continuation anterior inferiorly as a soft tissue Bankart. The inferior displacement of the superior labrum in the coronal plane constitutes the SLAP 3 component and development of bucket-handle pattern. The continuation into the anterior inferior labrum represents the Bankart component. A SLAP 5 can be formed from either a SLAP 2 or a SLAP 3 in combination with a Bankart lesion. (**A**) Coronal FS PD FSE. (**B**) Axial FS PD FSE.

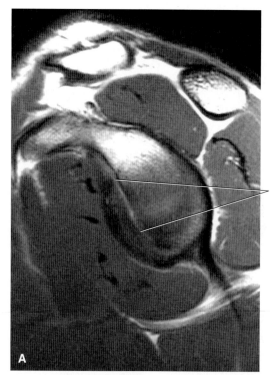

Superior
extension of
a Bankart
lesion

A

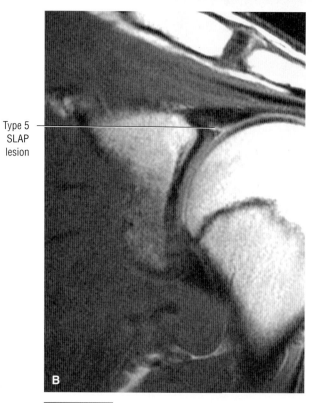

Type 5
SLAP
lesion

B

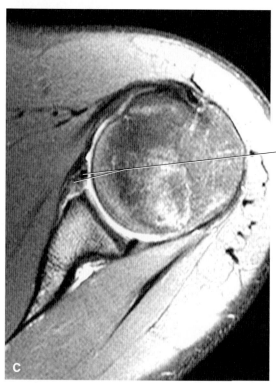

Osseous
Bankart
component
of type 5
SLAP lesion

C

FIGURE 8.67 Type 5 SLAP lesion with superior extension of a Bankart lesion into a superior SLAP lesion. The superior labral lesion may be type 2 or 3. (**A**) Sagittal PD FSE image showing an extensive anterior labral tear. (**B**) Coronal PD FSE image of inferior displacement of the superior labrum. (**C**) Axial FS PD FSE image of an anterior labral soft tissue Bankart lesion.

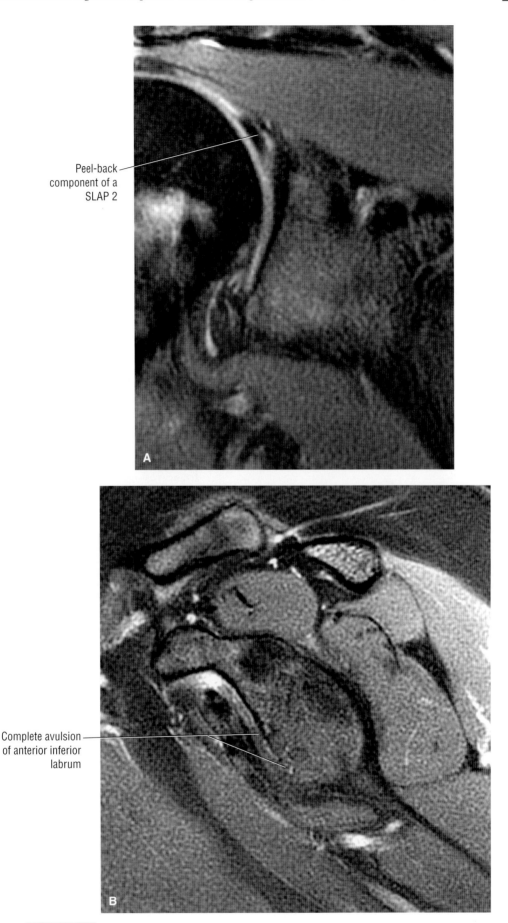

Peel-back
component of a
SLAP 2

Complete avulsion
of anterior inferior
labrum

FIGURE 8.68   SLAP 5 lesion with SLAP 2 component of the posterior aspect of the superior labrum (posterior to the 12 o'clock position) and complete avulsion of the anterior inferior labrum as assessed on sagittal images. Subtle flattening of the anterior inferior glenoid rim. (**A**) FS PD coronal. (**B**) FS PD sagittal.

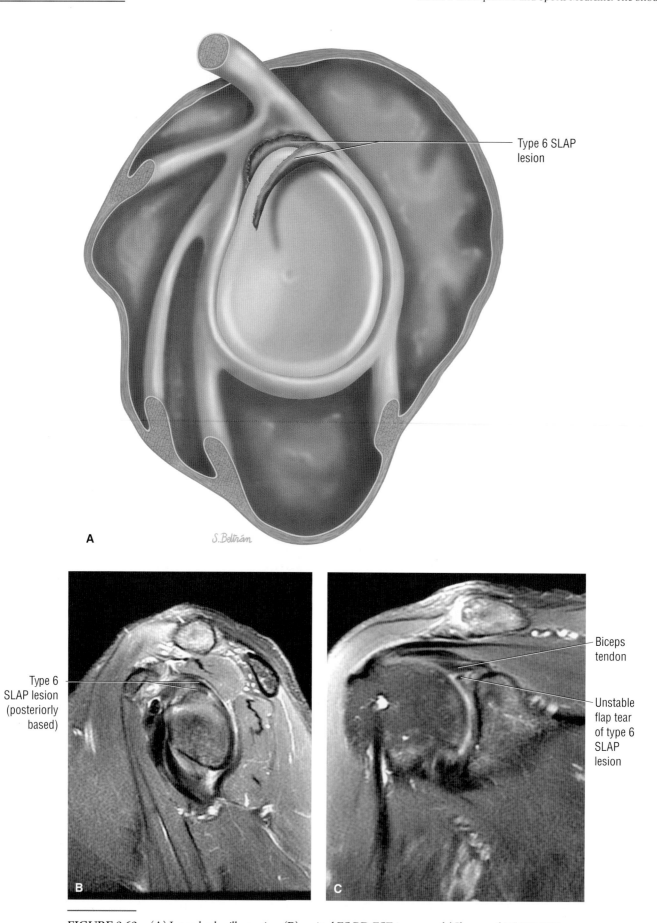

FIGURE 8.69 (**A**) Lateral color illustration, (**B**) sagittal FS PD FSE image, and (**C**) coronal FS PD FSE image of posterior-based superior flap SLAP 6 lesion. The sagittal plane is required for direct visualization of the flap morphology; otherwise, the coronal MR appearance is similar to a bucket-handle tear.

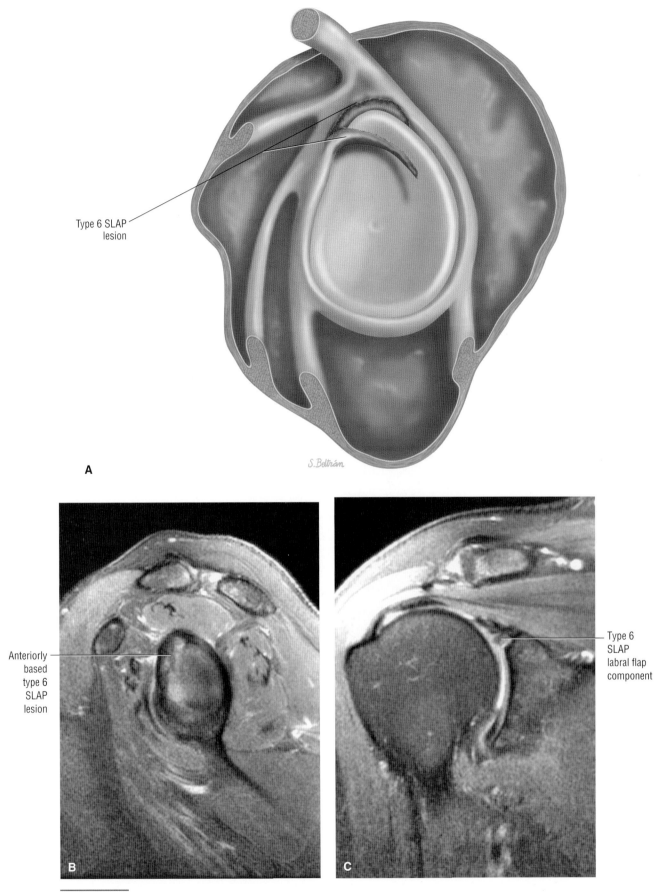

FIGURE 8.70   (**A**) Lateral color graphic, (**B**) sagittal FS PD FSE image, and (**C**) coronal FS PD FSE of anterior-based superior flap tear of a SLAP 6 lesion.

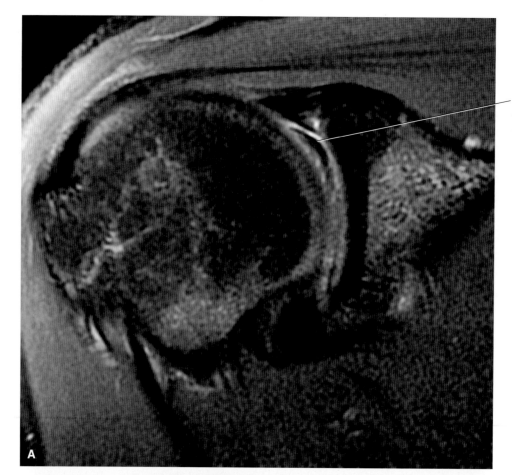

SLAP 3
component of a
SLAP 6 tear

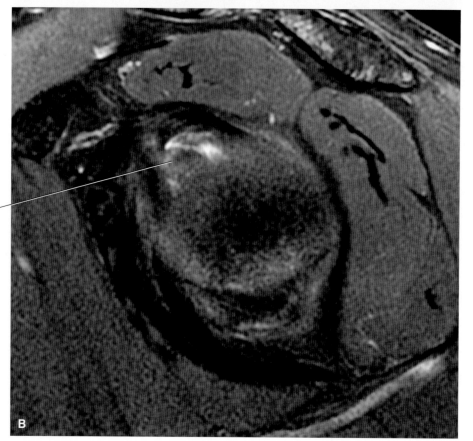

Flap of superior
labral tissue
producing a SLAP
6 pattern

FIGURE 8.71   SLAP 6 lesion with SLAP 3 component of the superior labrum as characterized by inferior displacement of labral tissue. The morphology of the flipped labral tissue creates a flap of tissue in the sagittal plane and the SLAP 6 pattern. (**A**) Coronal FS PD. (**B**) FS PD sagittal.

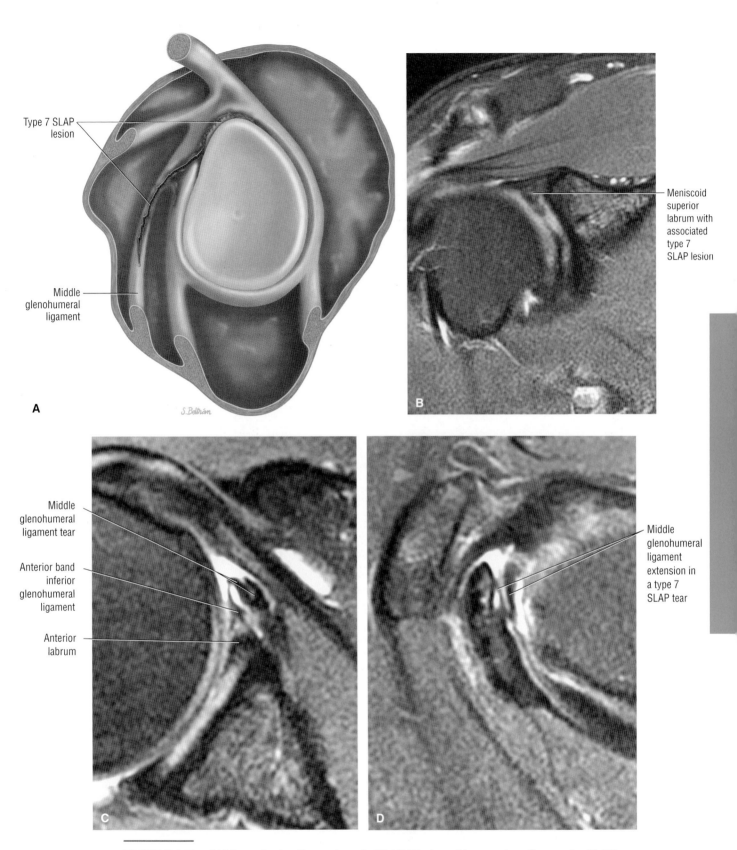

FIGURE 8.72 (**A**) Lateral color illustration of a SLAP 7 lesion with extension of a superior SLAP 2 or 3 into the middle glenohumeral ligament (MGL). (**B**) Coronal FS PD FSE image demonstrates anterior extension of a SLAP tear toward the MGL. (**C**) Axial T2*-weighted GRE image with fragmentation of the MGL. Normal MGL laxity with ligament redundancy may falsely appear as a torn ligament on axial images. Therefore, confirmation of pathology requires proper correlation with sagittal images. (**D**) Confirmation of MGL involvement on a sagittal FS PD FSE image.

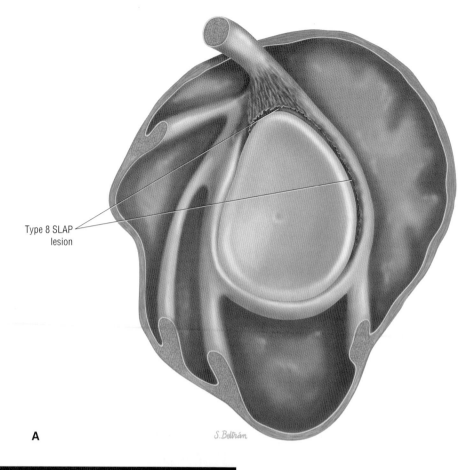

Type 8 SLAP
lesion

S. Beltrán

A

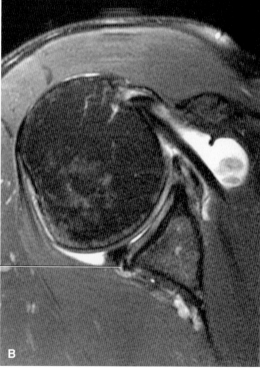

Posterior
labral
extension
of a type 8
SLAP tear

B

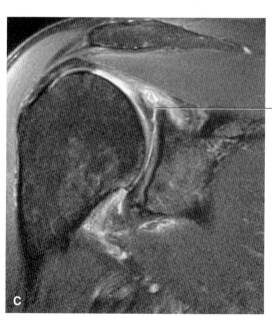

Type 8
SLAP lesion
(superior
labral
component)

C

FIGURE 8.73 (**A**) Lateral (sagittal) color illustration of a type 8 SLAP with extension of a SLAP 2 to involve the posterior labrum. (**B**) Coronal FS PD FSE image with a SLAP 2 component and paralabral cyst as part of the SLAP 8 lesion. (**C**) Axial FS PD FSE image documents posterior labral tear extension from the biceps labral complex.

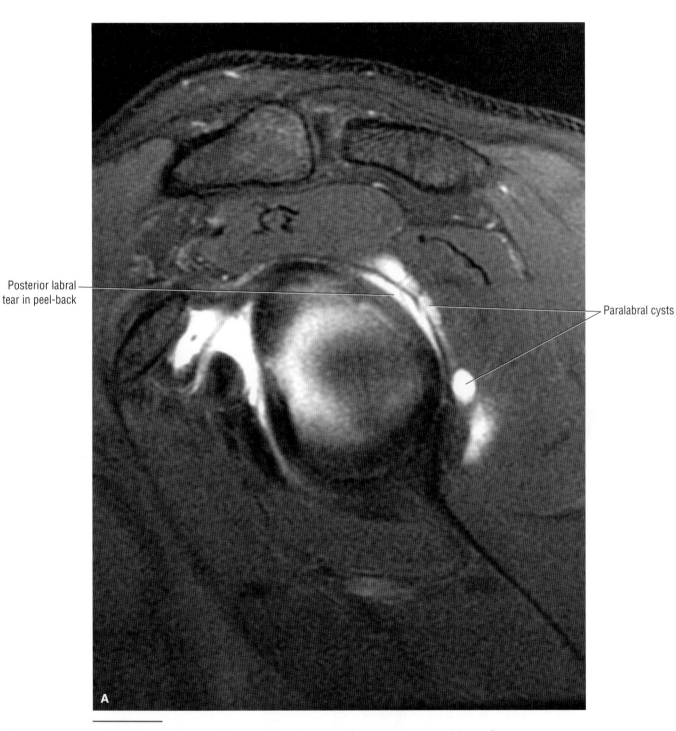

Posterior labral
tear in peel-back

Paralabral cysts

FIGURE 8.74   SLAP 8 lesion with involvement of the entire posterior labrum from posterior superior to posterior inferior quadrant with the development of communicating paralabral cysts. (**A**) Sagittal FS PD FSE MR arthrogram. The posterior paralabral cysts follow the course of the posterior labral tear.

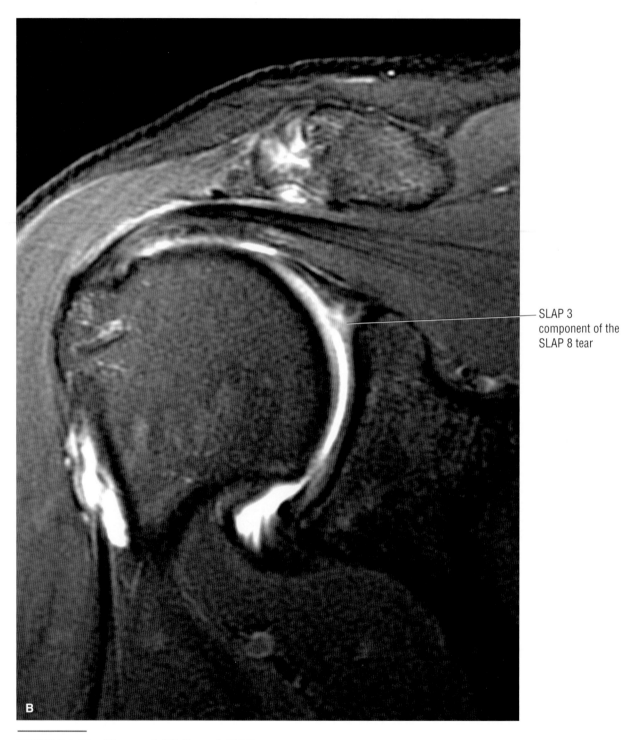

SLAP 3
component of the
SLAP 8 tear

FIGURE 8.74   (*Continued*) (**B**) Coronal FS PD.

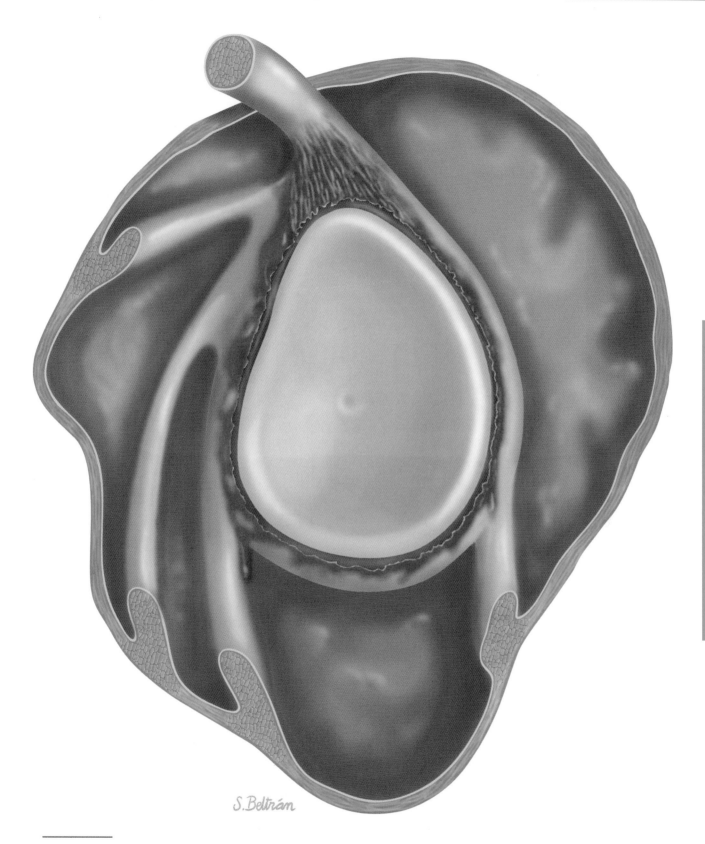

FIGURE 8.75 Lateral color graphic of a type 9 SLAP lesion with circumferential labral tearing of all glenoid quadrants.

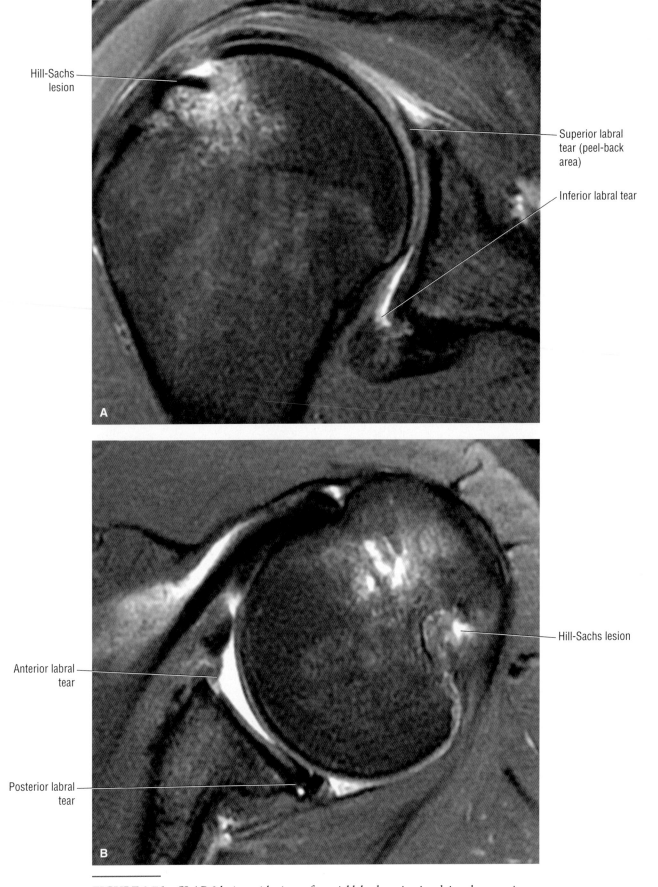

FIGURE 8.76   SLAP 9 lesion with circumferential labral tearing involving the superior labrum, inferior labrum, anterior labrum, and posterior labrum. Associated Hill-Sachs deformity is present because of the macroinstability event associated with this case. (**A**) Coronal FS PD. (**B**) Axial FS PD.

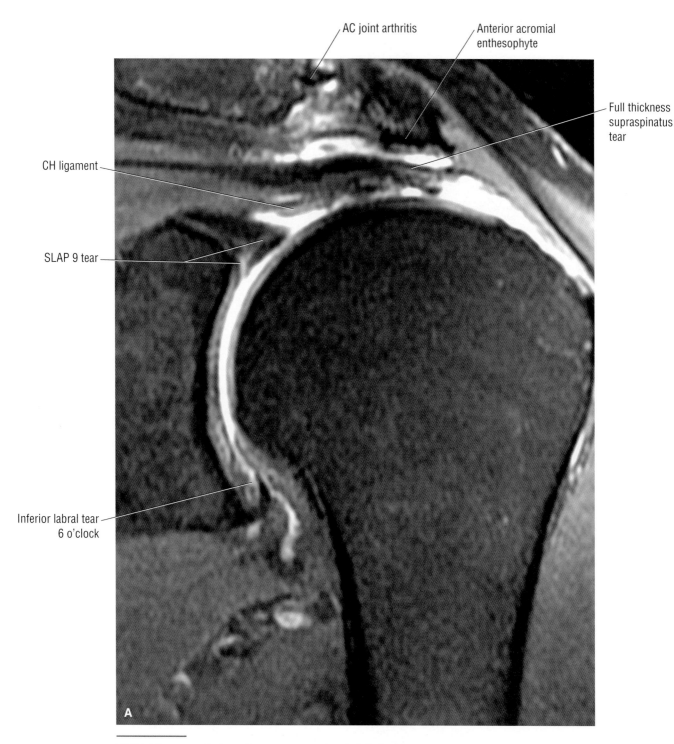

FIGURE 8.77 SLAP 9 lesion associated with full-thickness supraspinatus tendon tear. In the coronal plane, both the tear of the superior labrum and inferior labrum (6 o'clock position) are identified. Axial plane images show involvement of both the anterior inferior labrum and posterior labrum with separation from the underlying glenoid articular cartilage. (**A**) Coronal FS PD.

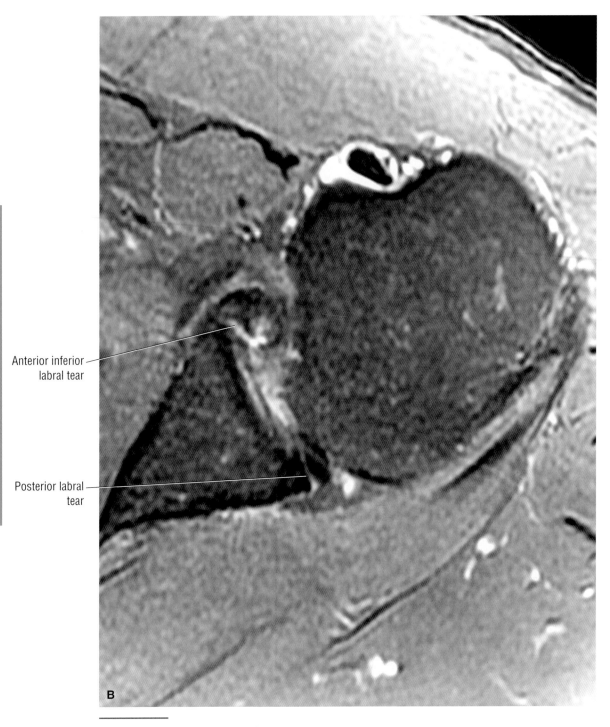

Anterior inferior
labral tear

Posterior labral
tear

B

FIGURE 8.77 (*Continued*) (**B**) Axial FS PD.

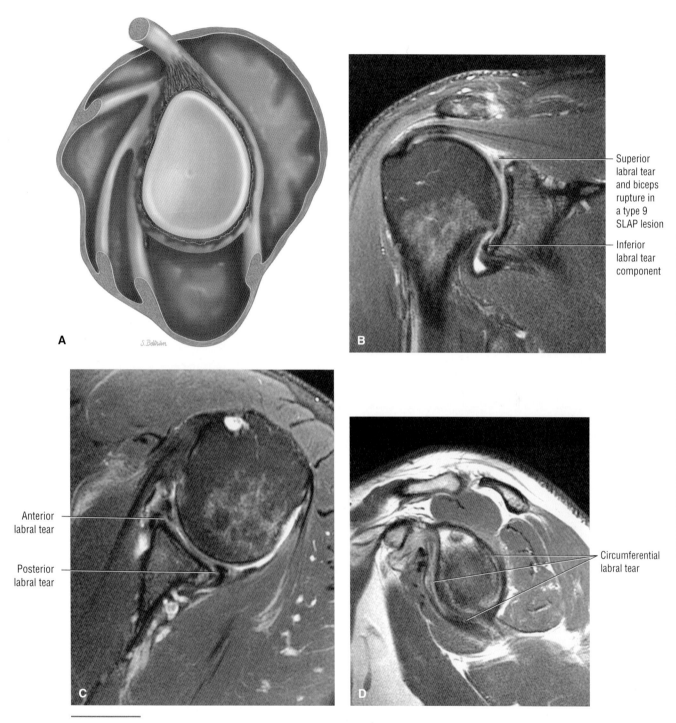

FIGURE 8.78 (**A**) Lateral color graphic of a type 9 SLAP lesion with circumferential labral tearing of all glenoid quadrants. (**B**) Coronal FS PD FSE image with a type 2 SLAP at the BLC and an inferior labral tear at the 6 o'clock position of the inferior pole. (**C**) Corresponding axial FS PD FSE image with anterior and posterior labral tears. (**D**) Sagittal PD FSE image of circumferential labral tear (around the entire glenoid "clock"). There is usually associated glenoid rim sclerosis.

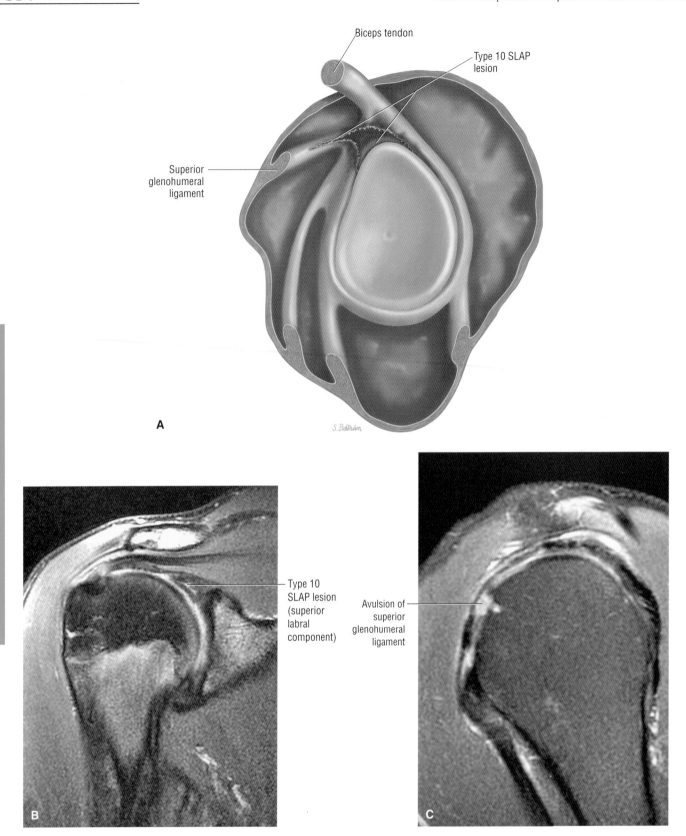

FIGURE 8.79   (**A**) A SLAP 10 lesion with associated rotator cuff interval involvement shown with extension in the superior glenohumeral ligament on a lateral glenoid color illustration. (**B**) Coronal FS PD FSE image with SLAP 2 component of the SLAP 10 lesion. (**C**) Sagittal FS PD FSE image with associated rupture of the superior glenohumeral ligament. A SLAP 10 lesion has also been used to designate a SLAP lesion in association with a posterior inferior labral tear. Description of the SLAP pattern along with is number will avoid any confusion regarding the specified pathology.

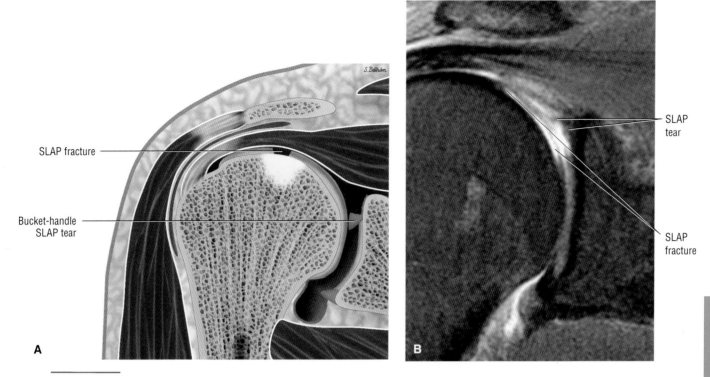

FIGURE 8.80 (**A**) Coronal color illustration and (**B**) coronal FS PD FSE image of a SLAP fracture with a chondral divot of the superior humeral head. This type of injury is caused by impaction, often occurring in the setting of a fall onto an outstretched arm that drives the humeral head against the superior labrum and biceps anchor. These chondral fractures are more anterior and medial than the posterolateral Hill-Sachs anterior instability lesion. The SLAP fracture is frequently associated with a type 3 or 4 SLAP lesion, especially in the presence of a meniscoid-type superior labrum, which is more susceptible to injury.

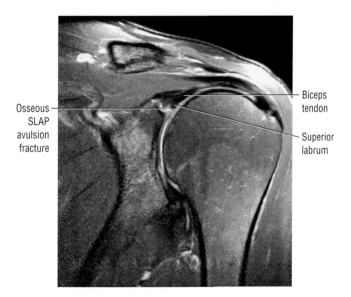

FIGURE 8.81 Coronal FS PD FSE image showing the unusual SLAP 2 avulsion fracture. This type of fracture is seen with osseous avulsion of the biceps and labrum from the superior glenoid as the biceps tendon is stretched over the humeral head during a fall onto an outstretched arm. The avulsion-type fracture is rare relative to the humeral head dome chondral "SLAP fracture."

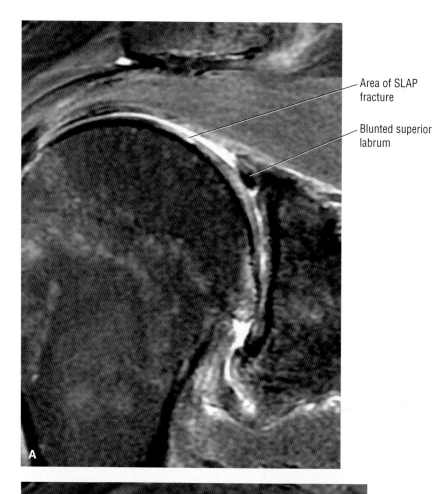

FIGURE 8.82 SLAP fracture with associated posterolabral tear. The chondral fracture of the superomedial humeral head is most frequently identified without reactive subchondral marrow edema. Careful inspection of the chondral surface must be performed to identify the defect in the articular cartilage surface. The SLAP lesion will usually be identified within one image of the SLAP fracture. The presence of chondral debris will serve as a synovial irritant and may be associated with synovitis in the axillary pouch, mid-rotator cuff interval, or subscapularis recess. This could lead to clinical findings of adhesive capsulitis. There is synovitis in the axillary pouch in this example. (**A,B**) Coronal FS PD.

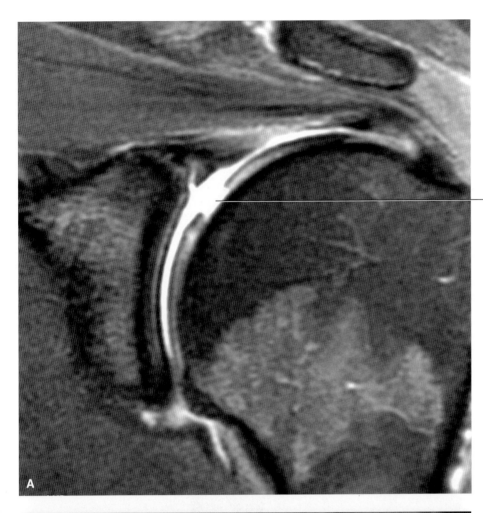

SLAP fracture

FIGURE 8.83 SLAP fracture with discreet grade 4 chondral defect opposite the superior labrum. The displaced chondral fragment occupies the posterior capsule in the axial plane. SLAP lesion should always be evaluated for the presence of humeral head chondral defects. The articular cartilage defect will secondarily insight a synovitis reaction within the glenohumeral joint that could lead to MR findings of adhesive capsulitis. (**A**) Coronal. (**B**) Axial FS PD.

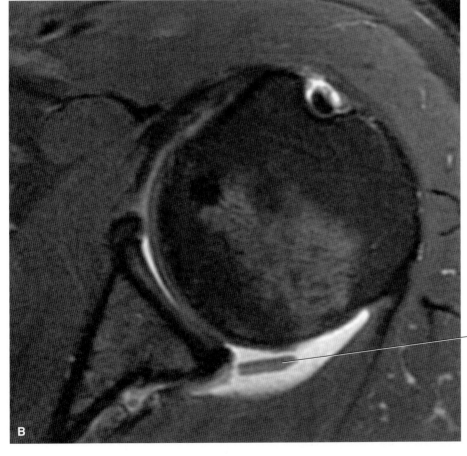

Chondral fragment posterior capsule

Treatment of SLAP Lesions

- Treatment of SLAP lesions is based on the type of labral lesion present.

  - A type 1 SLAP lesion is treated with arthroscopic débridement of the degenerative labrum.

  - Treatment of a type 2 SLAP lesion (which involves detachment of the superior labrum and biceps anchor) addresses the avulsed labrum and reattachment of the detached biceps anchor to the superior glenoid.

    - A suture anchor technique, for example, may be used for a type 2 SLAP tear.

  - Since there is no involvement of the biceps tendon in a type 3 SLAP lesion (a bucket-handle tear and a meniscoid-type superior labrum), arthroscopic débridement of the loose labral fragment may be sufficient to relieve symptoms of catching and snapping.

  - A type 4 SLAP lesion, which also involves a bucket-handle tear associated with a meniscoid-type superior labrum, additionally extends into the biceps tendon. Treatment of type 4 lesions ranges from resection of torn tissue to suture repair for bucket-handle tears associated with more extensive involvement of the biceps tendon.

  - Types 5 through 10 SLAP lesions require restoration of normal anatomy, including the MGHL and IGHLC. The labrum is stabilized and reattached.

- Although not all SLAP 2 lesions are symptomatic, patients with bucket-handle lesions (including type 3 or 4 SLAP tears, which produce a displaced labral fragment into the superior glenohumeral joint) benefit from early identification by MR or MR arthrography.

- Single-anchor, double-suture (SADS) technique to repair a type 2 SLAP lesion[558]

  - This technique creates a sling anterior and posterior to the biceps anchor point, allowing for stability and healing of the biceps labral complex.

  - Central anchor placement for biceps fixation is the key to a stable repair.

  - Posterior peel-back lesions may require an additional suture anchor in the posterosuperior corner.

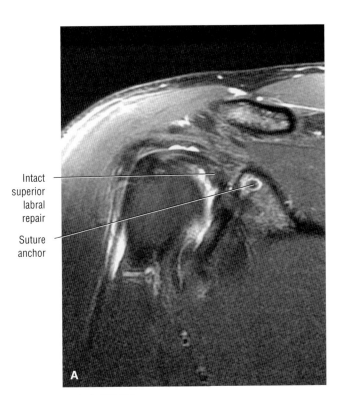

Intact
superior
labral
repair

Suture
anchor

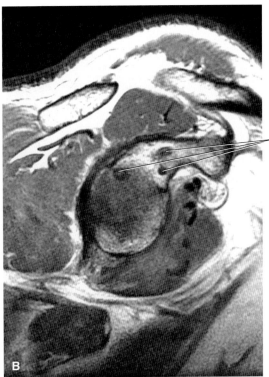

Suture
anchors
superior
quadrant
of glenoid

FIGURE 8.84 (**A**) Coronal FS PD FSE and (**B**) sagittal PD FSE images of a SLAP lesion treated with superior quadrant suture anchors. SLAP lesions have also been treated by a single-anchor, double-suture SLAP repair to form a sling around the biceps anchor. Techniques that drill across the glenoid or through the acromion or use an absorbable tacking device are less successful and may lead to implant failure, synovitis, and intraarticular loose fragments.

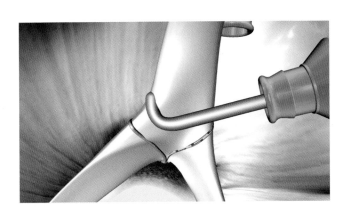

FIGURE 8.85 The SLAP repair is firmly secured to the superior glenoid, as confirmed with a probe. (© ConMed Linvatec. Reprinted from Miniaci A, Iannotti JP, Williams GR, Zuckerman, JD. *Disorders of the Shoulder: Sports Injuries.* 3rd ed. Philadelphia, PA: Lippincott Williams & Wilkins; 2014, with permission.)

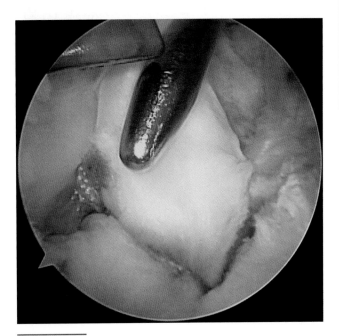

FIGURE 8.86 Final appearance of completed SLAP repair using the single-anchor, double-suture technique. (Reprinted from Miniaci A, Iannotti JP, Williams GR, Zuckerman, JD. *Disorders of the Shoulder: Sports Injuries.* 3rd ed. Philadelphia, PA: Lippincott Williams & Wilkins; 2014, with permission.)

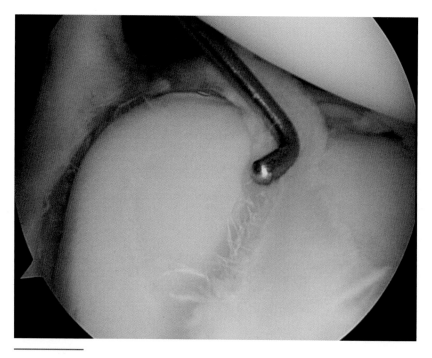

FIGURE 8.87   Type 3 SLAP lesion with bucket-handle tear of the superior labrum. (Reprinted from Miniaci A, Iannotti JP, Williams GR, Zuckerman, JD. *Disorders of the Shoulder: Sports Injuries.* 3rd ed. Philadelphia, PA: Lippincott Williams & Wilkins; 2014, with permission.)

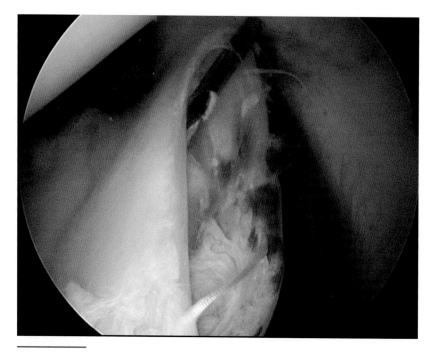

FIGURE 8.88   Type 4 SLAP lesion with tearing that extends into the biceps tendon. (Reprinted from Miniaci A, Iannotti JP, Williams GR, Zuckerman, JD. *Disorders of the Shoulder: Sports Injuries.* 3rd ed. Philadelphia, PA: Lippincott Williams & Wilkins; 2014, with permission.)

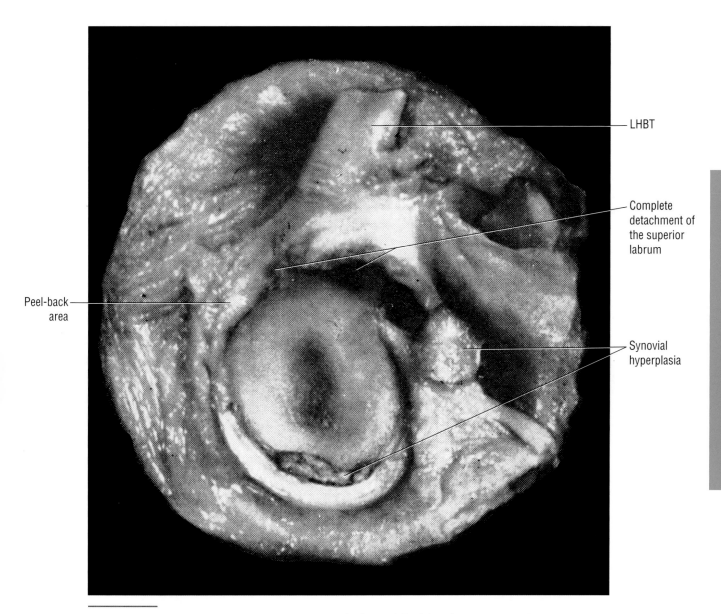

Peel-back
area

LHBT

Complete
detachment
of the superior
labrum

Synovial
hyperplasia

FIGURE 8.89   Synovial hyperplasia associated with chronic labral detachment. Synovial reaction (synovitis) is especially common when there is associated chondral pathology. (From DePalma AF. *Surgery of the Shoulder*. 3rd ed. Philadelphia, PA: JB Lippincott; 1983.)

MR Appearance of Labral Tears

Key Concepts

- The coronal oblique plane is used to assess both the superior labrum at the superior pole of the glenoid and the IGLLC at the inferior pole of the glenoid.

- The sagittal oblique plane is useful in identifying normal variations in the MGHL and the anterior band of the IGHL relative to the corresponding morphology of the anterior labrum in the axial plane.

  - The sagittal oblique plane demonstrates bucket-handle SLAP tear patterns.

- The inferior labrum, however, should be carefully evaluated on coronal MR images, which may be more accurate than the inferior-most axial images through the glenohumeral joint.

- The peripheral attachment of the labrum joins the capsule and glenohumeral ligaments, creating the capsulolabral complex.

- The central attachment of the labrum blends with the articular cartilage surface of the glenoid. A meniscoid appearance usually involves the superior labrum and is characterized by a free inner or central edge of the labrum.[635]

Intralabral Signal Intensity

- The labrum to be composed of bundles of fibrous tissue with a thin transitional zone of fibrocartilage between the labrum and articular cartilage.[138]

  - This transitional zone may be only a few cells in width and is variably visualized.

- This thin transitional cartilage may be over-read as a sublabral foramen or potentially as a SLAP lesion.

GLOM Sign

■ A glenoid ovoid mass (GLOM sign)[313] used by some as an indication of a labral tear is a term not used in orthopaedic surgery and is not that commonly assessed.

■ In fact, a low-signal-intensity mass anterior to the glenoid rim may represent a cord-like MGHL and should not be interpreted as a tear or avulsed anterior labrum.

IGHL Tears

■ Tears of the IGHL or IGL are usually associated with traumatic dislocation or subluxation.[88,138]

■ Labral tissue may be interposed between the humeral head and glenoid rim, most often due to a labral tear with a relatively discoid and hypermobile biceps labral configuration.

■ As the labrum becomes more meniscoid in shape, the likelihood of meniscal bucket-handle tears increases, and tissue may become interposed between the humeral head and glenoid surface.

SLAP Tears

■ The biceps labral sulcus or sublabral recess may exist throughout the superior glenoid labral complex and thus be identified posterior to the biceps anchor.

   ■ Hyperintense fluid in the BLC sulcus posterior to the biceps anchor is not necessarily pathologic.[559]

■ Distinguishing between a normal sulcus and a type 2 SLAP requires consideration of secondary and associated findings of a SLAP tear, including:[358]

   ■ Superior displacement of the labrum

   ■ Increased depth of the sulcus

   ■ Synovitis

   ■ Adjacent labral and chondral fraying

   ■ Micro-paralabral (early) cyst formation

■ Inferior displacement of the superior labrum, or a portion of the superior labrum, from its biceps attachment is associated with a displaced bucket-handle tear.

- Signal intensity seen between the biceps tendon and labrum indicates the presence of a SLAP lesion.

- Type 3 and type 4 SLAP lesions

  - Demonstrate an additional hypointense labral structure on sagittal images through the biceps labral complex (the triple structure sign of a displaced SLAP tear)

  - Three separate and distinct structures may also be appreciated on coronal images when there is fluid between the biceps tendon and the superior labrum and fluid between two separated labral fragments.[372]

- Type 5 SLAP lesions

  - In type 5 SLAP, the anterior labrum is torn in continuity with the SLAP tear (associated type 2 or type 3).

  - The Bankart component is identified on axial images, whereas the SLAP region is visualized in the coronal plane.

- Type 6 SLAP lesions

  - The type 6 SLAP is best identified on coronal images, although sagittal images are required to appreciate the flap component.

  - SLAP 6 lesions usually have the appearance of a SLAP 3 labral tear on coronal plane images because the labrum is either displaced or fragmented in the 12 o'clock position. On corresponding sagittal images, it is the morphology of the tear pattern of the superior labral tissue displaced as a flap that constitutes the classification of a type 6 SLAP.

    - On MR, the diagnosis of a SLAP 6 lesion is uncommon as the morphology of the flap component is usually not appreciated on sagittal images. Thus the majority of these cases are interpreted as SLAP 3 lesions.

- Type 7 SLAP lesions
  - Caution should be used in diagnosing a type 7 SLAP lesion because on axial images, the two separate portions of a normal lax MGHL may mistakenly appear like a torn ligament.
    - SLAP 7 lesions are less commonly diagnosed on MRI because of the normal variation pattern described for the glenohumeral ligament. Arthroscopy is more accurate in the direct identification of a SLAP 7 tear pattern. MRI, however, would be able to identify the associated superior labral tear of the biceps labral complex without difficulty.

- Type 8 SLAP lesions
  - Type 8 SLAP lesions involve the posterosuperior and posteroinferior labrum in continuity with a SLAP 2 tear.

- Type 9 SLAP lesions
  - Coronal images display superior and inferior labral tearing in type 9 SLAP.
  - Axial images demonstrate anterior and posterior labral tearing, and sagittal images show circumferential tearing with or without associated glenoid rim sclerosis.

- Type 10 SLAP lesions
  - The type 10 SLAP tear presents as a SLAP lesion plus injury to the biceps pulley associated with medial subluxation of the biceps tendon (medial relative to the bicipital groove).
  - Sagittal images demonstrate pathology of the superior glenohumeral ligament, whereas axial images are used to assess medial subluxation (instability) of the biceps tendon.
  - Alternative orthopaedic terminology for a type 10 SLAP is defined by the association of a SLAP (2 or 3) lesion and a posterior inferior labral tear (e.g., Kim lesion)

- Important to clinically differentiate traumatic symptomatic SLAP tears from asymptomatic degeneration.
  - Chronic SLAP lesions demonstrate intermediate signal synovium or granulation tissue without acute free fluid when associated with labral pathology. A chronic SLAP lesion may be present in an asymptomatic shoulder.

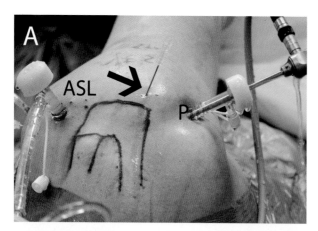

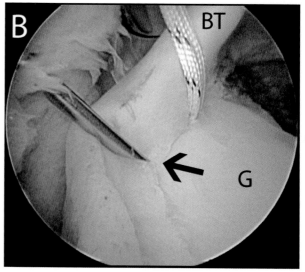

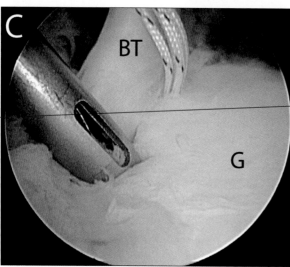

FIGURE 8.90   Port of Wilmington portal for posterior anchor in SLAP repair. (**A**) An external view shows placement of a spinal needle (*black arrow*) 1 cm lateral and 1 cm anterior the posterolateral corner of the acromion in a right shoulder. (**B**) Arthroscopic view from a posterior portal demonstrating the spinal needle's (*black arrow*) trajectory. (**C**) Placement of a posterior anchor for SLAP repair through the Port of Wilmington portal. ASL, anterosuperolateral portal; BT, biceps tendon; G, glenoid; P, posterior portal. (Reprinted from Burkhart S, Lo IK, Brady PC, Denard PJ. *The Cowboy's Companion: A Trail Guide for the Arthroscopic Shoulder Surgeon.* Philadelphia, PA: Lippincott Williams & Wilkins; 2012, with permission.)

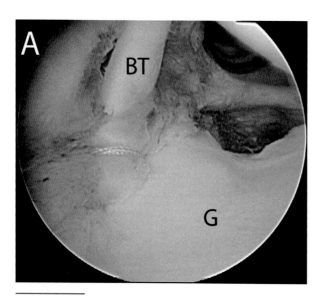

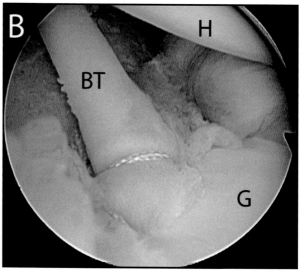

FIGURE 8.91   Final repair of a SLAP lesion in a right shoulder viewing from posterior. (**A**) Sutures encircle the labrum to stabilize the biceps root. (**B**) Retesting of the peel-back maneuver demonstrates a stable construct that does not displace medially. BT, biceps tendon; G, glenoid; H, humerus. (Reprinted from Burkhart S, Lo IK, Brady PC, Denard PJ. *The Cowboy's Companion: A Trail Guide for the Arthroscopic Shoulder Surgeon.* Philadelphia, PA: Lippincott Williams & Wilkins; 2012, with permission.)

9

Shoulder-Related Pathology Including Paralabral Cysts and Biceps Tendon

Shoulder-Related Pathology Including Paralabral Cysts and Biceps Tendon

Paralabral Cysts and Suprascapular Nerve Entrapment

Key Concepts

- ■ Paralabral cysts frequently communicate with a SLAP 2 or posterior-type SLAP 2 lesion.

- ■ A paralabral cyst usually coexists with a labral tear but may be associated with degenerative arthritis.

- ■ Suprascapular notch cysts are associated with edema or atrophy of the supraspinatus and infraspinatus.

- ■ Spinoglenoid notch cysts are associated with edema or atrophy of the infraspinatus.

- ■ Inferior paralabral cysts are associated with isolated denervation of the teres minor muscle.

■ Paralabral cysts may occur in any of the following locations:

- ■ Associated with the biceps labral complex in continuity with a SLAP 2 or posterior peel-back type SLAP 2 lesion involving the posterior superior labrum

- ■ The anterior labrum

- ■ The posterior labrum

- ■ The inferior labrum

■ Complex (anterior and posterior) paralabral cysts may be associated with multiple locations.

■ Paralabral cysts that extend to the spinoglenoid notch can produce atrophy of the infraspinatus and/or the supraspinatus muscles secondary to suprascapular nerve entrapment.[35,164,172]

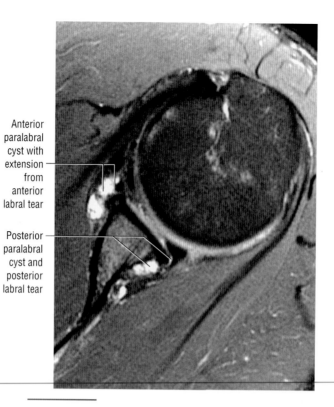

Anterior paralabral cyst with extension from anterior labral tear

Posterior paralabral cyst and posterior labral tear

FIGURE 9.1   Axial FS PD FSE image showing anterior and posterior paralabral cysts communicating with their respective labral tears.

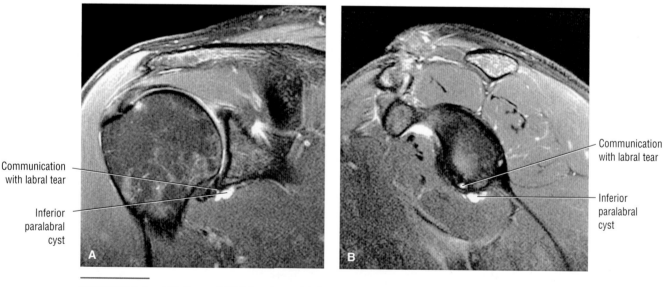

Communication with labral tear

Inferior paralabral cyst

Communication with labral tear

Inferior paralabral cyst

FIGURE 9.2   (**A**) Coronal FS PD FSE and (**B**) sagittal FS PD FSE images of an inferior paralabral cyst communicating with an anteroinferior-to-inferior labral tear.

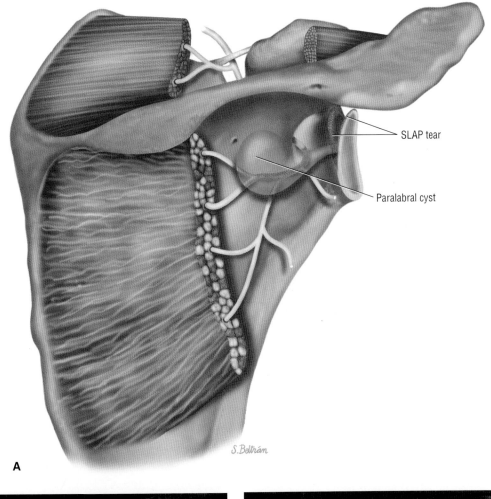

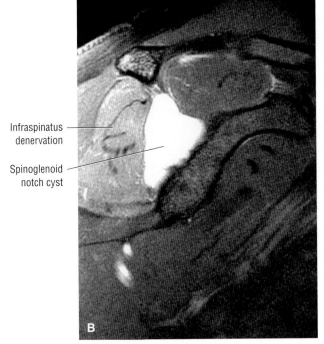

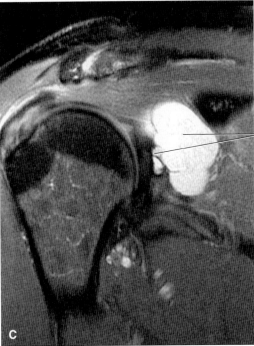

SLAP tear

Paralabral cyst

Infraspinatus denervation

Spinoglenoid notch cyst

Spinoglenoid notch paralabral cyst communicating with type 2 SLAP lesion

FIGURE 9.3 (**A**) Posterior coronal color illustration, (**B**) sagittal FS PD FSE image, and (**C**) coronal FS PD FSE image illustrate a spinoglenoid notch cyst in communication with a SLAP 2 tear and causing compression of the suprascapular nerve.

- ■ Intramuscular hemorrhage may mimic the appearance of a synovial ganglion.

- ■ There is a high correlation between paralabral cysts, which have a posterior location, and posterosuperior labral tears.[172,592]

    - ■ Cysts that communicate with and undermine the posterosuperior glenoid labrum or posterior SLAP 2 lesions may extend medially to the spinoglenoid notch

- ■ Anterior inferior paralabral cysts may be identified in communication with tears of the anterior inferior glenoid labrum.

    - ■ These small tears may not be appreciated on routine axial images and an abduction external rotation view may be necessary to display the IGLLC.

- ■ SLAP type 2 lesions may be visualized with fluid signal intensity communicating with a superiorly located paralabral cyst.

- ■ Anterior extension of a paralabral cyst through a labral tear can involve the subcoracoid space superior to the subscapularis bursa.

- ■ Posterosuperior paralabral cysts are thus commonly seen in association with posterior capsulolabral injuries including SLAP lesions[172,592] and typically involve the spinoglenoid notch.

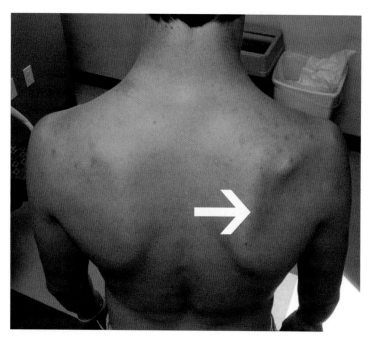

FIGURE 9.4 Clinical photo demonstrating infraspinatus atrophy (*white arrow*) in the right shoulder that resulted from a spinoglenoid cyst. Note the lack of supraspinatus atrophy on the right. The supraspinatus is preserved because the compression of the suprascapular nerve occurs at the spinoglenoid notch, distal to the supraspinatus innervation. (Reprinted from Burkhart S, Lo IK, Brady PC, Denard PJ. *The Cowboy's Companion: A Trail Guide for the Arthroscopic Shoulder Surgeon.* Philadelphia, PA: Lippincott Williams & Wilkins; 2012, with permission.)

- The spinoglenoid notch is located posterior to the suprascapular notch and is the location for the suprascapular nerve after it turns around the lateral edge of the scapular spine.[164]

- The inappropriate use of the term "suprascapular notch" to describe the location of all superior paralabral cysts may result in surgical exploration that is far anterior to the correct location of the cyst within the spinoglenoid notch.[553]

  - Most superior paralabral cysts originate in the spinoglenoid notch.

- At the level of the suprascapular fossa, the suprascapular nerve has passed through the suprascapular notch.

- Paralabral cysts that extend to the spinoglenoid notch can produce atrophy of the infraspinatus and/or the supraspinatus muscles secondary to suprascapular nerve entrapment.[35,164,172]

- Isolated infraspinatus atrophy is associated with more posteriorly located paralabral cysts of the spinoglenoid notch or occurs with spinoglenoid ligament entrapment.

- Proximal suprascapular nerve entrapment occurs with cysts located in the anterior suprascapular notch.

- Suprascapular nerve entrapment at the suprascapular notch also occurs secondary to a thickening or scarring of the transverse scapular ligament in conjunction with a tight, bony notch or by repetitive-use injuries at the shoulder.

- The suprascapular nerve has two motor branches that innervate the supraspinatus, in addition to sensory branches to the glenohumeral and acromioclavicular joints.

- Since the suprascapular nerve does not have a cutaneous sensory component, patients with isolated compression at the more posterior- and inferior-located spinoglenoid notch may experience painless muscle wasting of the infraspinatus.

- In contrast, compression of the suprascapular nerve proximally, at the suprascapular notch, is frequently associated with nonspecific shoulder pain involving both the supraspinatus and infraspinatus.

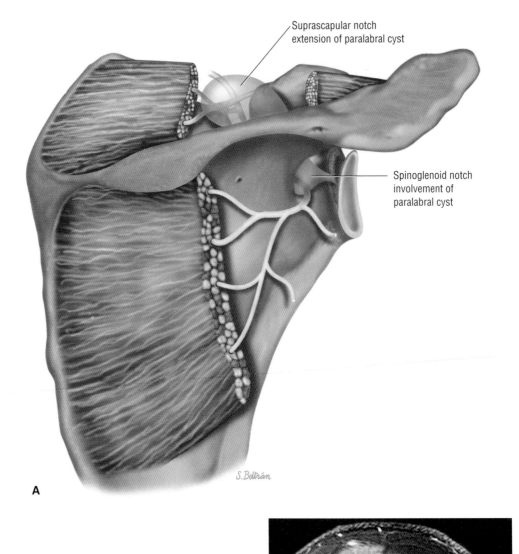

Suprascapular notch
extension of paralabral cyst

Spinoglenoid notch
involvement of
paralabral cyst

S.Beltrán

A

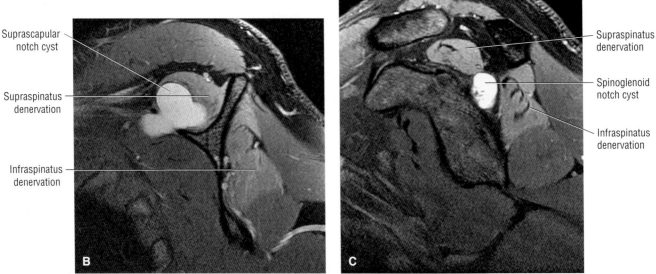

Suprascapular
notch cyst

Supraspinatus
denervation

Infraspinatus
denervation

B

Supraspinatus
denervation

Spinoglenoid
notch cyst

Infraspinatus
denervation

C

FIGURE 9.5   (**A**) Posterior coronal color graphic illustrating the combined denervation of the supraspinatus and infraspinatus muscles associated with paralabral cyst involvement affecting both the suprascapular notch anteriorly and the spinoglenoid notch posteriorly. MR characteristics can be seen on sagittal FS PD FSE images at the level of the suprascapular notch (**B**) and the spinoglenoid notch (**C**).

- This painful paralysis of both the supraspinatus and infraspinatus muscles occurs as the sensory fibers of the posterior glenohumeral joint capsule arise at the level of the suprascapular notch.

- The suprascapular nerve terminates by contributing two to four motor branches to the infraspinatus.

- Posterosuperior labral tears frequently develop paralabral cysts that extend into the spinoglenoid notch.

  - These cysts are located in proximity to the motor branches to the infraspinatus.

  - The suprascapular nerve is thus potentially constrained in one or two locations: the suprascapular notch (fixed by the transverse scapular ligament) and the spinoglenoid notch (fixed by the spinoglenoid ligament).[458]

- Paralabral cysts develop along the path of least resistance and therefore dissect along the fibrofatty tissue overlying the suprascapular nerve toward the spinoglenoid notch between the supraspinatus and infraspinatus muscles.[553]

  - They arise from interruptions in the integrity of the joint such as labral tears, capsular tears, or capsular diverticula.

- A paralabral cyst should be assumed to communicate with an adjacent labral tear unless it is far removed from the labrum.[602]

- As a result of compression of the suprascapular nerve, supraspinatus and infraspinatus muscle atrophy is seen in association with anteriorly located masses and proximal nerve entrapment.

- In the initial stage of suprascapular nerve compromise, edematous changes in the infraspinatus muscle are characterized by low to intermediate signal intensity on T1-weighted images and hyperintensity on fluid sensitive images.

- Chronic compression may lead to the development of fatty muscle atrophy.

- Paralabral cysts that are not directly related to the labrum may be associated with degenerative arthritis of the shoulder.

- They may also be associated with a symptomatic labral tear without nerve compression.

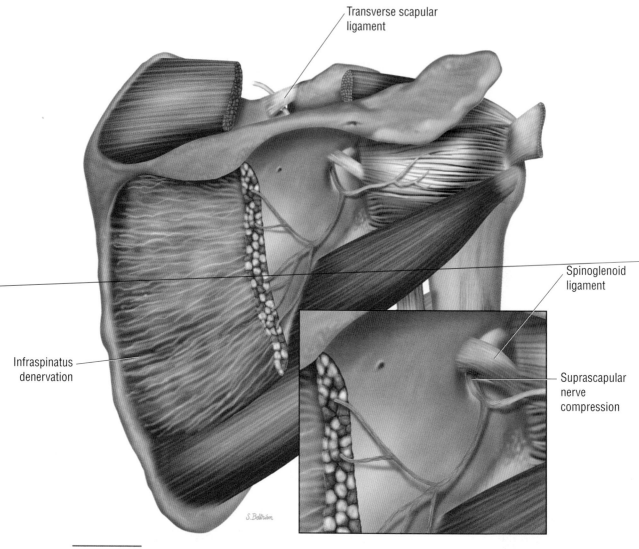

FIGURE 9.6   Selective or isolated infraspinatus denervation secondary to compression by a thickened spinoglenoid ligament. The suprascapular nerve and artery enter the supraspinatus fossa through the scapular notch by passing deep to the transverse scapular ligament. The suprascapular nerve enters the infraspinatus fossa by coursing lateral to the spinoglenoid notch. The lateral margin of the spinoglenoid notch is created by the fibrous band called the spinoglenoid ligament. The suprascapular nerve is relatively immobile in this area and thus susceptible to injury or compression by paralabral cysts. In extreme abduction and external rotation (in the throwing athlete, for example), the medial tendinous margin of the supraspinatus and infraspinatus can impinge against the lateral edge of the scapula spine. This results in compression of the infraspinatus branch of the suprascapular nerve. Painless atrophy of the infraspinatus muscle in volleyball players (attributed to contraction of the infraspinatus muscle during the volleyball serving action) involves neuropathy of the inferior branch of the suprascapular nerve.

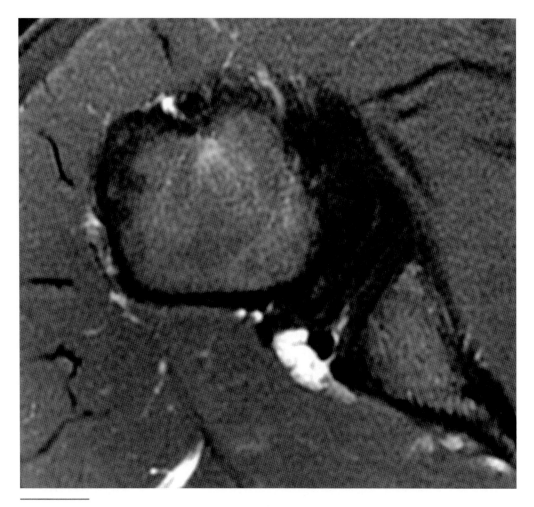

FIGURE 9.7   Discrete paralabral cyst in direct communication with the posterior inferior glenoid labral tear. The linear connection between the tear and the paralabral cyst is evident. Axial PD image.

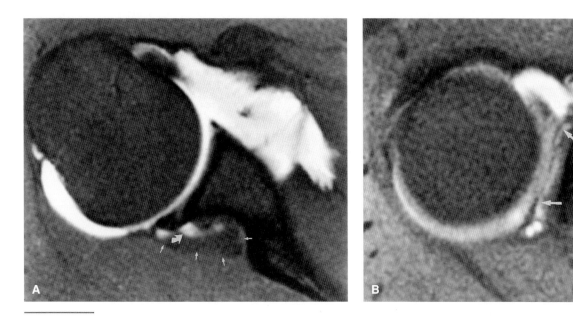

FIGURE 9.8   T1 FS axial MR arthrograms of paralabral cyst. (**A**) Partial filling (*curved arrow*) of a spinoglenoid notch cyst (*small straight arrows*) with intraarticular contrast. (**B**) Communication of the cyst with a SLAP type 2 lesion. The superior labrum is torn from anterior to posterior (*arrows*) as assessed on the axial image through the most superior aspect of the glenohumeral joint.

Clinical Profile of Paralabral Cysts

- Suprascapular nerve compression syndrome (pain and weakness of supraspinatus and infraspinatus muscles)

- SLAP lesions with associated anterosuperior, posterosuperior, or combined paralabral cysts

- Posterosuperior labral tears associated with spinoglenoid notch cysts, presenting as a deep ache or muscle tightness in the shoulder with progressive weakness

- Axillary nerve compression (weakness of the deltoid and teres minor associated with axillary nerve denervation), when the cyst extends inferiorly and dissects into the quadrilateral space

- Isolated teres minor muscle denervation exists when the teres minor branch of the axillary nerve is compressed by an inferior paralabral cyst.
    - Clicking or catching with pain in the cocking and acceleration phase of throwing (a deep ache in the posterior shoulder with progressive weakness indicates nerve compression)

Mechanisms of Injury in Paralabral Cysts Associated with SLAP Tears

- Trauma with a fall on the shoulder

- Traction injury

- Weight lifting (which is also associated with traction injury to the teres minor nerve branch of the axillary nerve, even in the absence of an inferior paralabral cyst)

- Sports emphasizing an overhead motion

- Initial treatment of a paraglenoid cyst is conservative, progressing to cyst aspiration or surgical release of the suprascapular ligament in symptomatic patients.

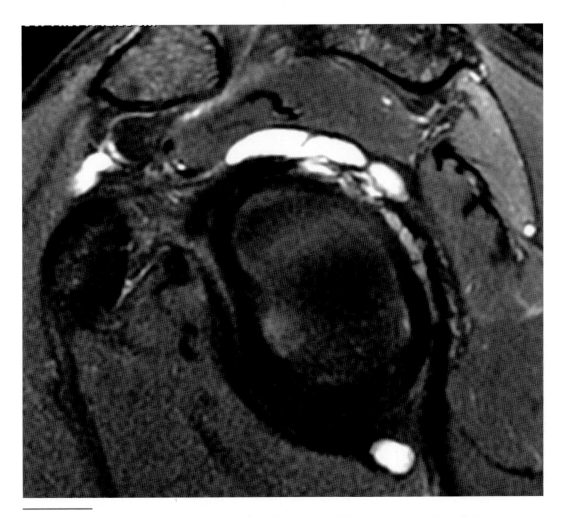

FIGURE 9.9 Continuity of paralabral cyst from the posterior labrum to the posterior inferior labrum in direct communication with the extension of a SLAP 8 lesion. The cysts occur adjacent to the underlying labral tear. There is subtle denervation of the infraspinatus muscle. The selective edema of the infraspinatus is the result of nerve involvement distal to the supraspinatus fossa as the suprascapular nerve passes around the base of the scapular spine or the spinoglenoid notch to supply the infraspinatus muscle. Sagittal FS PD DSE image.

Quadrilateral Space Syndrome

Key Concepts

- ■ The posterior branch of the axillary nerve courses adjacent to the inferior pole of the glenoid and inferior joint capsule and then divides into a branch to the teres minor muscle and a superolateral brachial cutaneous nerve branch.

- ■ The quadrilateral space syndrome is more commonly associated with denervation edema or atrophy restricted to the teres minor muscle, although the teres minor and deltoid are both supplied by the axillary nerve.

- ■ The quadrilateral space syndrome is an entrapment (compression) neuropathy of the axillary nerve in the quadrilateral space.[494,661]

  - ■ Fibrous bands more common cause compared to mass lesions or paralabral cysts for compression of the axillary nerve

- ■ Increased signal intensity within the teres minor and deltoid muscle indicates denervation on FS PD FSE or STIR images.

  - ■ The lateral cutaneous branch and the branch to the teres minor are closest to the glenoid rim and are most vulnerable.

- ■ Chronic fatty atrophy is best appreciated on T1- or PD-weighted images.

- ■ Compression of the distal branch of the axillary nerve and involvement of the posterior humeral circumflex artery is associated with:

  - ■ Proximal humeral and scapular fractures

  - ■ Posttraumatic fibrous bands

  - ■ Masses, including teres minor hypertrophy and lipomas

- ■ Posttraumatic axillary neuropathy

  - ■ Anterior shoulder dislocation with the compression of the nerve and the subscapularis muscle by the dislocated humeral head

  - ■ Proximal humeral fractures

  - ■ Direct trauma to the deltoid muscle

- ■ The axillary nerve normally innervates the teres minor, deltoid, and posterolateral cutaneous area of the upper arm and shoulder.

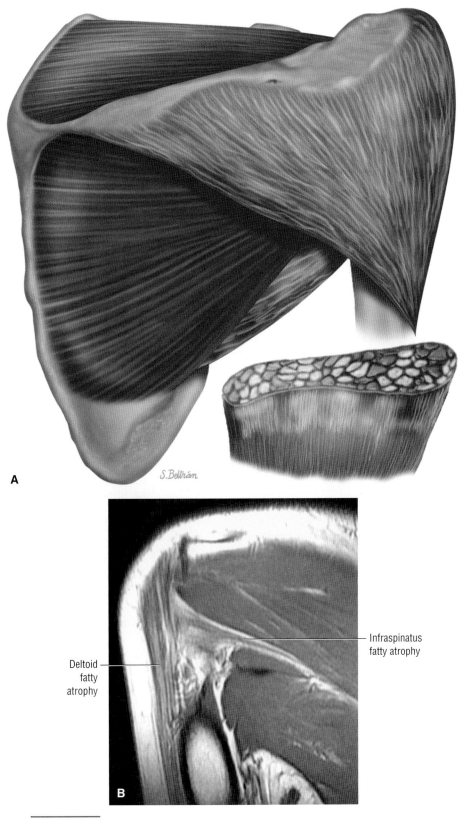

FIGURE 9.10 Quadrilateral space syndrome with denervation and fatty atrophy of the teres minor and deltoid in the throwing athlete. (**A**) Coronal illustration of teres minor and deltoid fatty atrophy. The axillary nerve is susceptible to entrapment by fibrous bands in the quadrilateral space when the arm is abducted and externally rotated. Selective involvement of the teres minor with posterior pain and tenderness may be present. (**B**) Coronal PD FSE image of fatty atrophy of both the deltoid and teres minor muscle groups.

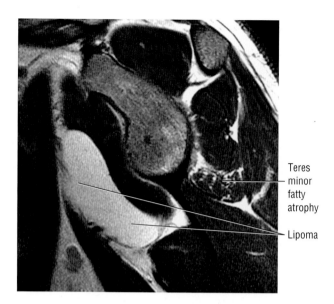

FIGURE 9.11   Sagittal PD FSE image of the quadrilateral space syndrome with isolated fatty atrophy of the teres minor associated with a space-occupying lipoma demonstrating fat signal intensity. The quadrilateral space, which contains the axillary nerve and posterior circumflex humeral artery, is bordered by the inferior border of the teres minor superiorly, the teres major inferiorly, the long head of the triceps brachii muscle medially, and the diaphysis of the humerus laterally.

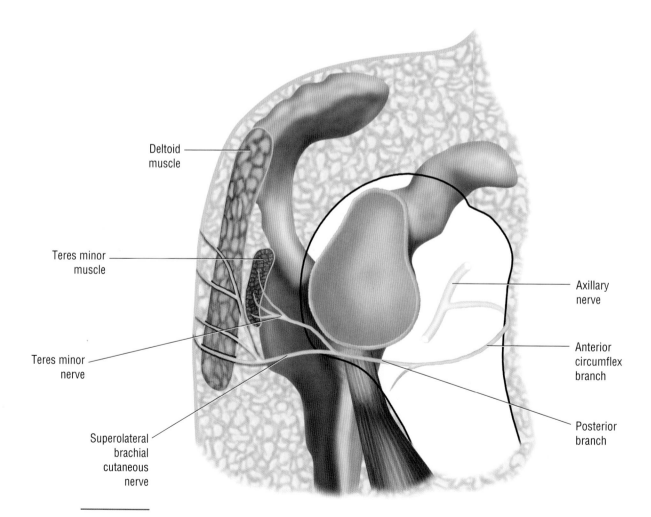

FIGURE 9.12   The normal course of the posterior branch of the axillary nerve, which divides into the nerve to the teres minor and a superolateral/brachial cutaneous nerve branch.

- Compression of the nerve and artery can result in ischemia and denervation. In the early and subacute phase, there may be an edematous muscle belly.

- Fatty atrophy of the deltoid and teres minor develops in the chronic phase.

- Athletes with pain on abduction and external rotation in the age range of 22 to 35 years are frequently affected.

- Associated abnormalities include:

    - Inferior labral tears with dissecting paralabral cysts

    - Lipomatous masses

    - Enlarged veins extending into the quadrilateral space

    - Fibrous bands

MR Findings

- The MR finding of chronic fatty atrophy of the teres minor and deltoid is not the most common presentation of imaging findings for quadrilateral space syndrome.

- The posterior branch of the axillary nerve course directly inferior and in close association with the inferior pole of the glenoid and shoulder joint capsule.

- The posterior branch divides into the nerve supplying the teres minor and superolateral brachial cutaneous nerve branch.

- The posterior branch of the axillary nerve is not only at risk for injury during capsular plication or internal shrinkage procedures but is also susceptible to compression by inferior paralabral cysts and axillary pouch pathology, including adhesive capsulitis and stretch injuries to the IGHL.

- Involvement of the superolateral brachial cutaneous nerve is associated with loss of sensation over the deltoid muscle.

- Isolated teres minor denervation may also be associated with nonstructural (relative to the axillary neurovascular structures) lesions, including rotator cuff injuries and traction of the axillary nerve of the of the teres minor branch resulting from a glenohumeral joint translation episode.

Treatment of Quadrilateral Space Syndrome

- ■ The treatment for neurapraxia (a transient episode of motor paralysis with little or no sensory or autonomic dysfunction) is conservative.

- ■ Relief of compression due to mass or fibrous bands, however, may be necessary.

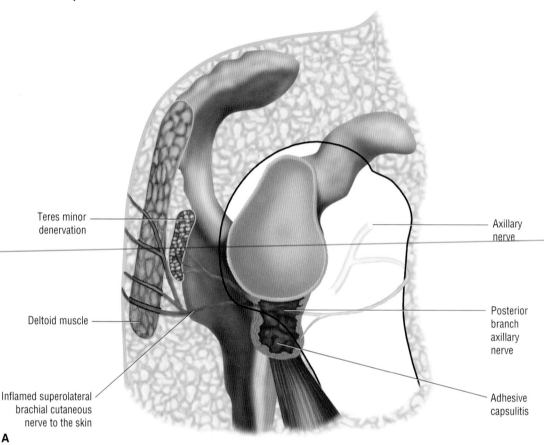

Teres minor denervation

Deltoid muscle

Inflamed superolateral brachial cutaneous nerve to the skin

Axillary nerve

Posterior branch axillary nerve

Adhesive capsulitis

A

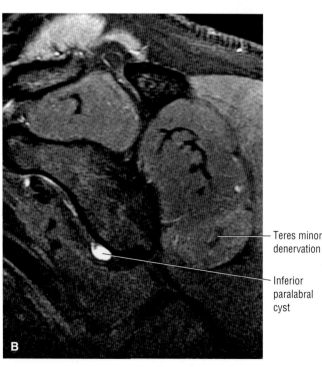

Teres minor denervation

Inferior paralabral cyst

B

FIGURE 9.13 (**A**) Teres minor denervation related to inferior capsular adhesive capsulitis. The thickened and inflamed inferior capsule is adjacent to the posterior branch of the axillary nerve. (**B**) Inferior paralabral cyst associated with teres minor hyperintensity on a sagittal FS PD FSE image.

Parsonage-Turner Syndrome

Key Concepts

- Parsonage-Turner syndrome is characterized by acute painful brachial neuritis.

- Supraspinatus and infraspinatus; supraspinatus, infraspinatus, and deltoid; and infraspinatus and teres minor are potential patterns of affected muscle groups.

- FS PD FSE images show all hyperintense muscles involved in the sagittal plane.

- The Parsonage-Turner syndrome is an acute brachial neuritis (acute shoulder pain described as intense and burning) or nontraumatic neuropathy involving an idiopathic denervation syndrome of the shoulder girdle musculature.[213]

- More than one nerve distribution may be involved, with denervation typically affecting mainly the lower motor neurons of the brachial plexus and/or individual nerves or nerve branches.

- The etiology is related to an immune-mediated inflammatory reaction against nerve fibers. Infection, surgery, trauma, childbirth, vaccinations, and systemic illness are all possible causes.

- In an associated rare digital form, the forearm, wrist, and hand may be involved.

- Denervation and swelling within the affected muscles are found in the early and subacute phase, which lasts 3 to 6 months.

- Fatty atrophy is seen in the chronic phase.

- Age range spans from 3 months to 74 years, with the majority of cases lasting up to 1 year.

- There is a 2 to 4:1 male predominance.

- Bilateral involvement may occur in up to one third of patients. Residual denervation is present in 10% to 20% of cases after 2 years.

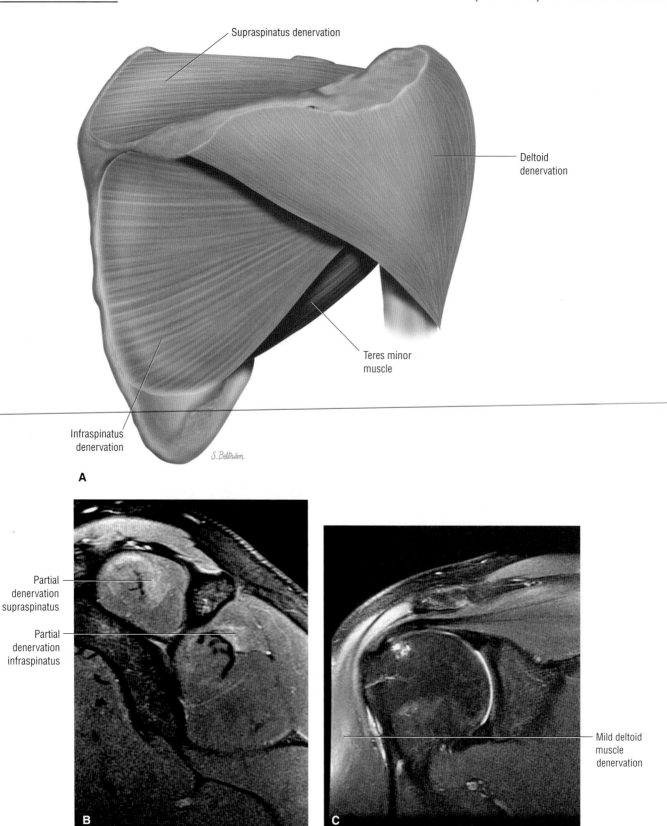

FIGURE 9.14 (**A**) Color posterior coronal illustration of Parsonage-Turner variation with denervation of the supraspinatus, infraspinatus, and deltoid (suprascapular and axillary nerve innervation). Sagittal (**B**) and coronal (**C**) FS PD FSE images showing subtle changes of Parsonage-Turner syndrome with denervation hyperintensity of the deltoid, supraspinatus, and infraspinatus muscles (**B**) and the deltoid muscle (**C**).

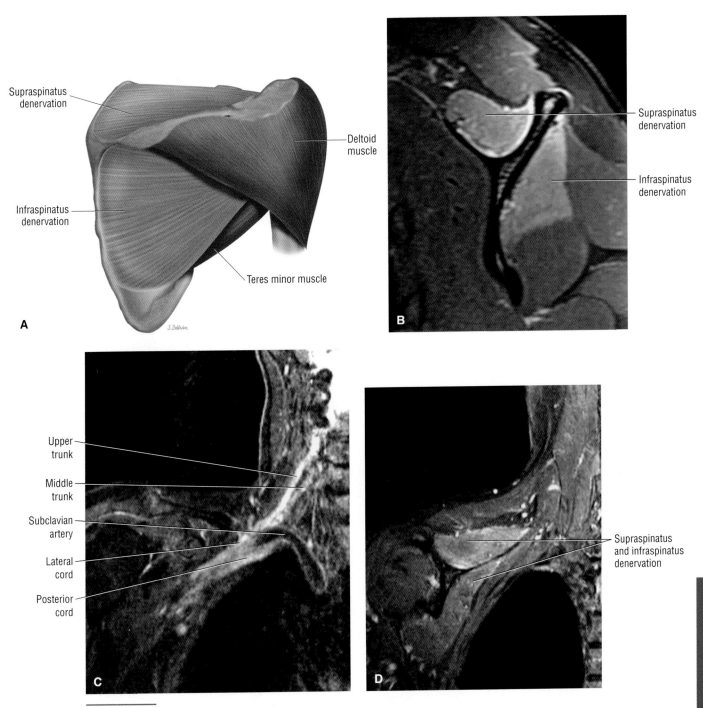

FIGURE 9.15 (**A**) Parsonage-Turner syndrome with denervation of the supraspinatus and infraspinatus muscles. (**B**) Sagittal FS PD FSE image with uniform supraspinatus and infraspinatus denervation without any associated suprascapular notch mass. The involvement of the supraspinatus and infraspinatus in idiopathic denervation is a common presentation of Parsonage-Turner. (**C**) Brachial plexus neuritis with hyperintensity of the upper and middle trunks. The suprascapular nerve is derived from the upper (superior) trunk. The upper or superior trunk is formed by the upper two roots (C5, C6). The brachial plexus network originates from the anterior primary rami of the C5 to T1 spinal nerves. (**D**) Corresponding coronal FS PD FSE sequence shows supraspinatus and infraspinatus denervation related to Parsonage-Turner syndrome as an acute brachial neuritis.

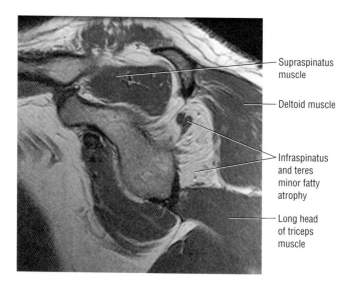

FIGURE 9.16 Chronic Parsonage-Turner syndrome with history of bilateral involvement. Fatty atrophy is demonstrated in the infraspinatus and teres minor on this sagittal PD FSE image. Parsonage-Turner syndrome is not usually associated with muscle fatty infiltration but more commonly demonstrates muscle atrophy with decreased muscle bulk.

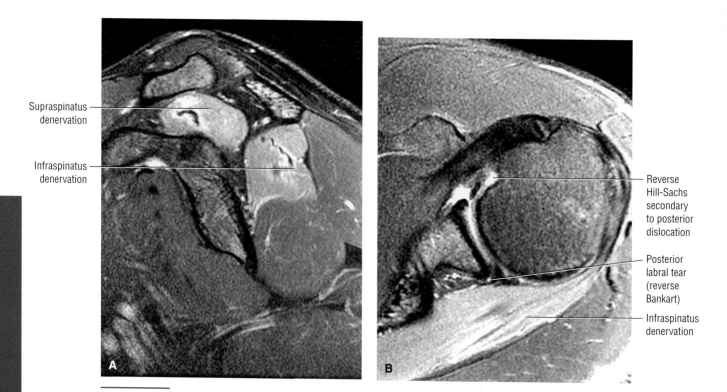

FIGURE 9.17 Posterior dislocation with suprascapular neurapraxia affecting the supraspinatus and infraspinatus muscles is seen on sagittal (**A**) and axial (**B**) FS PD FSE images. The MR appearance of supraspinatus and infraspinatus distribution could mimic Parsonage-Turner syndrome. The axillary nerve is usually at risk in anterior dislocations.

- MR examination of affected muscle groups demonstrates the following patterns:

    - Supraspinatus and infraspinatus muscles affected, indicating suprascapular nerve involvement

    - Supraspinatus, infraspinatus, and deltoid muscles affected, indicating suprascapular and axillary nerve involvement

    - Infraspinatus and teres minor muscles affected, indicating suprascapular and axillary nerve involvement

- In the acute and subacute phase, FS PD FSE and STIR images are helpful in identifying hyperintense diffuse muscle edema affecting the supraspinatus and infraspinatus muscles (suprascapular nerve involvement) and the deltoid muscle (axillary nerve involvement).

    - Chronic muscle changes may result in an overall decrease in muscle bulk in addition to fatty changes and/or atrophy within the muscle proper.

    - Resolving Parsonage-Turner may show patchy hyperintense signal in the involved muscle groups as assessed on sagittal images using fluid sensitive sequences.

- Rarely, denervation of the supraspinatus, infraspinatus, and teres minor muscles is caused by direct neurapraxia associated with a traumatic posterior dislocation, and this possibility should also be considered in the differential diagnosis of unilateral Parsonage-Turner syndrome.

- Parsonage-Turner syndrome can resemble a variety of other clinical entities:

    - Rotator cuff pathology

    - Cervical radiculopathy

    - Spinal cord tumor

    - Peripheral nerve compression

Biceps Tendon

Key Concepts

- The biceps tendon origin includes the posterosuperior labrum and supraglenoid tubercle medial to the BLC.

- The CHL–SGHL complex and not the transverse humeral ligament provides the stability of the biceps tendon in the intertubercular sulcus (groove).

- Intraarticular biceps tendinosis may be overestimated on sagittal images secondary to the magic-angle effect.

- Biceps tenosynovitis is visualized with hyperintense fluid or intermediate to hyperintense signal in the presence of thickened synovium.

- Biceps tendon ruptures occur at the biceps anchor or within the rotator cuff interval.

Related Anatomy

- The origin of the biceps tendon is most commonly at the posterosuperior glenoid labrum, although a variable portion may also be attached directly to the supraglenoid tubercle.[492]

- The primary attachment of the intraarticular biceps is to the superior portion of the labrum (at the BLC), prior to its attachment to the supraglenoid tubercle.

- Although the biceps tendon usually has a significant posterior superior labral attachment at the BLC, there are variations (in which the biceps may be attached equally to both the anterior and posterior aspects of the superior labrum or may have a major contribution to the anterosuperior labrum).

  - These variations may affect the relative anterior-to-posterior extent of the biceps labral sulcus when viewed on coronal MR images.[600]

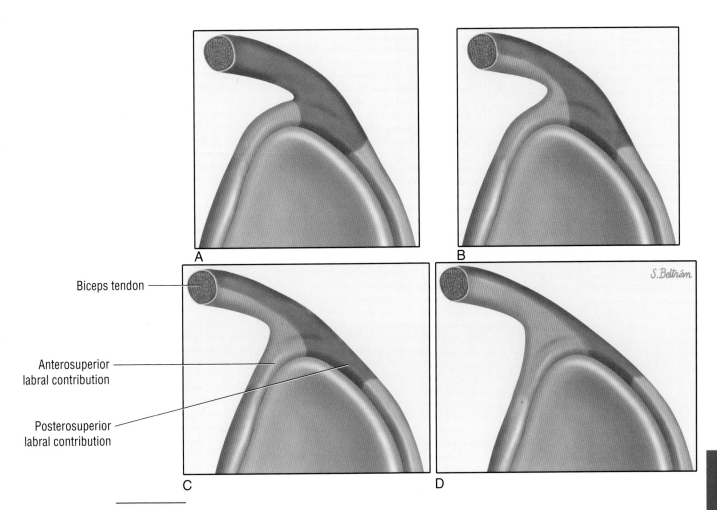

Biceps tendon

Anterosuperior labral contribution

Posterosuperior labral contribution

S. Beltrán

FIGURE 9.18 Variation in the biceps tendon contribution to the BLC. These variations include (**A**) an exclusive contribution to the posterosuperior labrum, (**B**) a primary contribution to the posterosuperior labrum and secondary involvement of the anterosuperior labrum, (**C**) equal contribution to the anterosuperior and posterosuperior labrum, and (**D**) a primary contribution to the anterosuperior labrum and secondary contribution to the posterosuperior labrum.

- The tendon of the long head of the biceps is divided into two zones, a traction zone of normal tendon and a sliding zone, which is the fibrocartilaginous portion of the biceps tendon in contact with the bicipital groove.

- The vascularity of the biceps tendon is decreased in the sliding zone, which has no vessels on the humeral side.

- A mesotendon may be present, arising from the posterolateral aspect of the groove, which is associated with the extra-articular biceps tendon.

- The position of the arm determines the extent of the intraarticular portion of the biceps tendon.

    - Intraarticular length of the LHBT is increased with the arm in adduction and neutral rotation.

- In adduction and extension, the maximal amount of biceps tendon is located intraarticularly.

    - With the arm in extreme abduction, the least amount of biceps tendon is located within the joint.

- The rotator interval between the supraspinatus and subscapularis tendons contains both the coracohumeral (CHL) and superior glenohumeral (SGHL) ligaments.

- The intraarticular biceps tendon is stabilized (preventing medial biceps dislocation) by the pulley or sling created by the CHL–SGHL complex.

    - The biceps pulley functions to protect the biceps tendon against anterior shearing stress.

■ **Components of the biceps pulley**

  ■ The CHL attachments include an origin from the lateral border of the coracoid and two bands of insertion: a lateral band that extends to the anterior edge of the supraspinatus and greater tuberosity and a medial band that extends to the superior edge of the subscapularis, transverse humeral ligament, and lesser tuberosity.

  ■ The SGHL attachments include an origin from the superior labrum, adjacent to the supraglenoid tubercle, and an insertion into the superolateral aspect of the lesser tuberosity, blending with the medial fibers of the CHL in the anterior aspect of the biceps sling.

  ■ The SGHL also crosses the floor of the interval, whereas the CHL forms the roof or bursal side of the rotator interval.

  ■ Both the supraspinatus and subscapularis tendons contribute to the formation of a sheath that surrounds the biceps at the proximal aspect of the bicipital groove.

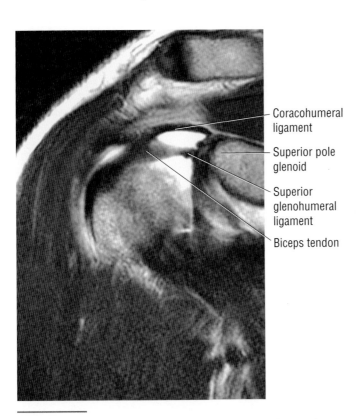

Coracohumeral ligament
Superior pole glenoid
Superior glenohumeral ligament
Biceps tendon

FIGURE 9.19 Coracohumeral and superior glenohumeral ligaments coursing laterally toward the entrance of the intertubercular groove, forming the stabilizing biceps pulley within the rotator cuff interval as seen on a coronal T2 FSE image.

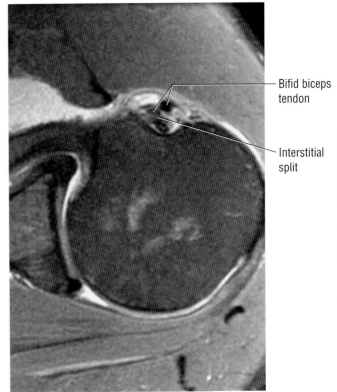

Bifid biceps tendon
Interstitial split

FIGURE 9.20 Axial FS PD FSE image showing the bifid biceps tendon with interstitial split of the posterior extra-articular component.

- In the intertubercular sulcus, the transverse humeral ligament is either absent or too weak to provide stability to the biceps.

- The transverse humeral ligament is not a distinct identifiable structure; instead, it represents a continuation of fibers of the subscapularis tendon with contributions from the supraspinatus tendon and the coracohumeral ligaments.[187]

- Within the groove itself, the falciform ligament, which is a tendinous expansion of the sternocostal portion of the pectoralis major muscle, helps to contain the biceps tendon.

- Interstitial splitting of a bifid biceps tendon may result in the appearance of three structures in the bicipital groove.

- The LHBT may end in two or, in rare cases, three tendons inserting onto the supraglenoid tubercle.

- The biceps brachii may also have three muscle bellies:
  - The long head
  - The short head
  - The third head

FIGURE 9.21 Inspection of the biceps tendon must include the intertubercular groove portion. This is inspected by placing a probe over the top of the biceps tendon and drawing the intertubercular groove portion into the joint. (**A**) Shows a normal-appearing biceps tendon. (**B**) When the intertubercular groove portion is drawn into the joint with a probe, a marked amount of synovitis is recognized. (**C**) Again, the biceps tendon appears to be normal in the intraarticular portion. (**D**) When a probe is used to draw in the intertubercular groove portion, a significant partial tear is detected. (Reprinted from Miniaci A, Iannotti JP, Williams GR, Zuckerman, JD. *Disorders of the Shoulder: Sports Injuries.* 3rd ed. Philadelphia, PA: Lippincott Williams & Wilkins; 2014, with permission.)

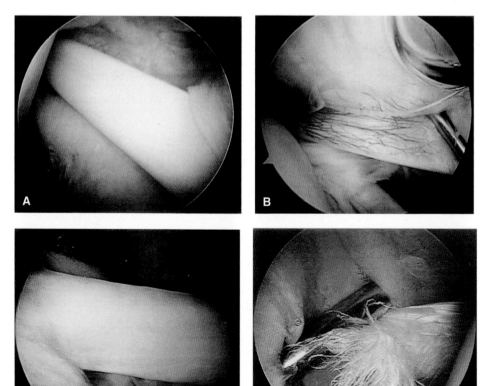

Biceps Tendinosis and Tenosynovitis

- Degeneration of the LHBT may occur as a result of chronic microtrauma or acute traumatic injury.[492]

- FS PD FSE images typically show thickening and increased signal intensity of the biceps tendon within the rotator interval or bicipital groove.

- Associated tenosynovitis may lead to an altered gliding mechanism of the biceps tendon sheath.

- In tenosynovitis, there is a disproportionate increase in the amount of fluid in the bicipital sheath relative to the volume of glenohumeral fluid.

- Tenosynovitis of the biceps is associated with a variety of inflammatory or infectious processes of the glenohumeral joint, including:
    - Rheumatoid arthritis
    - Osteoarthritis (or osteochondromatosis of the shoulder and biceps tendon sheath)
    - Hemodialysis arthropathy
    - Crystalline arthritis

- Biceps tendinosis accompanies rotator cuff disease, especially impingement.

- When the anterior cuff is torn, the biceps is impinged upon by exposure to the acromion through the rotator cuff tear gap.

- Biceps tendon degeneration may occur in conditions that cause biceps instability (the spectrum of pulley lesions of the rotator cuff interval) and in the throwing athlete with chronic microtrauma and shearing forces.

- Tendinosis of the biceps is associated with the following lesions:
    - Pulley lesions of the rotator interval
    - Anterosuperior impingement (ASI)
    - Posterior peel-back lesions in throwing athletes
    - SLAP lesions
    - Biceps tenosynovitis

- Patients with biceps tendinosis present with upper arm pain or shoulder pain often radiating into the upper arm, especially in overhead athletes.

- The typical complaint is of dull anterior shoulder pain especially with lifting and elevated pushing or pulling. Impingement signs are often positive.

- Pain can often be reproduced on physical examination with tests such as Yergason's test (bicipital groove pain with resisted supination), Speed's bicipital resistance test, and O'Brien's test (an active compression test to entrap the anterosuperior labrum and demonstrate SLAP lesions).

■ Biceps lesions have been classified into three types based on their pathoanatomy:[492]

    ■ Type A is impingement tendinitis (tendinosis).

    ■ Type B is subluxation and/or dislocation of the biceps tendon.

    ■ Type C is attritional tendinitis (tendinosis).

■ Impingement tendinitis is associated with impingement syndrome and rotator cuff disease.

■ The biceps is exposed to the rigid coracoacromial arch in the presence of a full thickness rotator cuff tear. Impingement tendinitis is the most common cause of biceps tendinitis (tendinosis).

■ Lesions of the rotator cuff interval that involve the CHL–SGHL complex (as isolated disorders or in combination with tears of the supraspinatus and subscapularis tendons) are associated with subluxation and dislocation of the biceps tendon. Inflammation and fraying of the biceps tendon occur with the spectrum of pulley lesions associated with biceps instability.

■ Attrition tendinitis is rare and represents a primary biceps tendon lesion that occurs within the bicipital groove.

■ Stenosis of the bicipital groove results in attrition and degeneration of the biceps tendon.

■ Inflammation of the biceps sheath is associated with hypertrophic spurs and further narrowing of a tight canal.

■ Biceps lesions have also been classified based on their anatomic location, including:

    ■ The biceps origin

    ■ The rotator interval

    ■ The rotator cuff (lesions associated with rotator cuff tears)

■ Biceps origin lesions include SLAP tears, which may be associated with extension into the biceps tendon (type 4).

■ Interval lesions have been subdivided into biceps instability lesions and isolated rupture of the biceps.

■ Both subluxation and dislocation (no contact between the LHBT and the bicipital groove) of the biceps tendon can occur in association with rotator cuff tears, in addition to tendinitis and tendon rupture.

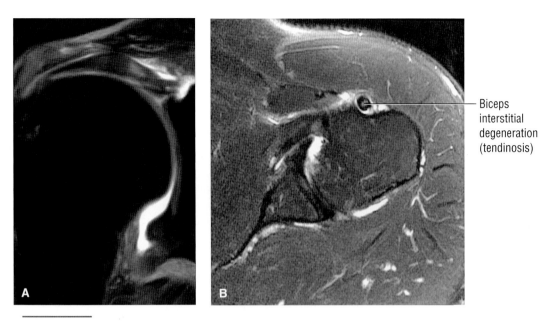

FIGURE 9.22   (**A**) Biceps tendinosis with thickening and increased signal intensity within the substance of the intraarticular biceps can be seen on this coronal FS PD FSE image. (**B**) Extra-articular biceps tendon with interstitial degeneration is seen on this axial FS PD FSE image.

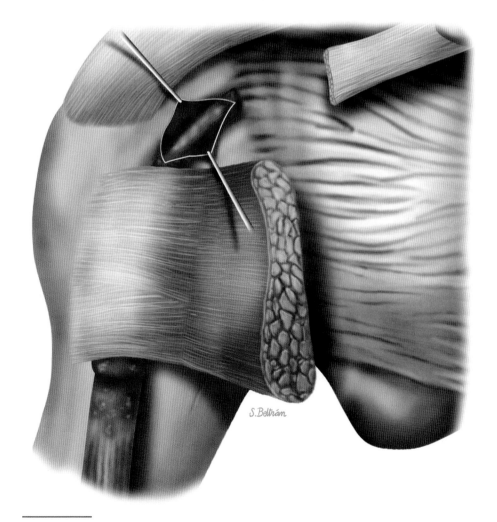

FIGURE 9.23   Biceps tenosynovitis with inflammation of the proximal biceps tendon sheath. A positive Speed's test (downward force applied to the arm with the elbow extended and forearm supinated) with upper anterior arm and shoulder pain is associated with biceps tendon inflammation.

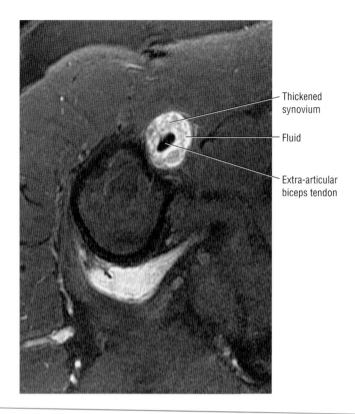

FIGURE 9.24 Axial FS PD FSE image showing thickened intermediate synovium with hyperintense fluid surrounding the biceps tendon in severe tenosynovitis. Disproportionate fluid in the biceps tendon sheath relative to the glenohumeral joint and or the presence of intermediate signal intensity synovium is associated with tenosynovitis.

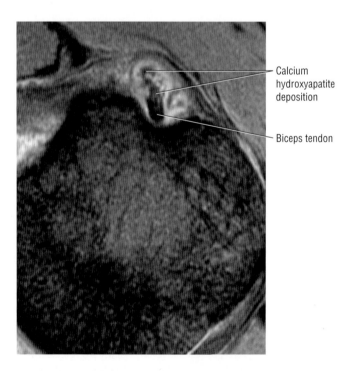

FIGURE 9.25 Calcium hydroxyapatite deposition involving the proximal biceps sheath. Calcific tendinitis may involve the biceps at its attachment to the superior pole of the glenoid or distal to the glenohumeral joint at the junction of the tendon and muscle. Small deposits are characteristic at the level of the proximal humeral diaphysis and occur anterior, medial, or lateral to the biceps tendon, as seen on this axial T2* GRE image.

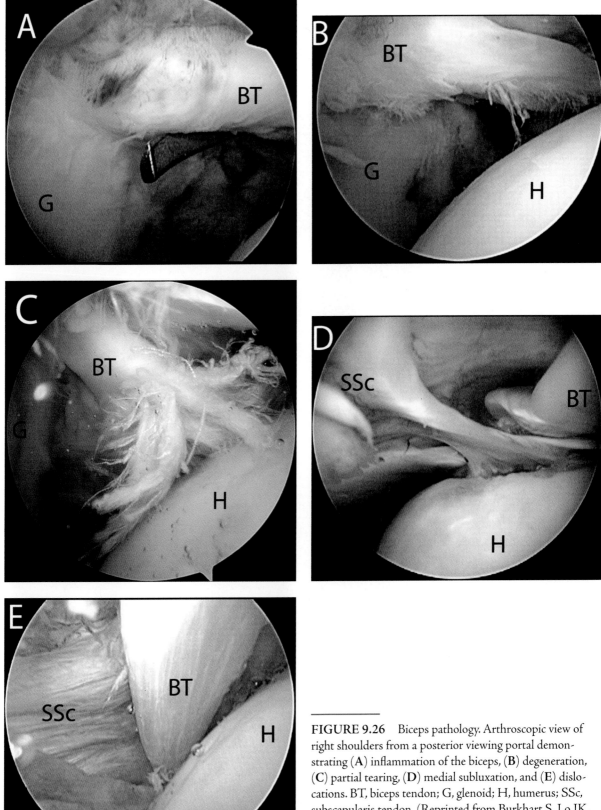

FIGURE 9.26 Biceps pathology. Arthroscopic view of right shoulders from a posterior viewing portal demonstrating (**A**) inflammation of the biceps, (**B**) degeneration, (**C**) partial tearing, (**D**) medial subluxation, and (**E**) dislocations. BT, biceps tendon; G, glenoid; H, humerus; SSc, subscapularis tendon. (Reprinted from Burkhart S, Lo IK, Brady PC, Denard PJ. *The Cowboy's Companion: A Trail Guide for the Arthroscopic Shoulder Surgeon*. Philadelphia, PA: Lippincott Williams & Wilkins; 2012, with permission.)

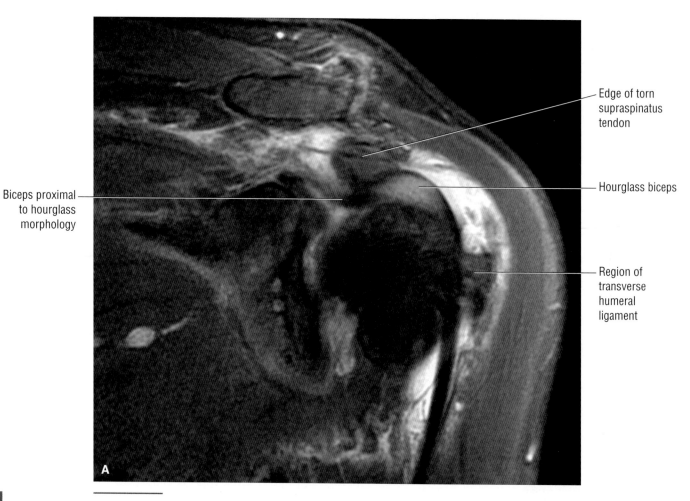

Biceps proximal to hourglass morphology

Edge of torn supraspinatus tendon

Hourglass biceps

Region of transverse humeral ligament

FIGURE 9.27   Hourglass biceps tendon with severe tendinosis of the intraarticular biceps occurring adjacent to the entrance of the bicipital groove. The biceps tendon immediately adjacent to the superior glenoid tubercle is tapered with normal morphology. The hourglass morphology is characterized by tendon enlargement and convexity to its margins with intrasubstance degeneration. These changes occur proximal to the transverse ligament. The hourglass biceps tendon represents a hypertrophic tendinopathy that may be associated with entrapment of the LHBT within the gleno-humeral joint. Locking of the shoulder may occur as the hourglass biceps no longer slides through the bicipital groove. (**A**) Coronal FS PD image.

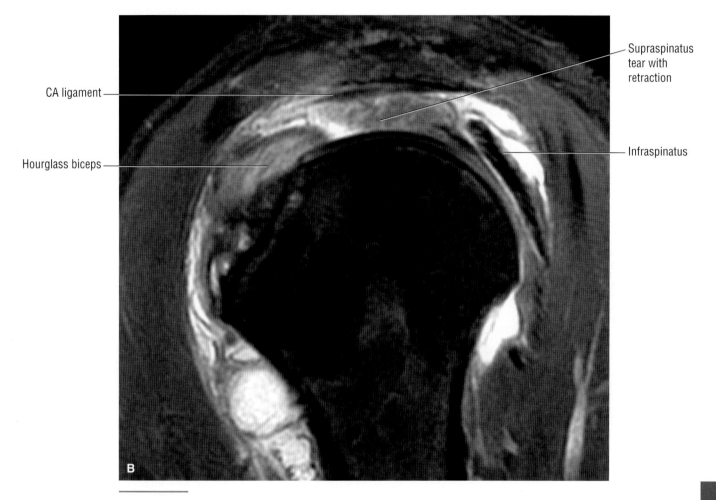

CA ligament

Hourglass biceps

Supraspinatus tear with retraction

Infraspinatus

FIGURE 9.27 *(Continued)* (**B**) Sagittal FS PD. With incarceration of the LHBT there may be associated SLAP lesions and chondral abrasions of the humeral head. The morphology of the bicipital groove (hypertrophy or stenosis) and associated inflammation are contributory to entrapment of the tendon. The sagittal image demonstrates the anterior to posterior elongation as well as the increased tendon diameter. Tendinosis signal intensity is intermediate and diffuse within the enlarged segment of the biceps tendon.

FIGURE 9.28   Empty bicipital groove resulting from distal retraction of the biceps tendon. Coronal FS PD.

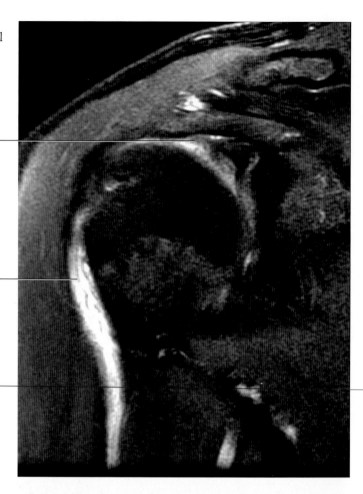

Stump of torn intraarticular biceps

Empty groove

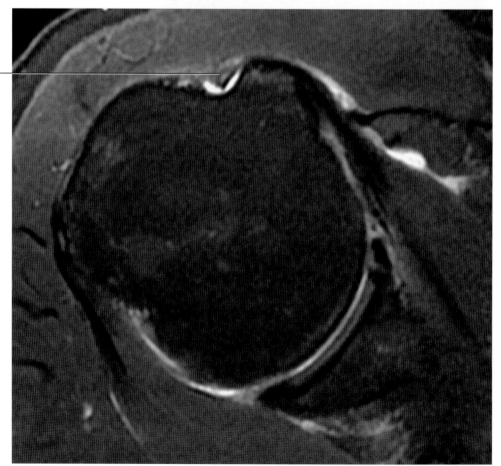

Reduced diameter of extra-articular biceps tendon

FIGURE 9.29   Partial tear of the biceps with attenuated cross-sectional diameter of the biceps tendon in its extra-articular course. Axial FS PD.

Biceps Tendon Rupture

- Biceps tendon rupture occurs at the top of the bicipital groove, usually in patients older than 40 years of age, and is often attributed to the spectrum of shoulder impingement.

  - Biceps degeneration and progression to biceps rupture can also exist as a primary pathology independent of subacromial impingement.

- Biceps tendon pathology is frequently associated with subscapularis tendon tears.

- Pure musculotendinous junction ruptures are rare and are associated with violent trauma.

- Biceps rupture may also occur as a complication of proximal humeral fractures, especially if impingement occurs at the osseous bicipital groove.

- Although biceps tendon tears are most common in the rotator interval, they may also occur adjacent to the biceps anchor.

- There may be a proximal stump extending from the supraglenoid tubercle.

- The biceps tendon tear may be associated with retraction of the tendon and absence of both the intraarticular portion and proximal extra-articular portion of the biceps.

- Posterior dislocation and entrapment of the long head of the biceps tendon is rare and is associated with anterior shoulder dislocation.[572]

  - Tears of the supraspinatus, infraspinatus, and subscapularis tendons allow the biceps to displace in a lateral direction over the greater tuberosity and posterior to the humeral head.

  - The entrapped biceps tendon may prevent reduction of the humeral head.

- LHBT rupture can be related to friction produced by the rough surface of the bicipital groove.

  - LHBT vulnerable proximally where the tendon courses medially, changing direction at a right angle over the sharp osseous edge of the inlet as it enters the glenohumeral joint

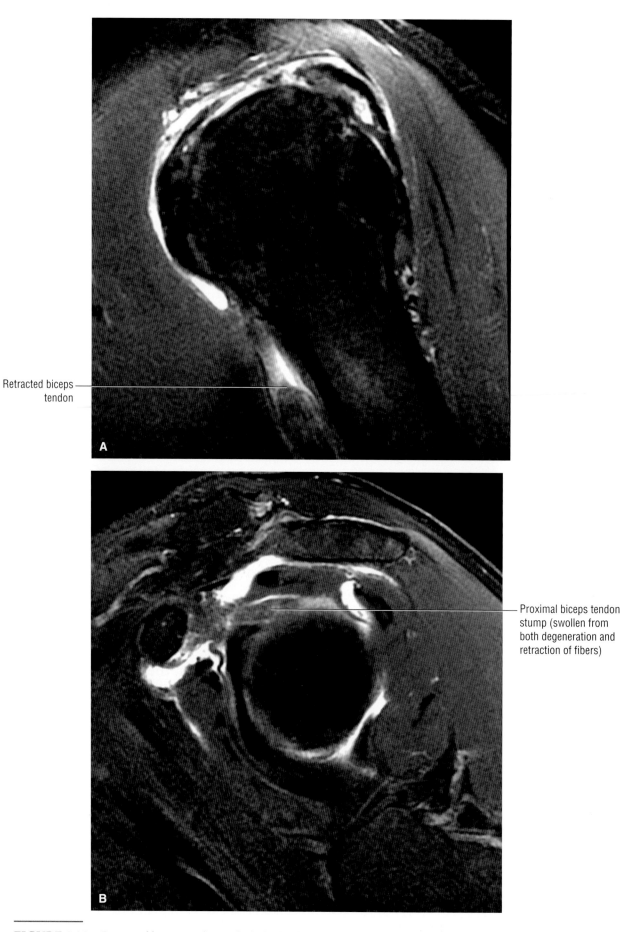

Retracted biceps
tendon

Proximal biceps tendon
stump (swollen from
both degeneration and
retraction of fibers)

FIGURE 9.30   Retracted biceps tendon with the bulk of the biceps identified below the subscapularis. The proximal stump is visualized deep to the supraspinatus tendon on the sagittal plane. (**A,B**) Sagittal FS PD. Prior to rupture the degenerative biceps tendon may become swollen as its tendon fibers breakdown within a sleeve of reactive surrounding synovium.

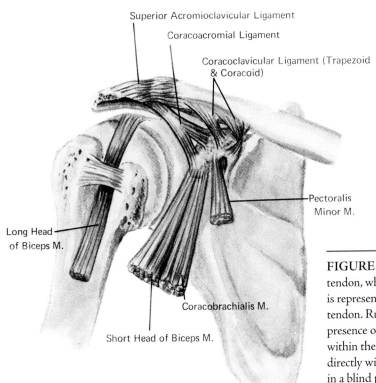

Superior Acromioclavicular Ligament

Coracoacromial Ligament

Coracoclavicular Ligament (Trapezoid & Coracoid)

Pectoralis Minor M.

Long Head of Biceps M.

Coracobrachialis M.

Short Head of Biceps M.

FIGURE 9.31 Color illustration of the long head of the biceps tendon, which is intraarticular but extra synovial. The proximal biceps is represented by both the short head and long head of the biceps tendon. Ruptures almost always involve the LHBT component. The presence of tenosynovitis as detected on MRI correlates with fluid within the synovial sheath of the biceps tendon which communicates directly with the glenohumeral joint. The biceps synovial sheath ends in a blind pouch at the distal end of the bicipital groove. (Modified from DePalma AF. *Surgery of the Shoulder*. 3rd ed. Philadelphia, PA: JB Lippincott; 1983.)

■ Neer classifies ruptures of the long head of the biceps tendon into three types:

   ■ Type 1 is tendon rupture without retraction.

   ■ Type 2 is tendon rupture with partial recession.

   ■ Type 3 is a self-attaching rupture without retraction.

■ Clinical diagnosis of a self-attaching long head rupture without retraction is difficult, and these types of injuries are usually identified at the time of rotator cuff repair.

■ Absence of the biceps tendon on axial images through the bicipital groove or on sagittal images is diagnostic.

■ A bifid biceps tendon may be mistaken for a tear that splits the biceps tendon longitudinally.

■ A bifid biceps tendon is more likely to be visualized throughout all axial images in the glenohumeral joint and extends below the bony glenoid.

■ A longitudinally split biceps tendon is more commonly restricted to a segment of the superior biceps tendon.

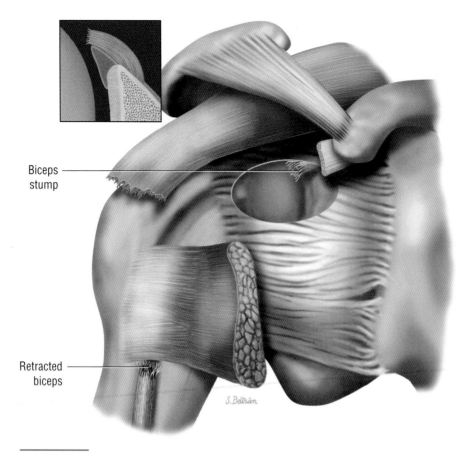

Biceps
stump

Retracted
biceps

S. Beltrán

FIGURE 9.32   Coronal anterior view color illustration of rupture of the intraarticular biceps at the BLC adjacent to the biceps anchor.

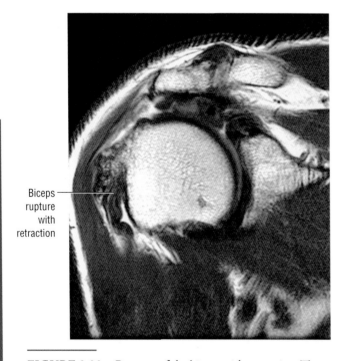

Biceps
rupture
with
retraction

FIGURE 9.33   Rupture of the biceps with retraction. The edge of the torn biceps tendon is visualized as a redundant structure in the groove. Coronal T2 FS MR is especially useful in distinguishing between retraction and partial recession (retraction) from a self-attaching but nonretracted biceps.

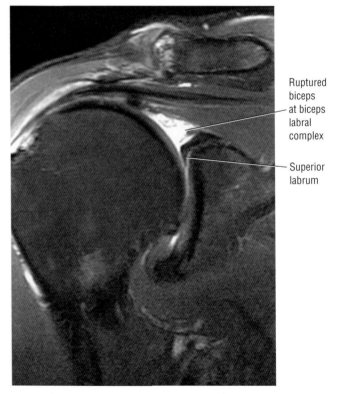

Ruptured
biceps
at biceps
labral
complex

Superior
labrum

FIGURE 9.34   Coronal FS PD FSE image with biceps rupture at the supraglenoid tubercle. The LHBT may rupture as part of the spectrum of SLAP lesions.

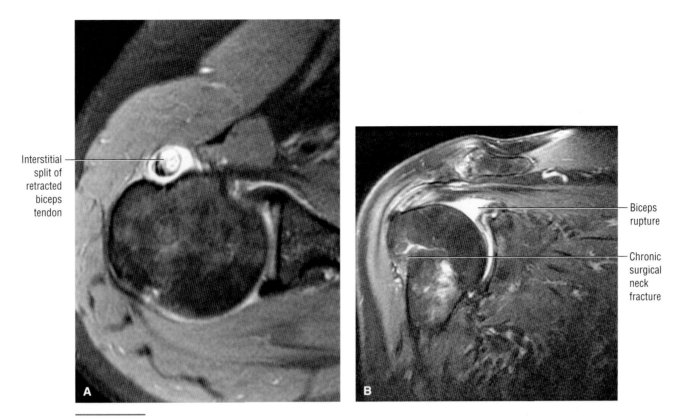

FIGURE 9.35 (**A**) Severe interstitial split of the biceps tendon involving the extra-articular course of the tendon split is hyperintense on this axial FS PD FSE image. (**B**) Corresponding biceps tendon rupture and retraction associated with chronic proximal humeral surgical neck fracture are seen on a coronal FS PD FSE image.

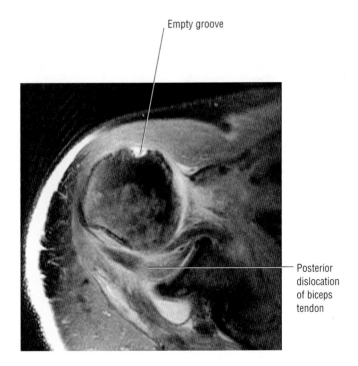

FIGURE 9.36 Axial FS PD FSE image of posterior dislocation of the biceps tendon posterior to the humeral head and biceps labral complex. There is an associated complete rupture of the rotator cuff. The bicipital groove is empty and the biceps tendon is posteriorly directed relative to the humeral head and entrapped.

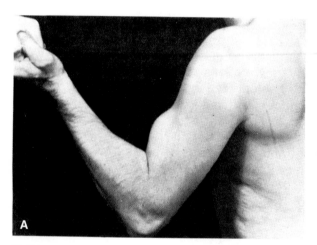
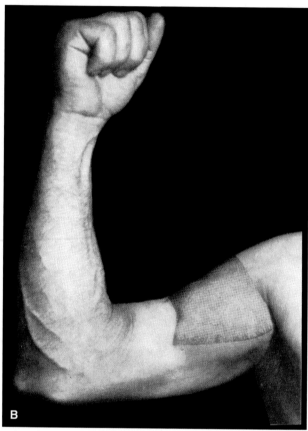

FIGURE 9.37 (**A**) Rupture of the long head of the biceps tendon; the rupture occurred at the supra-glenoid tubercle. When the supinated forearm is flexed against resistance, the biceps muscle mass forms a bulge in the lower part of the arm. The characteristic "popeye sign" is associated with proximal tendon rupture with the distal retraction of the biceps muscle. The retracted muscle may be mobile (unfixed) or fixed. (**B**) Rupture of the biceps muscle at the lower musculotendinous junction shown for comparison. When the muscle is contracted, the muscle mass moves proximally. Note the flattened areas in the lower part of the arm below the bulging muscle. (A and B modified from DePalma AF. *Surgery of the Shoulder.* 3rd ed. Philadelphia, PA: JB Lippincott; 1983.)

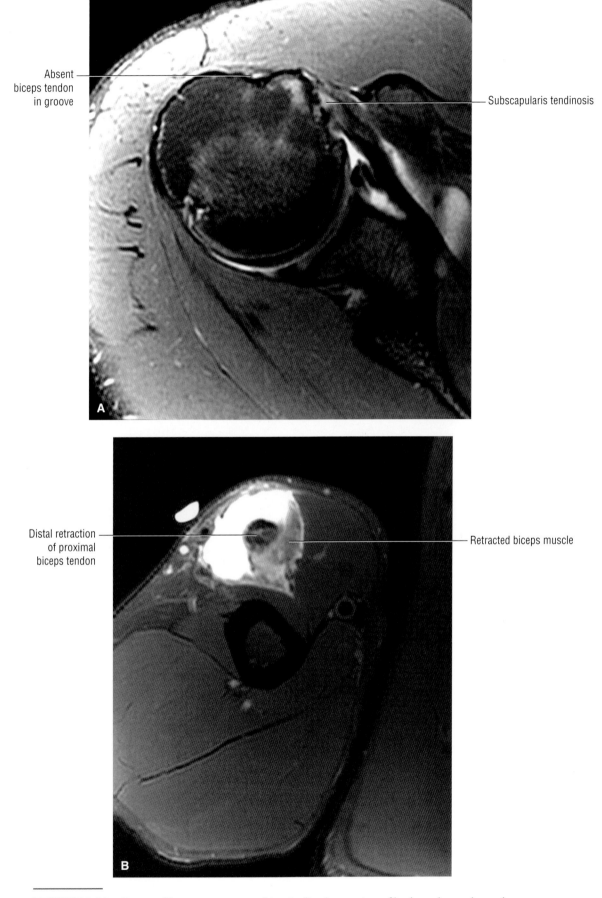

FIGURE 9.38 Proximal biceps rupture resulting in distal retraction of both tendon and muscle, producing convexity in the lower portion of the upper arm. (**A,B**) Axial FS PD.

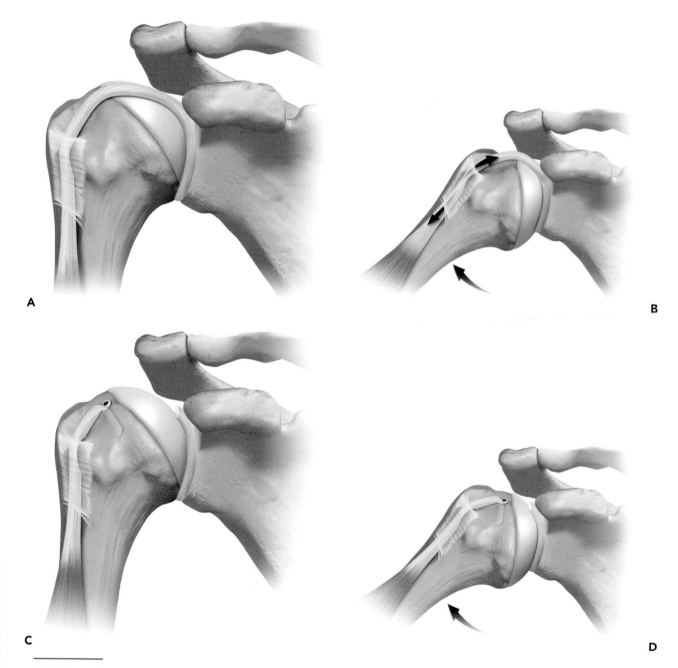

FIGURE 9.39 Schematic of a biceps tenodesis high in the bicipital groove. (**A**) Prior to tenodesis, the biceps tendon crosses the glenohumeral joint. (**B**) Movement of the glenohumeral joint results in relative motion of the biceps tendon within the bicipital groove. (**C**) Following a biceps tenodesis high in the bicipital groove, the tendon no longer crosses the glenohumeral joint. (**D**) Because the tendon no longer crosses the glenohumeral joint, movement of the joint does not result in any relative motion within the bicipital groove. Therefore, pain generation by movement of an inflamed tendon in the groove is eliminated. (Reprinted from Burkhart S, Lo IK, Brady PC, Denard PJ. *The Cowboy's Companion: A Trail Guide for the Arthroscopic Shoulder Surgeon.* Philadelphia, PA: Lippincott Williams & Wilkins; 2012, with permission.)

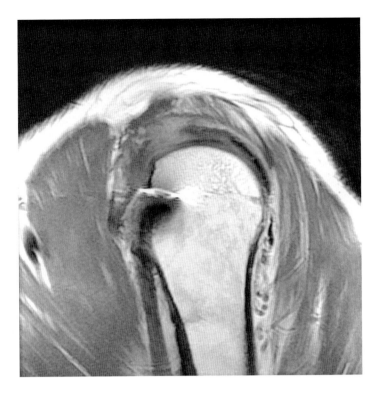

FIGURE 9.40   Management with arthroscopic biceps tenodesis is based on the ability to also repair an associated rotator cuff tear. Either a suture-only or suture anchor-to-bone fixation technique can be used. Anchor-to-bone fixation is used when the rotator interval tissues are deficient. Sagittal PD FSE image.

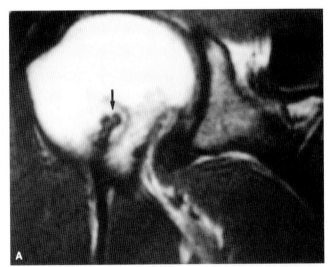

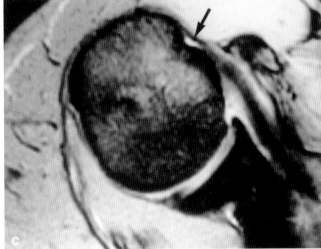

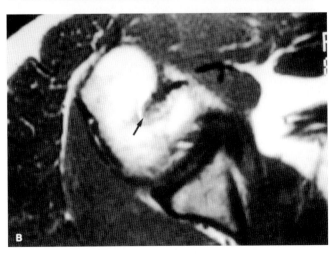

FIGURE 9.41   T1-weighted (**A**) coronal oblique and (**B**) axial images show biceps tenodesis (*arrow*). (**C**) The corresponding T2*-weighted axial image shows an absence of the biceps tendon in the bicipital groove (*arrow*).

Treatment of Biceps Lesions

- Biceps tenodesis in the bicipital groove is the treatment of choice in biceps tendinosis.
    - Location of tenodesis:
        - Upper, middle, and lower portions of the biceps groove
        - Subpectoral anterior humerus
        - Suprapectoral anterior humerus
            - Suprapectoral intraosseous biceps tenodesis (SPIBiT)
            - Excellent fixation (strong suture fixation to avoid tendon breakdown or shredding)
            - Anchors tendon within bone for improved healing
            - Suprapectoral and below the biceps groove ideal for removing all the pathologic tendon and to reduce the possibility of persistent postoperative groove pain[559]

- The criteria for biceps tenodesis[360,551] include:
    - Reversible tendon change with less than 25% partial thickness tear from a normal width biceps tendon
        - The biceps tendon size and groove location are normal.
    - Irreversible tendon change with partial thickness tear or fraying of greater than 25% of the normal biceps tendon width
        - There is associated biceps subluxation and disruption of the bicipital groove osseous or ligamentous anatomy.
    - Biceps tenodesis instead of tenotomy in patients < 70 years of age, males, laborers, or where preservation of biceps is important
    - Cosmesis favors tenodesis in patients including bodybuilders and females with thin arms.
    - Biceps tenotomy is used more commonly in patients over the age of 70.
        - Arthroscopic biceps tenotomy[559]
            - Results in relief of pain
            - Disadvantage of creating the "Popeye" cosmetic deformity plus loss of some elbow flexion and supination strength
            - Usually performed for older, less healthy, or less active patients

Adhesive Capsulitis

Key Concepts

- Acute adhesive capsulitis demonstrates a hyperintense and thickened IGHL on coronal FS PD FSE images.

    - Associated synovial hypertrophy is shown as intermediate signal intensity and occupies the space created by the axillary pouch.

- Residual or chronic thickening of the axillary pouch of the IGHL shown with intermediate signal intensity on coronal FS PD FSE images.

- Adhesive capsulitis is associated with synovitis in other joint locations, including the rotator cuff interval and subscapularis recess, in addition to the axillary pouch.

- The axillary nerve is susceptible to injury during transection of the axillary pouch in arthroscopic treatment of adhesive capsulitis.

- Arthroscopic capsular release should be considered when conservative management or manipulation is unsuccessful.

- Adhesive capsulitis is a clinical syndrome of pain and severely restricted joint motion (frozen shoulder) secondary to thickening and contraction of the joint capsule and synovium.[160,493,549]

- Produces painful restriction of active and passive shoulder and scapulothoracic motion

- Symptoms are usually present for at least 1 month.

- Clinical course can be divided into stable or progressive categories.

    - Three-stage process

        - Initial painful phase (pain with movement)

        - Stiffness phase (loss of motion)

        - Resolution phase (months to years with pain and motion progressively returns to normal)

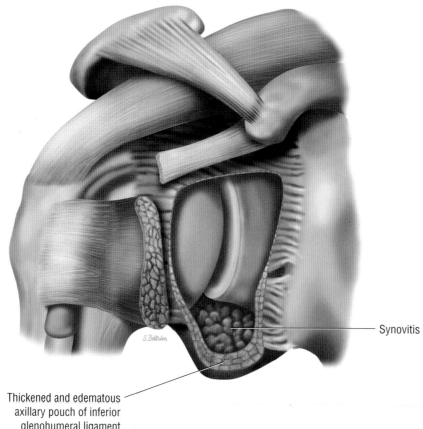

Synovitis

Thickened and edematous
axillary pouch of inferior
glenohumeral ligament

A

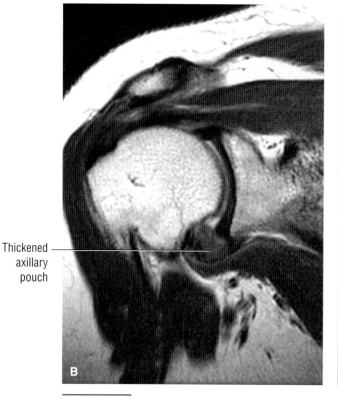

Thickened
axillary
pouch

B

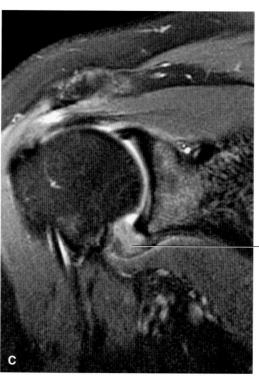

Hyperintense
axillary pouch

C

FIGURE 9.42 (**A**) Adhesive capsulitis or frozen shoulder with thickened inflamed IGHL and synovial thickening within the axillary pouch. Idiopathic adhesive capsulitis is more common than posttraumatic or secondary adhesive capsulitis, which occurs in only 10% of cases. Coronal PD FSE (**B**) and FS PD FSE (**C**) images of adhesive capsulitis. The thickened, hyperintense axillary pouch produces a soft tissue fullness in the anteroinferior capsule. Primary adhesive capsulitis has a 5:1 female-to-male prevalence. Patients may present with spontaneous insidious pain following a mild or trivial traumatic event including extension or lifting.

- Adhesive capsulitis can be primary (idiopathic).

    - With no predisposing history or cause

- Secondary adhesive capsulitis

    - With an antecedent event such as trauma or previous surgery

- Inflammation of the inferior shoulder capsule also causes a limited range of motion.

- Clinical pain worsens overtime with dull aching pain localized to the upper arm. Sharp pain with specific movements as in arm extension posteriorly. Parascapular aching and muscle soreness occur as glenohumeral motion is lost, leading to scapulothoracic muscle overload.[559]

- Association with other shoulder disorders, such as impingement, represents secondary adhesive capsulitis.

- The etiology of secondary adhesive capsulitis can be further subdivided into the following causes:[23]

    - Trauma

    - Surgery

    - Degenerative disease

    - Intrinsic rotator cuff and biceps tendinitis/tear

    - Inflammatory disease

    - Metabolic disease (including diabetes mellitus)

- An autoimmune theory is supported by increased C-reactive protein levels and the presence of HLA-B27 in adhesive capsulitis.

- History of hypothyrodism

- Ten percent to 20% of patients with diabetes (36% of those with type 1 or insulin-dependent diabetes) are affected.

- On MR arthrography, there is a decreased capacity to inject contrast material in a tight or resistant joint.[114]

- Articular fluid volumes are unreliable in the identification of adhesive capsulitis.

- ■ **Important MR findings in adhesive capsulitis include:**

  - ■ Synovitis (intermediate signal intensity)

  - ■ Capsular contraction, which may require validation with MR arthrography to appreciate loss of capsular volume and compliancy

  - ■ Effusion of the glenohumeral joint

  - ■ A hyperintense thickened IGHL and intermediate-signal-intensity synovial hypertrophy within the confines of the axillary pouch in symptomatic or active adhesive capsulitis

  - ■ A thickened IGHL without hyperintensity on FS PD FSE images in postinflammatory changes or scarring of the axillary pouch

    - ▨ Chronic changes of adhesive capsulitis may present with intermediate signal intensity of the IGHL on T1 and PD weighted images.

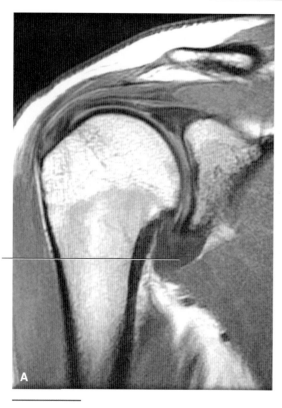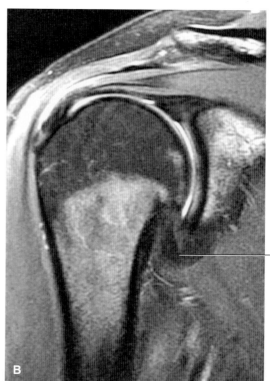

Thickened intermediate signal axillary pouch

Hypointense axillary pouch

FIGURE 9.43   Coronal PD FSE (**A**) and FS PD FSE (**B**) images show the chronic phase of adhesive capsulitis with a thickened IGHL without hyperintensity on the FS PD FSE image. The normally hypointense ligament will demonstrate intermediate signal intensity on PD or T1-weighted images in the chronic phase. MR arthrography is required to demonstrate loss of the inferior capsular recess with scarring.

- The hyperintense IGHL in the coronal plane is the most specific finding as the MR correlate for clinical adhesive capsulitis. In the presence of a hyperintense IGHL, synovitis should be evaluated in the axillary pouch, mid rotator cuff interval, and subscapularis recess.

  - If synovitis is present in the axillary pouch, rotator cuff interval, and subscapularis recess without an associated hyperintense IGHL, the diagnosis of adhesive capsulitis can still be raised in a differential diagnosis.

  - Isolated synovitis (one or two areas) to either the axillary pouch, rotator cuff interval, or subscapularis recess with a normal IGHL should be described without implying clinical adhesive capsulitis.

  - Subacute adhesive capsulitis may show intermediate synovial intensity of the IGHL on T1, PD and fluid sensitive sequences.

- Intravenous contrast MR imaging, used to enhance the acute changes of adhesive capsulitis, shows a hyperintense thickened IGHL.

- There is also thickening of the CHL and joint capsule in the rotator cuff interval and obliteration of the fat triangle between the CHL and the coracoid process (subcoracoid triangle sign).[351]

- Synovitis may be also observed at the superior border of the subscapularis tendon.

- Arthroscopic findings range from proliferative synovitis to capsular and intraarticular subscapularis tendon thickening to fibrosis.

- MR identification of adhesive capsulitis should always be reported and should not be assumed to be posttraumatic.

- Posttraumatic adhesive capsulitis is not common and is seen in only 10% of cases.

- A small percentage of patients may have persistent symptoms after conservative treatment.[549]

- Other treatment options include:

  - Brisement or distention arthrography leading to capsular rupture

  - Manipulation under anesthesia

  - Arthroscopic capsular release

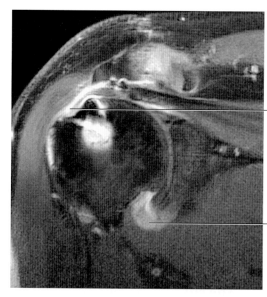

Supraspinatus tendon retear

Contrast-enhanced axillary pouch

FIGURE 9.44 Intravenous enhancement of the axillary pouch in adhesive capsulitis on a coronal FS T1-weighted MR image. Associated retear of the rotator cuff repair is seen.

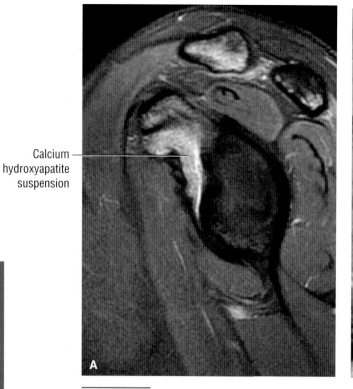

Calcium hydroxyapatite suspension

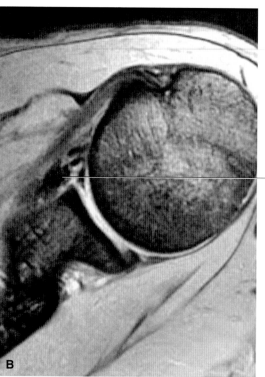

Susceptibility artifact from calcium hydroxyapatite

FIGURE 9.45 (**A**) Sagittal FS PD FSE and (**B**) axial T2* GRE images of calcific tendinitis subscapularis bursal variant with intermediate-signal-intensity paste-like thickening deep to the subscapularis tendon. GRE images are required to appreciate the susceptibility and hypointensity of the calcium hydroxyapatite crystals. Without the GRE images the MR findings might of been mistakened for subscapularis recess synovial thickening associated with adhesive capsulitis.

Calcific Tendinitis

Key Concepts

- Calcium (calcium hydroxyapatite) deposits in the soft tissues about the shoulder joint.

- Visualized with greater sensitivity and specificity as hypointensity on a T2* GRE sequence

- The semiliquid state of calcium hydroxyapatite may demonstrate heterogeneous hyperintensity on FS PD FSE images, although hypointensity is still characteristic on T2* GRE images.

- The supraspinatus and infraspinatus are the most commonly affected tendons.

- Calcification of the rotator cuff most commonly occurs in the supraspinatus tendon but can occur in any of the tendons of the rotator cuff.[35,495]

  - The involved tendons, from most to least likely, are:[545]

    - Supraspinatus

    - Infraspinatus

    - Teres minor

    - Subscapularis

- Periarticular soft tissues including the capsule, ligaments, and bursa are also potential sites of involvement.

- The size of the deposition varies from a few millimeters to several centimeters.

- Degenerative and reactive calcification theories

- Formation of calcific deposits in the tendinous portion of the rotator cuff is a degenerative process.

- The calcific buildup can be extremely painful and act almost as an internal furuncle.

  - The calcific buildup stage includes a formation phase (deposition and coalescence) which correlates with the chalk-like consistency. The resting phase has fibrocartilaginous tissue demarcating the border of the deposit. The resorptive phase includes vascular channels, macrophages, and multinucleated giant cells. The calcific deposit has a tootpaste-like or creamy characteristic and correlates with increased clinical symptoms.

Classification of Calcific Tendinitis (Three Phases)

- ■ An asymptomatic silent phase with calcium salts deposited in the critical zone of the tendon

- ■ A mechanical phase of enlarging deposits causing intratendinous stress pain associated with intrabursal or subbursal rupture

- ■ Adhesive periarthritis

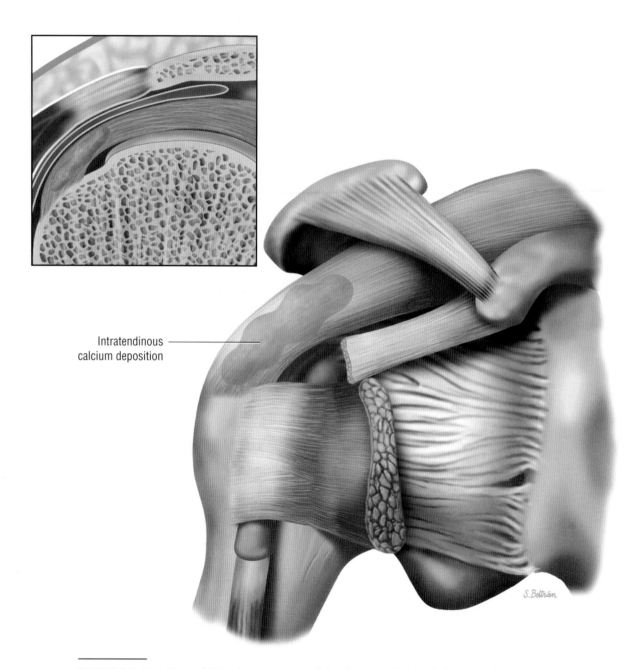

Intratendinous
calcium deposition

FIGURE 9.46   Coronal 3D color perspective of the silent or subclinical phase of calcium deposition within the substance of the rotator cuff tendons. A localized capillary or synovial blush (a "strawberry lesion") may be seen at arthroscopy during inspection of the articular surface of the supraspinatus or infraspinatus tendons in the area where the calcium deposit is suspected.[559]

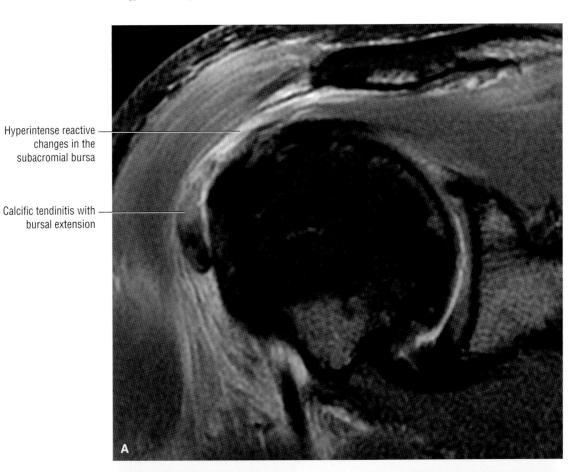

Hyperintense reactive changes in the subacromial bursa

Calcific tendinitis with bursal extension

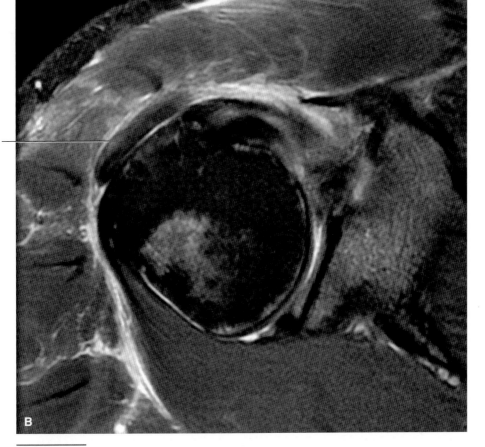

Calcific tendinitis with bursal extension and inflammation

FIGURE 9.47 Calcific tendinitis with calcium hydroxyapatite deposition in the subacromial bursa with secondary inflammatory reaction. (**A**) Coronal FS PD. (**B**) Axial FS PD.

- Adhesive periarthritis is associated with adhesive bursitis as a complication of tendinous calcific deposits.

  - The bursitis is an acute inflammatory reaction to the crystal deposits in a semiliquid state and demonstrates a more heterogeneous hyperintensity with associated scattered foci of signal void on T2, FS PD FSE, or T2*-weighted images.

Microscopic Features of Calcific Tendinitis

- Crystalline hydroxyapatite in the tendon

- Influx of inflammatory cells, especially in the resorptive phase

- Macrophages and multinucleate giant cells

- Fibroblasts, in the post-calcific phase

MR Examination of Calcific Tendinitis

- Calcium hydroxyapatite deposition disease located within the rotator cuff tendons is visualized as a globular area of decreased signal intensity or a mass.

  - The globular morphology may be hood-like, linear, angular, or round.

- Hyperintense perilesional edema and subacromial-subdeltoid fluid are seen on fluid sensitive images.

- Tendinosis or a partial rotator cuff tear are associated findings.

- Cuff tendon fiber injury occurs as the calcium hydroxyapatite infiltrates and replaces damaged tissue.

Treatment of Calcific Tendinitis

- Usually consists of a subacromial decompression, along with excision and removal of the calcific deposits by dissection and débridement

  - Tendon defect approximated with one or two sutures

- Suture anchor fixation in cases of full thickness tendon involvement which comprises the tendon footprint

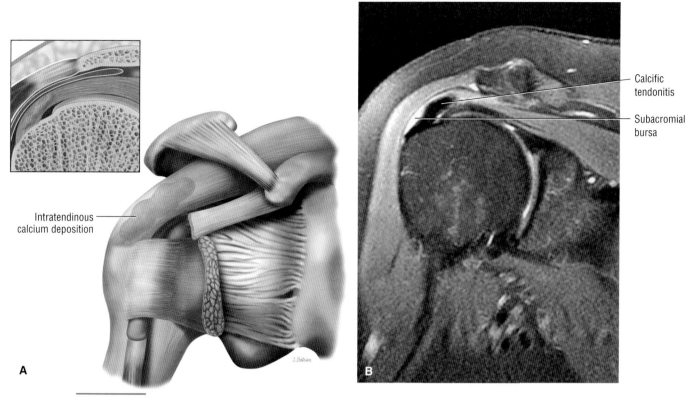

FIGURE 9.48 (**A**) Coronal 3D color perspective of the silent or subclinical phase of calcium deposition within the substance of the rotator cuff tendons. (**B**) Transition from the silent phase to the early mechanical phase is characterized by mild elevation of the subacromial bursal floor. Localized hyperintensity of the adjacent subacromial bursa can be seen on this coronal FS PD FSE image.

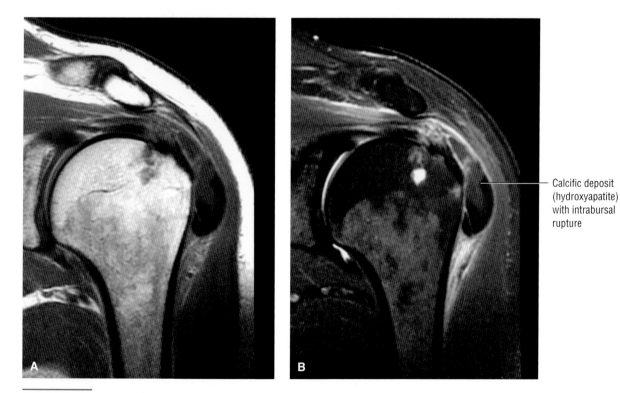

FIGURE 9.49 Coronal PD FSE (**A**) and FS PD FSE (**B**) images show the mechanical phase of intrabursal rupture with the bulk of the calcific deposit occupying the subacromial-subdeltoid bursal space. The mechanical phase is characterized by bursal floor elevation, subbursal rupture, or intrabursal rupture.

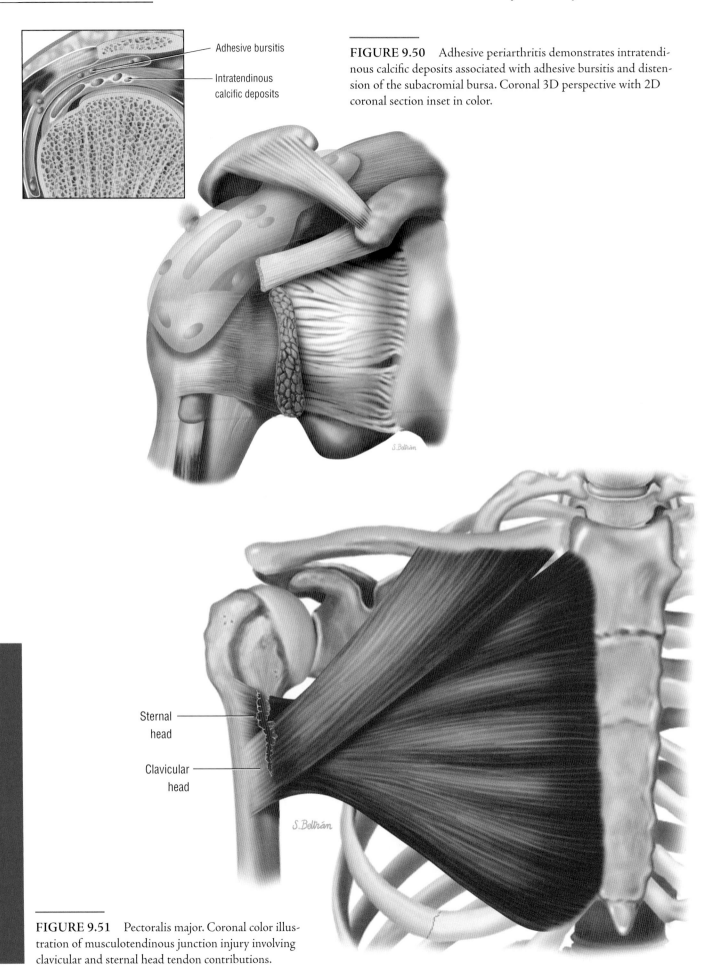

FIGURE 9.50 Adhesive periarthritis demonstrates intratendinous calcific deposits associated with adhesive bursitis and distension of the subacromial bursa. Coronal 3D perspective with 2D coronal section inset in color.

FIGURE 9.51 Pectoralis major. Coronal color illustration of musculotendinous junction injury involving clavicular and sternal head tendon contributions.

Pectoralis Major Tear

Key Concepts

■ The bilaminar pectoralis major tendon is formed from the sternocostal and clavicular heads of the pectoralis muscle.

■ Partial musculotendinous pectoralis major tears with combined sternal and clavicular head involvement are the most common presentation.

■ Axial MR images must include the humeral diaphyseal insertion of the lateral lip of the bicipital groove.

■ Coronal oblique images are prescribed parallel to the course of the pectoralis muscle as identified on axial images first.

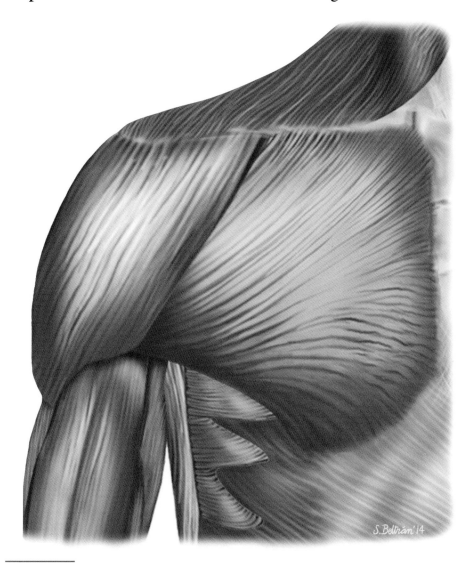

FIGURE 9.52   The pectoralis major and the lattisimus dorsi muscle work in concert to provide for glenohumeral stability. The pectoralis major muscle is active in internal rotation against resistance and is a powerful adductor of the glenohumeral joint.

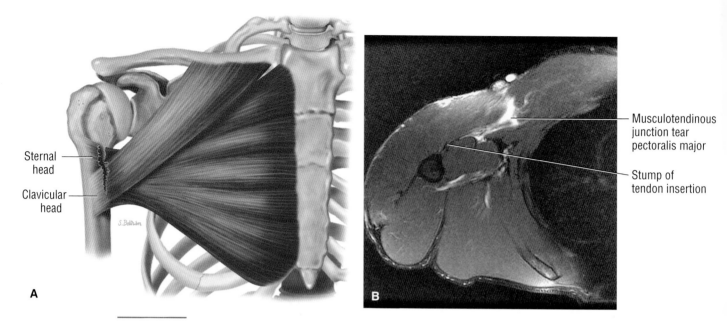

Sternal
head

Clavicular
head

S. Beltran

A

Musculotendinous
junction tear
pectoralis major

Stump of
tendon insertion

B

FIGURE 9.53   (**A**) Coronal color illustration of musculotendinous junction injury involving clavicular and sternal head tendon contributions. (**B**) Axial FS PD FSE image with hyperintensity and
retraction of the pectoralis major in a musculotendinous junction injury with intact remaining stump
of tendon insertion.

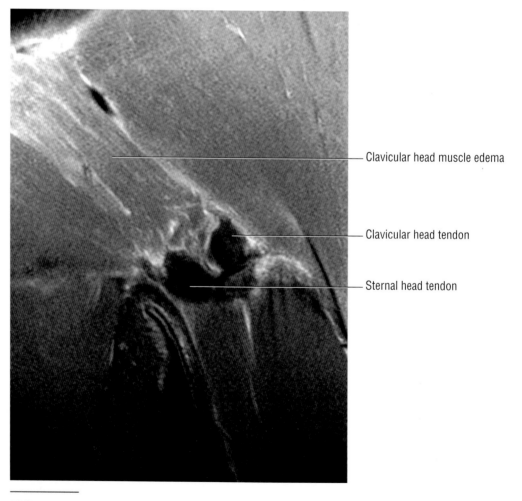

Clavicular head muscle edema

Clavicular head tendon

Sternal head tendon

FIGURE 9.54   Complete rupture of the pectoralis tendon with retraction of clavicular and sternal heads. The hypointense retracted tendons
are increased in cross-sectional diameter. Coronal oblique FS PD image.

- Pectoralis major tears may involve disruption of the pectoralis myotendinous unit or the humeral insertion site.[363]

- The broad, bilaminar tendon of the pectoralis major inserts into the lateral lip of the bicipital groove.

- The two heads of the pectoralis major muscle:
  - The sternocostal head
    - Forms the posterior tendon insertion
    - Produces the rounded anterior axillary fold prominence with spiral layering of muscle fibers
    - The most inferior fibers insert superiorly and the superior fibers insert inferiorly.
    - More susceptible to avulsion than the clavicular head
  - The clavicular head
    - Forms the anterior insertion

- The pectoralis major is innervated by the medial and lateral pectoral nerves from the medial and lateral cords of the brachial plexus.

- The pectoralis major functions in adduction and medial rotation of the humerus.

Common Causes of Pectoralis Major Tears

- Resisted forced abduction and external rotation

- Forceful contraction with the arm adducted, flexed, and internally rotated

- Tendon rupture in bench press weight lifting (muscle failure associated with bench press lifting is secondary to either overload of the short inferior fibers in the eccentric phase of lifting with sternal head failure or from a direct blow as sternoclavicular head failure)

- Most injuries involve the musculotendinous junction or the distal tendon insertion.[116]

- Partial tears are the most common presentation, with combined sternal and clavicular head injuries more frequent than individual head injuries.

- Silent injuries of the pectoralis muscle may occur in the elderly.

- In acute rupture, pain is severe and weakness is present in internal rotation.

- Deformity is also present, especially with attempted muscle contraction.

- The weight lifter usually has a history of injury during humeral extension at the beginning of a lift.
    - A hematoma then develops in the proximal medial arm or chest wall.
- Tendinous avulsions from the humerus are associated with ecchymosis.

MR Appearance of Pectoralis Major Tears

- MR findings on FSE PD FSE images include:
    - Hyperintense edema in the clavicle, sternum, or ribs
    - Increased signal intensity at the humeral insertion in the proximal humeral diaphysis (lateral lip of bicipital groove)
    - Hyperintense edema and hemorrhage within the muscle tear site, perifascial zone, and subcutaneous fat
- A complete tear of the pectoralis major may retract and undergo fibrosis, causing a visible deformity of the chest wall.
- In more than 90% of cases, both primary and delayed repair successfully restore strength and function.
- Complete rupture of the pectoralis major tendon is an indication for immediate surgical repair.
    - These injuries usually occur in young active individuals who would have persistent weakness without repair.
    - Chronic ruptures have also been successfully repaired in symptomatic athletes.

Pectoralis Major Complications and Latissimus Dorsi Avulsions

- Mature scar tissue formation in a failed repair can be used to perform a delayed repair of the avulsed tendon stump.
- Complications of pectoralis major injuries are:
    - Hematoma with pseudocyst
    - Infection
    - Rupture at the musculotendinous junction
- Latissimus dorsi avulsions are also evaluated by inspecting the tendon insertion along the humeral diaphysis.
    - These injuries are related to forceful resisted arm adduction and are associated with multiple sport activities including waterskiing, golf, pitching in baseball, rock climbing, volleyball, and gymnastics.

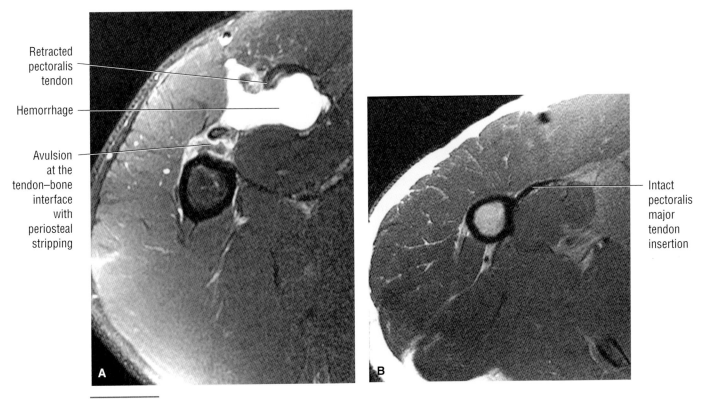

Retracted pectoralis tendon

Hemorrhage

Avulsion at the tendon–bone interface with periosteal stripping

Intact pectoralis major tendon insertion

FIGURE 9.55 (**A**) Axial FS PD FSE image shows complete avulsion of the tendon–bone interface with localized hemorrhage. The pectoralis major muscle may be injured at the tendon–bone interface or the tendon–musculotendinous junction or intramuscularly. Hematoma and periosteal stripping are associated with primary tendon avulsion. (**B**) Axial PD FSE image of normal pectoralis major tendon insertion shown for comparison. The hypointense pectoralis major tendon is located directly anterior to the coracobrachialis muscle.

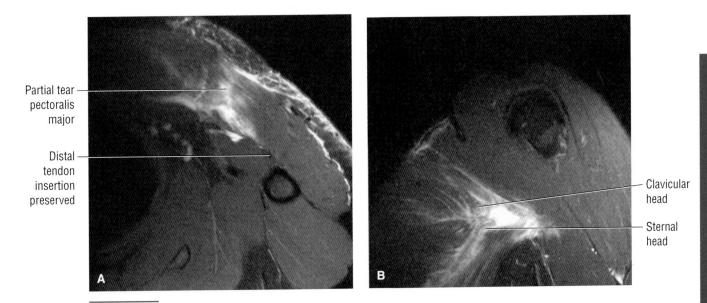

Partial tear pectoralis major

Distal tendon insertion preserved

Clavicular head

Sternal head

FIGURE 9.56 Partial tear involving both the clavicular and sternal head with preservation of the distal tendon insertion on axial FSE PD (**A**) and coronal oblique FS PD FSE (**B**) images. There is greater disruption of clavicular head muscle fibers appreciated on the coronal oblique image of the pectoralis muscle.

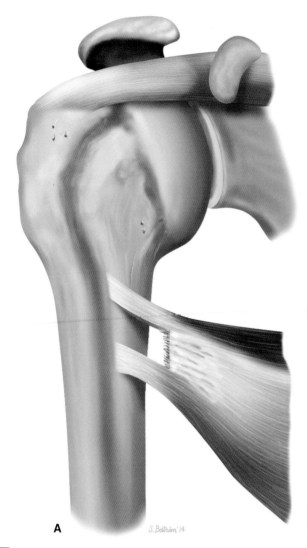

A

S.Beltrán'14

FIGURE 9.57 Partial tear of the latissimus dorsi tendon along the inferior aspect of the intertubercular groove anterior and lateral to the teres major insertion and medial to the pectoralis major insertion. On MRI, the edema is visible along the superior to inferior extent of the latissimus insertion on the proximal humeral diaphysis. It may difficult to differentiate between latissimus dorsi and teres major on coronal plane MR images (latissimus dorsi muscle extends more inferior). The latissimus dorsi tendon is anterior to the teres major muscle on sagittal images. (**A**) Color illustration. (**B**) Coronal FS PD. The normal insertion of the latissimus dorsi tendon is over a 7cm superior to inferior tendon attachment to the humerus.

Partial tear humeral attachment latissimus dorsi tendon with muscle edema

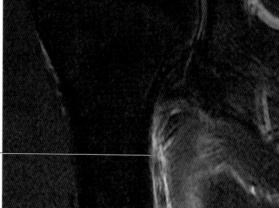

B

Acromioclavicular Separations

Key Concepts

- AC separations range from AC ligament sprains to complete disruption of the AC joint capsule and coracoclavicular ligaments.

- Displacement between the coracoid and clavicle and the position of the distal clavicle relative to the acromial facet are assessed on sagittal and coronal images.

- Associated fractures may occur in the coracoid, acromion, or clavicle.

- AC injuries range from separations (direct trauma) to distal clavicle osteolysis (overuse injury in weight lifters).

  - Most common mechanism of AC joint injury is direct trauma from a fall on the point of the shoulder with the arm adduction.[182]

- A direct fall onto the shoulder may result in a distal clavicle fracture or an AC separation.[361]

- The relevant anatomy of the AC joint is used to classify these injuries.

  - Diarthroidal joint

  - Articulation permits gliding, shearing, and rotational motion.

  - Static stabilizers are the acromioclavicular ligaments (superior, inferior, anterior, and posterior), the coracoclavicular ligaments (trapezoid and conoid), and the coracoacromial ligament.

  - Dynamic stabilizers represented by the deltoid and trapezius muscles

- The distal clavicle is stabilized in the anteroposterior direction by the AC ligament (capsule) and in the superior-to-inferior direction by the coracoclavicular ligaments (the cone-shaped conoid and the broad trapezoid ligament).

- The coracoacromial ligament can be used as a ligament substitute when transferred to the end of a recessed distal clavicle and thus functions as a coracoclavicular ligament.

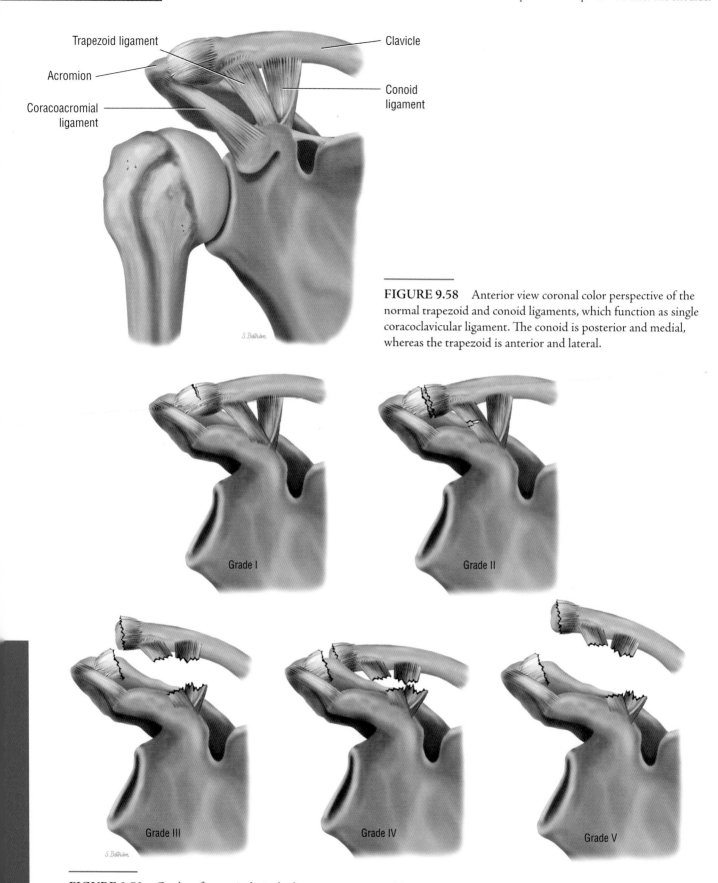

FIGURE 9.58 Anterior view coronal color perspective of the normal trapezoid and conoid ligaments, which function as single coracoclavicular ligament. The conoid is posterior and medial, whereas the trapezoid is anterior and lateral.

FIGURE 9.59 Grades of acromioclavicular ligamentous injuries. Type I: Intact acromioclavicular and coraco-clavicular ligaments. Type II: Disruption of acromioclavicular ligaments. Type III: Disruption of acromioclavicular and coracoclavicular ligaments. Type IV: Acromioclavicular and coracoclavicular ligament disruption and posterior displacement of the clavicle into or through the trapezius muscle. Type V: Acromioclavicular and coracoclavicular ligament disruption plus injury to the deltoid and trapezius muscle attachments. There is a significant separation between the clavicle and the acromion. In the rare type VI injury, there is inferior dislocation of the distal clavicle (not shown).

Classification of AC Joint Separation

■ AC separations are classed into six different types based on the degree of displacement and the location of the distal clavicle (also based on the extent of injury to the AC and coracoclavicular [CC] ligaments and the integrity of the fascia associated with the deltoid and trapezius muscles).

  ■ Type I: AC ligamentous sprain

  ■ Type II: AC joint disruption with intact coracoclavicular ligaments

  ■ Type III: AC joint and coracoclavicular ligament disruption. The coracoclavicular interspace is widened 25% to 100% and the distal clavicle is mobile in both superior to inferior and anteroposterior directions.

  ■ Type IV: Posterior displacement of the clavicle into or through the trapezius

  ■ Type V: Type III separation with greater displacement (100% to 300% compared to the contralateral side) between the coracoid and clavicle

  ■ Type VI: Inferior dislocation of the clavicle inferior to the acromion (subacromial) or coracoid (subcoracoid)

Treatment of AC Joint Separation

■ Indications for surgical intervention include types IV, V, and VI dislocations.

■ Treatment options for type III AC dislocations are more controversial and are often based on activity requirements.[559]

  ■ Needs of an athlete compared to those of a laborer or someone with a more sedentary lifestyle

  ■ Surgical intervention for types IV, V, and VI shoulder separations

  ■ Types I and II separations conservative treatment before consideration of a distal clavicle excision

  ■ Acute type III AC separations usually treated nonsurgically but evaluated on an individual case basis for the possible benefits of acute intervention.

  ■ Irreducible separations require open reduction if deltotrapezial muscle and fascia are entrapped under the clavicle.

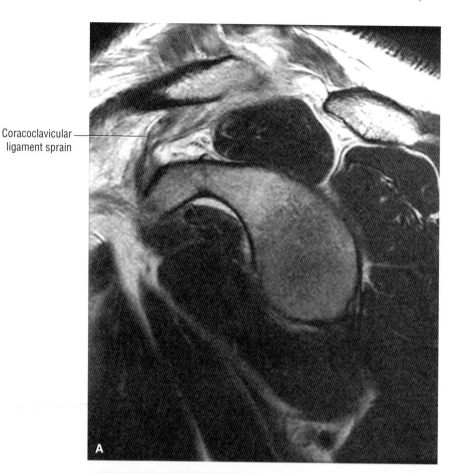

Coracoclavicular
ligament sprain

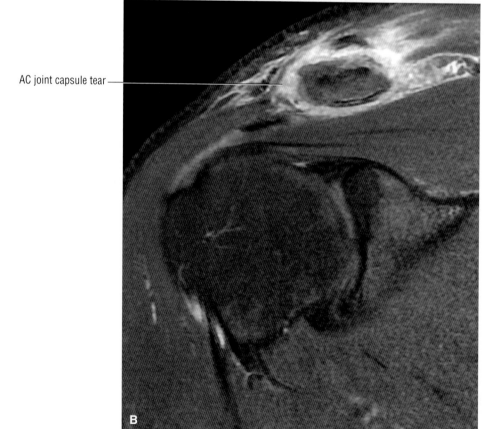

AC joint capsule tear

FIGURE 9.60   AC joint dislocation with rupture of the AC joint capsule (grade 2) with sprain (not disruption) of the CC ligaments. (**A**) Sagittal T2 FSE. (**B**) Coronal PD FSE.

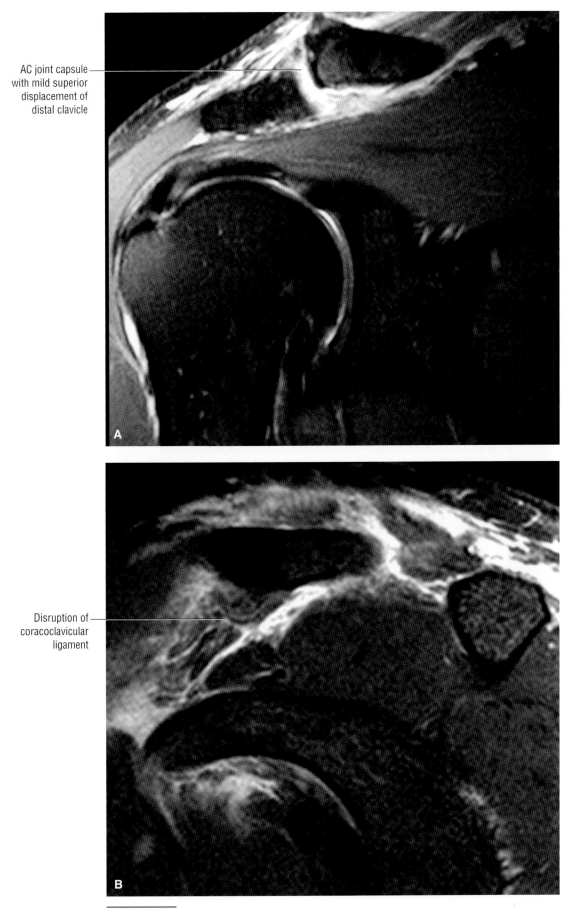

AC joint capsule with mild superior displacement of distal clavicle

Disruption of coracoclavicular ligament

FIGURE 9.61 Grade 3 AC joint separation with disruption of the AC joint and CC ligaments. The deltoid fascia is intact and the displacement of the coracoid compared to the clavicle is less than 100%. (**A**) Coronal FS PD. (**B**) Sagittal FS PD.

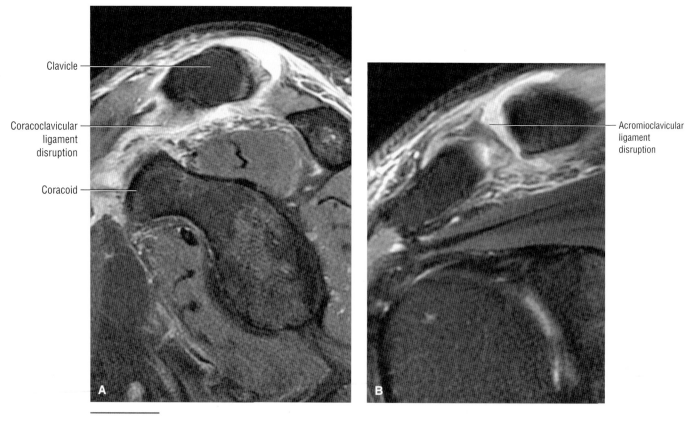

Clavicle

Coracoclavicular ligament disruption

Coracoid

Acromioclavicular ligament disruption

FIGURE 9.62 Type III AC separation with complete disruption of both the AC and CC ligaments. The distal clavicle is above the superior border of the acromion. The CC interspace is usually widened by 25% to 100%. The space between the coracoid and clavicle is normally between 1.1 and 1.3 cm. (**A**) Sagittal FS PD FSE image. (**B**) Coronal FS PD FSE image.

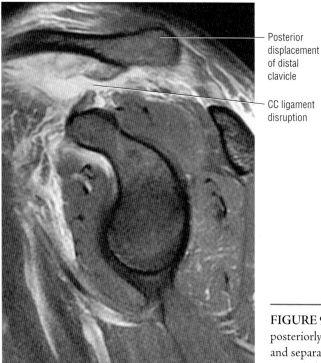

Posterior displacement of distal clavicle

CC ligament disruption

FIGURE 9.63 Type IV AC separation with the distal clavicle displaced posteriorly into the trapezius. There is a fluid-filled gap between the torn and separated CC ligaments and widening of the AC joint space in the coronal plane. Sagittal FS PD FSE image.

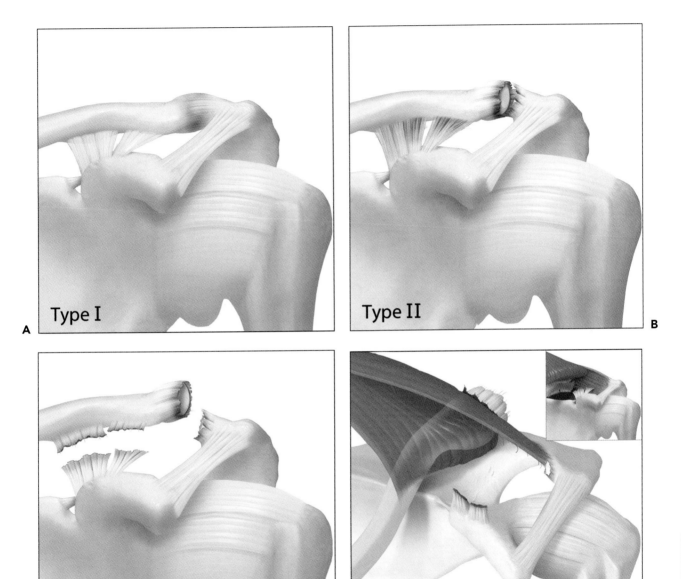

FIGURE 9.64 Schematic of the six types of AC joint separations. (**A**) A grade I injury involves a strain of the AC ligaments only. (**B**) A grade II injury includes disruption of the AC ligaments, but the CC ligaments are intact. (**C**) In a grade III injury, the AC and CC ligaments are disrupted, but the deltoid fascia remains intact and displacement of the coracoid relative to the clavicle is <100%. (**D**) In a grade IV injury, the AC and CC ligaments are disrupted and the clavicle is displaced posteriorly into or through (inset) the trapezius muscle.

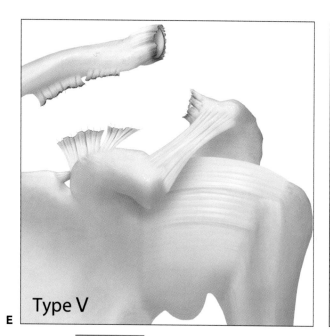
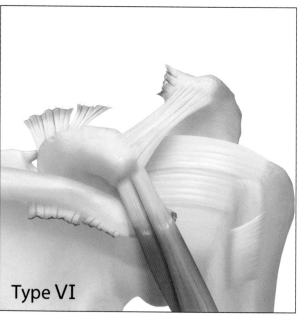

FIGURE 9.64 *(Continued)* (**E**) In a grade V injury, the AC and CC ligaments are disrupted and the CC displacement is >100% relative to the contralateral distance. (**F**) In a grade VI injury, the clavicle is displaced inferior to the coracoid. (Reprinted from Burkhart S, Lo IK, Brady PC, Denard PJ. *The Cowboy's Companion: A Trail Guide for the Arthroscopic Shoulder Surgeon*. Philadelphia, PA: Lippincott Williams & Wilkins; 2012, with permission.)

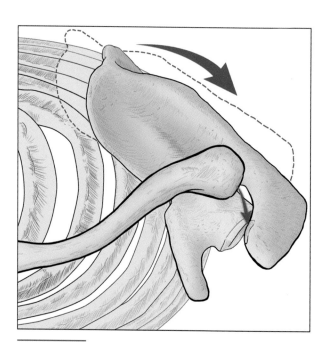

FIGURE 9.65 Following disruption of the acromioclavicular joint, the scapula protracts (*blue arrows*). This can result in impingement and scapular dyskinesis as well as coracoid tenderness as a result of pectoralis minor contracture. (Reprinted from Burkhart S, Lo IK, Brady PC, Denard PJ. *The Cowboy's Companion: A Trail Guide for the Arthroscopic Shoulder Surgeon*. Philadelphia, PA: Lippincott Williams & Wilkins; 2012, with permission.)

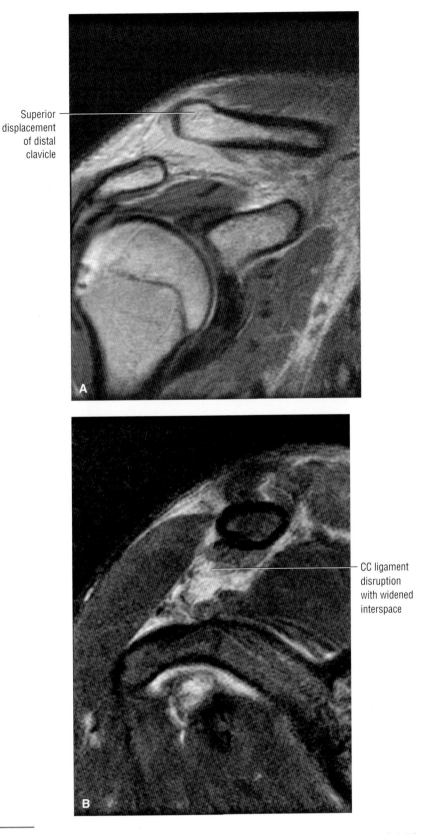

Superior displacement of distal clavicle

CC ligament disruption with widened interspace

FIGURE 9.66 (**A,B**) Type V AC separation with complete disruption of the AC and CC ligaments and severe superior displacement of the distal clavicle. The deltoid and trapezius aponeurosis is avulsed from the distal clavicle and the distal clavicle is displaced subcutaneously, with the CC interspace widened 100% to 300%. The type V injury is thus a more severe form a type III injury with the addition of the trapezius and deltoid fascia stripped from both the acromion and clavicle. Clinically, there is a severe droop secondary to downward displacement of the scapula and humerus. (**A**) Coronal PD FSE image. (**B**) Sagittal PD/T2 FSE image.[182]

Arthritis

Key Concepts

- Central and posterior glenoid wear with sclerosis and cartilage loss is typically seen in osteoarthritis.

- Loose bodies are frequently located in the subscapularis recess.

- Coronal images demonstrate the medial and inferior projection of humeral head osteophytes. Spurring is also present directed from the inferior pole of the glenoid.

  - Humeral head articular cartilage is carefully assessed from the superior aspect of the humeral head to the medial aspect of the humeral head at the level of the glenohumeral joint.

    - Blistering of humeral head articular cartilage is a sign of impending chondral breakdown.[559]

  - Intermediate signal articular cartilage can be attenuated or present as a full thickness grade 4 chondral defect when following the contour of the humeral head. Failure to recognize articular cartilage loss of the humeral head on coronal images will result in underestimating the degree of joint space narrowing and associated degenerative osteoarthritis when comparing MR studies with radiographs.

- Severe glenohumeral osteoarthritis may be associated with reactive subchondral marrow edema.

- Rheumatoid-related synovial hypertrophy or pannus is intermediate in signal intensity on FS PD FSE images and will enhance with intravenous contrast.

- Rotator cuff tears are commonly seen in association with rheumatoid arthritis.

- Rice bodies are hypointense on FS PD FSE images and represent detached fibrotic synovial villi.

Osteoarthritis

- Osteoarthritis is characterized by chondral erosions, osteophyte formation, subchondral cysts and sclerosis, and synovitis.[310]

- Degenerative arthritis may be:

  - Primary

    - Caused by chronic microtrauma

  - Secondary

    - Related to predisposing events of previous trauma, congenital deformity, infection, or metabolic disorder

- Treatment options other than shoulder replacement[75]:

  - Capsular release and osteophyte débridement in a stiff (capsular stiffness) and painful shoulder

  - Isolated chondral lesions in younger patients with a preserved joint space, options include labral advancement or microfracture.

  - Glenoid resurfacing in young patients with decreased joint space (chondrolysis and posttraumatic arthritis)

- The shoulder is predisposed to unique instabilities because of its non-weight-bearing anatomy.

- Compression of weakened bone occurs with subchondral fracture.

- Loose bodies are seen with fragmentation of osteochondral surfaces.

- Synovial hypertrophy and synovial fluid production correlate with joint pain and increased intraarticular pressure.

- MR is accurate in identifying both posterior glenoid wear and posterior humeral subluxation in primary degenerative joint disease.[340]

- Hypointense glenoid sclerosis is associated with loss of posterior glenoid articular cartilage on axial PD and FS PD FSE images.

  - Although anterior capsular contracture may be more difficult to visualize, with appropriate sequences, it can be seen as hypointense thickening of the anterior capsule.

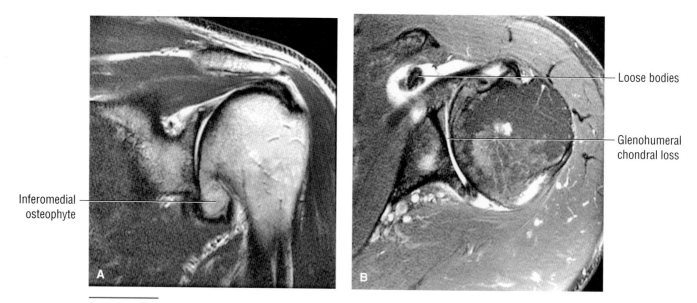

FIGURE 9.67   Coronal T2 FSE (**A**) and axial FS PD FSE (**B**) images of osteoarthritis with glenohumeral chondral loss, inferomedial osteophytes, and subscapularis bursa loose bodies.

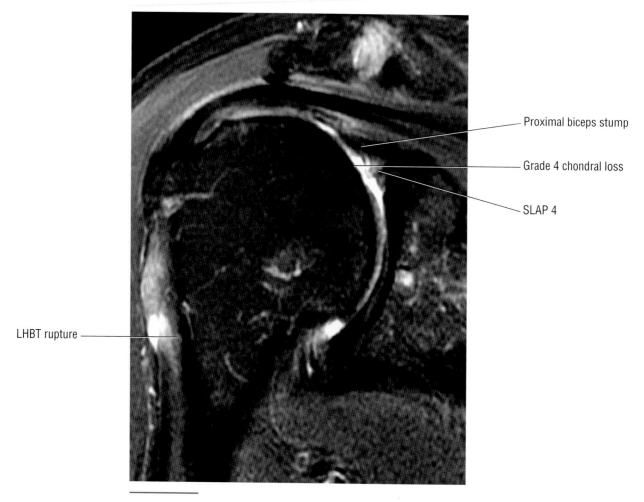

FIGURE 9.68   Grade 4 chondral loss of the humeral head associated with chronic SLAP lesion and biceps tendon rupture. Loss of articular cartilage of the humeral head on MRI correlates with joint space narrowing on radiographs. Coronal FS PD.

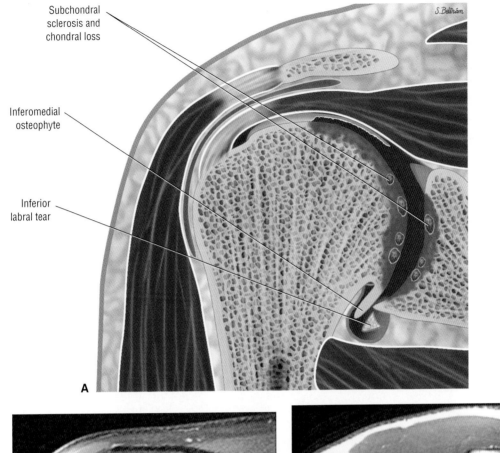

Subchondral sclerosis and chondral loss

Inferomedial osteophyte

Inferior labral tear

S.Beltrán

A

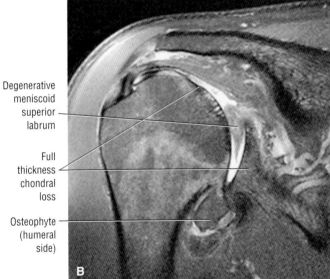

Degenerative meniscoid superior labrum

Full thickness chondral loss

Osteophyte (humeral side)

B

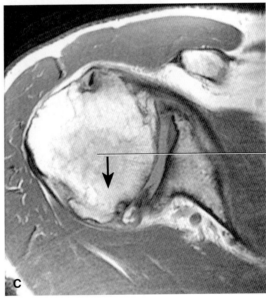

Posterior humeral subluxation associated with glenohumeral chondral loss

C

FIGURE 9.69 Advanced changes of osteoarthritis of the glenohumeral joint. Articular cartilage loss with sclerosis and subchondral cystic change is greatest in the area of the humeral head in contact with the glenoid between 60° and 100° of abduction. Characteristic large peripheral osteophytes develop inferiorly and limit rotation by effectively enlarging the diameter of the humeral head. (**A**) Coronal color section of degenerative osteoarthritis of the glenohumeral joint. (**B**) Coronal FS PD FSE image with full thickness glenohumeral articular cartilage loss, inferior osteophytes, and labral tearing shown at the BLC and inferior glenohumeral ligament labral complex. (**C**) Axial PD FSE with posterior glenoid wear advancing to involve the entire glenohumeral joint. Posterior glenoid wear is associated with an internal rotation contracture and posterior subluxation of the humeral head.

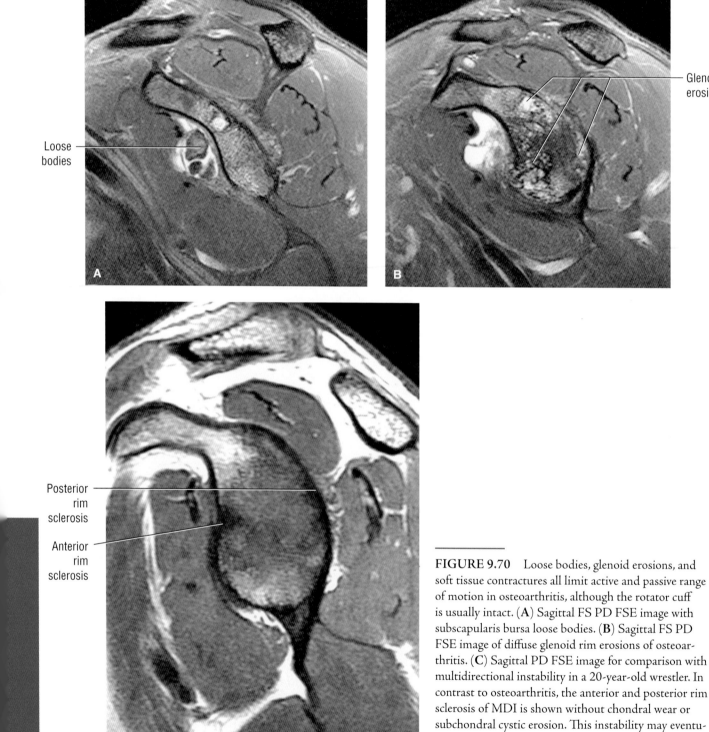

Loose bodies

Glenoid erosions

Posterior rim sclerosis

Anterior rim sclerosis

FIGURE 9.70 Loose bodies, glenoid erosions, and soft tissue contractures all limit active and passive range of motion in osteoarthritis, although the rotator cuff is usually intact. (**A**) Sagittal FS PD FSE image with subscapularis bursa loose bodies. (**B**) Sagittal FS PD FSE image of diffuse glenoid rim erosions of osteoarthritis. (**C**) Sagittal PD FSE image for comparison with multidirectional instability in a 20-year-old wrestler. In contrast to osteoarthritis, the anterior and posterior rim sclerosis of MDI is shown without chondral wear or subchondral cystic erosion. This instability may eventually be associated with glenohumeral arthritis but should be identified and differentiated at this stage.

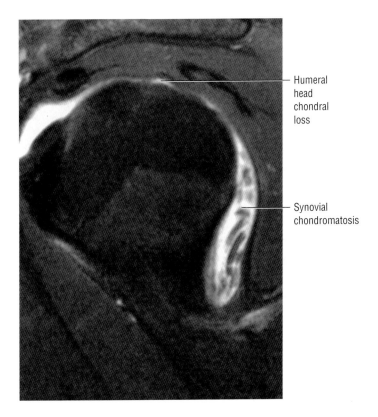

FIGURE 9.71   Secondary chondromatosis associated with full thickness chondral loss of the humeral head on a sagittal FS PD FSE image.

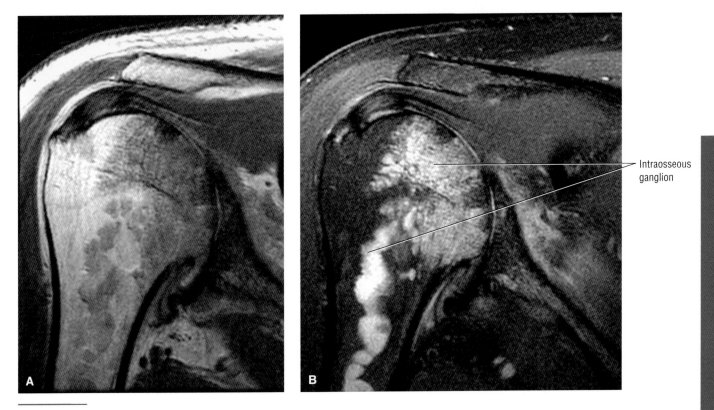

FIGURE 9.72   Atypical manifestation of osteoarthritis with intraosseous ganglion extending into the proximal humeral diaphysis as seen on a coronal PD FSE image (**A**) and a coronal FS PD FSE image (**B**).

- Rotator cuff tears are uncommon in primary degenerative joint disease.

- Humeral head sclerosis and cartilage loss are usually central or superior in glenohumeral osteoarthritis.

- Peripheral osteophytes projecting from the humeral head are directed inferiorly on coronal images.

- Subchondral cysts are seen in both the humeral head and glenoid.

- Glenoid cartilage loss and sclerosis is usually central or posterior, and there can be complete loss of the glenoid chondral surface.

- Glenoid peripheral osteophytes involve the lower two thirds of the glenohumeral joint.

- The inferior capsule may be enlarged and the anterior capsule contracted.

- Loose bodies occur within the glenohumeral joint or subscapularis bursa.

- Advanced glenoid arthrosis demonstrates subchondral erosions of the glenoid fossa on sagittal images in the posterosuperior, posteroinferior, inferior, and anteroinferior quadrants.

- A secondary chondromatosis is associated with full thickness chondral loss of the humerus or glenoid.

- An intraosseous ganglion is a less common finding in degenerative osteoarthritis and may be mistaken for an intraosseous hemangioma or infectious tract.

- If conservative treatment with physical therapy and NSAIDs is not successful, total shoulder replacement is considered.

- The major diagnostic indications for total shoulder replacement include:[537]
  - Rheumatoid arthritis
  - Osteoarthritis (primary and secondary)
  - Old trauma
  - Prosthetic revision
  - Arthritis after recurrent dislocation
  - Rotator cuff arthropathy

- Weight lifters and triathlon athletes (primarily from activities during the swimming phase of the competition) are subject to AC joint and posterosuperior labrum stress and are prone to this combination of arthrosis and posterosuperior labral tears.[571]

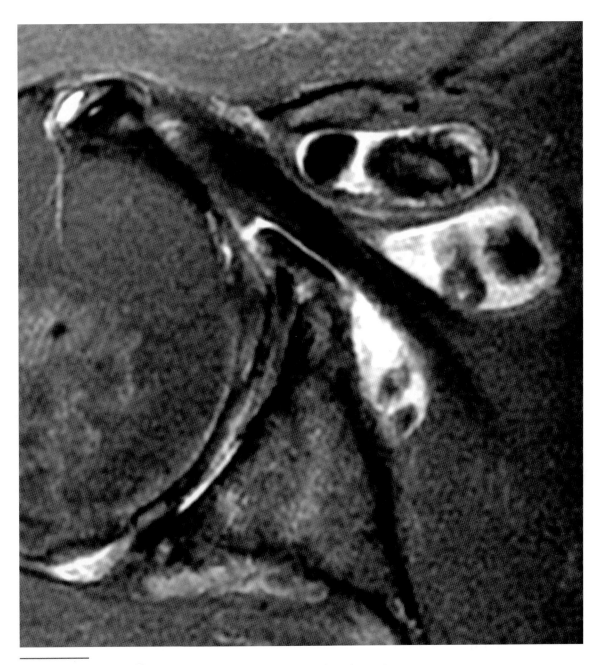

FIGURE 9.73   Multiple osteochondral loose bodies within the subscapularis recess as synovial chondromatosis. Axial FS PD. Typically not all of the loose bodies are ossified. Primary synovial chondromatosis is a monoarticular condition of unknown etiology and secondary synovial chondromatosis is associated with glenohumeral joint degenerative change.

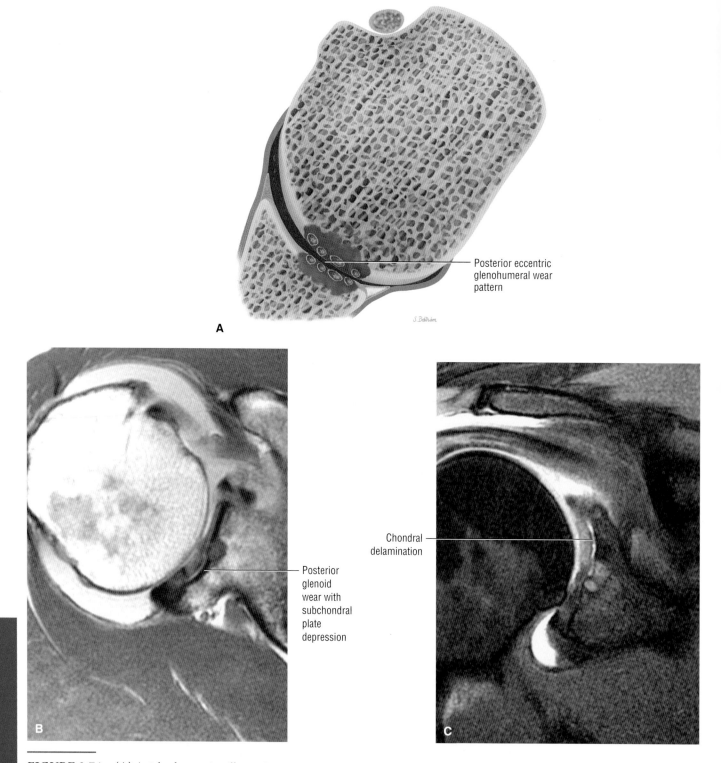

FIGURE 9.74 (**A**) Axial color section illustrating posterior or eccentric wear pattern of osteoarthritis with loss of posterior glenohumeral joint articular cartilage. Axial PD FSE (**B**) and coronal FS PD FSE (**C**) images showing posterior glenoid eccentric wear with subchondral fracture, chondral delamination, and joint space narrowing. MR is used to assess the wear pattern and glenoid bone stock, important in planning the resurfacing of the glenoid.

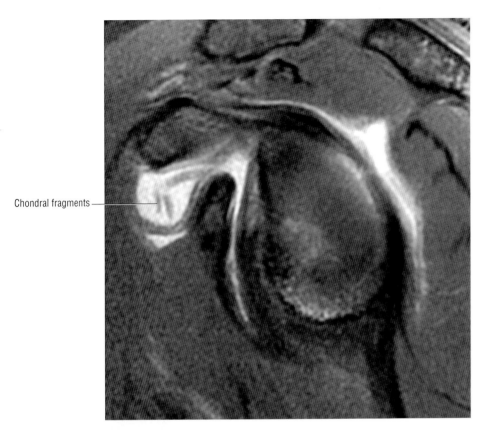

Chondral fragments

FIGURE 9.75 Discreet chondral fragments occupying the subscapularis recess. Chondral fragments are intermediate in signal of fluid sensitive sequences. In comparison, an osteochondral fragment would have a hypointense peripheral border or, if larger, would have marrow-containing elements. Sagittal FS PD.

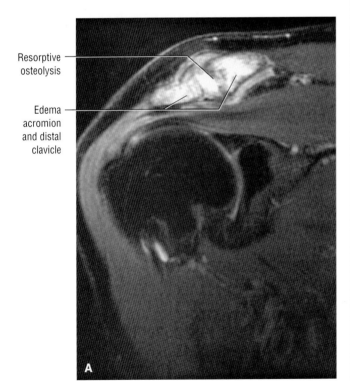

Resorptive osteolysis

Edema acromion and distal clavicle

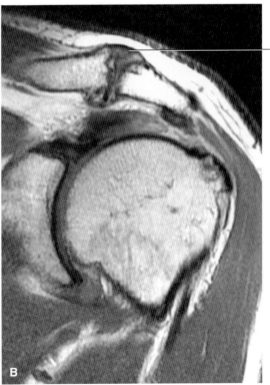

AC joint hypertrophy

FIGURE 9.76 (**A**) Coronal FS PD FSE image showing AC joint with hyperintense edema of the distal clavicle and adjacent acromion in a weight lifter. Repetitive microtrauma is associated with posttraumatic arthritis, including osteolysis. The "weight lifter's clavicle" represents subchondral injury with microfractures and resorptive osteolysis. (**B**) Coronal PD FSE image showing AC joint arthrosis associated with rotator cuff impingement. Characteristic AC joint hypertrophy, greater tuberosity squaring, inferior acromial spurs, and full thickness rotator cuff tear are shown.

Rheumatoid Arthritis

- Rheumatoid arthritis is a systemic inflammatory arthritic condition.[340]

- The glenoid articular cartilage is eroded medially, in contrast to the eccentric wear pattern of degenerative joint disease.

- The erosions of rheumatoid arthritis involves both cartilage and subchondral bone.[310]

- The superolateral articular surface of the humerus is commonly affected by erosive involvement.

- The glenohumeral, AC, and sternoclavicular shoulder articulations may be affected simultaneously.

- Bilateral disease and separate involvement of the elbow, wrist, and hand are not uncommon.

- Rheumatic disease of the shoulder is associated with full thickness rotator cuff tears in up to 50% in patients requiring total shoulder arthroplasty.

- Inflammation, fibrosis, and synovial hypertrophy involve both the subdeltoid bursa and synovial joint lining.

  - In addition, osseous erosions, resorption, sclerosis, and cysts may be found.

  - The synovial hypertrophy is often accompanied by decreased-signal-intensity rice bodies within the intermediate to hyperintense fluid/synovial complex.

  - Rice bodies are detached fibrotic synovial villi.

  - Uniform joint space narrowing often results.

  - The shoulder capsule may become thinned or stretch.

- Elevation or superior ascent of the humeral head is associated with rotator cuff defects.

- Surgical treatment includes:

  - Synovectomy

  - Arthroplasty

  - Arthrodesis

  - Osteotomy

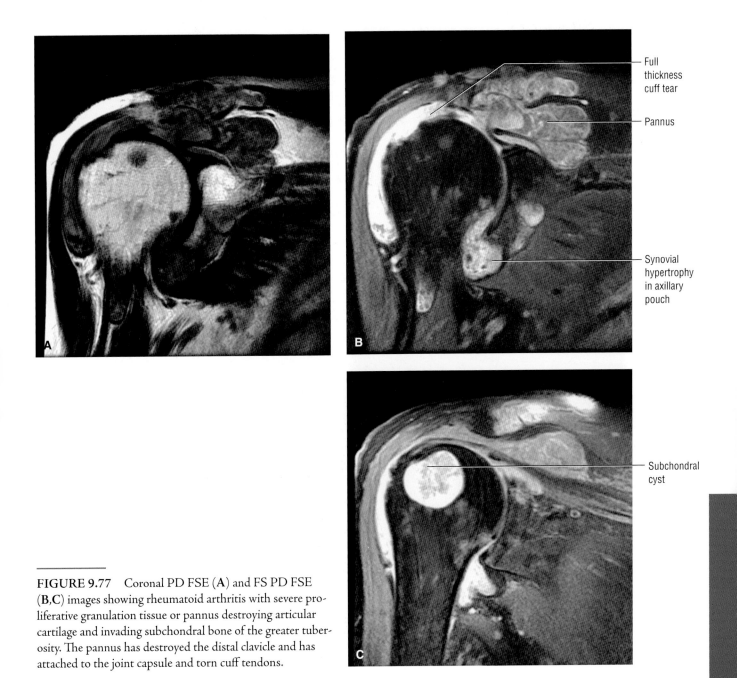

FIGURE 9.77 Coronal PD FSE (**A**) and FS PD FSE (**B,C**) images showing rheumatoid arthritis with severe proliferative granulation tissue or pannus destroying articular cartilage and invading subchondral bone of the greater tuberosity. The pannus has destroyed the distal clavicle and has attached to the joint capsule and torn cuff tendons.

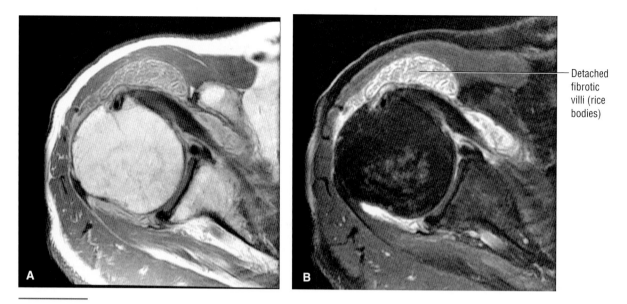

FIGURE 9.78   Intermediate-signal rice bodies or detached fibrotic villi of rheumatoid arthritis shown on axial PD FSE (**A**) and FS PD FSE (**B**) images.

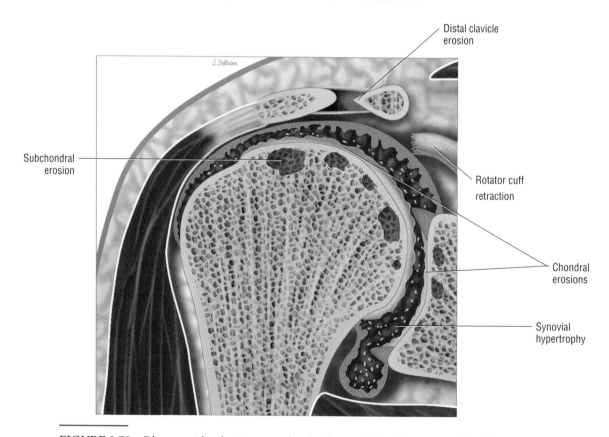

FIGURE 9.79   Rheumatoid arthritis targets the glenohumeral joint but may involve all synovial-lined joints, including the acromioclavicular and sternoclavicular joints. Marginal erosions and subchondral cysts may involve large areas of the humeral head. Glenoid destruction is associated with central or peripheral erosions. Sclerosis and osteophytosis are not common and represent the development of secondary osteoarthritis. Chondral loss, subchondral erosions, and synovial pannus are shown on this color coronal illustration. Erosion with tapering of the distal clavicle is also indicated.

Fractures of the Proximal Humerus and Osteochondral Lesions

Key Concepts

- Proximal humeral fractures have been grouped into involvement of the anatomic neck, greater tuberosity, lesser tuberosity, and surgical neck.

- Fracture displacement and angulation requires correlation of coronal and axial images.

- A chondral SLAP fracture involves the posteromedial superior humeral head.

- In acute fractures, T2* GRE images may be useful if hyperintense marrow edema obscures fracture site morphology or if a number of segments are involved.

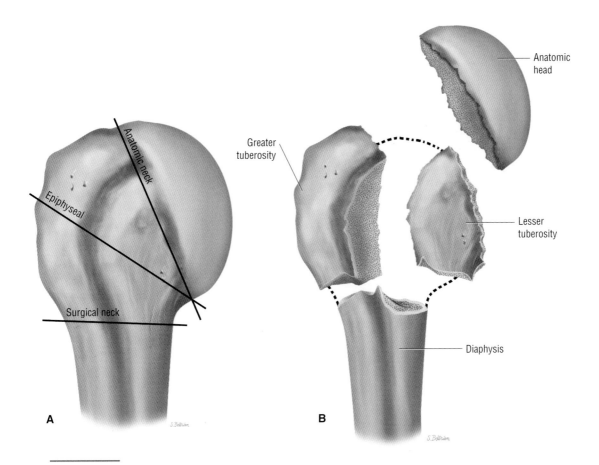

FIGURE 9.80 Fractures of the humeral head. (**A**) Original Kocher classification based on three different anatomic levels. This classification has been replaced by a description that included multiple fracture sites and differentiates between displaced and undisplaced fractures. (**B**) Division of the proximal humerus into four separate fragments based on anatomic lines of epiphyseal union. These distinct fragments are the greater tuberosity, the lesser tuberosity, the anatomic head, and the diaphysis.

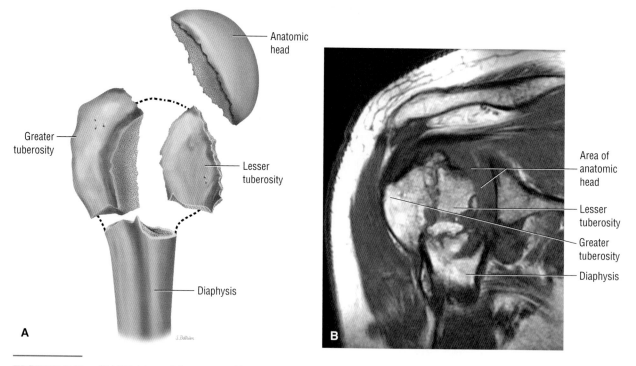

FIGURE 9.81 (A) Division of the proximal humerus into four separate fragments based on anatomic lines of epiphyseal union. These distinct fragments are the greater tuberosity, the lesser tuberosity, the anatomic head, and the diaphysis. (B) Coronal PD FSE image with fracture fragments involving the greater tuberosity, anatomic head, shaft, and lesser tuberosity identified.

Classification of Humeral Head Fractures

- Neer classifies upper humeral fractures into four types:[402]
    1. Those involving the anatomic neck of the humerus
    2. Those involving the greater tuberosity
    3. Those involving the lesser tuberosity
    4. Those involving the shaft or surgical neck of the humerus

- A one-part fracture has either no or minimal displacement or angulation of any of the segments.

- A two-part fracture involves displacement of one segment.

- A three-part fracture involves displacement of two segments with an associated unimpacted surgical neck fracture with rotatory displacement.

- A four-part fracture is characterized by displacement of all four segments.

- Displacement is defined by fracture segment displacement of greater than 1cm or angulation of more than 45°.

- Eight percent of proximal humeral fractures have minimal or no displacement and are held together by the rotator cuff, capsule, and periosteum.

MR Findings of Humeral Head Fractures

- Chondral lesions of the posteromedial superior humeral head are associated with SLAP tears and are referred to as SLAP fractures.[558]

  - These chondral injuries should not be mistaken for the more posterolateral Hill-Sachs deformity of the humeral head.

  - There may be a relative lack of subchondral edema in shearing chondral injuries.

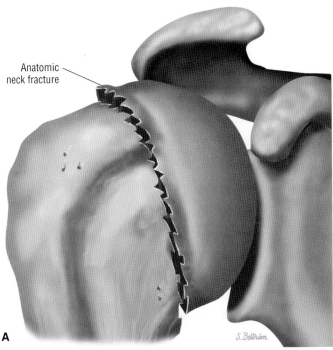

FIGURE 9.82 (**A**) Fracture of the anatomic neck at the articular segment. (A one-part fracture has no or minimal displacement or angulation. A two-part fracture has one segment displaced. A three-part fracture has two segments displaced with one tuberosity in continuity with the head. A four-part fracture has three segments displaced.) (**B**) Coronal PD FSE image of a displaced two-part fracture of the anatomic neck with proximal displacement of the diaphysis relative to the medial articular segment. (**C**) Axial PD FSE image showing the three-fragment sign of the shaft, anatomic neck, and glenoid visualized on a single axial image.

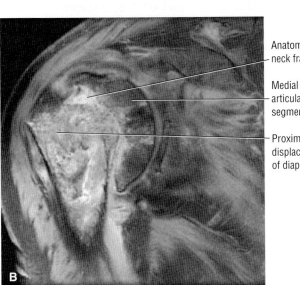

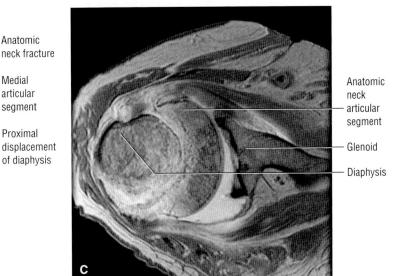

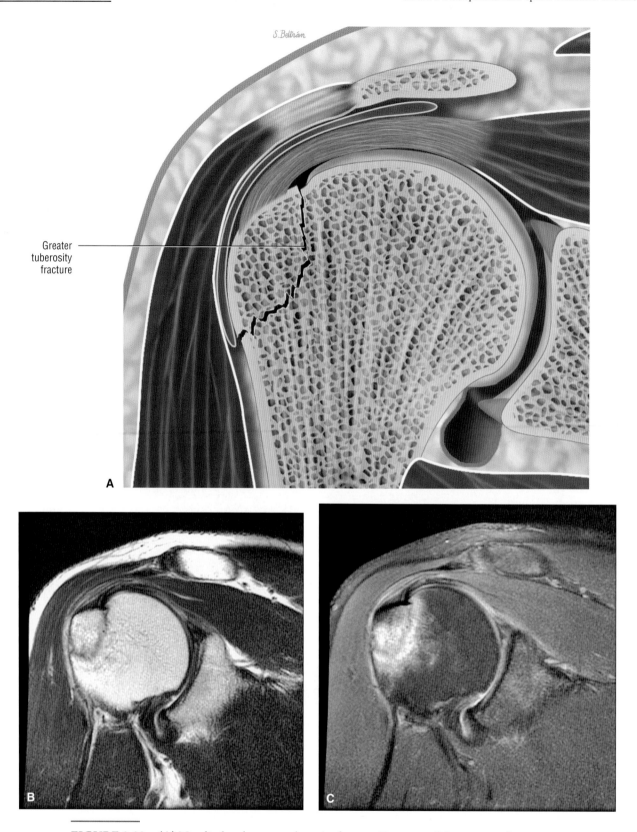

FIGURE 9.83 (**A**) Nondisplaced greater tuberosity fracture. Fractures of the greater tuberosity are associated with anterior dislocations. A greater tuberosity fracture usually reduces into an acceptable anatomic position but may displace underneath the acromial process or be directed posteriorly by the pull of the rotator cuff muscles. Impacted greater tuberosity fracture without superior displacement on coronal PD FSE (**B**) and FS PD FSE (**C**) images.

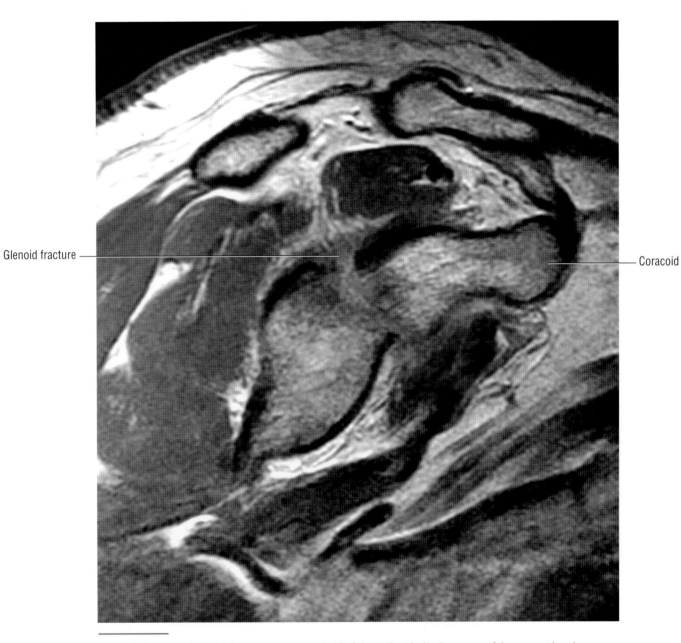

Glenoid fracture

Coracoid

FIGURE 9.84 Glenoid fracture upper one-half of glenoid with displacement of the coracoid and superior one-third of the glenoid fossa. Glenoid fossa fractures are associated with severe trauma. There is usually damage to the glenoid chondral surface. Glenohumeral alignment needs to be restored. Sagittal T2 FSE.

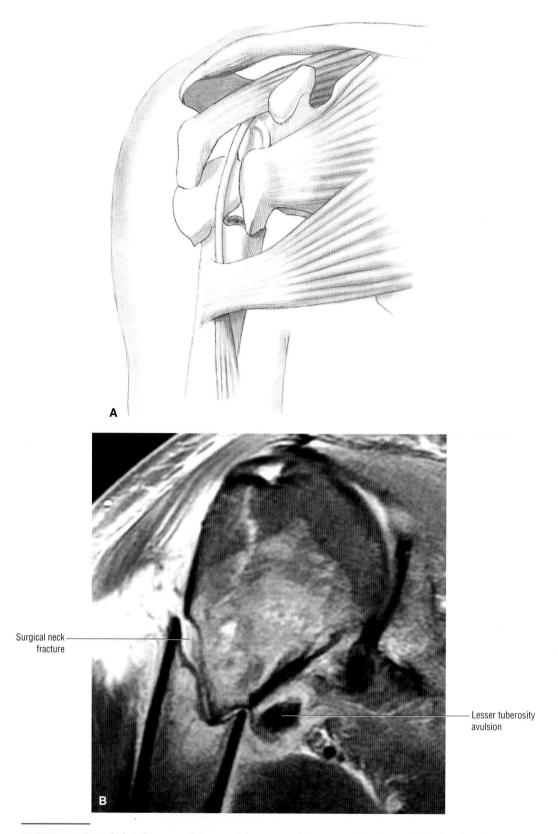

FIGURE 9.85 (**A**) A four-part fracture of the proximal humerus. The humeral head is free-floating and displaced from both tuberosities and the shaft. The lesser tuberosity fragment is pulled medially by the subscapularis, the greater tuberosity fragment is pulled posteriorly and superiorly by the supraspinatus and infraspinatus, and the shaft fragment is pulled medially by the pectoralis major. (Reprinted from Craig EV. *Master Techniques in Orthopaedic Surgery: Shoulder*. 3rd ed. Philadelphia, PA: Lippincott Williams & Wilkins; 2013, with permission.) (**B**) Unusual type of three-part fracture involving the avulsed lesser tuberosity and surgical neck of the humerus. Diaphyseal fracture component which would typically be pulled medially by the pectoralis major. There is medial displacement and angulation of the proximal humeral head and metaphyseal components. Coronal FS PD FSE.

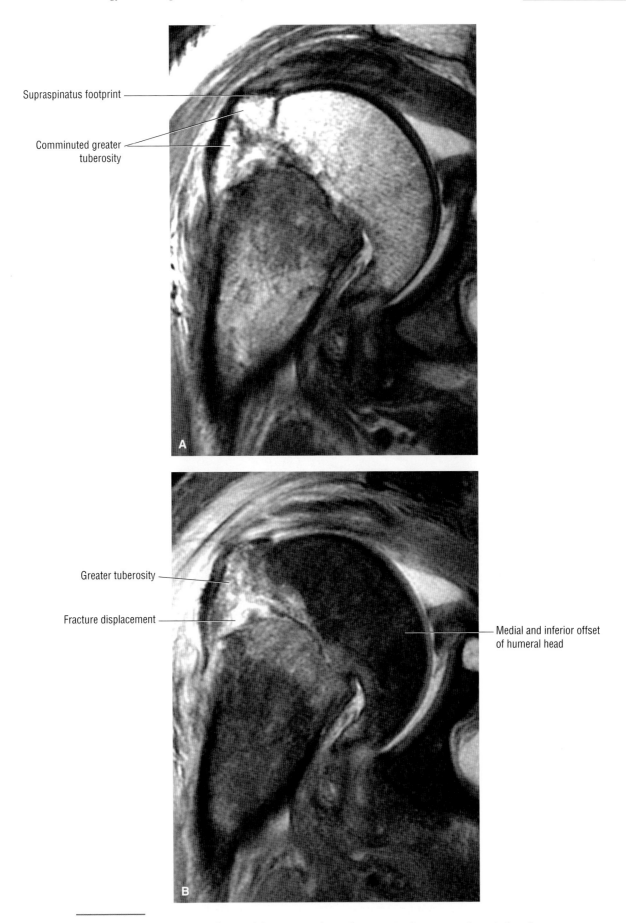

FIGURE 9.86 Three-part humeral fracture involving the greater tuberosity and surgical neck. The supraspinatus tendon is attached to the comminuted greater tuberosity fragment. The humeral head is displaced medially. If the lesser tuberosity was avulsed this would be a four-part fracture. (**A**) Coronal T2 FSE. (**B**) Coronal FS PD.

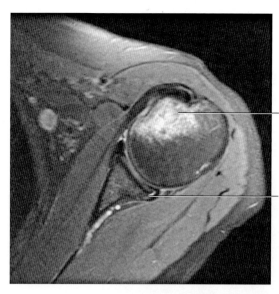

Nondisplaced lesser tuberosity fracture

Posterior labral tear

FIGURE 9.87 Axial FS PD FSE image showing a nondisplaced lesser tuberosity fracture associated with a posterior labral tear and dislocation. A fracture of the lesser tuberosity may be pulled anteriorly and medially by the subscapularis muscle.

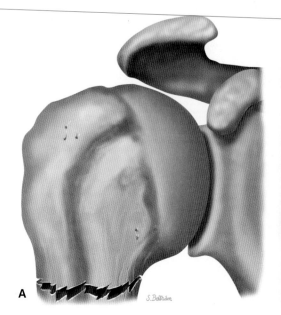

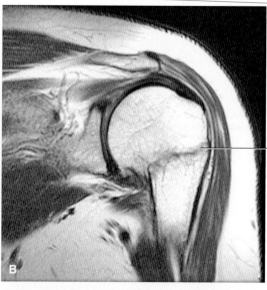

Surgical neck fracture

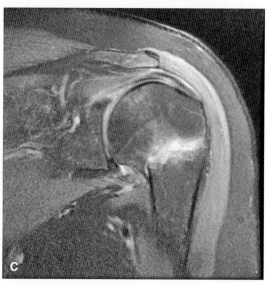

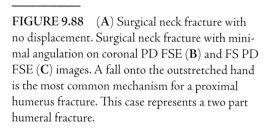

FIGURE 9.88 (**A**) Surgical neck fracture with no displacement. Surgical neck fracture with minimal angulation on coronal PD FSE (**B**) and FS PD FSE (**C**) images. A fall onto the outstretched hand is the most common mechanism for a proximal humerus fracture. This case represents a two part humeral fracture.

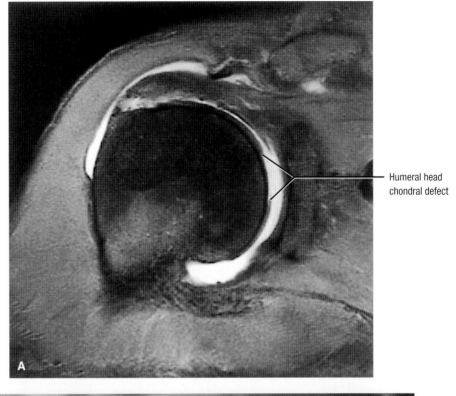

Humeral head
chondral defect

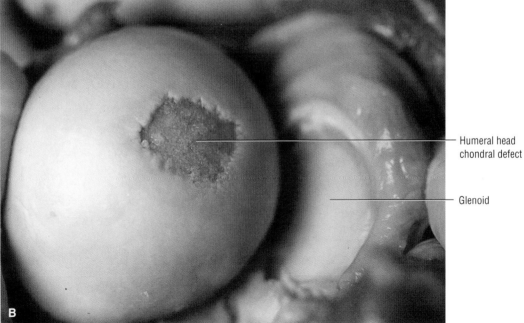

Humeral head
chondral defect

Glenoid

FIGURE 9.89 (**A**) Coronal FS T1-weighted MR arthrogram of the posteromedial location of a SLAP fracture of the articular surface of the superior humeral head caused by a fall onto an outstretched arm. A chondral divot can be seen in the superior dome of the humeral head. These chondral fractures are usually not associated with subchondral edema may be overlooked on review of coronal MR images. (**B**) Corresponding gross dissection of the SLAP fracture.

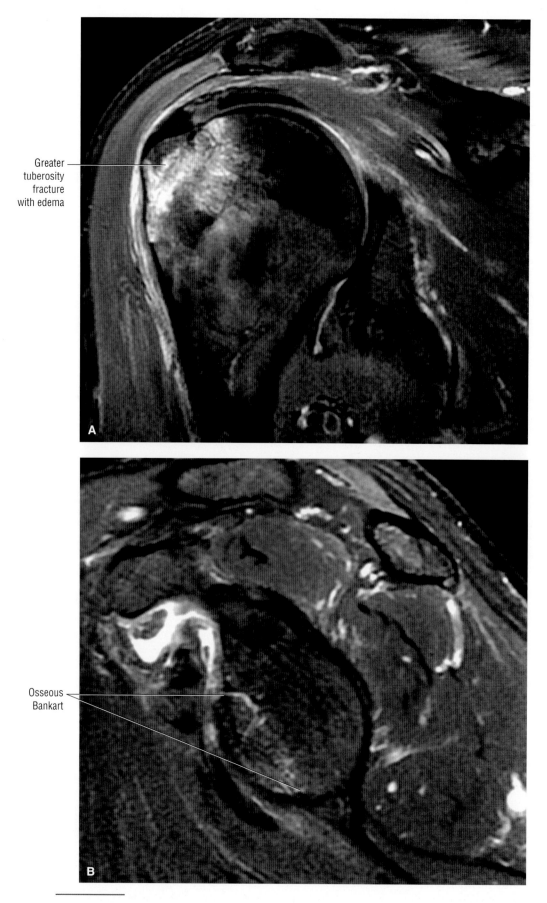

FIGURE 9.90 Greater tuberosity fracture associated with nondisplaced osseous Bankart fracture of the anterior inferior glenoid rim. In older patients, macroinstability episodes may be associated with a greater tuberosity fracture in place of a Hill-Sachs lesion. (**A**) Coronal FS PD. (**B**) Sagittal FS PD.

Avascular Necrosis (AVN)

Key Concepts

- ◼ Risk increases with three- and four-part fractures.

- ◼ MR findings of AVN may be subchondral or metaphyseal in location.

- ◼ Extended hyperintense marrow edema of the proximal humerus is often associated with the more acute stages of AVN.

- ◼ Sagittal images are helpful in assessing early subchondral collapse with a loss of sphericity of the humeral head contour.

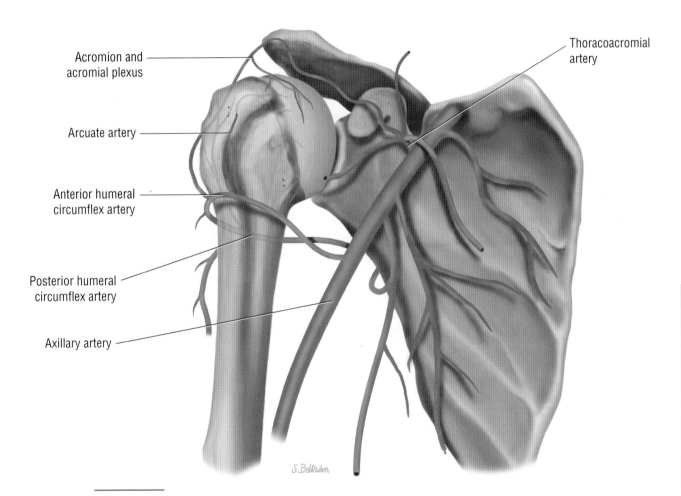

Acromion and acromial plexus

Arcuate artery

Anterior humeral circumflex artery

Posterior humeral circumflex artery

Axillary artery

Thoracoacromial artery

S. Beltrán

FIGURE 9.91 Coronal color graphic view of the blood supply of the humeral head. The major or primary vascular supply to the humeral head is from the anterior humeral circumflex artery. The arcuate artery, a continuation of the ascending branch of the anterior humeral circumflex, supplies the humeral head, including the greater and lesser tuberosities. A secondary or smaller contribution to the humeral head blood supply is derived from branches of the posterior circumflex artery and the tendinous-osseous anastomoses of the vascular rotator cuff.

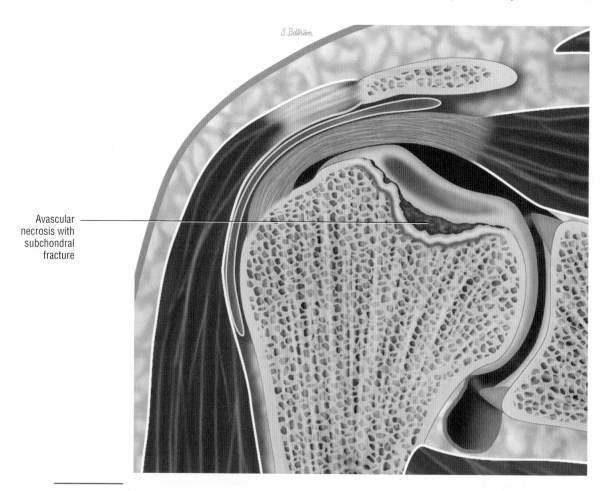

Avascular
necrosis with
subchondral
fracture

FIGURE 9.92   Localized nontraumatic AVN associated with systemic lupus erythematosus. Lupus patients who are not on glucocorticoids or immunosuppressive drugs are at increased risk for septic arthritis and osteonecrosis. Osteonecrosis occurs in 4% to 15% of lupus patients and affects the humeral head in 80% of cases. Color coronal illustration anterior view of osteonecrosis with subchondral fractures.

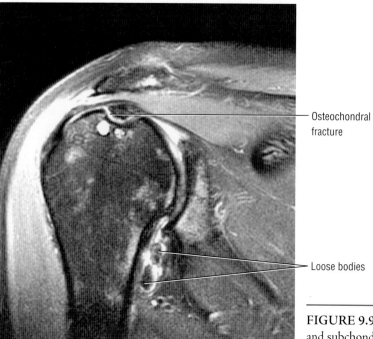

Osteochondral
fracture

Loose bodies

FIGURE 9.93   Focal osteochondral lesion involving the chondral and subchondral bone of the superior humeral head. Loose bodies are demonstrated in the axillary pouch on this coronal FS PD FSE image.

- AVN may occur in association with three- and four-part fractures in which the main arterial supply to the humeral head is at risk from injury to a branch of the anterior humeral circumflex artery[11] and its intraosseous anastomoses.

   - AVN may occur even in the absence of humeral head displacement.

- Nontraumatic AVN of the humeral head may be either idiopathic or secondary to a variety of systemic conditions, including:[497]

   - Steroid use, including posttransplantation therapy
   - Dysbaric disorders
   - Vasculitis
   - Alcoholism
   - Sickle cell disease
   - Hyperuricemia
   - Gaucher disease
   - Pancreatitis
   - Familial hyperlipidemia
   - Lymphoma

- Superior central area of the humeral head common (same location as glenohumeral contact joint)

- AVN of the humeral head can usually be differentiated from osteoarthritis by the involvement of subchondral low-signal-intensity ischemia limited to the humerus, without associated glenoid involvement (i.e., sclerosis).

   - AVN patients are younger than most glenohumeral degenerative joint patients.

- AVN demonstrates a serpiginous pattern of involvement that may be identified in both metaphyseal and subarticular locations.

Classification for AVN of the Humeral Head

- The Neer classification for AVN of the humeral head is similar to the Ficat staging for hip osteonecrosis:[406]

   - Stage 1: Asymptomatic; conventional radiographs produce negative results, whereas MR imaging results are positive for alterations in subchondral marrow.

- Stage 2: Clinically characterized by pain; the humeral head retains its specific shape, although mild depression of the articular cartilage may be present in an area of subchondral bone.

- Stage 3: Subchondral collapse or fracture with overlying articular cartilage irregularity is seen. No involvement of the glenohumeral joint articular cartilage at this stage.

  - Sagittal images should be evaluated for any contour flattening of the humeral head as a direct result of the subchondral fracture. The articular cartilage is secondary involved as a result of the collapse of the underlying subchondral bone.

- Stage 4: Incongruity of the glenohumeral joint with secondary chondral findings

- Paget's disease of the humerus also produces marrow changes, especially in the paratrabecular endosteal areas, which may be mistaken for ischemic disease.

- Patients frequently present at a lateral stage of AVN.

- Core decompression for nontraumatic early stage AVN.

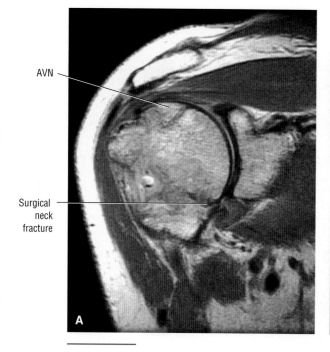
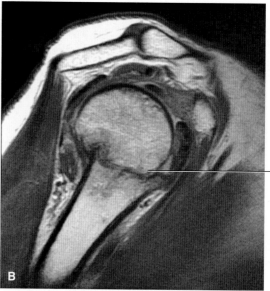

AVN

Surgical
neck
fracture

Minimally
displaced
fracture of
the surgical
neck

FIGURE 9.94   A minimally (<1cm) displaced surgical neck fracture with AVN of the humeral head on coronal PD FSE (**A**) and sagittal PD FSE (**B**) images.

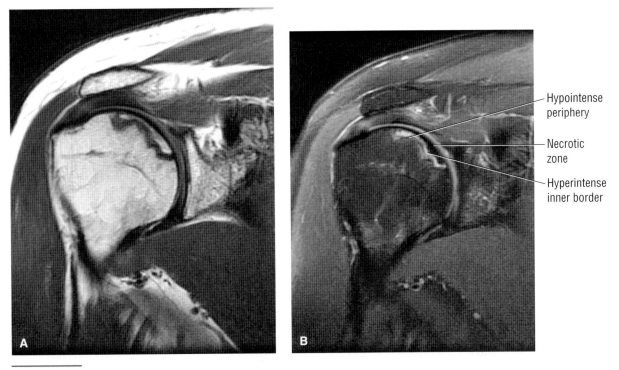

FIGURE 9.95 Localized nontraumatic AVN associated with systemic lupus erythematosus. Lupus patients who are not on glucocorticoids or immunosuppressive drugs are at increased risk for septic arthritis and osteonecrosis. Osteonecrosis occurs in 4% to 15% of lupus patients and affects the humeral head in 80% of cases. Coronal PD FSE (**A**) and FS PD FSE (**B**) images demonstrate AVN prior to subchondral collapse. The double line sign of osteonecrosis consists of a hyperintense inner border and a hypointense outer margin on the FS PD FSE image (**B**).

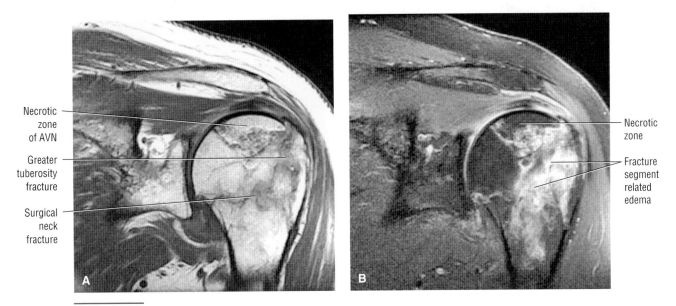

FIGURE 9.96 Nondisplaced surgical neck and greater tuberosity fracture with humeral head AVN on coronal PD FSE (**A**) and FS PD FSE (**B**) images.

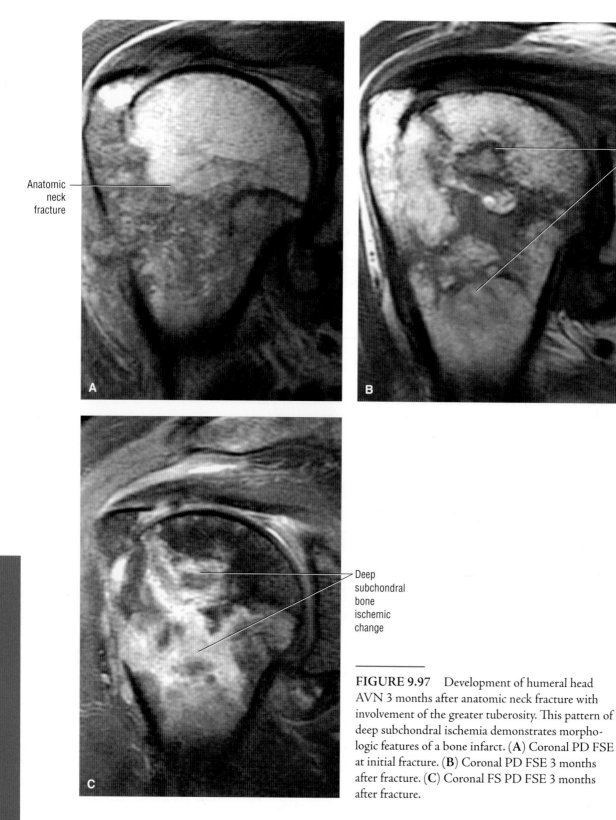

Anatomic neck fracture

Subchondral ischemia (osteonecrosis)

Deep subchondral bone ischemic change

FIGURE 9.97   Development of humeral head AVN 3 months after anatomic neck fracture with involvement of the greater tuberosity. This pattern of deep subchondral ischemia demonstrates morphologic features of a bone infarct. (**A**) Coronal PD FSE at initial fracture. (**B**) Coronal PD FSE 3 months after fracture. (**C**) Coronal FS PD FSE 3 months after fracture.

Infection

Key Concepts

■ T1-weighted images in at least one plane provide yellow marrow fat contrast relative to the patchy hypointensity of osseous osteomyelitis.

■ T2* GRE images, although not sensitive for infection, can increase specificity in the diagnosis of osteomyelitis if areas of trabecular hyperintensity are shown.

■ Evaluate other causes of non-infected fluid collections:

■ Scapulothoracic bursitis or "snapping scapula syndrome" as a fluid collection between the scapula and chest wall

■ Intravenous contrast, although not specific for osteomyelitis, is used to enhance soft tissue tracts and abscesses, which may communicate with adjacent osseous erosions.

■ Intraarticular sepsis[498] of the shoulder is classified as:

■ Hematogenous

■ Secondary to contiguous spread from osteomyelitis

■ Secondary to trauma, surgery, or intraarticular injection

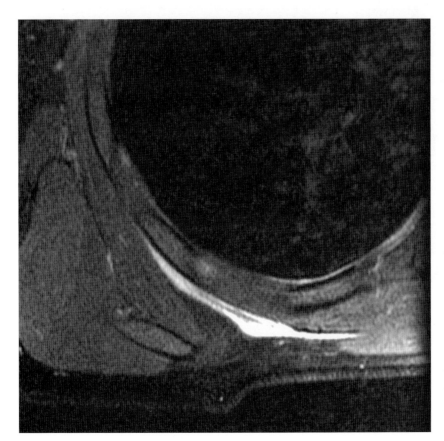

FIGURE 9.98   Scapulothrocic bursitis with curvilinear fluid signal hyperintensity postero-lateral to the chest between the scapula and the ribs. This collection should not be mistaken for an abscess. This is a diagnosis that requires larger coverage than typically provided by the geometry of a dedicated shoulder coil. Clinical patient may present with snapping scapula syndrome from overuse in sport activities. MR findings are usually uncommon even if clinical exam is positive. Axial FS PD.

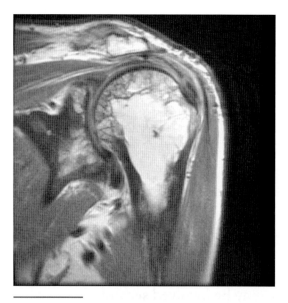

FIGURE 9.99   Coronal PD FSE image showing increased osseous resorption and bone formation, characteristic changes of Paget's disease. The osseous appearance may mimic fracture and metastatic carcinoma. The three phases of Paget's disease are lytic, mixed lytic and blastic, and blastic phases. Pagetoid marrow contains new bone formation and fibrovascular tissue and is at an increased risk for fracture. This should not be mistakened for infection.

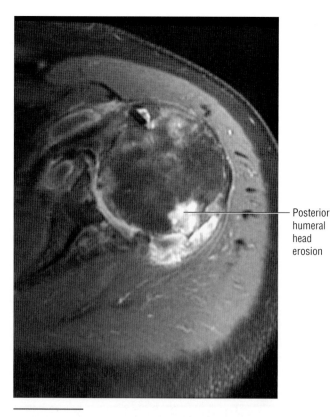

Posterior humeral head erosion

FIGURE 9.100   Axial FS PD FSE image of osteomyelitis secondary to injection of steroids with focal posterior humeral head erosion and soft tissue hyperintense complex fluid collection.

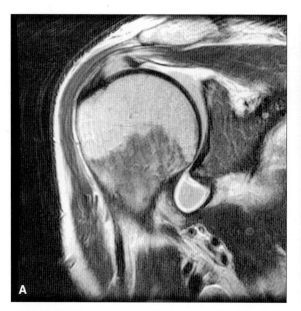

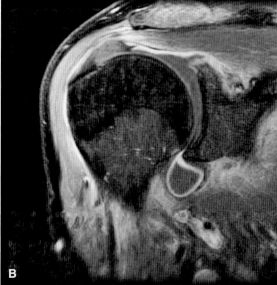

FIGURE 9.101   Septic shoulder with a hyperintense outline of inflammatory fluid within the axillary pouch as seen on coronal PD FSE (**A**) and FS PD FSE (**B**) images. There is no osseous involvement at this stage.

■ Osteomyelitis of the humerus may extend to involve the joint directly.

■ Septic arthritis of the shoulder commonly affects the glenohumeral joint.

■ Sarcoidosis of the shoulder frequently demonstrates a hypertrophic synovial inflammatory reaction simulating infection.

■ Hematogenous osteomyelitis is more frequent (80% to 90%) in children.

■ In adults, contiguous spread of osteomyelitis is usually secondary to surgery or direct inoculation.

■ In intravenous injection drug users, the clavicle may be involved secondary to hematogenous seeding.

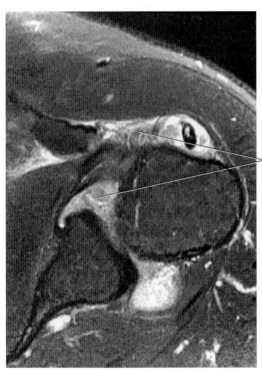

Sarcoid synovial reaction (granulomatous synovitis)

FIGURE 9.102 Sarcoid inflammatory reaction may be mistaken for a septic joint. Inflammatory arthropathy is a common feature of sarcoidosis.

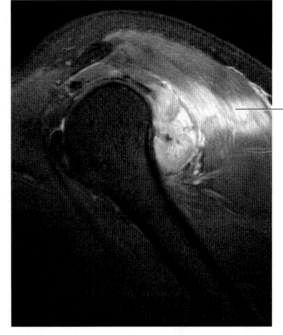

Inflammatory tract

FIGURE 9.103 Sagittal FS PD FSE image of an inflammatory tract with myositis that developed as a reaction to a flu inoculation.

- MR findings include synovial fluid inhomogeneity and non-rheumatoid-type synovial hypertrophy.

- Subtle osseous erosions of the humerus with adjacent reactive marrow edema are seen in the initial stages of osteomyelitis.

- Inhomogeneous or patchy areas of hypointense humeral head and glenoid marrow involvement frequently require a T1-weighted sequence to appreciate osseous involvement.

- Hyperintensity of marrow visualized on T2* GRE images is suspicious for involvement of osteomyelitis in the presence of intraarticular sepsis.

- Since GRE imaging is not a marrow-sensitive technique, any signs of destruction of trabecular bone and/or influx of free water are more serious indicators of contiguous spread.

- FS PD FSE and STIR images may be sensitive but are not nonspecific with respect to marrow hyperintensity and distinguishing reactive edema from infection.

- Enlarged axillary lymph nodes may be seen in malignancy and infection and are best assessed on sagittal images.

- Metastatic disease may be mistaken for infection.

  - In metastatic disease, there is bone marrow involvement with trabecular destruction and less tissue reaction.

- Fibrous dysplasia may present in multiple locations in the polyostotic form.

- Large B cell lymphoma (non-Hodgkin lyphoma) is a common shoulder neoplasm that may be a mimic of infection in the stage of fat marrow replacement.

- Upper extermity metastases (20% of bony metastases)

  - Fifty percent involve the humerus.

- Intravenous MR contrast agents are nonspecific for osseous bone lesions (for both infection, metastases, and primary lesions).

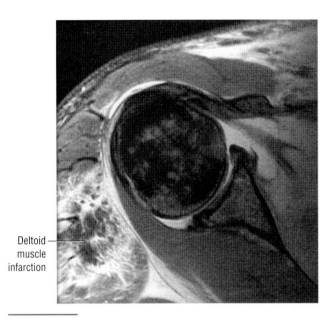

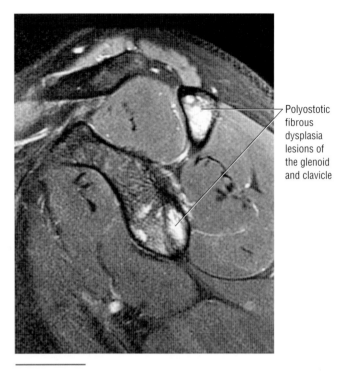

FIGURE 9.104 Rarely, infectious myositis is complicated by a muscle infarction. Fibrotic myopathy, which usually involves the deltoid and quadriceps, may produce similar muscle hypointensity as a complication of direct intramuscular injection of drugs, as seen on this axial FS PD FSE image.

FIGURE 9.105 Osseous involvement of the glenoid and clavicle in polyostotic fibrous dysplasia, which may be mistaken for infection or metastatic disease, is seen on this sagittal FS PD FSE image.

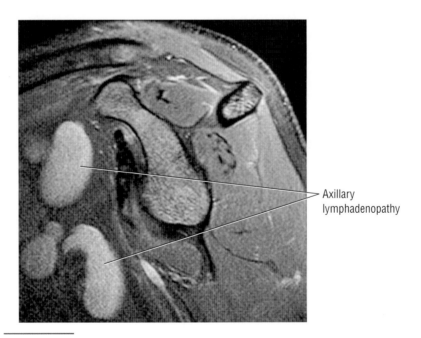

FIGURE 9.106 Sagittal FS PD FSE image showing enlarged axillary lymph nodes in chronic lymphocytic leukemia.

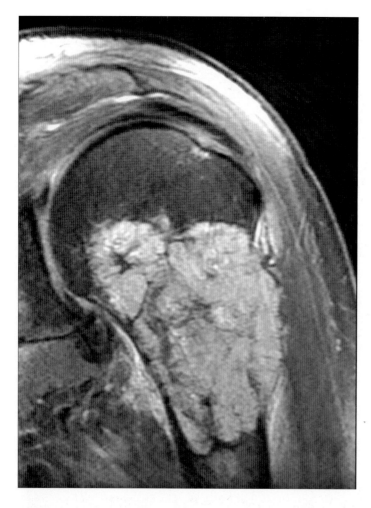

FIGURE 9.107 Metastatic renal cell carcinoma with characteristic medullary expansion and cortical disruption of the proximal humerus. Coronal FS PD.

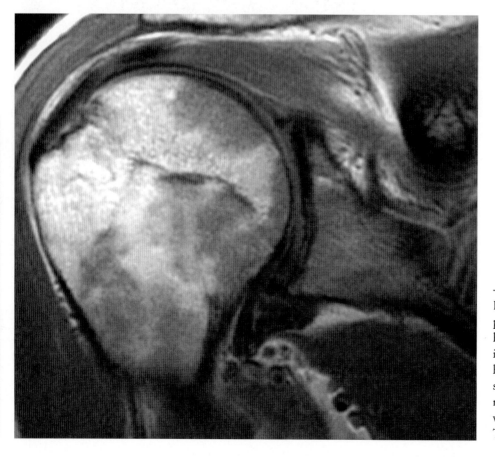

FIGURE 9.108 Osseous lymphoma with areas of abnormal hypointense marrow replacement that include the metaphysis and proximal humeral head proximal to the physeal scar. This irregular pattern of marrow replacement should never be confused with red marrow activation. Coronal T2 FSE.

FIGURE 9.109 Chondrosarcoma with expansile hyperintense lesion of the scapula to include the glenoid and coracoid. The chondrosarcoma has expanded beyond the confines of the ossesous scapular and involves soft tissue structures. After intravenous MR contrast, there is irregular nodular enhancement along the inner border of the periphery of the tumor. The hypointense center of the chondrosarcoma corresponds to the chondroid lates of the tumor matrix. Typically, however, intravenous MR contrast agents are unreliable in their ability to evaluate osseous lesions because of the unpredictable pattern of contrast enhancement. This is in sharp distinction to the useful application of contrast agents in the evaluation of soft tissue lesions where central versus peripheral enhancement can increase the specificity of diagnosis. (**A**) Axial FS PD. (**B**) Axial T1 FS contrast enhanced.

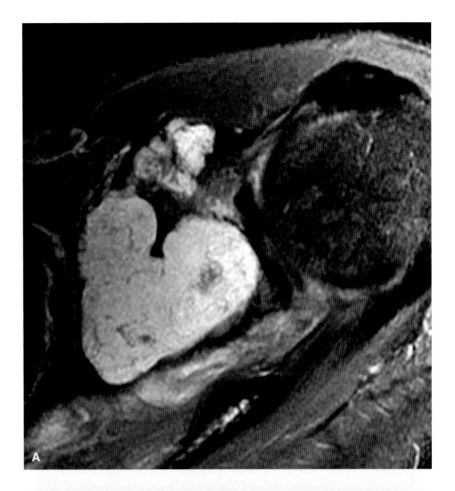

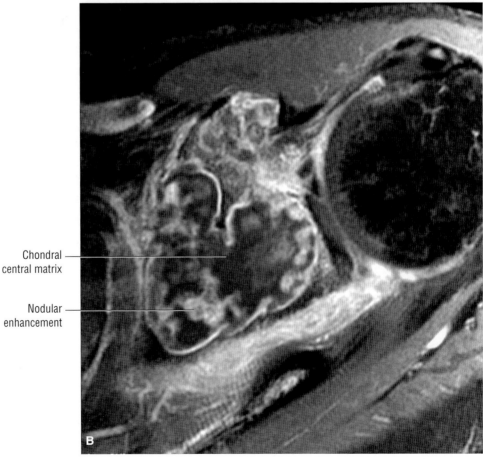

Chondral central matrix

Nodular enhancement

Shoulder Replacement

Glenohumeral Arthroplasty

- Glenohumeral arthroplasty[340] includes:
    - Nonprosthetic arthroplasty
    - Prosthetic humeral hemiarthroplasty
        - Often used in cases of combined arthritis and cuff deficiency
    - Total glenohumeral arthroplasty
        - Recommended in osteoarthritis and rheumatoid arthritis when the rotator cuff is intact

- MR evaluation is useful in selecting the most appropriate type of procedure by quantifying the rotator cuff integrity, fatty atrophy, and fracture union.
    - Further MR evaluation of the deltoid muscle is important since shoulder prostheses cannot function if the deltoid is atrophied.

Reverse Shoulder Replacement

- Reverse shoulder replacement designed for:[168,629]
    - Cases of deficient rotator cuff and arthritis (rotator cuff tear arthropathy)
    - Complex fractures
    - Revision of a failed joint replacement with a chronically torn and atrophied rotator cuff

- The glenoid socket is replaced with an artificial ball and the humeral head is replaced by a socket implant.
    - This configuration thus reverses the normal relationship of the humeral head to the glenoid.

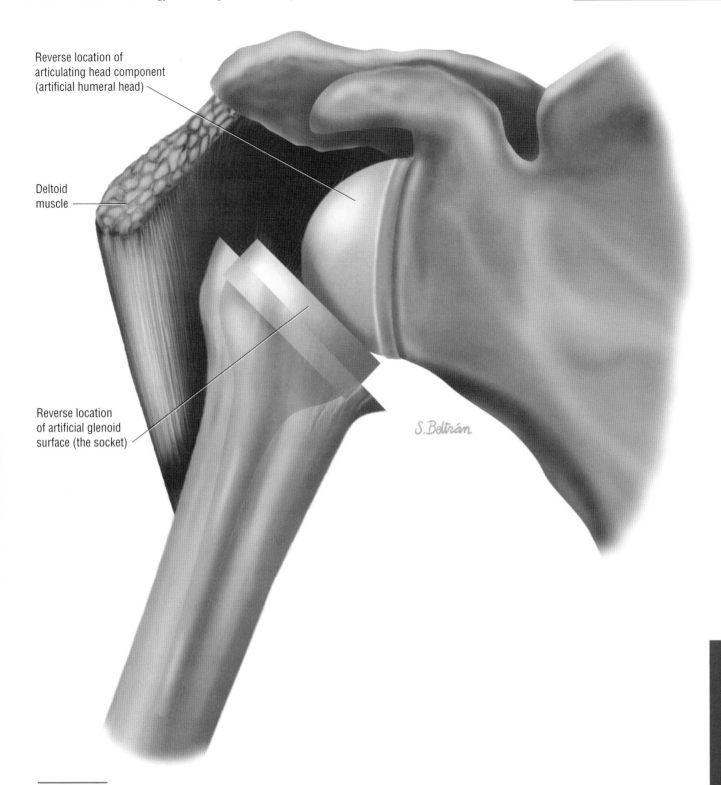

Reverse location of
articulating head component
(artificial humeral head)

Deltoid
muscle

Reverse location
of artificial glenoid
surface (the socket)

S. Beltrán

FIGURE 9.110   Reverse shoulder replacement optimizes the force of the deltoid (by increasing
the lever arm) and stabilizes the glenohumeral articulation by moving the center of rotation of the
glenohumeral joint medially and inferiorly. This provides an increased mechanical advantage for
raising the arm overhead. Reverse prosthesis may be used to direct forces through the glenosphere,
converting centrifugal or outward forces into centripetal or inward forces.

References

1. Abboud JA, Bartolozzi AR, Widmer BJ, DeMola PM. Bicipital groove morphology on MRI has no correlation to intra-articular biceps tendon pathology. *J Shoulder Elbow Surg* 2010;19(6):790–794. doi:10.1016/j.jse.2010.04.044.

2. Abella, HA. Imaging of shoulder opens new turf fight for radiologists. *Diag Imaging* 2006:37–40.

3. Ahearn N, McCann PA, Tasker A, Sarangi PP. The influence of rotator cuff pathology on functional outcome in total shoulder replacement. *Int J Shoulder Surg* 2013;7(4):127–131. doi:10.4103/0973-6042.123509.

4. Ahmed I, Ashton F, Robinson CM. Arthroscopic Bankart repair and capsular shift for recurrent anterior shoulder instability: functional outcomes and identification of risk factors for recurrence. *J Bone Joint Surg Am* 2012;94(14):1308–1315. doi:10.2106/JBJS.J.01983.

5. Alfonso DT. Causes of neonatal brachial plexus palsy. *Bull NYU Hosp Jt Dis* 2011;69(1):11–16.

6. Almeida GP, Silveira PF, Rosseto NP, Barbosa G, Ejnisman B, Cohen M. Glenohumeral range of motion in handball players with and without throwing-related shoulder pain. *J Shoulder Elbow Surg* 2013;22(5):602–607. doi:10.1016/j.jse.2012.08.027.

7. Alpert J, Flannery R, Epstein R, Monaco R, Prendergast N. Humeral stress edema: an injury in overhead athletes quarterback with humeral "shin" spints–a case report. *Clin J Sport Med* 2014;24(5):e59–e61.

8. Altan E, Ozbaydar MU, Tonbul M, Yalcin L. Comparison of two different measurement methods to determine glenoid bone defects: area or width? *J Shoulder Elbow Surg* 2014;23(8):1215–1222. doi:10.1016/j.jse.2013.11.029.

9. Amin MF, Youssef AO. The diagnostic value of magnetic resonance arthrography of the shoulder in detection and grading of SLAP lesions: comparison with arthroscopic findings. *Eur J Radiol* 2012;81(9):2343–2347. doi:10.1016/j.ejrad.2011.07.006.

10. Anakwenze OA, Hsu JE, Abboud JA, Levine WN, Huffman GR. Recurrent anterior shoulder instability associated with bony defects. *Orthopedics* 2011;34(7):538–544; quiz 545–546. doi:10.3928/01477447-20110526-21.

11. Andary JL, Petersen SA. The vascular anatomy of the glenohumeral capsule and ligaments: an anatomic study. *J Bone Joint Surg Am* 2002;84(12):2258.

12. Andersen LL, Andersen CH, Skotte JH, Suetta C, Søgaard K, Saltin B, Sjøgaard G. High-intensity strength training improves function of chronically painful muscles: case-control and RCT studies. *Biomed Res Int* 2014;2014:187324.doi:10.1155/2014/187324.

13. Andrews JR, Carson WG Jr, McLeod WD. Glenoid labrum tears related to the long head of the biceps. *Am J Sports Med* 1985;13(5):337.

14. Aoki M, Ishii S, Usui M. The slope of the acromion and rotator cuff impingement. *Orthop Trans* 1986;10:228.

15. Applegate GR, Hewitt M, Snyder SJ, et al. Chronic labral tears: value of magnetic resonance arthrography in evaluating the glenoid labrum and labral-bicipital complex. *Arthroscopy* 2004;20(9):959.

16. Arai R, Kobayashi M, Toda Y, Nakamura S, Miura T, Nakamura T. Fiber components of the shoulder superior labrum. *Surg Radiol Anat* 2012;34(1):49–56. doi:10.1007/s00276-011-0840-8.

17. Arai R, Mochizuki T, Yamaguchi K, Sugaya H, Kobayashi M, Nakamura T, Akita K. Functional anatomy of the superior glenohumeral and coracohumeral ligaments and the subscapularis tendon in view of stabilization of the long head of the biceps tendon. *J Shoulder Elbow Surg* 2010;19(1):58–64. doi:10.1016/j.jse.2009.04.001.

18. Arce G, Bak K, Bain G, Calvo E, Ejnisman B, Di Giacomo G, Gutierrez V, Guttmann D, Itoi E, Ben Kibler W, Ludvigsen T, Mazzocca A, de Castro Pochini A, Savoie F III, Sugaya H, Uribe J, Vergara F, Willems J, Yoo YS, McNeil JW II, Provencher MT. Management of disorders of the rotator cuff: proceedings of the ISAKOS upper extremity committee consensus meeting. *Arthroscopy* 2013;29(11):1840–1850. doi:10.1016/j.arthro.2013.07.265.

19. Armitage MS, Faber KJ, Drosdowech DS, Litchfield RB, Athwal GS. Humeral head bone defects: remplissage, allograft, and arthroplasty. *Orthop Clin North Am* 2010;41(3):417–425. doi:10.1016/j.ocl.2010.03.004.

20. Bak K, Wiesler ER, Poehling GG; ISAKOS Upper Extremity Committee. Consensus statement on shoulder instability. *Arthroscopy* 2010;26(2):249–255. doi:10.1016/j.arthro.2009.06.022.

21. Bancroft LW, Wasyliw C, Pettis C, Farley T. Postoperative shoulder magnetic resonance imaging. *Magn Reson Imaging Clin N Am* 2012;20(2):313–325, xi. doi:10.1016/j.mric.2012.01.010.

22. Barber F, Maki N. Posterior shoulder instability: arthroscopic repair. In: Gumpert E, Zurhellen O, Stewart D, eds. *Surgical Techniques for the Shoulder and Elbow.* New York, NY: Thieme; 2003:110.

23. Barber F, Nicholson G. Adhesive capsulitis: manipulation or arthroscopic capsular division. In: Gumpert E, Zurhellen O, Stewart D, eds. *Surgical Techniques for the Shoulder and Elbow.* New York, NY: Thieme; 2003:127.

24. Barber F, Wolf EM. Acromioclavicular separations: Rockwood screw technique for chronic problems. In: Gumpert E, Zurhellen O, Stewart D, eds. *Surgical Techniques for the Shoulder and Elbow.* New York, NY: Thieme; 2003:11.

25. Barber F, Wolf EM. Anterior shoulder instability: HAGL lesion repair. In: Gumpert E, Zurhellen O, Stewart D, eds. *Surgical Techniques for the Shoulder and Elbow.* New York, NY: Thieme; 2003:110–112.

26. Barber F, Wolf EM. Arthroscopic treatment of multidirectional instability. In: Gumpert E, Zurhellen O, Stewart D, eds. *Surgical Techniques for the Shoulder and Elbow.* New York, NY: Thieme; 2003:110.

27. Barile A, Lanni G, Conti L, Mariani S, Calvisi V, Castagna A, Rossi F, Masciocchi C. Lesions of the biceps pulley as cause of anterosuperior impingement of the shoulder in the athlete: potentials and limits of MR arthrography compared with arthroscopy. *Radiol Med* 2013;118(1): 112–122. doi:10.1007/s11547-012-0838-2.

28. Bartl C, Salzmann GM, Seppel G, Eichhorn S, Holzapfel K, Wörtler K, Imhoff AB. Subscapularis function and structural integrity after arthroscopic repair of isolated subscapularis tears. *Am J Sports Med* 2011;39(6):1255–1262. doi:10.1177/0363546510396317.

29. Baudi P, Rasia Dani E, Campochiaro G, Rebuzzi M, Serafini F, Catani F. The rotator cuff tear repair with a new arthroscopic transosseous system: the Sharc-FT(®). *Musculoskelet Surg* 2013;97(suppl 1): 57–61. doi:10.1007/s12306-013-0254-3.

30. Beall DP, Williamson EE, Ly JQ, et al. Association of biceps tendon tears with rotator cuff abnormalities: degree of correlation with tears of the anterior and superior portions of the rotator cuff. *AJR Am J Roentgenol* 2003;180(3):633.

31. Beeler S, Ek ET, Gerber C. A comparative analysis of fatty infiltration and muscle atrophy in patients with chronic rotator cuff tears and suprascapular neuropathy. *J Shoulder Elbow Surg* 2013;22(11):1537–1546. doi:10.1016/j.jse .2013.01.028.

32. Beitzel K, Kirchhoff C, Beitzel KI, Reiser MF, Kirchhoff S. In vivo evaluation of the kinematics of the long head of the biceps tendon within the pulley: a 3 T MRI motion analysis. *Arch Orthop Trauma Surg* 2013;133(12):1719–1725. doi:10.1007/s00402-013-1865-8.

33. Bell JE. Arthroscopic management of multidirectional instability. *Orthop Clin North Am* 2010;41(3): 357–365. doi:10.1016/j.ocl.2010.02.006.

34. Beltran J, Noto AM, Herman LJ, et al. Tendons: high-field-strength, surface coil MR imaging. *Radiology* 1987;162(3):735.

35. Beltran J, Rosenberg ZS. Diagnosis of compressive and entrapment neuropathies of the upper extremity: value of MR imaging. *AJR Am J Roentgenol* 1994;163(3):525.

36. Beltran LS, Nikac V, Beltran J. Internal impingement syndromes. *Magn Reson Imaging Clin N Am* 2012;20(2):201–211, ix–x. doi:10.1016/j. mric.2012.01.008.

37. Bercandino JT. *Update on the Shoulder. Magnetic Resonance Imaging Clinics of North America.* Philadelphia, PA: Saunders; 2012;20:2.

38. Bencardino JT, Beltran J, Rosenberg ZS, et al. Superior labrum anterior-posterior lesions: diagnosis with MR arthrography of the shoulder. *Radiology* 2000;214(1):267.

39. Bencardino JT, Gyftopoulos S, Palmer WE. Imaging in anterior glenohumeral instability. *Radiology* 2013;269(2):323–337. doi:10.1148 /radiol.13121926.

40. Bennett WF. Subscapularis, medial, and lateral head coracohumeral ligament insertion anatomy. Arthroscopic appearance and incidence of "hidden" rotator interval lesions. *Arthroscopy* 2001;17(2):173.

41. Berdusco R, Trantalis JN, Nelson AA, Sohmer S, More KD, Wong B, Boorman RS, Lo IK. Arthroscopic repair of massive, contracted, immobile tears using interval slides: clinical and MRI structural follow-up [published online ahead of print September 22, 2013]. *Knee Surg Sports Traumatol Arthrosc.*

42. Berquist T, Peterson J. Shoulder and arm. In: Berquist T, ed. *MRI of the Musculoskeletal System.* 5th ed. Philadelphia, PA: Lippincott Williams & Wilkins; 2006:557–656.

43. Bhatia S, Frank RM, Ghodadra NS, Hsu AR, Romeo AA, Bach BR Jr, Boileau P, Provencher MT. The outcomes and surgical techniques of the latarjet procedure. *Arthroscopy* 2014;30(2):227–235. doi:10.1016/j.arthro.2013.10.013.

44. Bhatia S, Ghodadra NS, Romeo AA, Bach BR, Verma NN, Vo ST, Provencher MT. The importance of the recognition and treatment of glenoid bone loss in an athletic population. *Sports Health* 2011;3(5):435–440.

45. Biberthaler P, Wiedemann E, Nerlich A, et al. Microcirculation associated with degenerative rotator cuff lesions. In vivo assessment with orthogonal polarization spectral imaging during arthroscopy of the shoulder. *J Bone Joint Surg Am* 2003;85(3):475.

46. Bigliani LU, Morrison DS. Subacromial impingement syndrome. In: Dee R, ed. *Principles of Orthopaedic Practice.* New York, NY: McGraw-Hill; 1989:627.

47. Bigliani LU. The morphology of the acromion and its relationship to rotator cuff tears. *Orthop Trans* 1986;10:216.

48. Bijlsma JW, Berenbaum F, Lafeber FP. Osteoarthritis: an update with relevance for clinical practice. *Lancet* 2011;377(9783):2115–2126. doi:10.1016/S0140-6736(11)60243-2.

49. Bilsel K, Erdil M, Elmadag M, Ozden VE, Celik D, Tuncay I. The effect of infraspinatus hypotrophy and weakness on the arthroscopic treatment of spinoglenoid notch cyst associated with superior labrum anterior-to-posterior lesions. *Knee Surg Sports Traumatol Arthrosc* 2014;22(9): 2209–2015.

50. Binder H, Schurz M, Aldrian S, Fialka C, Vécsei V. Physeal injuries of the proximal humerus: long-term results in seventy two patients. *Int*

Orthop 2011;35(10):1497–1502. doi:10.1007/s00264-011-1277-8.

51. Bishop JY, Jones GL, Rerko MA, Donaldson C; MOON Shoulder Group. 3-D CT is the most reliable imaging modality when quantifying glenoid bone loss. *Clin Orthop Relat Res* 2013;471(4):1251–1256. doi:10.1007/s11999-012-2607-x.

52. Blum A, Lecocq S, Louis M, Wassel J, Moisei A, Teixeira P. The nerves around the shoulder. *Eur J Radiol* 2013 82(1):2–16. doi:10.1016/j.ejrad.2011.04.033.

53. Boileau P, Brassart N, Watkinson DJ, et al. Arthroscopic repair of full-thickness tears of the supraspinatus: does the tendon really heal? *J Bone Joint Surg Am* 2005;87(6):1229.

54. Boileau P, Fourati E, Bicknell R. Neer modification of open Bankart procedure: what are the rates of recurrent instability, functional outcome, and arthritis? *Clin Orthop Relat Res* 2012;470(9):2554–2560. doi:10.1007/s11999-012-2296-5.

55. Boileau P, O'Shea K, Vargas P, Pinedo M, Old J, Zumstein M. Anatomical and functional results after arthroscopic Hill-Sachs remplissage. *J Bone Joint Surg Am* 2012;94(7):618–626. doi:10.2106/JBJS.K.00101.

56. Bois AJ, Fening SD, Polster J, Jones MH, Miniaci A. Quantifying glenoid bone loss in anterior shoulder instability: reliability and accuracy of 2-dimensional and 3-dimensional computed tomography measurement techniques. *Am J Sports Med* 2012;40(11):2569-2577. doi:0.1177/0363546512458247.

57. Bois AJ, Walker RE, Kodali P, Miniaci A. Imaging instability in the athlete: the right modality for the right diagnosis. *Clin Sports Med* 2013;32(4):653–684. doi:10.1016/j.csm.2013.07.004.

58. Bokor DJ, Fritsch BA. Posterior shoulder instability secondary to reverse humeral avulsion of the glenohumeral ligament. *J Shoulder Elbow Surg* 2010;19(6):853–858. doi:10.1016/j.jse.2010.01.026.

59. Bonutti PM, Norfray JF, Friedman RJ, et al. Kinematic MRI of the shoulder. *J Comput Assist Tomogr* 1993;17(4):666.

60. Borrero CG, Casagranda BU, Towers JD, Bradley JP. Magnetic resonance appearance of posterosuperior labral peel back during humeral abduction and external rotation. *Skeletal Radiol* 2010;39(1):19–26. doi:10.1007/s00256-009-0744-4.

61. Bossert M, Prati C, Bertolini E, Toussirot E, Wendling D. Septic arthritis of the acromioclavicular joint. *Joint Bone Spine* 2010;77(5):466–469. doi:10.1016/j.jbspin.2010.03.010.

62. Boughebri O, Kilinc A, Valenti P. Reverse shoulder arthroplasty combined with a latissimus dorsi and teres major transfer for a deficit of both active elevation and external rotation. Results of 15 cases with a minimum of 2-year follow-up. *Orthop Traumatol Surg Res* 2013;99(2):131–137. doi:10.1016/j.otsr.2012.11.014.

63. Bowen MK, Warren RF. Ligamentous control of shoulder stability based on selective cutting and static translation experiments. *Clin Sports Med* 1991;10(4):757.

64. Boykin RE, Friedman DJ, Higgins LD, Warner JJ. Suprascapular neuropathy. *J Bone Joint Surg Am* 2010;92(13):2348–2364. doi:10.2106/JBJS.I.01743.

65. Braun S, Horan MP, Elser F, Millett PJ. Lesions of the biceps pulley. *Am J Sports Med* 2011;39(4):790–795. doi:10.1177/0363546510393942.

66. Braun S, Millett PJ, Yongpravat C, Pault JD, Anstett T, Torry MR, Giphart JE. Biomechanical evaluation of shear force vectors leading to injury of the biceps reflection pulley: a biplane fluoroscopy study on cadaveric shoulders. *Am J Sports Med* 2010;38(5):1015–1024. doi:10.1177/0363546509355142.

67. Brems J. Rotator cuff tear: evaluation and treatment. 1988;11(1):69.

68. Brilakis E, Mataragas E, Deligeorgis A, Maniatis V, Antonogiannakis E. Midterm outcomes of arthroscopic remplissage for the management of recurrent anterior shoulder instability. [published online ahead of print February 1, 2014]. *Knee Surg Sports Traumatol Arthrosc.*

69. Budzik JF, Wavreille G, Pansini V, Moraux A, Demondion X, Cotten A. Entrapment neuropathies of the shoulder. *Magn Reson Imaging Clin N Am* 2012;20(2):373–391, xii. doi:10.1016/j.mric.2012.01.013.

70. Burk DL Jr, Karasick D, Kurtz AB, et al. Rotator cuff tears: prospective comparison of MR imaging with arthrography, sonography, and surgery. *AJR Am J Roentgenol* 1989;153(1):87.

71. Burkhart SS, Debeer JF, Tehrany AM, et al. Quantifying glenoid bone loss arthroscopically in shoulder instability. *Arthroscopy* 2002;18(5):488.

72. Burkhart SS, Morgan CD, Kibler WB. The disabled throwing shoulder: spectrum of pathology. Part I: pathoanatomy and biomechanics. *Arthroscopy* 2003;19(4):404.

73. Burkhart SS, Morgan CD, Kibler WB. The disabled throwing shoulder: spectrum of pathology Part III: the SICK scapula, scapular dyskinesis, the kinetic chain, and rehabilitation. *Arthroscopy* 2003;19(6):641.

74. Burkhart SS, Morgan CD, Kibler WB. The disabled throwing shoulder: spectrum of pathology. Part II: evaluation and treatment of SLAP lesions in throwers. *Arthroscopy* 2003;19(5):531.

75. Burkhart S, Lo IK, Brady PC, Denard PJ. *The Cowboy's Companion: A Trail Guide for the Arthroscopic Shoulder Surgeon*. Philadelphia, PA: Lippincott Williams & Wilkins; 2012.

76. Burkhead Jr W, Habermeyer P, Walch G. The biceps tendon and rotator cuff disease. In: Cooke D, Klass F, Sfarra S, eds. *Rotator Cuff Disorders*. Baltimore, MD: Williams & Wilkins, 1996:133.

77. Burkhead Jr W, Walch G. Posteriosuperior glenoid impingement. In: Cooke D, Klass F, Sfarra S, eds. *Rotator Cuff Disorders*. Baltimore, MD: Williams & Wilkins, 1996:193.

78. Butt U, Charalambous CP. Complications associated with open coracoid transfer procedures for shoulder instability. *J Shoulder Elbow Surg* 2012;21(8):1110–1119. doi:10.1016/j.jse.2012.02.008.

79. Butterfield TA. Eccentric exercise in vivo: strain-induced muscle damage and adaptation in a stable

system. *Exerc Sport Sci Rev* 2010;38(2):51–60. doi:10.1097/JES.0b013e3181d496eb.

80. Cadet ER. Evaluation of glenohumeral instability. *Orthop Clin North Am* 2010;41(3):287–295. doi:10.1016/j.ocl.2010.02.005.

81. Calderone M, Cereatti A, Conti M, Della Croce U. Comparative evaluation of scapular and humeral coordinate systems based on biomedical images of the glenohumeral joint. *J Biomech* 2014;47(3): 736–741. doi:10.1016/j.jbiomech.2013.10.045.

82. Callaghan J, McNiesh LM, DeHaven JR, et al. A prospective comparison of double contrast computed tomography: CT, arthrography and arthroscopy of the shoulder. *Am J Sports Med* 1988;16:13.

83. Cameron KL, Mountcastle SB, Nelson BJ, DeBerardino TM, Duffey ML, Svoboda SJ, Owens BD. History of shoulder instability and subsequent injury during four years of follow-up: a survival analysis. *J Bone Joint Surg Am* 2013;95(5): 439–445. doi:10.2106/JBJS.L.00252.

84. Campbell ST, Ecklund KJ, Chu EH, McGarry MH, Gupta R, Lee TQ. The role of pectoralis major and latissimus dorsi muscles in a biomechanical model of massive rotator cuff tear. *J Shoulder Elbow Surg* 2014;23(8):1136–1142. doi:10.1016/j.jse.2013.11.030.

85. Canella C, Demondion X, Abreu E, Marchiori E, Cotten H, Cotten A. Anatomical study of spinal accessory nerve using ultrasonography. *Eur J Radiol* 2013;82(1):56–61. doi:10.1016/j.ejrad.2011.04.038.

86. Carbone S, Napoli A, Gumina S. MRI of adhesive capsulitis of the shoulder: distension of the bursa in the superior subscapularis recess is a suggestive sign of the pathology. *Eur J Radiol* 2014;83(2):345–348. doi:10.1016/j.ejrad.2013.10.017.

87. Carroll KW, Helms CA, Speer KP. Focal articular cartilage lesions of the superior humeral head: MR imaging findings in seven patients. *AJR Am J Roentgenol* 2001;176(2):393.

88. Caspari RB. Shoulder arthroscopy: a review of the present state of the art. *Contemp Orthop* 1982;4:523.

89. Castagna A, Delle Rose G, Borroni M, Cillis BD, Conti M, Garofalo R, Ferguson D, Portinaro N. Arthroscopic stabilization of the shoulder in adolescent athletes participating in overhead or contact sports. *Arthroscopy* 2012;28(3): 309–315. doi:10.1016/j.arthro.2011.08.302.

90. Castagna A, Garofalo R, Cesari E, Markopoulos N, Borroni M, Conti M. Posterior superior internal impingement: an evidence-based review [corrected]. *Br J Sports Med* 2010;44(5): 382–388. doi:10.1136/bjsm.2009.059261.

91. Ceroni D, Cherkaoui A, Ferey S, Kaelin A, Schrenzel J. Kingella kingae osteoarticular infections in young children: clinical features and contribution of a new specific real-time PCR assay to the diagnosis. *J Pediatr Orthop* 2010;30(3): 301–304. doi:10.1097/BPO.0b013e3181d4732f.

92. Chahal J, Leiter J, McKee MD, Whelan DB. Generalized ligamentous laxity as a predisposing factor for primary traumatic anterior shoulder dislocation. *J Shoulder Elbow Surg* 2010;19(8):1238–1242. doi:10.1016/j.jse.2010.02.005.

93. Chambers L, Altchek DW. Microinstability and internal impingement in overhead athletes. *Clin Sports Med* 2013;32(4):697–707. doi:10.1016/j.csm.2013.07.006.

94. Chandnani V, Ho C, Gerharter J, et al. MR findings in asymptomatic shoulders: a blind analysis using symptomatic shoulders as controls. *Clin Imaging* 1992;16(1):25.

95. Chandnani VP, Gagliardi JA, Murnane TG, et al. Glenohumeral ligaments and shoulder capsular mechanism: evaluation with MR arthrography. *Radiology* 1995;196(1):27.

96. Chandnani VP, Yeager TD, DeBerardino T, et al. Glenoid labral tears: prospective evaluation with MRI imaging, MR arthrography, and CT arthrography. *AJR Am J Roentgenol* 1993;161(6):1229.

97. Chang EY, Fliszar E, Chung CB. Superior labrum anterior and posterior lesions and microinstability. *Magn Reson Imaging Clin N Am* 2012;20(2):277–294, x–xi. doi:10.1016/j.mric.2012.01.002.

98. Chang EY, Hoenecke HR Jr, Fronek J, Huang BK, Chung CB. Humeral avulsions of the inferior glenohumeral ligament complex involving the axillary pouch in professional baseball players. *Skeletal Radiol* 2014;43(1):35–41. doi:10.1007/s00256-013-1744-y.

99. Chauvin NA, Jaimes C, Laor T, Jaramillo D. Magnetic resonance imaging of the pediatric shoulder. *Magn Reson Imaging Clin N Am* 2012;20(2):327–347, xi. doi:10.1016/j.mric.2012.01.009.

100. Chhadia AM, Goldberg BA, Hutchinson MR. Abnormal translation in SLAP lesions on magnetic resonance imaging abducted externally rotated view. *Arthroscopy* 2010;26(1):19–25. doi:10.1016/j.arthro.2009.06.028.

101. Cho CH. Complicated acromioclavicular joint cyst with massive rotator cuff tear. *Am J Orthop (Belle Mead NJ)* 2014;43(2):70–73.

102. Cho HL, Lee CK, Hwang TH, Suh KT, Park JW. Arthroscopic repair of combined Bankart and SLAP lesions: operative techniques and clinical results. *Clin Orthop Surg* 2010;2(1): 39–46. doi:10.4055/cios.2010.2.1.39.

103. Cho NS, Lee BG, Rhee YG. Radiologic course of the calcific deposits in calcific tendinitis of the shoulder: does the initial radiologic aspect affect the final results? *J Shoulder Elbow Surg* 2010;19(2):267–272. doi:10.1016/j.jse.2009.07.008.

104. Cho NS, Yi JW, Lee BG, Rhee YG. Retear patterns after arthroscopic rotator cuff repair: single-row versus suture bridge technique. *Am J Sports Med* 2010;38(4):664–671. doi:10.1177/0363546509350081.

105. Cho SH, Cho NS, Rhee YG. Preoperative analysis of the Hill-Sachs lesion in anterior shoulder instability: how to predict engagement of the lesion. *Am J Sports Med* 2011;39(11):2389–2395. doi:10.1177/0363546511398644.

106. Choo HJ, Lee SJ, Kim DW, Park YM, Kim JH. Assessment of the rotator cable in various rotator cuff conditions using indirect MR arthrography. *Acta Radiol* 2014;55(9):1104–1011.

107. Choo HJ, Lee SJ, Kim JH, Cha SS, Park YM, Park JS, Lee JW, Oh M. Can symptomatic acromioclavicular joints be differentiated from

asymptomatic acromioclavicular joints on 3-T MR imaging? *Eur J Radiol* 2013;82(4): e184–e191. doi:10.1016/j.ejrad.2012.10.027.

108. Christie A, Dagfinrud H, Ringen HO, Hagen KB. Beneficial and harmful effects of shoulder arthroplasty in patients with rheumatoid arthritis: results from a Cochrane review. *Rheumatology (Oxford)* 2011;50(3):598–602. doi:10.1093/rheumatology/keq345.

109. Chun KA, Kim MS, Kim YJ. Comparisons of the various partial-thickness rotator cuff tears on MR arthrography and arthroscopic correlation. *Korean J Radiol* 2010;11(5):528–535. doi:10.3348/kjr.2010.11.5.528.

110. Chung CB, Sorenson S, Dwek JR, et al. Humeral avulsion of the posterior band of the inferior glenohumeral ligament: MR arthrography and clinical correlation in 17 patients. *AJR Am J Roentgenol* 2004;183(2):355.

111. Clark JM, Harryman DT II. Tendons, ligaments, and capsule of the rotator cuff. Gross and microscopic anatomy. *J Bone Joint Surg Am* 1992;74(5):713.

112. Clarke SE, Chafetz RS, Kozin SH. Ossification of the proximal humerus in children with residual brachial plexus birth palsy: a magnetic resonance imaging study. *J Pediatr Orthop* 2010;30(1): 60–66. doi:10.1097/BPO.0b013e3181c6c344.

113. Codman EA. *The Shoulder: Rupture of the Supraspinatus Tendon and Other Lesions in or About the Subacromial Bursa.* Boston, MA: Thomas Todd; 1934.

114. Cohn RM, Jazrawi LM. The throwing shoulder: the orthopedist perspective. *Magn Reson Imaging Clin N Am* 2012;20(2):261–275, x. doi:10.1016/j.mric.2012.01.001.

115. Conaghan PG, McQueen FM, Bird P, Peterfy CG, Haavardsholm EA, Gandjbakhch F, Bøyesen P, Coates L, Ejbjerg B, Eshed I, Foltz V, Hermann KG, Freeston J, Lillegraven S, Lassere M, Wiell C, Anandarajah A, Duer-Jensen A, O'Connor P, Genant HK, Emery P, Ostergaard M. Update on research and future directions of the OMERACT MRI inflammatory arthritis group. *J Rheumatol* 2011;38(9):2031–2033. doi:10.3899/jrheum.110419.

116. Connell DA, Potter HG, Sherman MF, et al. Injuries of the pectoralis major muscle: evaluation with MR imaging. *Radiology* 1999;210(3):785.

117. Connolly KP, Schwartzberg RS, Reuss B, Crumbie D Jr, Homan BM. Sensitivity and specificity of noncontrast magnetic resonance imaging reports in the diagnosis of type-II superior labral anterior-posterior lesions in the community setting. *J Bone Joint Surg Am* 2013;95(4):308–313. doi:10.2106/JBJS.K.01115.

118. Cooles FA, Isaacs JD. Pathophysiology of rheumatoid arthritis. *Curr Opin Rheumatol* 2011;23(3): 233–240. doi:10.1097/BOR.0b013e32834518a3.

119. Cooper D, Warner JP, Deng X. Anatomy and function of the coracohumeral ligament. Presented at the Annual Meeting of the Orthopaedic Research Society, Anaheim, CA, 1991.

120. Cooper DE, Arnoczky SP, O'Brien SJ, et al. Anatomy, histology, and vascularity of the glenoid labrum. An anatomical study. *J Bone Joint Surg Am* 1992;74(1):46.

121. Cothran RL Jr, Helms C. Quadrilateral space syndrome: incidence of imaging findings in a population referred for MRI of the shoulder. *AJR Am J Roentgenol* 2005;184(3):989.

122. Cotton RE, Rideout DF. Tears of the humeral rotator cuff; a radiological and pathological necropsy survey. *J Bone Joint Surg Br* 1964;46:314.

123. Craig EV, Habermeyer P, Lichtenberg S. Arthroscopic repair of anterior instability. In: Craig EV, ed. *The Shoulder.* 2nd ed. Philiadelphia, PA: Lippincott Williams & Wilkins, 2004:83.

124. Craig EV. *Master Techniques in Orthopaedic Surgery: Shoulder.* Philadelphia, PA: Lippincott Williams & Wilkins; 2013.

125. Crall TS, Bishop JA, Guttman D, Kocher M, Bozic K, Lubowitz JH. Cost-effectiveness analysis of primary arthroscopic stabilization versus nonoperative treatment for first-time anterior glenohumeral dislocations. *Arthroscopy* 2012;28(12):1755–1765. doi:10.1016/j.arthro.2012.05.885.

126. Crass JR, Craig EV, Feinberg SB. Sonography of the postoperative rotator cuff. *AJR Am J Roentgenol* 1986;146(3):561.

127. Crim J, Burks R, Manaster BJ, Hanrahan C, Hung M, Greis P. Temporal evolution of MRI findings after arthroscopic rotator cuff repair. *AJR AJR Am J Roentgenol* 2010;195(6):1361–1366. doi:10.2214/AJR.10.4436.

128. Crockett HC, Wingert NC, Wright JM, Bonner KF. Repair of SLAP lesions associated with a Buford complex: a novel surgical technique. *Arthroscopy* 2011;27(3):314–321. doi:10.1016/j.arthro.2010.09.005.

129. Cueff F, Ropars M, Chagneau F, Thomazeau H, Berton E, Nourissat G; French Arthroscopy Society. Interest of complementary inferior glenohumeral ligament fixation in capsulo-labral repair for shoulder instability: a biomechanical study. *Orthop Traumatol Surg Res* 2010; 96(8 Suppl):S94–S98. doi:10.1016/j.otsr.2010.09.012.

130. Daley EL, Bajaj S, Bisson LJ, Cole BJ. Improving injection accuracy of the elbow, knee, and shoulder: does injection site and imaging make a difference? A systematic review. *Am J Sports Med* 2011;39(3):656–662. doi:10.1177/0363546510390610.

131. Davis SJ, Teresi LM, Bradley WG, et al. Effect of arm rotation on MR imaging of the rotator cuff. *Radiology* 1991;181(1):265.

132. de Beer JF, Roberts C. Glenoid bone defects—open latarjet with congruent arc modification. *Orthop Clin North Am* 2010;41(3):407–415. doi:10.1016/j.ocl.2010.02.008.

133. De Maeseneer M, Van Roy F, Lenchik L, et al. CT and MR arthrography of the normal and pathologic anterosuperior labrum and labral-bicipital complex. *Radiographics* 2000;20 Spec No:S67.

134. Degen RM, Giles JW, Thompson SR, Litchfield RB, Athwal GS. Biomechanics of complex shoulder instability. *Clin Sports Med* 2013;32(4):625–636. doi:10.1016/j.csm.2013.07.002.

135. Dehaan A, Munch J, Durkan M, Yoo J, Crawford D. Reconstruction of a bony bankart lesion: best fit based on radius of curvature. *Am J Sports Med* 2013;41(5):1140–1145. doi:10.1177/0363546513478578.

136. DePalma AF, White JB, Callery G. Degenerative lesions of the shoulder joint at various age groups which are compatible with good function. *AAOS Intr Course Lecture* 1950;7:168.

137. DePalma AF. *Surgery of the Shoulder*. Philadelphia, PA: JB Lippincott; 1983.

138. Detrisac DJ, Johnson LL. *Arthroscopic Shoulder Anatomy: Pathologic and Surgical Implications*. Thorofare, NJ: Slack; 1986.

139. Dierckman BD, Shah NR, Larose CR, Gerbrandt S, Getelman MH. Non-insertional tendinopathy of the subscapularis. *Int J Shoulder Surg* 2013;7(3): 83–90. doi:10.4103/0973-6042.118876.

140. Dilisio MF, Noble JS, Bell RH, Noel CR. Postarthroscopic humeral head osteonecrosis treated with reverse total shoulder arthroplasty. *Orthopedics* 2013;36(3):e377–e380. doi:10.3928/01477447-20130222-30.

141. Dodson C, Dines D, Dines JS, Walch G, Williams G. *Controversies in Shoulder Instability*. Philadelphia, PA: Lippincott Williams & Wilkins; 2014.

142. Dubrow SA, Streit JJ, Shishani Y, Robbin MR, Gobezie R. Diagnostic accuracy in detecting tears in the proximal biceps tendon using standard non-enhancing shoulder MRI. *Open Access J Sports Med* 2014;5:81–87. doi:10.2147/OAJSM.S58225.

143. Dumont GD, Russell RD, Browne MG, Robertson WJ. Area-based determination of bone loss using the glenoid arc angle. *Arthroscopy* 2012;28(7): 1030–1035. doi:10.1016/j.arthro.2012.04.147.

144. Dumont GD, Russell RD, Robertson WJ. Anterior shoulder instability: a review of pathoanatomy, diagnosis and treatment. *Curr Rev Musculoskelet Med* 2011;4(4):200–207. doi:10.1007/s12178-011-9092-9.

145. Dunham KS, Bencardino JT, Rokito AS. Anatomic variants and pitfalls of the labrum, glenoid cartilage, and glenohumeral ligaments. *Magn Reson Imaging Clin N Am* 2012;20(2):213–228, x. doi:10.1016/j .mric.2012.01.014.

146. Dunteman R, Snyder S. Arthroscopic repair of the PASTA lesion. In: Barber FA, Fischer SP, eds. *Surgical Techniques for the Shoulder and Elbow*. New York, NY: Thieme; 2003:55.

147. Dwek JR. The periosteum: what is it, where is it, and what mimics it in its absence? *Skeletal Radiol* 2010;39(4):319–323. doi:10.1007/s00256-009 -0849-9.

148. Dwyer T, Razmjou H, Henry P, Gosselin-Fournier S, Holtby R. Association between pre-operative magnetic resonance imaging and reparability of large and massive rotator cuff tears [published online ahead of print October 30, 2013]. *Knee Surg Sports Traumatol Arthrosc*.

149. Dwyer T, Petrera M, Bleakney R, Theodoropoulos JS. Shoulder instability in ice hockey players: incidence, mechanism, and MRI findings. *Clin Sports Med* 2013;32(4):803–813. doi:10.1016/j.csm .2013.07.013.

150. Edelson JG, Luchs J. Aspects of coracoacromial ligament anatomy of interest to the arthroscopic surgeon. *Arthroscopy* 1995;11(6):715.

151. Edwards TB, Walch G, Sirveaux F, et al. Repair of tears of the subscapularis. *J Bone Joint Surg Am* 2005;87(4):725.

152. Ekelund A, Nyberg R. Can reverse shoulder arthroplasty be used with few complications in rheumatoid arthritis? *Clin Orthop Relat Res* 2011;469(9):2483–2488. doi:10.1007/s11999 -010-1654-4.

153. El-Azab H, Buchmann S, Beitzel K, Waldt S, Imhoff AB. Clinical and structural evaluation of arthroscopic double-row suture-bridge rotator cuff repair: early results of a novel technique. *Knee Surg Sports Traumatol Arthrosc* 2010;18(12): 1730–1737. doi:10.1007/s00167-010-1257-3.

154. Elkinson I, Giles JW, Boons HW, Faber KJ, Ferreira LM, Johnson JA, Athwal GS. The shoulder remplissage procedure for Hill-Sachs defects: does technique matter? *J Shoulder Elbow Surg* 2013;22(6):835–841. doi:10.1016/j.jse .2012.08.015.

155. Elkinson I, Giles JW, Faber KJ, Boons HW, Ferreira LM, Johnson JA, Athwal GS. The effect of the remplissage procedure on shoulder stability and range of motion: an in vitro biomechanical assessment. *J Bone Joint Surg Am* 2012;94(11): 1003–1012. doi:10.2106/JBJS.J.01956.

156. Ellenbecker TS, Cools A. Rehabilitation of shoulder impingement syndrome and rotator cuff injuries: an evidence-based review. *Br J Sports Med* 2010;44(5):319–327. doi:10.1136/bjsm.2009 .058875.

157. Ellman H. Diagnosis and treatment of incomplete rotator cuff tears. *Clin Orthop* 1990;(254):64.

158. Ellman H. Shoulder arthroscopy: current indications and techniques. *Orthopedics* 1988;11(1):45.

159. Elser F, Braun S, Dewing CB, Giphart JE, Millett PJ. Anatomy, function, injuries, and treatment of the long head of the biceps brachii tendon. *Arthroscopy* 2011;27(4):581–592. doi:10.1016/j.arthro.2010.10.014.

160. Emig EW, Schweitzer ME, Karisick D, et al. Adhesive capsulitis of the shoulder: MR diagnosis. *AJR Am J Roentgenol* 1995;164:1457.

161. Encalada-Diaz I, Cole BJ, Macgillivray JD, Ruiz-Suarez M, Kercher JS, Friel NA, Valero-Gonzalez F. Rotator cuff repair augmentation using a novel polycarbonate polyurethane patch: preliminary results at 12 months' follow-up. *J Shoulder Elbow Surg* 2011;20(5):788–794. doi:10.1016/j.jse.2010.08.013.

162. Esch J, Yergler M. Partial-thickness rotator cuff tears. In: Barber FA, Fischer SP, eds. *Surgical Techniques for the Shoulder and Elbow*. New York, NY: Thieme; 2003:50.

163. Evancho AM, Stiles RG, Fajman WA, et al. MR imaging diagnosis of rotator cuff tears. *AJR Am J Roentgenol* 1988;151(4):751.

164. Fehrman DA, Orwin JF, Jennings RM. Suprascapular nerve entrapment by ganglion cysts: a report of 6 cases with arthroscopic findings and review of the literature. *Arthroscopy* 1995;11:727.

165. Feller JF, Tirman PF, Steinbach LS, et al. Magnetic resonance imaging of the shoulder: review. *Semin Roentgenol* 1995;30(3):224.

166. Ferrari JD, Ferrari DA, Coumas J, et al. Posterior ossification of the shoulder: the Bennett lesion. Etiology, diagnosis, and treatment. *Am J Sports Med* 1994;22(2):171.

167. Flannigan B, Kursunoglu-Brahme S, Snyder S, et al. MR arthrography of the shoulder: comparison with conventional MR imaging. *AJR Am J Roentgenol* 1990;155(4):829.

168. Frank RM, Mall NA, Gupta D, Shewman E, Wang VM, Romeo AA, Cole BJ, Bach BR Jr, Provencher MT, Verma NN. Inferior suture anchor placement during arthroscopic bankart repair: influence of portal placement and curve

drill guide. *Am J Sports Med* 2014;42(5): 1182–1189.

169. Frankle M, Kumar A. Reverse total shoulder replacement for arthritis with an irreparable rotator cuff tear. *Tech Shoulder Elbow Surg* 2003;4(2):77.

170. Friedman LG, Griesser MJ, Miniaci AA, Jones MH. Recurrent instability after revision anterior shoulder stabilization surgery. *Arthroscopy*. 2014; 30(3):372–381. doi:10.1016/j.arthro.2013 .11.019.

171. Frisch KE, Marcu D, Baer G, Thelen DG, Vanderby R. The influence of partial and full thickness tears on infraspinatus tendon strain patterns. *J Biomech Eng* 2014;136(5):051004. doi:10.1115/1.4026643.

172. Fritz RC, Helms CA, Steinback LS, et al. Suprascapular nerve entrapment: evaluation with MR imaging. *Radiology* 1992;182:437.

173. Fukuda H, Hamada K, Yamanaka K. Pathology and pathogenesis of bursal-side rotator cuff tears viewed from en bloc histologic sections. *Clin Orthop* 1990;(254):75.

174. Gallino M, Battiston B, Annaratone G, et al. Coracoacromial ligament: a comparative arthroscopic and anatomic study. *Arthroscopy* 1995;11(5):564.

175. Gamulin A, Dayer R, Lübbeke A, Miozzari H, Hoffmeyer P. Primary open anterior shoulder stabilization: a long-term, retrospective cohort study on the impact of subscapularis muscle alterations on recurrence. *BMC Musculoskelet Disord* 2014;15:45. doi:10.1186/1471-2474-15-45.

176. Gandjbakhch F, Conaghan PG, Ejbjerg B, Haavardsholm EA, Foltz V, Brown AK, Møller Døhn U, Lassere M, Freeston J, Bøyesen P, Bird P, Fautrel B, Hetland ML, Emery P, Bourgeois P, Hørslev-Petersen K, Kvien TK, McQueen F, Ostergaard M. Synovitis and osteitis are very frequent in rheumatoid arthritis clinical remission: results from an MRI study of 294 patients in clinical remission or low disease activity state. *J Rheumatol* 2011;38(9):2039–2044. doi:10 .3899/jrheum.110421.

177. Gaskill TR, Braun S, Millett PJ. Multimedia article. The rotator interval: pathology and management. *Arthroscopy* 2011;27(4):556–567. doi:10.1016/j.arthro.2010.10.004.

178. Gee AO, Angeline ME, Dines JS, Dines DM. Shoulder instability after total arthroplasty: a case of arthroscopic repair. *HSS J* 2014;10(1): 88–91. doi:10.1007/s11420-013-9373-5.

179. George MS, Khazzam M, Kuhn JE. Humeral avulsion of glenohumeral ligaments. *J Am Acad Orthop Surg* 2011;19(3):127–133.

180. Gheno R, Zoner CS, Buck FM, Nico MA, Haghighi P, Trudell DJ, Resnick D. Accessory head of biceps brachii muscle: anatomy, histology, and MRI in cadavers. *AJR Am J Roentgenol* 2010;194(1):W80–W83. doi:10.2214 /AJR.09.3158.

181. Ghodadra N, Gupta A, Romeo AA, Bach BR Jr, Verma N, Shewman E, Goldstein J, Provencher MT. Normalization of glenohumeral articular contact pressures after Latarjet or iliac crest bone-grafting. *J Bone Joint Surg Am* 2010;92(6):1478–1489. doi:10.2106/JBJS .I.00220.

182. Giacomo GD, Pouliart N, Constantini A, de Vita A. *Atlas of Functional Shoulder Anatomy*. Milan, Italy: Springer-Verlag; 2008.

183. Giaconi JC, Link TM, Vail TP, Fisher Z, Hong R, Singh R, Steinbach LS. Morbidity of direct MR arthrography. *AJR Am J Roentgenol* 2011;196(4):868–874. doi:10.2214/AJR.10.5145.

184. Giaroli EL, Major NM, Higgins LD. MRI of internal impingement of the shoulder. *AJR Am J Roentgenol* 2005;185(4):925.

185. Gibson ME, Gurley D, Trenhaile S. Traumatic subscapularis tendon tear in an adolescent american football player. *Sports Health* 2013;5(3): 267–269. doi:10.1177/1941738112470912.

186. Giles JW, Elkinson I, Ferreira LM, Faber KJ, Boons H, Litchfield R, Johnson JA, Athwal GS. Moderate to large engaging Hill-Sachs defects: an in vitro biomechanical comparison of the remplissage procedure, allograft humeral head reconstruction, and partial resurfacing arthroplasty. *J Shoulder Elbow Surg* 2012;21(9):1142–1151. doi:10.1016/j.jse.2011.07.017.

187. Gleason PD, Beall DP, Sanders TG, et al. The transverse humeral ligament: a separate anatomical structure or a continuation of the osseous attachment of the rotator cuff? *Am J Sports Med* 2006;34(1):72.

188. Godin J, Sekiya JK. Systematic review of arthroscopic versus open repair for recurrent anterior shoulder dislocations. *Sports Health* 2011;3(4):396–404.

189. Gokalp G, Algin O, Yildirim N, Yazici Z. Adhesive capsulitis: contrast-enhanced shoulder MRI findings. *J Med Imaging Radiat Oncol* 2011;55(2):119–125. doi:10.1111/j.1754-9485 .2010.02215.x.

190. Goudie EB, Murray IR, Robinson CM. Instability of the shoulder following seizures. *J Bone Joint Surg Br* 2012;94(6):721–728. doi:10.1302 /0301-620X.94B6.28259.

191. Grantham C, Heckmann N, Wang L, Tibone JE, Struhl S, Lee TQ. A biomechanical assessment of a novel double endobutton technique versus a coracoid cerclage sling for acromioclavicular and coracoclavicular injuries [published online ahead of print July 30, 2014]. *Knee Surg Sports Traumatol Arthrosc*.

192. Griffin JW, Brockmeier SF. Shoulder instability with concomitant bone loss in the athlete. *Clin Sports Med* 2013;32(4):741–760. doi:10.1016 /j.csm.2013.07.008.

193. Gulotta LV, Lobatto D, Delos D, Coleman SH, Altchek DW. Anterior shoulder capsular tears in professional baseball players. *J Shoulder Elbow Surg* 2014;23(8):e173–178. doi:10.1016/j.jse.2013 .11.027.

194. Guo JB, Zhang JD, Zhao YM, Yang Y. Fracture separation of the proximal humeral epiphyses in neonate: a case report and literature review. *Chin J Traumatol* 2010;13(1):62–64.

195. Gusmer PB, Potter HG, Schatz JA, et al. Labral injuries: accuracy of detection with unenhanced MR imaging of the shoulder. *Radiology* 1996; 200(2):519.

196. Gyftopoulos S, Bencardino J, Nevsky G, Hall G, Soofi Y, Desai P, Jazrawi L, Recht MP. Rotator cable: MRI study of its appearance in the intact rotator cuff with anatomic and histologic correlation. *AJR Am J Roentgenol* 2013;200(5):1101–1105. doi:10.2214/AJR.12.9312.

197. Gyftopoulos S, Bencardino JT, Immerman I, Zuckerman JD. The rotator cable: magnetic resonance evaluation and clinical correlation. *Magn*

Reson Imaging Clin N Am 2012;20(2):173–185, ix. doi:10.1016/j.mric.2012.01.007.

198. Gyftopoulos S, Yemin A, Beltran L, Babb J, Bencardino J. Engaging Hill-Sachs lesion: is there an association between this lesion and findings on MRI? *AJR Am J Roentgenol* 2013;201(4):W633–W638. doi:10.2214/AJR.12.10206.

199. Habermeyer P, Magosch P, Pritsch M, et al. Anterosuperior impingement of the shoulder as a result of pulley lesions: a prospective arthroscopic study. *J Shoulder Elbow Surg* 2004;13(1):5.

200. Habibian A, Stauffer A, Resnick D, et al. Comparison of conventional and computed arthrotomography with MR imaging in the evaluation of the shoulder. *J Comput Assist Tomogr* 1989;13(6):968.

201. Hanchard NC, Lenza M, Handoll HH, Takwoingi Y. Physical tests for shoulder impingements and local lesions of bursa, tendon or labrum that may accompany impingement. *Cochrane Database Syst Rev* 2013;(4):CD007427. doi:10.1002/14651858.CD007427.pub2.

202. Haneveld H, Hug K, Diederichs G, Scheibel M, Gerhardt C. Arthroscopic double-row repair of the rotator cuff: a comparison of bio-absorbable and non-resorbable anchors regarding osseous reaction. *Knee Surg Sports Traumatol Arthrosc* 2013;21(7):1647–1654. doi:10.1007/s00167-013-2510-3.

203. Hantes ME, Karidakis GK, Vlychou M, Varitimidis S, Dailiana Z, Malizos KN. A comparison of early versus delayed repair of traumatic rotator cuff tears. *Knee Surg Sports Traumatol Arthrosc* 2011;19(10):1766–1770. doi:10.1007/s00167-011-1396-1.

204. Hariharan P, Kabrhel C. Sensitivity of erythrocyte sedimentation rate and C-reactive protein for the exclusion of septic arthritis in emergency department patients. *J Emerg Med* 2011;40(4):428–431. doi:10.1016/j.jemermed.2010.05.029.

205. Harper KW, Helms CA, Haystead CM, et al. Glenoid dysplasia: incidence and association with posterior labral tears as evaluated on MRI. *AJR Am J Roentgenol* 2005;184(3):984.

206. Harris JD, Gupta AK, Mall NA, Abrams GD, McCormick FM, Cole BJ, Bach BR Jr, Romeo AA, Verma NN. Long-term outcomes after Bankart shoulder stabilization. *Arthroscopy* 2013;29(5):920–933. doi:10.1016/j.arthro.2012.11.010.

207. Harris JD, Romeo AA. Arthroscopic management of the contact athlete with instability. *Clin Sports Med* 2013;32(4):709–730. doi:10.1016/j.csm.2013.07.007.

208. Harryman DT II, Sidles JA, Harris SL, et al. The role of the rotator interval capsule in passive motion and stability of the shoulder. *J Bone Joint Surg Am* 1992;74(1):53.

209. Hawkins RJ, Belle RM. Posterior instability of the shoulder. *AAOS Instr Course Lect* 1989;38:211.

210. Hawkins RJ, Kennedy JC. Impingement syndrome in athletes. *Am J Sports Med* 1980;8(3):151.

211. Hayes ML, Collins MS, Morgan JA, Wenger DE, Dahm DL. Efficacy of diagnostic magnetic resonance imaging for articular cartilage lesions of the glenohumeral joint in patients with instability. *Skeletal Radiol* 2010;39(12):1199–1204. doi:10.1007/s00256-010-0922-4.

212. Hayter CL, Koff MF, Shah P, Koch KM, Miller TT, Potter HG. MRI after arthroplasty: comparison of MAVRIC and conventional fast spin-echo techniques. *AJR Am J Roentgenol* 2011;197(3):W405–W411. doi:10.2214/AJR.11.6659.

213. Helms CA, Martinez S, Speer KP. Acute brachial neuritis (Parsonage-Turner syndrome): MR imaging appearance—report of three cases. *Radiology* 1998;207(1):255.

214. Helms CA, McGonegle SJ, Vinson EN, Whiteside MB. Magnetic resonance arthrography of the shoulder: accuracy of gadolinium versus saline for rotator cuff and labral pathology. *Skeletal Radiol* 2011;40(2):197–203. doi:10.1007/s00256-010-0978-1.

215. Hibberd EE, Oyama S, Myers JB. Increase in humeral retrotorsion accounts for age-related increase in glenohumeral internal rotation deficit in youth and adolescent baseball players. *Am J Sports Med* 2014;42(4):851–858.

216. Hitchon CA, Chandad F, Ferucci ED, Willemze A, Ioan-Facsinay A, van der Woude D, Markland J, Robinson D, Elias B, Newkirk M, Toes RM, Huizinga TW, El-Gabalawy HS. Antibodies to porphyromonas gingivalis are associated with anticitrullinated protein antibodies in patients with rheumatoid arthritis and their relatives. *J Rheumatol* 2010;37(6):1105–1112. doi:10.3899/jrheum.091323.

217. Hodler J, Kursunoglu-Brahme S, Snyder SJ, et al. Rotator cuff disease: assessment with MR arthrography versus standard MR imaging in 36 patients with arthroscopic confirmation. *Radiology* 1992;182(2):431.

218. Hogendoorn S, van Overvest KL, Watt I, Duijsens AH, Nelissen RG. Structural changes in muscle and glenohumeral joint deformity in neonatal brachial plexus palsy. *J Bone Joint Surg Am* 2010;92(4):935–942. doi:10.2106/JBJS.I.00193.

219. Hollister MS, Mack LA, Patten RM, et al. Association of sonographically detected subacromial/subdeltoid bursal effusion and intra-articular fluid with rotator cuff tear. *AJR Am J Roentgenol* 1995;165(3):605.

220. Holt RG, Helms CA, Steinbach L, et al. Magnetic resonance imaging of the shoulder: rationale and current applications. *Skeletal Radiol* 1990;19(1):5.

221. Holzapfel K, Waldt S, Bruegel M, Paul J, Heinrich P, Imhoff AB, Rummeny EJ, Woertler K. Inter- and intraobserver variability of MR arthrography in the detection and classification of superior labral anterior posterior (SLAP) lesions: evaluation in 78 cases with arthroscopic correlation. *Eur Radiol* 2010;20(3):666–673. doi:10.1007/s00330-009-1593-1.

222. Horst K, Von Harten R, Weber C, Andruszkow H, Pfeifer R, Dienstknecht T, Pape HC. Assessment of coincidence and defect sizes in Bankart and Hill-Sachs lesions after anterior shoulder dislocation: a radiological study. *Br J Radiol* 2014;87(1034):20130673. doi:10.1259/bjr.20130673.

223. Horwitz TM, Tocantins LM. An anatomical study of the role of the long thoracic nerve and the related scapular bursae in the pathogenesis of local paralysis of the serratus anterior muscle. *Anat Rec* 1938;71:375.

224. Hovelius L, Sandström B, Olofsson A, Svensson O, Rahme H. The effect of capsular repair, bone block healing, and position on the results of the Bristow-Latarjet procedure (study III): long-term follow-up in 319 shoulders. *J Shoulder Elbow Surg* 2012;21(5):647–660. doi:10.1016/j.jse.2011 .03.020.

225. Howell SM, Galinat BJ. The glenoid-labral socket. A constrained articular surface. *Clin Orthop* 1989;(243):122.

226. Huang BK, Resnick D. Novel anatomic concepts in magnetic resonance imaging of the rotator cuff tendons and the footprint. *Magn Reson Imaging Clin N Am* 2012;20(2):163–172, ix. doi:10.1016/j.mric.2012.01.006.

227. Huber DJ, Sauter R, Mueller E, et al. MR imaging of the normal shoulder. *Radiology* 1986;158(2):405.

228. Huijsmans PE, de Witte PB, de Villiers RV, Wolterbeek DW, Warmerdam P, Kruger NR, de Beer JF. Recurrent anterior shoulder instability: accuracy of estimations of glenoid bone loss with computed tomography is insufficient for therapeutic decision-making. *Skeletal Radiol* 2011;40(10):1329–1334. doi:10.1007/s00256 -011-1184-5.

229. Hurley JA. Anatomy of the shoulder. In: Nicholas JA, Hershman EB, eds. *The Upper Extremity in Sports Medicine*. 2nd ed. St. Louis, MO: Mosby Year Book; 1995:23.

230. Hutchinson MR, Veenstra MA. Arthroscopic decompression of shoulder impingement secondary to os acromiale. *Arthroscopy* 1993;9(1):28.

231. Hwang E, Carpenter JE, Hughes RE, Palmer ML. Effects of biceps tension and superior humeral head translation on the glenoid labrum. *J Orthop Res* 201432(11):1424–1429.doi:10.1002/jor .22688.

232. Iannotti JP, Deutsch A, Green A, Rudicel S, Christensen J, Marraffino S, Rodeo S. Time to failure after rotator cuff repair: a prospective imaging study. *J Bone Joint Surg Am* 2013;95(11):965– 971. doi:10.2106/JBJS.L.00708.

233. Iannotti JP, Zlatkin MB, Esterhai JL, et al. Magnetic resonance imaging of the shoulder. Sensitivity, specificity, and predictive value. *J Bone Joint Surg Am* 1991;73(1):17.

234. Iannotti JP, Williams GR, Miniaci A, Zuckerman, JD. *Disorders of the Shoulder: Diagnosis and Management*. 3rd ed. Philadelphia, PA: Lippincott Williams & Wilkins; 2014.

235. Ishihara Y, Mihata T, Tamboli M, Nguyen L, Park KJ, McGarry MH, Takai S, Lee TQ. Role of the superior shoulder capsule in passive stability of the glenohumeral joint. *J Shoulder Elbow Surg* 2014;23(5):642–648. doi:10.1016/j.jse.2013 .09.025.

236. Itoi E, Tabata S. Incomplete rotator cuff tears. Results of operative treatment. *Clin Orthop* 1992;(284):128.

237. Iyer RS, Thapa MM, Chew FS. Chronic recurrent multifocal osteomyelitis: review. *AJR Am J Roentgenol* 2011;196(6 Suppl):S87–S91. doi:10.2214/AJR.09.7212.

238. Izadpanah K, Winterer J, Vicari M, Jaeger M, Maier D, Eisebraun L, Ute Will J, Kotter E, Langer M, Südkamp NP, Hennig J, Weigel M. A stress MRI of the shoulder for evaluation of ligamentous stabilizers in acute and chronic acromio-

clavicular joint instabilities. *J Magn Reson Imaging* 2013;37(6):1486–1492. doi:10.1002/jmri.23853.

239. Jacobson JA, Duquin TR, Sanchez-Sotelo J, Schleck CD, Sperling JW, Cofield RH. Anatomic shoulder arthroplasty for treatment of proximal humerus malunions. *J Shoulder Elbow Surg* 2014;23(8):1232 –1239. doi:10.1016/j.jse.2013.11.015.

240. Jacobson JA, Miller B, Bedi A, Morag Y. Imaging of the postoperative shoulder. *Semin Musculoskelet Radiol* 2011;15(4):320–339. doi:10.1055/s-0031-1286014.

241. Jaggi A, Lambert S. Rehabilitation for shoulder instability. *Br J Sports Med* 2010;44(5): 333–340. doi:10.1136/bjsm.2009.059311.

242. Jankauskas L, Rüdiger HA, Pfirrmann CW, Jost B, Gerber C. Loss of the sclerotic line of the glenoid on anteroposterior radiographs of the shoulder: a diagnostic sign for an osseous defect of the anterior glenoid rim. *J Shoulder Elbow Surg* 2010;19(1):151–156. doi:10.1016/j.jse.2009 .04.013.

243. Jaramillo D. Infection: musculoskeletal. *Pediatr Radiol* 2011;41(suppl 1):S127–S134. doi:10.1007/s00247-011-2001-y.

244. Jazrawi LM, Alaia MJ, Chang G, Fitzgerald EF, Recht MP. Advances in magnetic resonance imaging of articular cartilage. *J Am Acad Orthop Surg* 2011;19(7):420–429.

245. Jee WH, McCauley TR, Katz LD, et al. Superior labral anterior posterior (SLAP) lesions of the glenoid labrum: reliability and accuracy of MR arthrography for diagnosis. *Radiology* 2001;218(1):127.

246. Ji JH, Shafi M, Jeong JJ, Park SE. Arthroscopic repair of large and massive rotator cuff tears using the biceps-incorporating technique: mid-term clinical and anatomical results [published online ahead of print October 2, 2013]. *Eur J Orthop Surg Traumatol*.

247. Ji JH, Shafi M, Moon CY, Park SE, Kim YJ, Kim SE. Arthroscopic suture bridge technique for intratendinous tear of rotator cuff in chronically painful calcific tendinitis of the shoulder. *Orthop Surg* 2013;5(4):289–292. doi:10.1111/os.12070.

248. Jia X, Ji JH, Pannirselvam V, Petersen SA, McFarland EG. Does a positive neer impingement sign reflect rotator cuff contact with the acromion? *Clin Orthop Relat Res* 2011;469(3):813–818. doi:10.1007/s11999-010-1590-3.

249. Jin W, Ryu KN, Park YK, et al. Cystic lesions in the posterosuperior portion of the humeral head on MR arthrography: correlations with gross and histologic findings in cadavers. *AJR Am J Roentgenol* 2005;184(4):1211.

250. Jo CH, Shin JS, Park IW, Kim H, Lee SY. Multiple channeling improves the structural integrity of rotator cuff repair. *Am J Sports Med* 2013;41(11):2650–2657. doi:10.1177 /0363546513499138.

251. Jobe CM. Posterior superior glenoid impingement: expanded spectrum. *Arthroscopy* 1995;11(5):530.

252. Johnson LL. *Diagnostic and Surgical Arthroscopy of the Shoulder* St. Louis, MO: Mosby Year Book; 1993:365.

253. Johnson SM, Robinson CM. Shoulder instability in patients with joint hyperlaxity. *J Bone Joint Surg Am* 2010;92(6):1545–1557. doi:10.2106/JBJS .H.00078.

254. Jones KJ, Kahlenberg CA, Dodson CC, Nam D, Williams RJ, Altchek DW. Arthroscopic capsular plication for microtraumatic anterior shoulder instability in overhead athletes. *Am J Sports Med* 2012;40(9):2009–2014. doi:10.1177/0363546512453299.

255. Jung JY, Ha DH, Lee SM, Blacksin MF, Kim KA, Kim JW. Displaceability of SLAP lesion on shoulder MR arthrography with external rotation position. *Skeletal Radiol* 2011;40(8):1047–1055. doi:10.1007/s00256-011-1134-2.

256. Jung JY, Jee WH, Chun HJ, Ahn MI, Kim YS. Magnetic resonance arthrography including ABER view in diagnosing partial-thickness tears of the rotator cuff: accuracy, and inter- and intra-observer agreements. *Acta Radiol* 2010;51(2):194–201. doi:10.3109/02841850903300298.

257. Kaar SG, Fening SD, Jones MH, Colbrunn RW, Miniaci A. Effect of humeral head defect size on glenohumeral stability: a cadaveric study of simulated Hill-Sachs defects. *Am J Sports Med* 2010;38(3):594–599. doi:10.1177/0363546509350295.

258. Kanavaki A, Ceroni D, Tchernin D, Hanquinet S, Merlini L. Can early MRI distinguish between Kingella kingae and Gram-positive cocci in osteoarticular infections in young children? *Pediatr Radiol* 2012;42(1):57–62. doi:10.1007/s00247-011-2220-2.

259. Kaplan KM, Elattrache NS, Jobe FW, Morrey BF, Kaufman KR, Hurd WJ. Comparison of shoulder range of motion, strength, and playing time in uninjured high school baseball pitchers who reside in warm- and cold-weather climates. *Am J Sports Med* 2011;39(2):320–328. doi:10.1177/0363546510382230.

260. Karzel RP, Nuber G, Lautenschlager E. Contact stresses during compression loading of the glenohumeral joint: the role of the glenoid labrum. *Proc Inst Med* 1989;42:64.

261. Kask K, Põldoja E, Lont T, Norit R, Merila M, Busch LC, Kolts I. Anatomy of the superior glenohumeral ligament. *J Shoulder Elbow Surg* 2010;19(6):908–916. doi:10.1016/j.jse.2010.01.019.

262. Kassarjian A, Torriani M, Ouellette H, et al. Intramuscular rotator cuff cysts: association with tendon tears on MRI and arthroscopy. *AJR Am J Roentgenol* 2005;185(1):160.

263. Katthagen JC, Hennecke D, Jensen G, Ellwein A, Voigt C, Lill H. Arthroscopy Arthroscopy after locked plating of proximal humeral fractures: implant removal, capsular release, and intra-articular findings. *Arthroscopy* 2014;30(9):1061–1067. doi:10.1016/j.arthro.2014.04.092.

264. Kerr ZY, Collins CL, Pommering TL, Fields SK, Comstock RD. Dislocation/separation injuries among US high school athletes in 9 selected sports: 2005–2009. *Clin J Sport Med* 2011;21(2):101–108. doi:10.1097/JSM.0b013e31820bd1b6.

265. Khan A, Samba A, Pereira B, Canavese F. Anterior dislocation of the shoulder in skeletally immature patients: comparison between non-operative treatment versus open Latarjet's procedure. *Bone Joint J* 2014;96-B(3):354–359. doi:10.1302/0301-620X.96B3.32167.

266. Kibler WB, Dome D. Internal impingement: concurrent superior labral and rotator cuff injuries. *Sports Med Arthrosc* 2012;20(1):30–33. doi:10.1097/JSA.0b013e318243240c.

267. Kibler WB, Kuhn JE, Wilk K, Sciascia A, Moore S, Laudner K, Ellenbecker T, Thigpen C, Uhl T. The disabled throwing shoulder: spectrum of pathology-10-year update. *Arthroscopy* 2013;29(1):141–161.e26. doi:10.1016/j.arthro.2012.10.009.

268. Kibler WB, Sciascia A, Thomas SJ. Glenohumeral internal rotation deficit: pathogenesis and response to acute throwing. *Sports Med Arthrosc* 2012;20(1):34–38. doi:10.1097/JSA.0b013e318244853e.

269. Kibler WB, Wilkes T, Sciascia A. Mechanics and pathomechanics in the overhead athlete. *Clin Sports Med* 2013;32(4):637–651. doi:10.1016/j.csm.2013.07.003.

270. Kieft GJ, Bloem JL, Obermann WR, et al. Normal shoulder: MR imaging. *Radiology* 1986;159(3):741.

271. Kieft GJ, Bloem JL, Rozing PM, et al. MR imaging of recurrent anterior dislocation of the shoulder: comparison with CT arthrography. *AJR Am J Roentgenol* 1988;150(5):1083.

272. Kieft GJ, Bloem JL, Rozing PM, et al. Rotator cuff impingement syndrome: MR imaging. *Radiology* 1988;166(1 Pt 1):211.

273. Kieft GJ, Sartoris DJ, Bloem JL, et al. Magnetic resonance imaging of glenohumeral joint diseases. *Skeletal Radiol* 1987;16(4):285.

274. Kijowski R, Farber JM, Medina J, et al. Comparison of fat-suppressed T2-weighted fast spin-echo sequence and modified STIR sequence in the evaluation of the rotator cuff tendon. *AJR Am J Roentgenol* 2005;185(2):371.

275. Kijowski R, Gold GE. Routine 3D magnetic resonance imaging of joints. *J Magn Reson Imaging* 2011;33(4):758–771. doi:10.1002/jmri.22342.

276. Kikukawa K, Ide J, Kikuchi K, Morita M, Mizuta H, Ogata H. Hypertrophic changes of the teres minor muscle in rotator cuff tears: quantitative evaluation by magnetic resonance imaging. [published online ahead of print June 4, 2014] *J Shoulder Elbow Surg.* doi:10.1016/j.jse.2014.03.014.

277. Kim HK, Emery KH, Salisbury SR. Bare spot of the glenoid fossa in children: incidence and MRI features. *Pediatr Radiol* 2010;40(7):1190–1196. doi:10.1007/s00247-009-1494-0.

278. Kim HM, Dahiya N, Teefey SA, Middleton WD, Stobbs G, Steger-May K, Yamaguchi K, Keener JD. Location and initiation of degenerative rotator cuff tears: an analysis of three hundred and sixty shoulders. *J Bone Joint Surg Am* 2010;92(5):1088–1096. doi:10.2106/JBJS.I.00686.

279. Kim KC, Rhee YG, Park JY, Shin HD, Cha SM, Park JY, Han SC, Yang JH. Anteroposterior translation of the glenohumeral joint in various pathologies: differences between shoulder MRI in the adducted neutral rotation and abducted externally rotated positions [published online ahead of print September 27, 2013]. *Knee Surg Sports Traumatol Arthrosc.*

280. Kim KC, Shin HD, Cha SM, Park JY. Comparisons of retear patterns for 3 arthroscopic rotator cuff repair methods. *Am J Sports Med* 2014;42(3):558–565. doi:10.1177/0363546514521577.

281. Kim SH, Noh KC, Park JS, et al. Loss of chondrolabral containment of the glenohumeral joint in atraumatic posteroinferior multidirectional instability. *J Bone Joint Surg Am* 2005;87(1):92.

282. Kim SH, Oh JH, Lee OS, Lee HR, Hargens AR. Postoperative imaging of bioabsorbable anchors in rotator cuff repair. *Am J Sports Med* 2014;42(3):552–557. doi:10.1177/0363546513517538.

283. Kim SJ, Hong SH, Jun WS, Choi JY, Myung JS, Jacobson JA, Lee JW, Choi JA, Kang HS. MR imaging mapping of skeletal muscle denervation in entrapment and compressive neuropathies. *Radiographics* 2011;31(2):319–332. doi:10.1148/rg.312105122.

284. Kim TK, Queale WS, Cosgarea AJ, et al. Clinical features of the different types of SLAP lesions: an analysis of one hundred and thirty-nine cases. Superior labrum anterior posterior. *J Bone Joint Surg Am* 2003;85(1):66.

285. Kim YJ, Choi JA, Oh JH, Hwang SI, Hong SH, Kang HS. Superior labral anteroposterior tears: accuracy and interobserver reliability of multidetector CT arthrography for diagnosis. *Radiology* 2011;260(1):207–215. doi:10.1148/radiol.11101176.

286. Kirchhoff C, Imhoff AB. Posterosuperior and anterosuperior impingement of the shoulder in overhead athletes-evolving concepts. *Int Orthop* 2010;34(7):1049–1058. doi:10.1007/s00264-010-1038-0.

287. Kjellin I, Ho CP, Cervilla V, et al. Alterations in the supraspinatus tendon at MR imaging: correlation with histopathologic findings in cadavers. *Radiology* 1991;181(3):837.

288. Klein MA, Miro PA, Spreitzer AM, et al. MR imaging of the normal sternoclavicular joint: spectrum of findings. *AJR Am J Roentgenol* 1995;165(2):391.

289. Klinger HM, Baums MH, Freche S, Nusselt T, Spahn G, Steckel H. Septic arthritis of the shoulder joint: an analysis of management and outcome. *Acta Orthop Belg* 2010;76(5):598–603.

290. Kluger R, Bock P, Mittlböck M, Krampla W, Engel A. Long-term survivorship of rotator cuff repairs using ultrasound and magnetic resonance imaging analysis. *Am J Sports Med* 2011;39(10):2071–2081. doi:10.1177/0363546511406395.

291. Ko SH, Shin SM, Jo BG. Outcomes of minimally 1 year follow-up for the arthroscopic Remplissage technique with Hill-Sachs lesion. *J Orthop* 2013;10(1):41–45. doi:10.1016/j.jor.2013.01.009.

292. Koch KM, Brau AC, Chen W, Gold GE, Hargreaves BA, Koff M, McKinnon GC, Potter HG, King KF. Imaging near metal with a MAVRIC-SEMAC hybrid. *Magn Reson Med* 2011;65(1):71–82. doi:10.1002/mrm.22523.

293. Kodali P, Jones MH, Polster J, Miniaci A, Fening SD. Accuracy of measurement of Hill-Sachs lesions with computed tomography. *J Shoulder Elbow Surg* 2011;20(8):1328–1334. doi:10.1016/j.jse.2011.01.030.

294. Koh KH, Kang KC, Lim TK, Shon MS, Yoo JC. Prospective randomized clinical trial of single- versus double-row suture anchor repair in 2- to 4-cm rotator cuff tears: clinical and magnetic resonance imaging results. *Arthroscopy* 2011;27(4):453–462. doi:10.1016/j.arthro.2010.11.059.

295. Koh KH, Laddha MS, Lim TK, Park JH, Yoo JC. Serial structural and functional assessments of rotator cuff repairs: do they differ at 6 and 19 months postoperatively? *J Shoulder Elbow Surg* 2012;21(7):859–866. doi:10.1016/j.jse.2011.05.027.

296. Koh KH, Lim TK, Park YE, Lee SW, Park WH, Yoo JC. Preoperative factors affecting footprint coverage in rotator cuff repair. 2014;42(4):869–876.

297. Koh KH, Shon MS, Lim TK, Yoo JC. Clinical and magnetic resonance imaging results of arthroscopic full-layer repair of bursal-side partial-thickness rotator cuff tears. *Am J Sports Med* 2011;39(8):1660–1667. doi:10.1177/0363546511412165.

298. Kopka L, Funke M, Fischer V, Keating D. MR arthrography of the shoulder with gadopentetate dimeglumine: influence of concentration, iodinated contrast material, and time of signal intensity. *AJR Am J Roentgenol* 1994;163:621.

299. Kovacs M, Ellenbecker T. An 8-stage model for evaluating the tennis serve: implications for performance enhancement and injury prevention. *Sports Health* 2011;3(6):504–513.

300. Koziak A, Chuang MJ, Jancosko JJ, Burnett KR, Nottage WM. Magnetic resonance arthrography assessment of the superior labrum using the BLC system: age-related changes mimicking SLAP-2 lesions. *Skeletal Radiol* 2014;43(8):1065–1070. doi:10.1007/s00256-014-1889-3.

301. Krief OP. MRI of the rotator interval capsule. *AJR Am J Roentgenol* 2005;184(5):1490.

302. Kuhn JE, Helmer TT, Dunn WR, Throckmorton V TW. Development and reliability testing of the frequency, etiology, direction, and severity (FEDS) system for classifying glenohumeral instability. *J Shoulder Elbow Surg* 2011;20(4):548–556. doi:10.1016/j.jse.2010.10.027.

303. Kuhn JE. A new classification system for shoulder instability. *Br J Sports Med* 2010;44(5):341–346. doi:10.1136/bjsm.2009.071183.

304. Kukkonen J, Joukainen A, Lehtinen J, Mattila KT, Tuominen EK, Kauko T, Äärimaa V. Treatment of non-traumatic rotator cuff tears: a randomised controlled trial with one-year clinical results. *Bone Joint J* 2014;96-B(1):75–81. doi:10.1302/0301-620X.96B1.32168.

305. Kurokawa D, Yamamoto N, Nagamoto H, Omori Y, Tanaka M, Sano H, Itoi E. The prevalence of a large Hill-Sachs lesion that needs to be treated. *J Shoulder Elbow Surg* 2013 Sep;22(9):1285 -9. doi:10.1016/j.jse.2012.12.033.

306. La Rocca Vieira R, Rybak LD, Recht M. Technical update on magnetic resonance imaging of the shoulder. *Magn Reson Imaging Clin N Am* 2012;20(2):149–161, ix. doi:10.1016/j.mric.2012.01.005.

307. Lapner PL, Lapner MA, Uhthoff HK. The anatomy of the superior labrum and biceps origin in the fetal shoulder. *Clin Anat* 2010;23(7):821–828. doi:10.1002/ca.21014.

308. Lee BG, Cho NS, Rhee YG. Anterior labroligamentous periosteal sleeve avulsion lesion in arthroscopic capsulolabral repair for anterior shoulder instability. *Knee Surg Sports Traumatol Arthrosc* 2011;19(9):1563–1569. doi:10.1007/s00167-011-1531-z.

309. Lee DH, Lee KH, Lopez-Ben R, et al. The double-density sign: a radiographic finding

suggestive of an os acromiale. *J Bone Joint Surg Am* 2004;86(12):2666.

310. Lee E, Flatow E. The shoulder and arm. In: Weinstein S, Buckwalter J, eds. Turek's Orthopaedics (Principles and Their Application)., 6th ed. Philadelphia, PA: Lippincott Williams & Wilkins;2005:345.

311. Lee SY, Cheng B, Grimmer-Somers K. The midterm effectiveness of extracorporeal shockwave therapy in the management of chronic calcific shoulder tendinitis. *J Shoulder Elbow Surg* 2011;20(5):845–854. doi:10.1016/j.jse.2010.10.024.

312. Lee SY, Lee JK. Horizontal component of partial-thickness tears of rotator cuff: imaging characteristics and comparison of ABER view with oblique coronal view at MR arthrography initial results. *Radiology* 2002;224(2):470.

313. Legan JM, Burkhard TK, Goff WB, II, et al. Tears of the glenoid labrum: MR imaging of 88 arthroscopically confirmed cases. *Radiology* 1991;179(1):241.

314. Lenza M, Buchbinder R, Takwoingi Y, Johnston RV, Hanchard NC, Faloppa F. Magnetic resonance imaging, magnetic resonance arthrography and ultrasonography for assessing rotator cuff tears in people with shoulder pain for whom surgery is being considered. *Cochrane Database Syst Rev* 2013;(9):CD009020. doi:10.1002/14651858.CD009020.pub2.

315. Lesniak BP, Baraga MG, Jose J, Smith MK, Cunningham S, Kaplan LD. Glenohumeral findings on magnetic resonance imaging correlate with innings pitched in asymptomatic pitchers. *Am J Sports Med* 2013;41(9):2022–2027. doi:10.1177/0363546513491093.

316. Li X, Fallon J, Egge N, Curry EJ, Patel K, Owens BD, Busconi BD. MRI study of associated shoulder pathology in patients with full-thickness subscapularis tendon tears. *Orthopedics.* 2013;36(1):e44–e50. doi:10.3928/01477447-20121217-17.

317. Liavaag S, Brox JI, Pripp AH, Enger M, Soldal LA, Svenningsen S. Immobilization in external rotation after primary shoulder dislocation did not reduce the risk of recurrence: a randomized controlled trial. *J Bone Joint Surg Am* 2011;93(10):897–904. doi:10.2106/JBJS.J.00416.

318. Liem D, Buschmann VE, Schmidt C, Gosheger G, Vogler T, Schulte TL, Balke M. The prevalence of rotator cuff tears: is the contralateral shoulder at risk? *Am J Sports Med* 2014;42(4):826–830.

319. Lindauer KR, Major NM, Rougier-Chapman DP, et al. MR imaging appearance of 180–360 degrees labral tears of the shoulder. *Skeletal Radiol* 2005;34(2):74.

320. Linker CS, Helms CA, Fritz RC. Quadrilateral space syndrome: findings at MR imaging. *Radiology* 1993;188(3):675.

321. Longo UG, Forriol F, Loppini M, Lanotte A, Salvatore G, Maffulli N, Denaro V. The safe zone for avoiding suprascapular nerve injury in bone block procedures for shoulder instability. A cadaveric study [published online ahead of print February 15, 2014]. *Knee Surg Sports Traumatol Arthrosc.*

322. Longo UG, Huijsmans PE, Maffulli N, Denaro V, De Beer JF. Video analysis of the mechanisms of shoulder dislocation in four elite rugby players. *J Orthop Sci* 2011;16(4):389–397. doi:10.1007/s00776-011-0087-6.

323. Loredo R, Longo C, Salonen D, et al. Glenoid labrum: MR imaging with histologic correlation. *Radiology* 1995;196(1):33.

324. Ly JQ, Beall DP, Sanders TG. MR imaging of glenohumeral instability. *AJR Am J Roentgenol* 2003;181(1):203.

325. Ma HL, Chiang ER, Wu HT, Hung SC, Wang ST, Liu CL, Chen TH. Clinical outcome and imaging of arthroscopic single-row and double-row rotator cuff repair: a prospective randomized trial. *Arthroscopy* 2012;28(1):16–24. doi:10.1016/j.arthro.2011.07.003.

326. Macarini L, Muscarella S, Lelario M, Stoppino L, Scalzo G, Scelzi A, Armillotta M, Sforza N, Vinci R. Rotator cable at MR imaging: considerations on morphological aspects and biomechanical role. *Radiol Med* 2011;116(1):102–113. doi:10.1007/s11547-010-0571-7.

327. Mack LA, Matsen FA, III, Kilcoyne RF, et al. US evaluation of the rotator cuff. *Radiology* 1985;157(1):205.

328. Macmahon PJ, Palmer WE. Magnetic resonance imaging in glenohumeral instability. *Magn Reson Imaging Clin N Am* 2012;20(2):295–312, xi. doi:10.1016/j.mric.2012.01.003.

329. Magarelli N, Milano G, Baudi P, Santagada DA, Righi P, Spina V, Leone A, Amelia R, Fabbriciani C, Bonomo L. Comparison between 2D and 3D computed tomography evaluation of glenoid bone defect in unilateral anterior gleno-humeral instability. *Radiol Med* 2012 Feb;117(1):102–111. doi:10.1007/s11547-011-0712-7.

330. Magee T, Shapiro M, Hewell G, et al. Complications of rotator cuff surgery in which bioabsorbable anchors are used. *AJR Am J Roentgenol* 2003;181(5):1227.

331. Major NM, Browne J, Domzalski T, Cothran RL, Helms CA. Evaluation of the glenoid labrum with 3-T MRI: is intraarticular contrast necessary? *AJR Am J Roentgenol* 2011;196(5):1139–1144. doi:10.2214/AJR.08.1734.

332. Marder RA, Heiden EA, Kim S. Calcific tendonitis of the shoulder: is subacromial decompression in combination with removal of the calcific deposit beneficial? *J Shoulder Elbow Surg* 2011;20(6):955–960. doi:10.1016/j.jse.2010.10.038.

333. Markenstein JE, Jaspars KC, van der Hulst VP, Willems WJ. The quantification of glenoid bone loss in anterior shoulder instability; MR-arthro compared to 3D-CT. *Skeletal Radiol* 2014;43(4):475–483. doi:10.1007/s00256-013-1780-7.

334. Martetschläger F, Padalecki JR, Millett PJ. Modified arthroscopic McLaughlin procedure for treatment of posterior instability of the shoulder with an associated reverse Hill-Sachs lesion. *Knee Surg Sports Traumatol Arthrosc* 2013;21(7):1642–1646. doi:10.1007/s00167-012-2237-6.

335. Martínez-Morillo M, Mateo Soria L, Riveros Frutos A, Tejera Segura B, Holgado Pérez S, Olivé Marqués A. Septic arthritis of the acromioclavicular joint: an uncommon location. *Reumatol Clin* 2014;10(1):37–42. doi:10.1016/j.reuma.2013.06.002.

336. Martinoli C, Bianchi S, Prato N, et al. US of the shoulder: non-rotator cuff disorders. *RadioGraphics* 2003;23(2):381.

337. Masciocchi C, Barile A, Fascetti E, et al. Magnetic resonance of the shoulder: technic, anatomy ana clinical results[in Italian]. *Radiol Med* 1989;78(5):485.

338. Matsen F III, Titelman R, Lippitt S, et al. Glenoinstability. In: Rockwood CA Jr, Matsen FA III, Wirth M, et al, eds. *The Shoulder*. 3rd ed. Philadelphia, PA: WB Saunders; 2004:655.

339. Matsen F III, Titelman R, Lippitt S, et al. Rotator cuff. In: Rockwood CA Jr, Matsen FA III, Wirth MA, et al, eds. *The Shoulder*. 3rd ed. Philadelphia, PA: WB Saunders; 2004:791–878.

340. Matsen FA III, Rockwood CA Jr, Wirth MA, et al. Glenohumeral arthritis and its management. In: Rockwood CA Jr, Matsen FA III, Wirth MA, et al, eds. *The Shoulder*. 3rd ed. Philadelphia, PA: WB Saunders; 2004:879.

341. Mayerhoefer ME, Breitenseher MJ, Roposch A, et al. Comparison of MRI and conventional radiography for assessment of acromial shape. *AJR Am J Roentgenol* 2005;184(2):671.

342. McArthur C, Welsh F, Campbell C. Posterior dislocation of long head of biceps tendon following traumatic anterior shoulder dislocation: imaging and intra-operative findings. *J Radiol Case Rep* 2013;7(9):19–26. doi:10.3941/jrcr.v7i9.1516.

343. McCarty LP III, Buss DD, Datta MW, Freehill MQ, Giveans MR. Complications observed following labral or rotator cuff repair with use of poly-L-lactic acid implants. *J Bone Joint Surg Am* 2013;95(6):507–511. doi:10.2106/JBJS.L.00314.

344. McCormick F, Bhatia S, Chalmers P, Gupta A, Verma N, Romeo AA. The management of type II superior labral anterior to posterior injuries. *Orthop Clin North Am* 2014 Jan;45(1):121–128. doi:10.1016/j.ocl.2013.08.008.

345. McCormick F, Nwachukwu B, Solomon D, Dewing C, Golijanin P, Gross DJ, Provencher MT. The efficacy of biceps tenodesis in the treatment of failed superior labral anterior posterior repairs. *Am J Sports Med* 2014;42(4):820–825.

346. McFarland EG, Garzon-Muvdi J, Jia X, Desai P, Petersen SA. Clinical and diagnostic tests for shoulder disorders: a critical review. *Br J Sports Med* 2010;44(5):328–332. doi:10.1136/bjsm.2009.067314.

347. McMahon PJ. Surgery and science of the rotator cuff: editorial comment. Clin Orthop Relat Res 2014;472(8):2425–2426.

348. McMinn RMH. *Last's Anatomy: Regional and Applied*. 8th ed. Edinburgh, United Kingdom: Churchill Livingstone;1990:53.

349. McNab I. Rotator cuff tendinitis. *Cal Med Assoc J* 1968;99 (3):91.

350. Mellado JM, Calmet J, Olona M, et al. Surgically repaired massive rotator cuff tears: MRI of tendon integrity, muscle fatty degeneration, and muscle atrophy correlated with intraoperative and clinical findings. *AJR Am J Roentgenol* 2005;184(5):1456.

351. Mengiardi B, Pfirrmann CW, Gerber C, et al. Frozen shoulder: MR arthrographic findings. *Radiology* 2004;233(2):486.

352. Meyer SJ, Dalinka MK. Magnetic resonance imaging of the shoulder. *Semin Ultrasound CT MR* 1990;11(4):253.

353. Middleton WD, Edelstein G, Reinus WR, et al. Sonographic detection of rotator cuff tears. *AJR Am J Roentgenol* 1985;144(2):349.

354. Middleton WD, Macrander S, Lawson TL, et al. High-resolution surface coil magnetic resonance imaging of the joints: anatomic correlation. *RadioGraphics* 1987;7(4):645.

355. Middleton WD. High-resolution MR imaging of the normal rotator cuff. *AJR Am J Roentgenol* 1987;148 (3):559.

356. Mihata T, Jun BJ, Bui CN, Hwang J, McGarry MH, Kinoshita M, Lee TQ. Effect of scapular orientation on shoulder internal impingement in a cadaveric model of the cocking phase of throwing. *J Bone Joint Surg Am* 2012;94(17):1576–1583.

357. Mihata T, McGarry MH, Kinoshita M, Lee TQ. Excessive glenohumeral horizontal abduction as occurs during the late cocking phase of the throwing motion can be critical for internal impingement. *Am J Sports Med* 2010;38(2):369–374. doi:10.1177/0363546509346408.

358. Mihata T, McGarry MH, Tibone JE, et al. Type II SLAP lesions: a new scoring system—the sulcus score. *J Shoulder Elbow Surg* 2005;14(1) (suppl S):19S.

359. Milano G, Saccomanno MF, Careri S, Taccardo G, De Vitis R, Fabbriciani C. Efficacy of marrow-stimulating technique in arthroscopic rotator cuff repair: a prospective randomized study. *Arthroscopy* 2013;29(5):802–810. doi:10.1016/j.arthro.2013.01.019.

360. Miller M. Biceps tenodesis. In: Miller MD, Howard RF, Plancher KD, eds. *Surgical Atlas of Sports Medicine*. Philadelphia, PA: Saunders; 2003:315.

361. Miller M. Treatment of acromioclavicular injuries. In: Miller MD, Howard RF, Plancher KD, eds. *Surgical Atlas of Sports Medicine*. Philadelphia, PA: Saunders; 2003:353.

362. Miller M. Treatment of subscapularis tendon avulsion. In: Miller MD, Howard RF, Plancher KD, eds. *Surgical Atlas of Sports Medicine*. Philadelphia, PA: Saunders; 2003:334.

363. Miller MD. Treatment of pectoralis major rupture. In: Miller MD, Howard RF, Plancher KD, eds. *Surgical Atlas of Sports Medicine*. Philadelphia, PA: Saunders; 2003:341.

364. Millett PJ, Horan MP, Martetschläger F. The "bony Bankart bridge" technique for restoration of anterior shoulder stability. *Am J Sports Med* 2013;41(3):608–614. doi:10.1177/0363546512472880.

365. Miniaci A, Dowdy PA, Willits KR, et al. Magnetic resonance imaging evaluation of the rotator cuff tendons in the asymptomatic shoulder. *Am J Sports Med* 1995;23(2):142.

366. Miniaci A, Dowdy PA. Rotator cuff disorders. In: Hawkins RJ, Misamore GW, eds. *Shoulder Injuries in the Athlete* New York: Churchill Livingstone; 1996:103.

367. Mink JH, Harris E, Rappaport M. Rotator cuff tears: evaluation using double-contrast shoulder arthrography. *Radiology* 1985;157(3):621.

368. Mirowitz SA. Normal rotator cuff: MR imaging with conventional and fat-suppression techniques. *Radiology* 1991;180(3):735.

369. Mizuno N, Yoneda M, Hayashida K, et al. Recurrent anterior shoulder dislocation caused by a midsubstance complete capsular tear. *J Bone Joint Surg Am* 2005;87(12):2717.

370. Modi CS, Karthikeyan S, Marks A, Saithna A, Smith CD, Rai SB, Drew SJ. Accuracy of abduction-external rotation MRA versus standard

MRA in the diagnosis of intra-articular shoulder pathology. *Orthopedics* 2013;36(3):e337–e342. doi:10.3928/01477447-20130222-23.

371. Mohana-Borges AV, Chung CB, Resnick D. MR imaging and MR arthrography of the postoperative shoulder: spectrum of normal and abnormal findings. *RadioGraphics* 2004;24(1):69.

372. Mohana-Borges AV, Chung CB, Resnick D. Superior labral anteroposterior tear: classification and diagnosis on MRI and MR arthrography. *AJR Am J Roentgenol* 2003;181(6):1449.

373. Mohtadi NG, Chan DS, Hollinshead RM, Boorman RS, Hiemstra LA, Lo IK, Hannaford HN, Fredine J, Sasyniuk TM, Paolucci EO. A randomized clinical trial comparing open and arthroscopic stabilization for recurrent trauanterior shoulder instability: two-year follow-up with disease-specific quality-of-life outcomes. *J Bone Joint Surg Am* 2014;96(5):353–360. doi:10.2106/JBJS.L.01656.

374. Montgomery SR, Chen NC, Rodeo SA. Arthroscopic capsular plication in the treatment of shoulder pain in competitive swimmers. *HSS J* 2010;6(2):145–149. doi:10.1007/s11420-009-9153-4.

375. Monu JU, Pope TL Jr, Chabon SJ, et al. MR diagnosis of superior labral anterior posterior (SLAP) injuries of the glenoid labrum: value of routine imaging without intra-articular injection of contrast material. *AJR Am J Roentgenol* 1994;163(6):1425.

376. Moon YL, Singh H, Yang H, Chul LK. Arthroscopic rotator interval closure by purse string suture for symptomatic inferior shoulder instability. *Orthopedics* 2011;34(4):269. doi:10.3928/01477447-20110228-02.

377. Moosikasuwan JB, Miller TT, Burke BJ. Rotator cuff tears: clinical, radiographic, and US findings. *Radiographics* 2005;25(6):1591.

378. Moosmayer S, Tariq R, Stiris M, Smith HJ. The natural history of asymptomatic rotator cuff tears: a three-year follow-up of fifty cases. *J Bone Joint Surg Am* 2013;95(14):1249–1255. doi:10.2106/JBJS.L.00185.

379. Morag Y, Bedi A, Jamadar DA. The rotator interval and long head biceps tendon: anatomy, function, pathology, and magnetic resonance imaging. *Magn Reson Imaging Clin N Am* 2012;20(2):229–237, x. doi:10.1016/j.mric.2012.01.012.

380. Morag Y, Jacobson JA, Shields G, et al. MR arthrography of rotator interval, long head of the biceps brachii, and biceps pulley of the shoulder. *Radiology* 2005;235(1):21.

381. Moran CJ, Pascual-Garrido C, Chubinskaya S, Potter HG, Warren RF, Cole BJ, Rodeo SA. Restoration of articular cartilage. *J Bone Joint Surg Am* 2014;96(4):336–344. doi:10.2106/JBJS.L.01329.

382. Morgan C, Rames RD, Snyder SJ. Anatomical variations of the glenohumeral ligaments. Presented at the Annual Meetings of the American Academy of Orthopedic Surgeons; 1991; Anaheim, CA.

383. Mori D, Funakoshi N, Yamashita F. Arthroscopic surgery of irreparable large or massive rotator cuff tears with low-grade fatty degeneration of the infraspinatus: patch autograft procedure versus partial repair procedure. *Arthroscopy* 2013;29(12):1911–1921. doi:10.1016/j.arthro.2013.08.032.

384. Morrison DS, Ofstein R. The use of magnetic resonance imaging in the diagnosis of rotator cuff tears. *Orthopedics* 1990;13(6):633.

385. Morrison OS, Bigilani LU. The clinical significance of variations in acromial morphology. *Orthop Trans* 1987;11:234.

386. Moseley HF. The anterior capsular mechanism in recurrent anterior dislocation of the shoulder. *J Bone Joint Surg Br* 1962;44:913.

387. Munk PL, Holt RG, Helms CA, et al. Glenoid labrum: preliminary work with use of radial-sequence MR imaging. *Radiology* 1989;173(3):751.

388. Murachovsky J, Bueno RS, Nascimento LG, Almeida LH, Strose E, Castiglia MT, de Oliveira HC, Ikemoto RY. Calculating anterior glenoid bone loss using the Bernageau profile view. *Skeletal Radiol* 2012;41(10):1231–1237. doi:10.1007/s00256-012-1439-9.

389. Murray IR, Ahmed I, White NJ, Robinson CM. Traumatic anterior shoulder instability in the athlete. *Scand J Med Sci Sports* 2013;23(4):387–405. doi:10.1111/j.1600-0838.2012.01494.x.

390. Murray IR, Goudie EB, Petrigliano FA, Robinson CM. Functional anatomy and biomechanics of shoulder stability in the athlete. *Clin Sports Med* 2013;32(4):607–624. doi:10.1016/j.csm.2013.07.001.

391. Murrell GA, Warren RF. The surgical treatment of posterior shoulder instability. *Clin Sports Med* 1995;14(4):903.

392. Myers JB, Oyama S, Clarke JP. Ultrasonographic assessment of humeral retrotorsion in baseball players: a validation study. *Am J Sports Med* 2012;40(5):1155–1160. doi:10.1177/0363546512436801.

393. Nadarajah CV, Weichert I. Milwaukee shoulder syndrome. *Case Rep Rheumatol* 2014;2014:458708. doi:10.1155/2014/458708.

394. Naimark A, Baum A. Injection of the subcoracoid bursa: a cause of technical failure in shoulder arthrography. *Can Assoc Radiol J* 1989;40(3):170.

395. Nakata W, Katou S, Fujita A, Nakata M, Lefor AT, Sugimoto H. Biceps pulley: normal anatomy and associated lesions at MR arthrography. *Radiographics* 2011;31(3):791–810. doi:10.1148/rg.313105507.

396. Narváez JA, Narváez J, De Lama E, De Albert M. MR imaging of early rheumatoid arthritis. *Radiographics* 2010;30(1):143–163; discussion 163–165. doi:10.1148/rg.301095089.

397. Neer CS II, Foster CR. Inferior capsular shift for involuntary inferior and multidirectional instability of the shoulder. A preliminary report. *J Bone Joint Surg Am* 1980;62(6):897.

398. Neer CS II, Welsh RP. The shoulder in sports. *Orthop Clin North Am* 1977;8(3):583.

399. Neer CS II. Anterior acromioplasty for the chronic impingement syndrome in the shoulder: a preliminary report. *J Bone Joint Surg Am* 1972;54(1):41.

400. Neer CS, II. Impingement lesions. *Clin Orthop Relat Res* 1983;(173):70.

401. Neer CS, Craig EU, Fukuda H. Cuff-tear arthropathy. *J Bone Joint Surg Am* 1985;65:1232.

402. Neer CS. *Shoulder Reconstruction*. Philadelphia, PA; WB Saunders; 1990:363.

403. Neer CS. Rupture of the long head of the biceps related to subacromial impingement. *Orthop Trans* 1977;1:111.

404. Neer CS. *Shoulder Reconstruction*. Philadelphia, PA: WB Saunders; 1990:41.

405. Neer CS. *Shoulder Reconstruction*. Philadelphia, PA: WB Saunders; 1990:273.

406. Neer CS. *Shoulder Reconstruction*. Philadelphia, PA: WB Saunders; 1990:194.

407. Neer CS. *Shoulder Reconstruction*. Philadelphia, PA: WB Saunders; 1990:1.

408. Neumann CH, Holt RG, Steinbach LS, et al. MR imaging of the shoulder: appearance of the supraspinatus tendon in asymptomatic volunteers. *AJR Am J Roentgenol* 1992;158(6):1281.

409. Neviaser TJ. The anterior labroligamentous periosteal sleeve avulsion lesion: a cause of anterior instability of the shoulder. *Arthroscopy* 1993;9(1):17.

410. Neviaser TJ. The GLAD lesion: another cause of anterior shoulder pain. *Arthroscopy* 1993;9(1):22.

411. Neyton L, Godenèche A, Nové-Josserand L, Carrillon Y, Cléchet J, Hardy MB. Arthroscopic suture-bridge repair for small to medium size supraspinatus tear: healing rate and retear pattern. *Arthroscopy* 2013;29(1):10–17. doi:10.1016/j.arthro.2012.06.020.

412. Nho SJ, Strauss EJ, Lenart BA, Provencher MT, Mazzocca AD, Verma NN, Romeo AA. Long head of the biceps tendinopathy: diagnosis and management. *J Am Acad Orthop Surg* 2010;18(11):645–656.

413. Nikulka C, Goldmann A, Schroeder RJ. Magnetic resonance imaging analysis of the subscapularis muscle after arthroscopic and open shoulder stabilization. *Clin Imaging* 2010;34(4):269–276. doi:10.1016/j.clinimag.2009.06.030.

414. Nimura A, Kato A, Yamaguchi K, Mochizuki T, Okawa A, Sugaya H, Akita K. The superior capsule of the shoulder joint complements the insertion of the rotator cuff. *J Shoulder Elbow Surg* 2012;21(7):867–872. doi:10.1016/j.jse.2011.04.034.

415. Nirschl RP. Rotator cuff tendinitis: basic concepts of pathoetiology. *AAOS Instr Course Lect* 1989;38:439.

416. Nofsinger C, Browning B, Burkhart SS, Pedowitz RA. Objective preoperative measurement of anterior glenoid bone loss: a pilot study of a computer-based method using unilateral 3-dimensional computed tomography. *Arthroscopy* 2011;27(3):322–329. doi:10.1016/j.arthro.2010.09.007.

417. Noonan B, Hollister SJ, Sekiya JK, Bedi A. Comparison of reconstructive procedures for glenoid bone loss associated with recurrent anterior shoulder instability. *J Shoulder Elbow Surg* 2014;23(8):1113–1119. doi:10.1016/j.jse.2013.11.011.

418. Norwood LA, Terry GC. Shoulder posterior subluxation. *Am J Sports Med* 1984;12(1):25.

419. Nourissat G, Radier C, Aim F, Lacoste S. Arthroscopic classification of posterior labrum glenoid insertion. *Orthop Traumatol Surg Res* 2014;100(2):167–170. doi:10.1016/j.otsr.2013.09.015.

420. O'Brien SJ, Neves MC, Arnoczky SP, et al. The anatomy and histology of the inferior glenohumeral ligament complex of the shoulder. *Am J Sports Med* 1990;18(5):449.

421. Obeidat MM, Omari A. Osteomyelitis of the scapula with secondary septic arthritis of the shoulder joint. *Singapore Med J* 2010;51(1):e1–e2.

422. Oberlander MA, Morgan BE, Visotsky JL. The BHAGL lesion: a new variant of anterior shoulder instability. *Arthroscopy* 1996;12(5):627.

423. Ogata S, Uhthoff HK. Acromial enthesopathy and rotator cuff tear. A radiologic and histologic postmortem investigation of the coracoacromial arch. *Clin Orthop* 1990;(254):39.

424. Ogul H, Karaca L, Can CE, Pirimoglu B, Tuncer K, Topal M, Okur A, Kantarci M. Anatomy, variants, and pathologies of the superior glenohumeral ligament: magnetic resonance imaging with three-dimensional volumetric interpolated breath-hold examsequence and conventional magnetic resonance arthrography. *Korean J Radiol* 2014;15(4):508–522.

425. Oh JH, Kim JY, Choi JA, Kim WS. Effectiveness of multidetector computed tomography arthrography for the diagnosis of shoulder pathology: comparison with magnetic resonance imaging with arthroscopic correlation. *J Shoulder Elbow Surg* 2010;19(1):14–20. doi:10.1016/j.jse.2009.04.012.

426. Oh JH, Shin SJ, McGarry MH, Scott JH, Heckmann N, Lee TQ. Biomechanical effects of humeral neck-shaft angle and subscapularis integrity in reverse total shoulder arthroplasty. *J Shoulder Elbow Surg* 2014;23(8):1091–1098. doi:10.1016/j.jse.2013.11.003.

427. Omoumi P, Teixeira P, Lecouvet F, Chung CB. Glenohumeral joint instability. *J Magn Reson Imaging* 2011;33(1):2–16. doi:10.1002/jmri.22343.

428. Ortmaier R, Resch H, Hitzl W, Mayer M, Blocher M, Vasvary I, Mattiassich G, Stundner O, Tauber M. Reverse shoulder arthroplasty combined with latissimus dorsi transfer using the bone-chip technique. *Int Orthop* 2014;38(3):553–559. doi:10.1007/s00264-013-2139-3.

429. Osti L, Buda M, Buono AD. Fatty infiltration of the shoulder: diagnosis and reversibility. *Muscles Ligaments Tendons J* 2014;3(4):351–354.

430. Ostör AJ, Richards CA, Tytherleigh-Strong G, Bearcroft PW, Prevost AT, Speed CA, Hazleman BL. Validation of clinical examination versus magnetic resonance imaging and arthroscopy for the detection of rotator cuff lesions. *Clin Rheumatol* 2013;32(9):1283–1291. doi:10.1007/s10067-013-2260-0.

431. Ovesen J, Nielsen S. Anterior and posterior shoulder instability. A cadaver study. *Acta Orthop Scand* 1986;57(4):324.

432. Owen RS, Iannotti JP, Kneeland JB, et al. Shoulder after surgery: MR imaging with surgical validation. *Radiology* 1993;186(2):443.

433. Owens BD, Nelson BJ, Duffey ML, Mountcastle SB, Taylor DC, Cameron KL, Campbell S, DeBerardino TM. Pathoanatomy of first-time, traumatic, anterior glenohumeral subluxation events. *J Bone Joint Surg Am* 2010;92(7):1605–1611. doi:10.2106/JBJS.I.00851.

434. Owens BD, Dickens JF, Kilcoyne KG, Rue JP. Management of mid-season traumatic anterior shoulder instability in athletes. *J Am Acad Orthop Surg* 2012;20(8):518–526. doi:10.5435/JAAOS-20-08-518.

435. Ozaki J, Fujimoto S, Nakagawa Y, et al. Tears of the rotator cuff of the shoulder associated with pathological changes in the acromion. A study in cadavera. *J Bone Joint Surg Am* 1988;70(8):1224.

436. Ozaki J. Tears of the rotator cuff of the shoulder associated with pathologic changes in the acromion. *J Bone Joint Surg Am* 1988;70:1124.

437. Paavolainen P, Ahovuo J. Ultrasonography and arthrography in the diagnosis of tears of the rotator cuff. *J Bone Joint Surg Am* 1994;76(3):335.

438. Pahlavan S, Baldwin KD, Pandya NK, Namdari S, Hosalkar H. Proximal humerus fractures in the pediatric population: a systematic review. *J Child Orthop* 2011;5(3):187–194. doi:10.1007/s11832-011-0328-4.

439. Palmer WE, Brown JH, Rosenthal DI. Labral-ligamentous complex of the shoulder: evaluation with MR arthrography. *Radiology* 1994;190(3):645.

440. Palmer WE, Brown JH, Rosenthal DI. Rotator cuff: evaluation with fat-suppressed MR arthrography. *Radiology* 1993;188(3):683.

441. Palmer WE, Caslowitz PL, Chew FS. MR arthrography of the shoulder: normal intra-articular structures and common abnormalities. *AJR Am J Roentgenol* 1995;164(1):141.

442. Palmer WE, Caslowitz PL. Anterior shoulder instability: diagnostic criteria determined from prospective analysis of 121 MR arthrograms. *Radiology* 1995;197(3):819.

443. Pape G, Bruckner T, Loew M, Zeifang F. Treatment of severe cuff tear arthropathy with the humeral head resurfacing arthroplasty: two-year minimum follow-up. *J Shoulder Elbow Surg* 2013;22(1):e1–e7. doi:10.1016/j.jse.2012.04.006.

444. Park HB, Yokota A, Gill HS, et al. Diagnostic accuracy of clinical tests for the different degrees of subacromial impingement syndrome. *J Bone Joint Surg Am* 2005;87(7):1446.

445. Park JG, Lee JK, Phelps CT. Os acromiale associated with rotator cuff impingement: MR imaging of the shoulder. *Radiology* 1994;193(1):255.

446. Park JY, Jung SW, Jeon SH, Cho HW, Choi JH, Oh KS. Arthroscopic repair of large U-shaped rotator cuff tears without margin convergence versus repair of crescent- or L-shaped tears. *Am J Sports Med* 2014;42(1):103–111. doi:10.1177/0363546513505425.

447. Park KJ, Tamboli M, Nguyen LY, McGarry MH, Lee TQ. A large humeral avulsion of the glenohumeral ligaments decreases stability that can be restored with repair. *Clin Orthop Relat Res* 2014;472(8):2372–2379. doi:10.1007/s11999-014-3476-2.

448. Park SY, Lee IS, Park SK, Cheon SJ, Ahn JM, Song JW. Comparison of three-dimensional isotropic and conventional MR arthrography with respect to the diagnosis of rotator cuff and labral lesions: focus on isotropic fat-suppressed proton density and VIBE sequences. *Clin Radiol* 2014;69(4):e173–e182. doi:10.1016/j.crad.2013.11.019.

449. Pascarelli L, Righi LC, Bongiovanni RR, Imoto RS, Teodoro RL, Ferro HF. Technique and results after distal braquial biceps tendon reparation, through two anterior mini-incisions. *Acta Ortop Bras* 2013;21(2):76–79. doi:10.1590/S1413-78522013000200002.

450. Paterson WH, Throckmorton TW, Koester M, Azar FM, Kuhn JE. Position and duration of immobilization after primary anterior shoulder dislocation: a systematic review and meta-

analysis of the literature. *J Bone Joint Surg Am* 2010;92(18):2924–2933. doi:10.2106/JBJS.J.00631.

451. Patten RM. Tears of the anterior portion of the rotator cuff (the subscapularis tendon): MR imaging findings. *AJR Am J Roentgenol* 1994;162(2):351.

452. Patten RM. Vacuum phenomenon: a potential pitfall in the interpretation of gradient-recalled-echo MR images of the shoulder. *AJR Am J Roentgenol* 1994;162(6):1383.

453. Patzer T, Kircher J, Lichtenberg S, Sauter M, Magosch P, Habermeyer P. Is there an association between SLAP lesions and biceps pulley lesions? *Arthroscopy* 2011;27(5):611–618. doi:10.1016/j.arthro.2011.01.005.

454. Peh WC, Farmer TH, Totty WG. Acromial arch shape: assessment with MR imaging. *Radiology* 1995;195(2):501.

455. Petrera M, Patella V, Patella S, Theodoropoulos J. A meta-analysis of open versus arthroscopic Bankart repair using suture anchors. *Knee Surg Sports Traumatol Arthrosc* 2010;18(12):1742–1747. doi:10.1007/s00167-010-1093-5.

456. Petrie MJ, Ismaiel AH. Treatment of massive rotator-cuff tears with a polyester ligament (LARS) patch. *Acta Orthop Belg* 2013;79(6):620–625.

457. Pillai G, Baynes JR, Gladstone J, Flatow EL. Greater strength increase with cyst decompression and SLAP repair than SLAP repair alone. *Clin Orthop Relat Res* 2011;469(4):1056–1060. doi:10.1007/s11999-010-1661-5.

458. Plancher KD, Peterson RK, Johnston JC, et al. The spinoglenoid ligament. Anatomy, morphology, and histological findings. *J Bone Joint Surg Am* 2005;87(2):361.

459. Pollock RG, Bigliani LU. The mechanical properties of the inferior glenohumeral ligament. Presented at the American Shoulder and Elbow Surgeons, 6th Opening Meeting; February 11, 1990; New Orleans, LA.

460. Polster JM, Schickendantz MS. Shoulder MRI: what do we miss? *AJR Am J Roentgenol* 2010;195(3):577–584. doi:10.2214/AJR.10.4683.

461. Ponce BA, Thompson KJ, Rosenzweig SD, Tate JP, Sarver DB, Thorpe JB II, Sheppard ED, Lopez RR. Re-evaluation of pectoralis major height as an anatomic reference for humeral height in fracture hemiarthroplasty. *J Shoulder Elbow Surg* 2013;22(11):1567–1572. doi:10.1016/j.jse.2013.01.039.

462. Pöyhiä TH, Lamminen AE, Peltonen JI, Kirjavainen MO, Willamo PJ, Nietosvaara Y. Brachial plexus birth injury: US screening for glenohumeral joint instability. *Radiology* 2010;254(1):253–260. doi:10.1148/radiol.09090570.

463. Provencher MT, Bhatia S, Ghodadra NS, Grumet RC, Bach BR Jr, Dewing CB, LeClere L, Romeo AA. Recurrent shoulder instability: current concepts for evaluation and management of glenoid bone loss. *J Bone Joint Surg Am* 2010;(suppl 2):133–151. doi:10.2106/JBJS.J.00906.

464. Provencher MT, Ghodadra N, Romeo AA. Arthroscopic management of anterior instability: pearls, pitfalls, and lessons learned. *Orthop Clin North Am* 2010;41(3):325–337. doi:10.1016/j.ocl.2010.02.007.

465. Provencher MT, LeClere LE, King S, McDonald LS, Frank RM, Mologne TS, Ghodadra NS, Romeo AA. Posterior instability of the shoulder: diagnosis and management. *Am J Sports Med* 2011;39(4):874–886. doi:10.1177/0363546510384232.

466. Provencher MT, Frank RM, Leclere LE, Metzger PD, Ryu JJ, Bernhardson A, Romeo AA. The Hill-Sachs lesion: diagnosis, classification, and management. *J Am Acad Orthop Surg* 2012;20(4):242–252. doi:10.5435/JAAOS-20-04-242.

467. Putz R, Reichelt A. Structural findings of the coraco-acromial ligament in rotator cuff rupture, tendinosis calcarea and supraspinatus syndrome [in German]. *Z Orthop Ihre Grenzgeb* 1990;128(1):46.

468. Quinn SF, Sheley RC, Demlow TA, et al. Rotator cuff tendon tears: evaluation with fat-suppressed MR imaging with arthroscopic correlation in 100 patients. *Radiology* 1995;195(2):497.

469. Rafii M, Firooznia H, Bonamo JJ, et al. Athlete shoulder injuries: CT arthrographic findings. *Radiology* 1987;162(2):559.

470. Rafii M, Firooznia H, Golimbu C, et al. CT arthrography of capsular structures of the shoulder. *AJR Am J Roentgenol* 1986;146(2):361.

471. Rafii M, Firooznia H, Sherman O, et al. Rotator cuff lesions: signal patterns at MR imaging. *Radiology* 1990;177(3):817.

472. Rafii M. Non-contrast MR imaging of the glenohumeral joint. Part II. Glenohumeral instability and labrum tears. *Skeletal Radiol* 2004;33(11):617.

473. Rafii M. Non-contrast MR imaging of the glenohumeral joint. Part I. Normal anatomy. *Skeletal Radiol* 2004;33(10):551.

474. Rafii M. The painful shoulder. In: Firooznia HF, Goliumbu C, Rafii M, eds. *MRI and CT of the Musculoskeletal System*. St. Louis, MO: Mosby Year Book; 1992:465.

475. Ramirez Ruiz FA, Baranski Kaniak BC, Haghighi P, Trudell D, Resnick DL. High origin of the anterior band of the inferior glenohumeral ligament: MR arthrography with anatomic and histologic correlation in cadavers. *Skeletal Radiol* 2012;41(5):525–530. doi:10.1007/s00256-011-1201-8.

476. Randelli P, Compagnoni R, Aliprandi A, Cannaò PM, Ragone V, Tassi A, Cabitza P. Long-term degradation of poly-lactic co-glycolide/β-tricalcium phosphate biocomposite anchors in arthroscopic Bankart repair: a prospective study. *Arthroscopy* 2014;30(2):165–171 doi:10.1016/j.arthro.2013.09.082.

477. Randelli P, Ragone V, Carminati S, Cabitza P. Risk factors for recurrence after Bankart repair a systematic review. *Knee Surg Sports Traumatol Arthrosc* 2012;20(11):2129–2138. doi:10.1007/s00167-012-2140-1.

478. Rashid MS, Crichton J, Butt U, Akimau PI, Charalambous CP. Arthroscopic "Remplissage" for shoulder instability: a systematic review. Knee Surg Sports Traumatol Arthrosc. 2014 [published online ahead of print February 6, 2014]. *Knee Surg Sports Traumatol Arthrosc.*

479. Rathbun JB, Macnab I. The microvascular pattern of the rotator cuff. *J Bone Joint Surg Br* 1970;52(3):540.

480. Recht MP, Kramer J, Petersilge CA, et al. Distribution of normal and abnormal fluid collections in the glenohumeral joint: implications for MR arthrography. *J Magn Reson Imaging* 1994;4(2):173.

481. Reinus WR, Shady KL, Mirowitz SA, et al. MR diagnosis of rotator cuff tears of the shoulder: value of using T2-weighted fat-saturated images. *AJR Am J Roentgenol* 1995;164(6):1451.

482. Rerko MA, Pan X, Donaldson C, Jones GL, Bishop JY. Comparison of various imaging techniques to quantify glenoid bone loss in shoulder instability. *J Shoulder Elbow Surg* 2013;22(4):528–534. doi:10.1016/j.jse.2012.05.034.

483. Resnick CS. Contemporary issues in computed tomography: CT of the musculoskeletal system. In: Scott WW Jr, Majid D, Fishman EK, eds. *The Shoulder*. New York, NY: Churchill; 1987.

484. Resnick D. Internal derangements of joints. In: Resnick D, ed. *Diagnosis of Bone and Joint Disorders*. 3rd ed. Philadelphia, PA: WB Saunders; 1995:2899–3228

485. Ricchetti ET, Ciccotti MC, Ciccotti MG, Williams GR Jr, Lazarus MD. Sensitivity of preoperative magnetic resonance imaging and magnetic resonance arthrography in detection of panlabral tears of the glenohumeral joint. *Arthroscopy* 2013 Feb;29(2):274–279. doi:10.1016/j.arthro.2012.10.005.

486. Richards RD, Sartoris DJ, Pathria MN, et al. Hill-Sachs lesion and normal humeral groove: MR imaging features allowing their differentiation. *Radiology* 1994;190(3):665.

487. Richardson ML, Patten RM. Age-related changes in marrow distribution in the shoulder: MR imaging findings. *Radiology* 1994;192(1):209.

488. Robb AJ, Fleisig G, Wilk K, Macrina L, Bolt B, Pajaczkowski J. Passive ranges of motion of the hips and their relationship with pitching biomechanics and ball velocity in professional baseball pitchers. *Am J Sports Med* 2010;38(12):2487–2493. doi:10.1177/0363546510375535.

489. Robertson PL, Schweitzer ME, Mitchell DG, et al. Rotator cuff disorders: interobserver and intraobserver variation in diagnosis with MR imaging. *Radiology* 1995;194(3):831.

490. Robinson CM, Aderinto J. Recurrent posterior shoulder instability. *J Bone Joint Surg Am* 2005;87(4):883.

491. Robinson CM, Seah M, Akhtar MA. The epidemiology, risk of recurrence, and functional outcome after an acute traumatic posterior dislocation of the shoulder. *J Bone Joint Surg Am* 2011;93(17):1605–1613. doi:10.2106/JBJS.J.00973.

492. Rockwood C, Burkhead W Jr, Arcand M, et al. The biceps tendon. In: Rockwood CA Jr, Matsen FA III, Wirth MA, et al, eds. *The Shoulder*. 3rd ed. Philadelphia, PA: WB Saunders; 2004:1059.

493. Rockwood C, Harryman DT II, Lazarus M. The stiff shoulder. In: Rockwood CA Jr, Matsen FA III, Wirth MA, et al, eds. *The Shoulder*. 3rd ed. Philadelphia, PA: WB Saunders; 2004:1121.

494. Rockwood C, Steinmann S, Spinner R. Nerve problems about the shoulder. In: Rockwood CA Jr, Matsen FA III, Wirth MA, et al, eds. *The Shoulder*. 3rd ed. Philadelphia, PA: WB Saunders; 2004:1009.

495. Rockwood C, Uhthoff HK, Dervin G, et al. Calcifying tendinitis. In: Rockwood CA Jr, Matsen

FA III, Wirth MA, et al, eds. *The Shoulder*. 3rd ed. Philadelphia, PA: WB Saunders; 2004:1033.

496. Rockwood C, Uhthoff HK, Dervin G, et al. Clinical evaluation of shoulder problems. In: Rockwood CA Jr, Matsen FA III, Wirth MA, et al, eds. *The Shoulder*. 3rd ed. Philadelphia, PA: WB Saunders; 2004:145.

497. Rockwood C, Uhthoff HK, Dervin G, et al. Fractures of the proximal humerus. In: Rockwood CA Jr, Matsen FA III, Wirth MA, et al, eds. *The Shoulder*. 3rd ed. Philadelphia, PA: WB Saunders; 2004:355.

498. Rockwood C, Uhthoff HK, Dervin G, et al. Sepsis of the shoulder: molecular mechanisms and pathogenesis. In: Rockwood CA Jr, Matsen FA III, Wirth MA, et al, eds. *The Shoulder*. 3rd ed. Philadelphia, PA: WB Saunders; 2004:1233.

499. Rockwood C Jr, Williams GR Jr, Young DC. Disorders of the acromioclavicular joint. In: Rockwood CA Jr, Matsen FA III, Wirth MA, et al, eds. *The Shoulder*. 3rd ed. Philadelphia, PA: WB Saunders; 2004:521.

500. Rodosky MW, Harner CD, Fu FH. The role of the long head of the biceps muscle and superior glenoid labrum in anterior stability of the shoulder. *Am J Sports Med* 1994;22(1):121.

501. Rouleau DM, Hebert-Davies J, Robinson CM. Acute traumatic posterior shoulder dislocation. *J Am Acad Orthop Surg* 2014;22(3):145–152. doi:10.5435/JAAOS-22-03-145.

502. Rowe C. Dislocations of the shoulder. In: Rowe C, ed. *The Shoulder*. New York, NY: Churchill Livingstone; 1988:165.

503. Rozing PM, Nagels J, Rozing MP. Prognostic factors in arthroplasty in the rheumatoid shoulder. *HSS J* 2011;7(1):29–36. doi:10.1007/s11420-010-9172-1.

504. Ruchelsman DE, Grossman JA, Price AE. Glenohumeral deformity in children with brachial plexus birth injuries. *Bull NYU Hosp Jt Dis.* 2011;69(1):36–43.

505. Rulewicz GJ, Beaty S, Hawkins RJ, Kissenberth MJ. Supraspinatus atrophy as a predictor of rotator cuff tear size: an MRI study utilizing the tangent sign. *J Shoulder Elbow Surg* 2013;22(6):e6–e10. doi:10.1016/j.jse.2012.10.048.

506. Russell RD, Knight JR, Mulligan E, Khazzam MS. Structural integrity after rotator cuff repair does not correlate with patient function and pain: a meta-analysis. *J Bone Joint Surg Am* 2014;96(4):265–271. doi:10.2106/JBJS.M.00265.

507. Safran O, Milgrom C, Radeva-Petrova DR, Jaber S, Finestone A. Accuracy of the anterior apprehension test as a predictor of risk for redislocation after a first traumatic shoulder dislocation. *Am J Sports Med* 2010;38(5):972–975. doi:10.1177/0363546509357610.

508. Sanders B, Lavery KP, Pennington S, Warner JJ. Clinical success of biceps tenodesis with and without release of the transverse humeral ligament. *J Shoulder Elbow Surg* 2012;21(1):66–71. doi:10.1016/j.jse.2011.01.037.

509. Sanders BS, Wilcox RB III, Higgins LD. Heterotopic ossification of the deltoid muscle after arthroscopic rotator cuff repair. *Am J Orthop (Belle Mead NJ)* 2010;39(7):E67–E71.

510. Sanders TG, Zlatkin M, Montgomery J. Imaging of glenohumeral instability. *Semin Roentgenol* 2010;45(3):160–179. doi:10.1053/j.ro.2009.12.008.

511. Sano H, Mineta M, Kita A, Itoi E. Tendon patch grafting using the long head of the biceps for irreparable massive rotator cuff tears. *J Orthop Sci* 2010;15(3):310–316. doi:10.1007/s00776-010-1453-5.

512. Scarpinato DF, Bramhall JP, Andrews JR. Arthroscopic management of the throwing athlete's shoulder: indications, techniques, and results. *Clin Sports Med* 1991;10(4):913.

513. Schaeffeler C, Mueller D, Kirchhoff C, Wolf P, Rummeny EJ, Woertler K. Tears at the rotator cuff footprint: prevalence and imaging characteristics in 305 MR arthrograms of the shoulder. *Eur Radiol* 2011;21(7):1477–1484. doi:10.1007/s00330-011-2066-x.

514. Schalamon J, Dampf S, Singer G, Ainoedhofer H, Petnehazy T, Hoellwarth ME, Saxena AK. Evaluation of fractures in children and adolescents in a level I trauma center in Austria. *J Trauma* 2011;71(2):E19–E25. doi:10.1097/TA.0b013e3181f8a903.

515. Scheibel M, Martinek V, Imhoff AB. Arthroscopic reconstruction of an isolated avulsion fracture of the lesser tuberosity. *Arthroscopy* 2005;21(4):487.

516. Schnaser E, Toussaint B, Gillespie R, Lefebvre Y, Gobezie R. Arthroscopic treatment of anterosuperior rotator cuff tears. *Orthopedics* 2013;36(11):e1394–e1400. doi:10.3928/01477447-20131021-20.

517. Schulze-Borges J, Agneskirchner JD, Bobrowitsch E, Patzer T, Struck M, Smith T, Wellmann M Biomechanical comparison of open and arthroscopic Latarjet procedures. *Arthroscopy* 2013;29(4):630–637. doi:10.1016/j.arthro.2012.12.003.

518. Schwartz E, Warren RF, O'Brien SJ, et al. Posterior shoulder instability. *Orthop Clin North Am* 1987;18(3):409.

519. Schwartz RE, O'Brien SJ, Warren RF. Capsular restraints to anterior-posterior motion of the abducted shoulder; a biomechanical study. *Orthop Trans* 1988;12:727.

520. Schwartz RE. Capsular restraints to anterior-posterior motion of the shoulder. *Trans Orthop Res Soc* 1987;12:78.

521. Schweitzer ME, Magbalon MJ, Fenlin JM, et al. Effusion criteria and clinical importance of glenohumeral joint fluid: MR imaging evaluation. *Radiology* 1995;194(3):821.

522. Schweitzer ME, Magbalon MJ, Frieman BG, et al. Acromioclavicular joint fluid: determination of clinical significance with MR imaging. *Radiology* 1994;192(1):205.

523. Sciascia A, Thigpen C, Namdari S, Baldwin K. Kinetic chain abnormalities in the athletic shoulder. *Sports Med Arthrosc* 2012;20(1):16–21. doi:10.1097/JSA.0b013e31823a021f.

524. Seeger LL, Gold RH, Bassett LW, et al. Shoulder impingement syndrome: MR findings in 53 shoulders. *AJR Am J Roentgenol* 1988;150(2):343.

525. Seeger LL, Gold RH, Bassett LW. Shoulder instability: evaluation with MR imaging. *Radiology* 1988;168(3):695.

526. Seeger LL, Ruszkowski JT, Bassett LW, et al. MR imaging of the normal shoulder: anatomic correlation. *AJR Am J Roentgenol* 1987;148(1):83.

527. Seeger LL. Magnetic resonance imaging of the shoulder. *Clin Orthop* 1989;(244):48.

528. Sela Y, Eshed I, Shapira S, Oran A, Vogel G, Herman A, Perry Pritsch M. Rotator cuff tears: correlation between geometric tear patterns on MRI and arthroscopy and pre- and postoperative clinical findings. [published online ahead of print January 20, 2014]. *Acta Radiol.*

529. Seroyer ST, Nho SJ, Provencher MT, Romeo AA. Four-quadrant approach to capsulolabral repair: an arthroscopic road map to the glenoid. *Arthroscopy* 2010;26(4):555–562. doi:10.1016/j.arthro.2009.09.019.

530. Sethi PM, Noonan BC, Cunningham J, Shreck E, Miller S. Repair results of 2-tendon rotator cuff tears utilizing the transosseous equivalent technique. *J Shoulder Elbow Surg* 2010;19(8):1210–1217. doi:10.1016/j.jse.2010.03.018.

531. Sharkey NA, Marder RA. The rotator cuff opposes superior translation of the humeral head. *Am J Sports Med* 1995;23:270.

532. Sharma P, Morrison WB, Cohen S. Imaging of the shoulder with arthroscopic correlation. *Clin Sports Med* 2013;32(3):339–359. doi:10.1016/j.csm.2013.03.009.

533. Shellock FG, Stoller D, Crues JV. MRI of the shoulder: a rational approach to the reporting of findings. *J Magn Reson Imaging* 1996;6(1):268.

534. Sher JS, Uribe JW, Posada A, et al. Abnormal findings on magnetic resonance images of asymptomatic shoulders. *J Bone Joint Surg Am* 1995;77(1):10.

535. Shibano K, Koishi H, Futai K, Yoshikawa H, Sugamoto K. Effect of Bankart repair on the loss of range of motion and the instability of the shoulder joint for recurrent anterior shoulder dislocation. *J Shoulder Elbow Surg* 2014;23(6):888–894. doi:10.1016/j.jse.2013.09.004.

536. Shin SJ. A comparison of 2 repair techniques for partial-thickness articular-sided rotator cuff tears. *Arthroscopy* 2012;28(1):25–33. doi:10.1016/j.arthro.2011.07.005.

537. Simone JP, Streubel PH, Athwal GS, Sperling JW, Schleck CD, Cofield RH. Anatomical total shoulder replacement with rotator cuff repair for osteoarthritis of the shoulder. *Bone Joint J* 2014;96-B(2):224–228. doi:10.1302/0301-620X.96B.32890.

538. Skendzel JG, Sekiya JK. Diagnosis and management of humeral head bone loss in shoulder instability. *Am J Sports Med* 2012;40(11):2633–2644. doi:10.1177/0363546512437314.

539. Skinner HA. Anatomical considerations relative to rupture of the supraspinatus tendon. *J Bone Joint Surg Br* 1937;18:137.

540. Smark CT, Barlow BT, Vachon TA, Provencher MT. Arthroscopic and magnetic resonance arthrogram features of Kim's lesion in posterior shoulder instability. *Arthroscopy* 2014;30(7):781–784. doi:10.1016/j.arthro.2014.02.038.

541. Smith DK, Chopp TM, Aufdemorte TB, et al. Sublabral recess of the superior glenoid labrum: study of cadavers with conventional nonenhanced MR imaging, MR arthrography, anatomic dissection, and limited histologic examination. *Radiology* 1996;201(1):251.

542. Smith III JP, Savoie III FH, Nottage WM, et al. SLAC lesions: diagnosis and treatment. In: Barber FA, Fischer SP, eds. *Surgical Techniques for the Shoulder and Elbow.* New York, NY: Thieme;

543. Smith T, Pastor MF, Goede F, Struck M, Wellmann M. Arthroscopic posterior shoulder stabilization with an iliac bone graft and capsular repair. [published online ahead of print July 25, 2014]. *Oper Orthop Traumatol.*

544. Snyder S. Arthroscopic classification of rotator cuff lesions and surgical decision making. In: Snyder SJ, ed. *Shoulder Arthroscopy.* 2nd ed. Philadelphia, PA: Lippincott Williams & Wilkins; 2003:201.

545. Snyder S. Calcium deposits about the shoulder. In: Snyder SJ, ed. *Shoulder Arthroscopy.* 2nd ed. Philadelphia, PA: Lippincott Williams & Wilkins; 2003:284.

546. Snyder S. Diagnositic arthroscopy of the shoulder: normal anatomy and variations. In: Snyder SJ, ed. *Shoulder Arthroscopy.* 2nd ed. Philadelphia, PA: Lippincott Williams & Wilkins; 2003:22.

547. Snyder S. Multidirectional instability of the shoulder or loose shoulder. In: Snyder SJ, ed. *Shoulder Arthroscopy.* 2nd ed. Philadelphia, PA: Lippincott Williams & Wilkins; 2003:132.

548. Snyder SJ, Karzel RP, Del Pizzo W, et al. SLAP lesions of the shoulder. *Arthroscopy* 1990;6(4):274.

549. Snyder SJ. Adhesive capsulitis or frozen shoulder. In: Snyder SJ, ed. *Shoulder Arthroscopy.* 2nd ed. Philadelphia, PA: Lippincott Williams & Wilkins; 2003:66.

550. Snyder SJ. Arthroscopic treatment of massive rotator cuff tears. In: Snyder SJ, ed. *Shoulder Arthroscopy.* 2nd ed. Philadelphia, PA: Lippincott Williams & Wilkins; 2003:251.

551. Snyder SJ. Biceps tendon. In: Snyder SJ, ed. *Shoulder Arthroscopy.* 2nd ed. Philadelphia, PA: Lippincott Williams & Wilkins; 2003:74.

552. Snyder SJ. Diagnostic arthroscopy: normal anatomy and variations. In: Snyder SJ, ed. *Shoulder Arthroscopy.* New York, NY: McGraw-Hill; 1994.

553. Snyder SJ. Ganglion cysts of the shoulder. In: Snyder SJ, ed. *Shoulder Arthroscopy.* 2nd ed. Philadelphia, PA: Lippincott Williams & Wilkins; 2003.

554. Snyder SJ. Posterior instability. In: Snyder SJ, ed. *Shoulder Arthroscopy.* 2nd ed. Philadelphia, PA: Lippincott Williams & Wilkins; 2003:121

555. Snyder SJ. Repair of full-thickness rotator cuff tendon and bursal flap tears. In: Snyder SJ, ed. *Shoulder Arthroscopy.* 2nd ed. Philadelphia, PA: Lippincott Williams & Wilkins; 2003:230.

556. Snyder SJ. Rotator cuff: introduction, evaluation, and imaging. In: Snyder SJ, ed. *Shoulder Arthroscopy.* 2nd ed. Philadelphia, PA: Lippincott Williams & Wilkins; 2003:184.

557. Snyder SJ. Subscapularis tendon injury. In: Snyder SJ, ed. *Shoulder Arthroscopy.* 2nd ed. Philadelphia, PA: Lippincott Williams & Wilkins; 2003:262.

558. Snyder SJ. Superior labrum, anterior to posterior lesions of the shoulder. In: Snyder SJ, ed. *Shoulder Arthroscopy.* 2nd ed. Philadelphia, PA: Lippincott Williams & Wilkins; 2003:147.

559. Snyder S, Karzel R, Getelman M, Burns J, Bahk M, Auerbach D. *Scoi Shoulder Arthroscopy.* 3rd ed. Wolters Kluwer/Lippincott Williams & Wilkins; 2015.

560. Sodl JF, McGarry MH, Campbell ST, Tibone JE, Lee TQ. Biomechanical effects of anterior capsular plication and rotator interval closure in simulated anterior shoulder instability. [published online ahead of print February 9, 2014]. *Knee Surg Sports Traumatol Arthrosc.*

561. Sofka CM, Lin J, Feinberg J, et al. Teres minor denervation on routine magnetic resonance imaging of the shoulder. *Skeletal Radiol* 2004;33(9):514.

562. Sommaire C, Penz C, Clavert P, Klouche S, Hardy P, Kempf JF. Recurrence after arthroscopic Bankart repair: is quantitative radiological analysis of bone loss of any predictive value? *Orthop Traumatol Surg Res* 2012;98(5):514–519. doi:10.1016/j.otsr.2012.03.015.

563. Speer KP. Anatomy and pathomechanics of shoulder instability. *Clin Sports Med* 1995;14(4):751.

564. Spencer BA, Dolinskas CA, Seymour PA, Thomas SJ, Abboud JA. Glenohumeral articular cartilage lesions: prospective comparison of non-contrast magnetic resonance imaging and findings at arthroscopy. *Arthroscopy* 2013;29(9):1466–1470. doi:10.1016/j.arthro.2013.05.023.

565. Sperer A, Wredmark T. Capsular elasticity and joint volume in recurrent anterior shoulder instability. *Arthroscopy* 1994;10:598.

566. Sternheim A, Chechik O, Freedman Y, Steinberg EL. Transient sternoclavicular joint arthropathy, a self-limited disease. *J Shoulder Elbow Surg* 2014;23(4):548–552. doi:10.1016/j.jse.2013.08.013.

567. Stetson WB, Phillips T, Deutsch A. The use of magnetic resonance arthrography to detect partial-thickness rotator cuff tears. *J Bone Joint Surg Am* 2005;87(suppl 2):81

568. Strauss EJ, McCormack RA, Onyekwelu I, Rokito AS. Management of failed arthroscopic rotator cuff repair. *J Am Acad Orthop Surg* 2012;20(5):301–309. doi:10.5435/JAAOS-20-05-301.

569. Streubel PN, Simone JP, Sperling JW, Cofield R. Thirty and ninety-day reoperation rates after shoulder arthroplasty. *J Bone Joint Surg Am* 2014;96(3):e17. doi:10.2106/JBJS.M.00127.

570. Strizak AM, Danzig L, Jackson DW, et al. Subacromial bursography. An anatomical and clinical study. *J Bone Joint Surg Am* 1982;64(2):196.

571. Strobel K, Pfirrmann CW, Zanetti M, et al. MRI features of the acromioclavicular joint that predict pain relief from intra-articular injection. *AJR Am J Roentgenol* 2003;181(3):755.

572. Strobel K, Treumann TC, Allgayer B. Posterior entrapment of the long biceps tendon after traumatic shoulder dislocation: findings on MR imaging. *AJR Am J Roentgenol* 2002;178(1):238.

573. Sugalski MT, Wiater JM, Levine WN, et al. An anatomic study of the humeral insertion of the inferior glenohumeral capsule. *J Shoulder Elbow Surg* 2005;14(1):91.

574. Sugaya H, Moriishi J, Kanisawa I, et al. Arthroscopic osseous Bankart repair for chronic recurrent traumatic anterior glenohumeral instability. *J Bone Joint Surg Am* 2005;87(8):1752.

575. Sugaya H. Techniques to evaluate glenoid bone loss. *Curr Rev Musculoskelet Med* 2014;7(1):1–5.

576. Sussmann AR, Cohen J, Nomikos GC, Schweitzer ME. Magnetic resonance imaging of shoulder arthropathies. *Magn Reson Imaging Clin N Am* 2012;20(2):349–371, xi–xii. doi:10.1016/j.mric.2012.01.004.

577. Tae SK, Oh JH, Kim SH, Chung SW, Yang JY, Back YW. Evaluation of fatty degeneration of the supraspinatus muscle using a new measuring tool and its correlation between multidetector computed tomography and magnetic resonance imaging. *Am J Sports Med* 2011;39(3):599–606. doi:10.1177/0363546510384791.

578. Takubo Y, Horii M, Kurokawa M, et al. Magnetic resonance imaging evaluation of the inferior glenohumeral ligament: non-arthrographic imaging in abduction and external rotation. *J Shoulder Elbow Surg* 2005;14(5):511.

579. Tasaki A, Nimura A, Nozaki T, Yamakawa A, Niitsu M, Morita W, Hoshikawa Y, Akita K. Quantitative and qualitative analyses of subacromial impingement by kinematic open MRI. [published online ahead of print February 9, 2014]. *Knee Surg Sports Traumatol Arthrosc.*

580. Tashjian RZ, Hung M, Burks RT, Greis PE. Influence of preoperative musculotendinous junction position on rotator cuff healing using single-row technique. *Arthroscopy* 2013;29(11):1748–1754. doi:10.1016/j.arthro.2013.08.014.

581. Tauber M. Management of acute acromioclavicular joint dislocations: current concepts. *Arch Orthop Trauma Surg* 2013;133(7):985–995. doi:10.1007/s00402-013-1748-z.

582. Tawfik AM, El-Morsy A, Badran MA. Rotator cuff disorders: how to write a surgically relevant magnetic resonance imaging report? *World J Radiol* 2014;6(6):274–283. doi:10.4329/wjr.v6.i6.274.

583. Teefey SA, Middleton WD, Payne WT, et al. Detection and measurement of rotator cuff tears with sonography: analysis of diagnostic errors. *AJR Am J Roentgenol* 2005;184(6):1768.

584. Tena-Arregui J, Barrio-Asensio C, Puerta-Fonolla J, et al. Arthroscopic study of the shoulder joint in fetuses. *Arthroscopy* 2005;21(9):1114.

585. Teoh KH, Watts AC, Chee YH, Reid R, Porter DE. Predictive factors for recurrence of simple bone cyst of the proximal humerus. *J Orthop Surg (Hong Kong)* 2010;18(2):215–219.

586. The MOON Shoulder Group:, Unruh KP, Kuhn JE, Sanders R, An Q, Baumgarten KM, Bishop JY, Brophy RH, Carey JL, Holloway BG, Jones GL, Ma BC, Marx RG, McCarty EC, Poddar SK, Smith MV, Spencer EE, Vidal AF, Wolf BR, Wright RW, Dunn WR. The duration of symptoms does not correlate with rotator cuff tear severity or other patient-related features: a cross-sectional study of patients with atraumatic, full-thickness rotator cuff tears. *J Shoulder Elbow Surg* 2014;23(7):1052–1058. doi:10.1016/j.jse.2013.10.001.

587. Thomas PR, Parks BG, Douoguih WA. Anterior shoulder instability with Bristow procedure versus conjoined tendon transfer alone in a simple soft-tissue model. *Arthroscopy* 2010;26(9):1189–1194. doi:10.1016/j.arthro.2010.01.033.

588. Tian CY, Cui GQ, Zheng ZZ, Ren AH. The added value of ABER position for the detection and classification of anteroinferior labroligamentous lesions in MR arthrography of the shoulder. *Eur J Radiol* 2013;82(4):651–657. doi:10.1016/j.ejrad.2012.11.038.

589. Timins ME, Erickson SJ, Estkowski LD, et al. Increased signal in the normal supraspinatus tendon on MR imaging: diagnostic pitfall caused by the magic-angle effect. *AJR Am J Roentgenol* 1995;165(1):109.

590. Tirman PF, Bost FW, Steinbach LS, et al. MR arthrographic depiction of tears of the rotator cuff: benefit of abduction and external rotation of the arm. *Radiology* 1994;192(3):851.

591. Tirman PF, Stauffer AE, Crues JV III, et al. Saline magnetic resonance arthrography in the evaluation of glenohumeral instability. *Arthroscopy* 1993;9(5):550.

592. Tirman PFJ, Feller JF, Janzen DL. Association of glenoid labral cysts with labral tears and glenohumeral instability: radiologic findings and clinical significance. *Radiology* 1994;190:653.

593. Tischer T, Vogt S, Kreuz PC, Imhoff AB. Arthroscopic anatomy, variants, and pathologic findings in shoulder instability. *Arthroscopy* 2011;27(10):1434–1443. doi:10.1016/j.arthro.2011.05.017.

594. Tjoumakaris FP, Bradley JP. The rationale for an arthroscopic approach to shoulder stabilization. *Arthroscopy* 2011;27(10):1422–1433. doi:10.1016/j.arthro.2011.06.006.

595. Totterman SM, Miller RJ, Kwok E. MR imaging of the shoulder rotator cuff. In: *Book of Abstracts*. Chicago, IL: Radiologic Society of North America; 1992:240.

596. Toussaint B, Schnaser E, Bosley J, Lefebvre Y, Gobezie R. Early structural and functional outcomes for arthroscopic double-row transosseous-equivalent rotator cuff repair. *Am J Sports Med* 2011;39(6):1217–1225. doi:10.1177/0363546510397725.

597. Tsai JC, Zlatkin MB. Magnetic resonance imaging of the shoulder. *Radiol Clin North Am* 1990;28(2):279.

598. Tshering Vogel DW, Steinbach LS, Hertel R, et al. Acromioclavicular joint cyst: nine cases of a pseudotumor of the shoulder. *Skeletal Radiol* 2005;34(5):260.

599. Tuite MJ, Cirillo RL, De Smet AA, et al. Superior labrum anterior-posterior (SLAP) tears: evaluation of three MR signs on T2-weighted images. *Radiology* 2000;215(3):841.

600. Tuite MJ, Rutkowski A, Enright T, et al. Width of high signal and extension posterior to biceps tendon as signs of superior labrum anterior to posterior tears on MRI and MR arthrography. *AJR Am J Roentgenol* 2005;185(6):1422.

601. Tuite MJ. Magnetic resonance imaging of rotator cuff disease and external impingement. *Magn Reson Imaging Clin N Am* 2012;20(2):187–200, ix. doi:10.1016/j.mric.2012.01.011.

602. Tung GA, Entzian D, Stern JB, et al. MR imaging and MR arthrography of paraglenoid labral cysts. *AJR Am J Roentgenol* 2000;174(6):1707.

603. Tung GA, Hou DD. MR arthrography of the posterior labrocapsular complex: relationship with glenohumeral joint alignment and clinical posterior instability. *AJR Am J Roentgenol* 2003;180(2):369.

604. Turkel SJ, Panio MW, Marshall JL, et al. Stabilizing mechanisms preventing anterior dislocation of the glenohumeral joint. *J Bone Joint Surg Am* 1981;63(8):1208.

605. Turkel SJ, Panio MW, Marshall JL. Stabilizing mechanisms preventing anterior dislocation of the glenohumeral joint. *J Bone Joint Surg Br* 1981;67:1208.

606. Tyson LL, Crues JV III. Pathogenesis of rotator cuff disorders. Magnetic resonance imaging characteristics. *Magn Reson Imaging Clin North Am* 1993;1(1):37.

607. Uchiyama Y, Hamada K, Khruekarnchana P, Handa A, Nakajima T, Shimpuku E, Fukuda H. Surgical treatment of confirmed intratendinous rotator cuff tears: retrospective analysis after an average of eight years of follow-up. *J Shoulder Elbow Surg* 2010;19(6):837–846. doi:10.1016/j.jse.2010.01.013.

608. Uhthoff AK, Sarkar K, Hammond DI. The subacromial bursa: a clinico-pathological study. In: Bateman JE, Welsh RP, eds. *Surgery of the Shoulder*. Philadelphia, PA: BC Decker; 1984:121.

609. Uhthoff HK, Sarkar K. Classification and definition of tendinopathies. *Clin Sports Med* 1991;10(4):707.

610. Uri O, Barmpagiannis K, Higgs D, Falworth M, Alexander S, Lambert SM. Clinical outcome after reconstruction for sternoclavicular joint instability using a sternocleidomastoid tendon graft. *J Bone Joint Surg Am* 2014;96(5):417–422. doi:10.2106/JBJS.M.00681.

611. Vahlensieck M, Pollack M, Lang P, et al. Two segments of the supraspinous muscle: cause of high signal intensity at MR imaging? *Radiology* 1993;186(2):449.

612. van Eijk J, van Alfen N. Neuralgic amyotrophy. *AJR Am J Roentgenol* 2011 Jun;196(6):W858; author reply W859. doi:10.2214/AJR.10.5995.

613. van Holsbeeck M, Strouse PJ. Sonography of the shoulder: evaluation of the subacromial-subdeltoid bursa. *AJR Am J Roentgenol* 1993;160(3):561.

614. van Holsbeeck MT, Kolowich PA, Eyler WR, et al. US depiction of partial-thickness tear of the rotator cuff. *Radiology* 1995;197(2):443.

615. Van Tongel A, Karelse A, Berghs B, Verdonk R, De Wilde L. Posterior shoulder instability: current concepts review. *Knee Surg Sports Traumatol Arthrosc* 2011;19(9):1547–1553. doi:10.1007/s00167-010-1293-z. Epub 2010 Oct 17.

616. Vanarthos WJ, Mono JUV. Type 4 acromion: a new classification. *Contemp Orthop* 1995;30:227.

617. Virk MS, Arciero RA. Superior labrum anterior to posterior tears and glenohumeral instability. *Instr Course Lect.* 2013;62:501–514.

618. Walch G, Nove-Josserand L, Boileau P, et al. Subluxation and dislocations of the tendon of the long head of the biceps. *J Shoulder Elbow Surg* 1998;7(2):100–108.

619. Walch G, Nove-Josserand L, Levigne C, et al. Complete ruptures of the supraspinatus tendon assoicated with "hidden lesions" of the rotator interval. *J Shoulder Elbow Surg* 1994;3(6):353.

620. Walch G. Patholgie de la longue portion du biceps. *Cahiers Enseignements de la SOFCOT, Expansion Scientifique* 1993;45:57.

621. Waldt S, Burkart A, Imhoff AB, et al. Anterior shoulder instability: accuracy of MR arthrography in the classification of anteroinferior labroligamentous injuries. *Radiology* 2005;237(2):578.

622. Waldt S, Burkart A, Lange P, et al. Diagnostic performance of MR arthrography in the assessment of superior labral anteroposterior lesions of the shoulder. *AJR Am J Roentgenol* 2004; 182(5):1271.

623. Wall MS, O'Brien SJ. Arthroscopic evaluation of the unstable shoulder. *Clin Sports Med* 1995;14(4):817.

624. Ward JP, Bradley JP. Decision making in the in-season athlete with shoulder instability. *Clin Sports Med* 2013;32(4):685–696. doi:10.1016/j.csm.2013.07.005.

625. Warner JJ, McMahon PJ. The role of the long head of the biceps brachii in superior stability of the glenohumeral joint. *J Bone Joint Surg Am* 1995;77(3):366.

626. Warner JP, Deng X, Warren RF. Static capsuloligamentous restraints to superior-inferior

translation of the glenohumeral joint. Presented at the Annual Meeting of the Orthopaedic Research Society; 1991; Anaheim, CA.

627. Waterman BR, Langston J, Slade DL. Allograft distal biceps reconstruction after closed intramuscular transection with delayed presentation. J Shoulder Elbow Surg 2013;22(5):e10–e13. doi:10.1016/j.jse.2013.01.007.

628. Wellmann M, de Ferrari H, Smith T, Petersen W, Siebert CH, Agneskirchner JD, Hurschler C. Biomechanical investigation of the stabilization principle of the Latarjet procedure. Arch Orthop Trauma Surg 2012;132(3):377–386. doi:10.1007/s00402-011-1425-z.

629. Werner CM, Steinmann PA, Gilbart M, et al. Treatment of painful pseudoparesis due to irreparable rotator cuff dysfunction with the Delta III reverse-ball-and-socket total shoulder prosthesis. J Bone Joint Surg Am 2005;87(7):1476.

630. White JJ, Titchener AG, Fakis A, Tambe AA, Hubbard RB, Clark DI. An epidemiological study of rotator cuff pathology using The Health Improvement Network database. Bone Joint J 2014;96-B(3):350–353. doi:10.1302/0301-620X.96B3.32336.

631. Wiater JM, Moravek JE Jr, Budge MD, Koueiter DM, Marcantonio D, Wiater BP. Clinical and radiographic results of cementless reverse total shoulder arthroplasty: a comparative study with 2 to 5 years of follow-up. J Shoulder Elbow Surg 2014;23(8):1208–114. doi:10.1016/j.jse.2013.11.032.

632. Wilk KE, Macrina LC, Arrigo C. Passive range of motion characteristics in the overhead baseball pitcher and their implications for rehabilitation. Clin Orthop Relat Res 2012;470(6):1586–1594. doi:10.1007/s11999-012-2265-z.

633. Wilk KE, Macrina LC, Fleisig GS, Porterfield R, Simpson CD II, Harker P, Paparesta N, Andrews JR. Correlation of glenohumeral internal rotation deficit and total rotational motion to shoulder injuries in professional baseball pitchers. Am J Sports Med 2011;39(2):329–335. doi:10.1177/0363546510384223.

634. Willems WJ. Reconstruction of glenoid bone defects in shoulder instability with autologous bone. Curr Rev Musculoskelet Med 2014;7(1):12–15.

635. Williams MM, Karzel RP, Snyder SJ. Labral disorders. In: Hawkins RJ, ed. Shoulder injuries in athlete, New York, NY: Churchill Livingstone; 1991:291.

636. Williams MM, Snyder SJ, Buford D Jr. The Buford complex—the "cord-like" middle glenohumeral ligament and absent anterosuperior labrum complex: a normal anatomic capsulolabral variant. Arthroscopy 1994;10(3):241.

637. Wilson AJ. Shoulder joint: arthrographic CT and long-term follow-up with surgical correlation. Radiology 1989;173:329.

638. Wischer TK, Bredella MA, Genant HK, et al. Perthes lesion (a variant of the Bankart lesion): MR imaging and MR arthrographic findings with surgical correlation. AJR Am J Roentgenol 2002;178(1):233.

639. Wise JN, Daffner RH, Weissman BN, Bancroft L, Bennett DL, Blebea JS, Bruno MA, Fries IB, Jacobson JA, Luchs JS, Morrison WB, Resnik CS, Roberts CC, Schweitzer ME, Seeger LL, Stoller DW, Taljanovic MS. ACR Appropriateness Criteria® on acute shoulder pain. J Am Coll Radiol 2011;8(9):602–609. doi:10.1016/j.jacr.2011.05.008.

640. Wolf BR, Britton CL, Vasconcellos DA, Spencer EE; MOON Shoulder Group. Agreement in the classification and treatment of the superior labrum. Am J Sports Med 2011;39(12):2588–2594. doi:10.1177/0363546511422869.

641. Wolf EM, Cheng JC, Dickson K. Humeral avulsion of glenohumeral ligaments as a cause of anterior shoulder instability. Arthroscopy 1995;11(5):600.

642. Wong I, Burns J, Snyder S. Arthroscopic GraftJacket repair of rotator cuff tears. J Shoulder Elbow Surg 2010;19(2)(suppl):104–109. doi:10.1016/j.jse.2009.12.017.

643. Wooten C, Klika B, Schleck CD, Harmsen WS, Sperling JW, Cofield RH. Anatomic shoulder arthroplasty as treatment for locked posterior dislocation of the shoulder. J Bone Joint Surg Am 2014;96(3):e19. doi:10.2106/JBJS.L.01588.

644. Workman TL, Burkhard TK, Resnick D, et al. Hill-Sachs lesion: comparison of detection with MR imaging, radiography, and arthroscopy. Radiology 1992;185(3):847.

645. Wu PT, Jou IM, Yang CC, Lin CJ, Yang CY, Su FC, Su WR. The severity of the long head biceps tendinopathy in patients with chronic rotator cuff tears: macroscopic versus microscopic results. J Shoulder Elbow Surg 2014;23(8):1099–1106. doi:10.1016/j.jse.2013.11.013.

646. Yamaguchi H, Suenaga N, Oizumi N, Hosokawa Y, Kanaya F. Open repair for massive rotator cuff tear with a modified transosseous-equivalent procedure: preliminary results at short-term follow-up. J Orthop Sci 2011;16(4):398–404. doi:10.1007/s00776-011-0092-9.

647. Yamamoto N, Muraki T, Sperling JW, Steinmann SP, Cofield RH, Itoi E, An KN. Stabilizing mechanism in bone-grafting of a large glenoid defect. J Bone Joint Surg Am 2010;92(11):2059–2066. doi:10.2106/JBJS.I.00261.

648. Yanny S, Toms AP. MR patterns of denervation around the shoulder. AJR Am J Roentgenol 2010;195(2):W157–W163. doi:10.2214/AJR.09.4127.

649. Yazici M, Kopuz C, Gulman B. Morphologic variants of acromion in neonatal cadavers. J Pediatr Orthop 1995;15(5):644.

650. Young AA, Baba M, Neyton L, Godeneche A, Walch G. Coracoid graft dimensions after harvesting for the open Latarjet procedure. J Shoulder Elbow Surg 2013;22(4):485–488. doi:10.1016/j.jse.2012.05.036.

651. Zacchilli MA, Owens BD. Epidemiology of shoulder dislocations presenting to emergency departments in the United States. J Bone Joint Surg Am 2010;92(3):542–549. doi:10.2106/JBJS.I.00450.

652. Zappia M, Reginelli A, Russo A, D'Agosto GF, Di Pietto F, Genovese EA, Coppolino F, Brunese L. Long head of the biceps tendon and rotator interval. Musculoskelet Surg 2013;97(suppl 2):S99–S108. doi:10.1007/s12306-013-0290-z.

653. Zhang AL, Gates CH, Link TM, Ma CB. Abnormal origins of the long head of the biceps tendon can lead to rotator cuff pathology: a report of two cases. Skeletal Radiol 2014;43(11):1621–1626.

654. Zhao J, Huangfu X, Yang X, Xie G, Xu C. Arthroscopic glenoid bone grafting with nonfixation for anterior shoulder instability:

52 patients with 2- to 5-year follow-up. *Am J Sports Med.* 2014;42(4):831–839.

655. Zhu YM, Lu Y, Zhang J, Shen JW, Jiang CY. Arthroscopic Bankart repair combined with remplissage technique for the treatment of anterior shoulder instability with engaging Hill-Sachs lesion: a report of 49 cases with a minimum 2-year follow-up. *Am J Sports Med* 2011;39(8):1640–1647. doi:10.1177/0363546511400018.

656. Ziegler D, Matsen F III, Harrington R. The superior rotator cuff tendon and acromion provide passive superior stability to the shoulder. *J Bone Joint Surg* 1996.

657. Zlatkin MB, Dalinka MK, Kressel HY. Magnetic resonance imaging of the shoulder. *Magn Reson Q* 1989;5(1):3.

658. Zlatkin MB, Iannotti JP, Roberts MC, et al. Rotator cuff tears: diagnostic performance of MR imaging. *Radiology* 1989;172(1):223.

659. Zlatkin MB, Reicher MA, Kellerhouse LE, et al. The painful shoulder: MR imaging of the glenohumeral joint. *J Comput Assist Tomogr* 1988;12(6):995.

660. Zlatkin MB, Sanders TG. Magnetic resonance imaging of the glenoid labrum. *Radiol Clin North Am* 2013;51(2):279–297. doi:10.1016/j.rcl.2012.11.003.

661. Zlatkin MB. Biceps tendon and miscellaneous shoulder lesion. In: Zlatkin MB, ed. *MRI of the Shoulder.* 2nd ed. Philadelphia, PA: Lippincott Williams & Wilkins; 2003:225.

662. Zlatkin MB. Cross-sectional imaging of the capsular mechanism of the glenohumeral joint. *AJR Am J Roentgenol* 1988;160:151.

663. Zlatkin MB. Evaluation of rotator cuff disease and glenohumeral instability with MR imaging: correlation with arthroscopy and arthrotomy in a large population of patients [abstract]. *Magn Reson Imagin* 1990;8(suppl 1):78.

664. Zlatkin MB. MR imaging of the shoulder: current experience and future trends. In: Kressel HY, Modic MT, Murphy WA, eds. *Syllabus Special Course MR.* Oak Brook, IL: RSNA Publications; 1990:225.

665. Zlatkin MB. Rotator cuff disease, In: Zlatkin MB, ed. *MRI of the Shoulder.* 2nd ed. Philadelphia, PA: Lippincott Williams & Wilkins; 2003:117.

666. Zlatkin MB. Shoulder instability. In: Zlatkin MB, ed. MRI of the shoulder, 2nd ed. Philadelphia, PA: Lippincott Williams & Wilkins; 2003.

667. Zoga AC, Schweitzer ME. Indirect magnetic resonance arthrography: applications in sports imaging. *Top Magn Reson Imaging* 2003;14(1):25–33.

668. Zubler V, Mamisch-Saupe N, Pfirrmann CW, Jost B, Zanetti M. Detection and quantification of glenohumeral joint effusion: reliability of ultrasound. *Eur Radiol* 2011;21(9):1858–1864. doi:10.1007/s00330-011-2127-1.

Index

Page numbers followed by "*f*" denote figures.